SANFORD GUIDE 熱病

THE SANFORD GUIDE
To Antimicrobial Therapy
2025

55th Edition

David N. Gilbert, M.D.
Henry F. Chambers, M.D.
Michael S. Saag, M.D.
Andrew T. Pavia, M.D.
Helen W. Boucher, M.D.

Douglas Black, Pharm.D.
David O. Freedman, M.D.
Kami Kim, M.D.
Brian S. Schwartz, M.D.

THE SANFORD GUIDE

To Antimicrobial Therapy
2025

55th Edition

Editors

David N. Gilbert, M.D.
Chief of Infectious Diseases,
Providence Portland Medical Center, Oregon
Professor of Medicine,
Oregon Health Sciences University

Henry F. Chambers, M.D.
San Francisco General Hospital
Professor of Medicine Emeritus
University of California, San Francisco

Michael S. Saag, M.D.
Professor of Medicine,
Division of Infectious Diseases,
University of Alabama, Birmingham

Andrew T. Pavia, M.D.
George & Esther Gross Presidential Professor
Chief, Division of Pediatric Infectious Diseases,
University of Utah, Salt Lake City

Helen W. Boucher, M.D.
Dean & Professor of Medicine,
Tufts University School of Medicine
Chief Academic Officer, Tufts Medicine
Boston, Massachusetts

Contributing Editors

Douglas Black, Pharm.D.
Professor of Pharmacy,
University of Washington, Seattle

Brian S. Schwartz, M.D.
Associate Professor of Medicine,
University of California, San Francisco

David O. Freedman, M.D.
Emeritus Professor of Medicine,
University of Alabama, Birmingham

Kami Kim, M.D.
Professor of Internal Medicine,
Division of Infectious Diseases
and International Medicine,
Morsani College of Medicine,
University of South Florida, Tampa

Managing Editor

Jeb C. Sanford

Publisher

Antimicrobial Therapy, Inc.

The SANFORD GUIDE TO ANTIMICROBIAL THERAPY is published by:

ANTIMICROBIAL THERAPY, INC.
11771 Lee Highway, P.O. Box 276
Sperryville, VA 22740-0276 USA
Tel 540-987-9480
Email: info@sanfordguide.com
www.sanfordguide.com

Acknowledgements
Thanks to Silvina Trapé, Jonatan Bohman and their team for manuscript design and layout of this edition of the SANFORD GUIDE.

Note to Readers
Since 1969, the SANFORD GUIDE has been independently prepared and published. Decisions regarding the content of the SANFORD GUIDE are solely those of the editors and the publisher. We welcome questions, comments and feedback concerning the SANFORD GUIDE. All of your feedback is reviewed and taken into account in updating the content of the SANFORD GUIDE.

Every effort is made to ensure accuracy of the content of this guide. However, current full prescribing information available in the package insert for each drug should be consulted before prescribing any product. The editors and publisher are not responsible for errors or omissions or for any consequences from application of the information in this book and make no warranty, express or implied, with respect to the currency, accuracy, or completeness of the contents of this publication. Application of this information in a particular situation remains the professional responsibility of the practitioner.

For the most current information, download the Sanford Guide mobile app or access web.sanfordguide.com and subscribe.

Printed in the United States of America
ISBN 978-1-944272-29-6
Pocket Edition (English)

—TABLE OF CONTENTS—

ABBREVIATIONS

3TC = lamivudine
AB,% = percent absorbed
ABC = abacavir
ABCD = amphotericin B colloidal dispersion
ABLC = ampho B lipid complex
ABSSSI = acute bacterial skin & skin structure infection
AD = after dialysis
ADF = adefovir
AG = aminoglycoside
AIDS = Acquired Immune Deficiency Syndrome
Amox-clav = amoxicillin-clavulanate
AM-CL-ER = amoxicillin-clavulanate extended release
AMK = amikacin
Amox = amoxicillin
AMP = ampicillin
Ampho B = amphotericin B
Amp-sulb = ampicillin-sulbactam
AP = atovaquone proguanil
APAG = antipseudomonal aminoglycoside
ARDS = acute respiratory distress syndrome
ARF = acute rheumatic fever
ASA = aspirin
ATS = American Thoracic Society
ATV = atazanavir
AUC = area under the curve
Azithro = azithromycin
BCRP = Breast Cancer Resistance Protein
bid = 2x per day
BL/BLI = beta-lactam/beta-lactamase inhibitor
BSA = body surface area
BW = body weight
C&S = culture & sensitivity
C/S = culture & sensitivity
CABP = community-acquired bacterial pneumonia
CAPD = continuous ambulatory peritoneal dialysis
CARB = carbapenems
CDC = U.S. Centers for Disease Control
Cefpodox = cefpodoxime proxetil
Ceftaz = ceftazidime
Ceftolo-tazo = ceftolozane-tazobactam
Ceph = cephalosporin
CFB = ceftobiprole
CFP = cefepime
Chloro = chloramphenicol
CIP = ciprofloxacin; **CIP-ER** = CIP extended release
Clarithro = clarithromycin; **ER** = extended release
Clav = clavulanate
Clinda = clindamycin
CLO = clofazimine
Clot = clotrimazole
CMV = cytomegalovirus
Cobi = cobicistat
CQ = chloroquine phosphate
CrCl = creatinine clearance
CrCln = CrCl normalized for BSA
CRBSI = catheter-related bloodstream infection
CRE = carbapenem resistant enteric
CRRT = continuous renal replacement therapy
CSD = cat-scratch disease
CSF = cerebrospinal fluid
CXR = chest x-ray
d4T = stavudine
Dapto = daptomycin
DBPCT = double-blind placebo-controlled trial
dc = discontinue
ddC = zalcitabine
ddI = didanosine
DIC = disseminated intravascular coagulation
Diclox = dicloxacillin
div = divided
DLV = delavirdine
DOR = doravirine
DORI = doripenem
DOT = directly observed therapy
Doxy = doxycycline
DR = delayed release
DRSP = drug-resistant S. pneumoniae
DBRPCT = Double blind, randomized, placebo-controlled trial
DS = double strength
EBV = Epstein-Barr virus
EES = erythromycin ethyl succinate
EFZ = efavirenz
ELV = elvitegravir
EMB = ethambutol
ENT = entecavir
ER = extended release
ERTA = ertapenem
Erythro = erythromycin
ESBLs = extended spectrum β-lactamases
ESR = erythrocyte sedimentation rate
ESRD = endstage renal disease
Flu = fluconazole
Flucyt = flucytosine
FOS-APV = fosamprenavir
FOS = fostemsavir
FQ = fluoroquinolone
FTC = emtricitabine
G = generic
GAS = Group A Strep
Gati = gatifloxacin
GC = gonorrhea
Gemi = gemifloxacin
Gent = gentamicin
gm = gram
GNB = gram-negative bacilli
Grazo = grazoprevir
Griseo = griseofulvin
Gtts = drops
H/O = history of
HAT = Human African Trypanosomiasis
HEMO = hemodialysis
HHV = human herpesvirus
HIV = human immunodeficiency virus
HLR = high-level resistance
HSCT = hematopoietic stem cell transplant
HSV = herpes simplex virus
IA = injectable agent/anti-inflammatory drugs
IDV = indinavir
IFN = interferon
IM = intramuscular
IMP = imipenem-cilastatin
IMP-rele = imipenem-cilastatin-relebactam
INH = isoniazid

ABBREVIATIONS (2)

Inv = investigational
IP = intraperitoneal
IT = intrathecal
Itra = itraconazole
IV = intravenous
IVDU = intravenous drug user
IVIG = intravenous immune globulin
Keto = ketoconazole
kg = kilogram
KPC = serine carbapenemase
LAB = liposomal ampho B
LCM = lymphocytic choriomeningitis virus
LCR = ligase chain reaction
LD = Loading Dose
LEN = lenacapavir
Levo = levofloxacin
LP/R = lopinavir/ ritonavir
MATE = Multidrug And Toxin Extrusion
MBL = metallo beta lactamase
mcg (or µg) = microgram
MD = Maintenance Dose
MDA = Mass Drug Administration
MDR = multi-drug resistant
MER = meropenem
MER-vabor = meropenem-vaborbactam
Metro = metronidazole
Mino = minocycline
mL = milliliter
MOL = molnupiravir
Moxi = moxifloxacin
MQ = mefloquine
MSM = men who have sex with men
MSSA/MRSA = methicillin-sensitive/resistant S. aureus
MTB = Mycobacterium tuberculosis
NAF = Nafcillin
NAI = not FDA-approved (indication or dose)
NB = name brand
NIR-RTV = nirmatrelvir + ritonavir
NF = nitrofurantoin
NFR = nelfinavir
NNRTI = non-nucleoside reverse transcriptase inhibitor
NOS = not otherwise specified mechanism of resistance
NRTI = nucleoside reverse transcriptase inhibitor
NSAIDs = non-steroidal
NUS = not available in the U.S.
NVP = nevirapine
OAT = Organic Anion Transporter
OATP = Organic Anion Transporter Polypeptide
O Ceph = oral cephalosporins
OCT = Organic Cation Transporter
Oflox = ofloxacin
P Ceph = parenteral cephalosporins
PCR = polymerase chain reaction
PEP = post-exposure prophylaxis
PGP = P-glycoprotein
PI = protease inhibitor
Pip-tazo = piperacillin-tazobactam
po = oral dosing
PQ = primaquine
PRCT = Prospective randomized controlled trials
PTLD = post-transplant lymphoproliferative disease
Pts = patients
Pyri = pyrimethamine
PZA = pyrazinamide
PZQ = Praziquantel
q wk = dose weekly
q[x]h = every [x] hours, e.g., q8h = every 8 hrs
qid = 4x per day
QS = quinine sulfate
R = resistant
RDBPCT = randomized double blind placebo controlled trial
RFB = rifabutin
RFP = rifapentine
Rick = Rickettsia
RIF = rifampin
RSV = respiratory syncytial virus
RTI = respiratory tract infection
RTV = ritonavir
rx = treatment
SA = Staph. aureus
sc = subcutaneous
SLED = Sustained Low Efficiency Dialysis
SSPE = Subacute sclerosing panencephalitis
SD = serum drug level after single dose
Sens = sensitive (susceptible)
SM = streptomycin
Sofos = sofosbuvir
SQV = saquinavir
SS = steady state serum level
STD = sexually transmitted disease
STH = Soil-Transmitted Helminth
subcut = subcutaneous
Sulb = sulbactam
Sx = symptoms
TAF = tenofovir alafenamide
Tazo = tazobactam
TBc = tuberculosis
TDF = tenofovir
TEE = transesophageal echocardiography
Teico = teicoplanin
Telithro = telithromycin
Tetra = tetracycline
tid = 3x per day
TMP-SMX = trimethoprim-sulfamethoxazole
TNF = tumor necrosis factor
Tobra = tobramycin
TPV = tipranavir
TST = tuberculin skin test
UGT = Uridine Diphosphate Glucuronosyltransferase
UTI = urinary tract infection
Vanco = vancomycin
Velpat = velpatasvir
VISA = vancomycin intermediately resistant S. aureus
VL = viral load
Vori = voriconazole
VZV = varicella-zoster virus
WHO = World Health Organization
ZDV = zidovudine

ABBREVIATIONS OF JOURNAL TITLES

AAC: Antimicrobial Agents & Chemotherapy
Adv PID: Advances in Pediatric Infectious Diseases
AHJ: American Heart Journal
AIDS Res Hum Retrovir: AIDS Research & Human Retroviruses
AAP: American Academy of Pediatrics
AJG: American Journal of Gastroenterology
AJM: American Journal of Medicine
AJRCCM: American Journal of Respiratory Critical Care Medicine
AJTMH: American Journal of Tropical Medicine & Hygiene
Aliment Pharmacol Ther: Alimentary Pharmacology & Therapeutics
Am J Hlth Pharm: American Journal of Health-System Pharmacy
Amer J Transpl: American Journal of Transplantation
AnEM: Annals of Emergency Medicine
AnIM: Annals of Internal Medicine
Ann Pharmacother: Annals of Pharmacotherapy
AnSurg: Annals of Surgery
Antivir Ther: Antiviral Therapy
ArDerm: Archives of Dermatology
ArIM: Archives of Internal Medicine
ARRD: American Review of Respiratory Disease
BMJ: British Medical Journal
BMT: Bone Marrow Transplantation
Brit J Derm: British Journal of Dermatology
Can JID: Canadian Journal of Infectious Diseases
Canad Med J: Canadian Medical Journal
CCM: Critical Care Medicine
CCTID: Current Clinical Topics in Infectious Disease
CDSR: Cochrane Database of Systematic Reviews
CID: Clinical Infectious Diseases
Clin Micro Inf: Clinical Microbiology and Infection
CMN: Clinical Microbiology Newsletter
Clin Micro Rev: Clinical Microbiology Reviews
CMAJ: Canadian Medical Association Journal
COID: Current Opinion in Infectious Disease
Curr Med Res Opin: Current Medical Research and Opinion
Derm Ther: Dermatologic Therapy
Dermatol Clin: Dermatologic Clinics
Dig Dis Sci: Digestive Diseases and Sciences
DMID: Diagnostic Microbiology and Infectious Disease
EID: Emerging Infectious Diseases
EJCMID: European Journal of Clin. Micro. & Infectious Diseases
Eur J Neurol: European Journal of Neurology
Exp Mol Path: Experimental & Molecular Pathology
Exp Rev Anti Infect Ther: Expert Review of Anti-Infective Therapy
Gastro: Gastroenterology
Hpt: Hepatology
ICHE: Infection Control and Hospital Epidemiology
IDC No. Amer: Infectious Disease Clinics of North America
IDCP: Infectious Diseases in Clinical Practice
IJAA: International Journal of Antimicrobial Agents
Inf Med: Infections in Medicine
J AIDS & HR: Journal of AIDS and Human Retrovirology
J All Clin Immun: Journal of Allergy and Clinical Immunology
J Am Ger Soc: Journal of the American Geriatrics Society
J Chemother: Journal of Chemotherapy
J Clin Micro: Journal of Clinical Microbiology
J Clin Virol: Journal of Clinical Virology
J Derm Treat: Journal of Dermatological Treatment
J Hpt: Journal of Hepatology
J Inf: Journal of Infection
J Med Micro: Journal of Medical Microbiology
J Micro Immunol Inf: Journal of Microbiology, Immunology, & Infection
J Ped: Journal of Pediatrics
J Viral Hep: Journal of Viral Hepatitis
JAC: Journal of Antimicrobial Chemotherapy
JACC: Journal of American College of Cardiology
JAIDS: JAIDS Journal of Acquired Immune Deficiency Syndromes
JAMA: Journal of the American Medical Association
JAVMA: Journal of the Veterinary Medicine Association
JCI: Journal of Clinical Investigation
JCM: Journal of Clinical Microbiology
JIC: Journal of Infection and Chemotherapy
JID: Journal of Infectious Diseases
JNS: Journal of Neurosurgery
JPIDS: Journal of Pediatric Infectious Diseases Society
JTMH: Journal of Tropical Medicine and Hygiene
Ln: Lancet
LnID: Lancet Infectious Disease
Mayo Clin Proc: Mayo Clinic Proceedings
Med Lett: Medical Letter
Med Mycol: Medical Mycology
MMWR: Morbidity & Mortality Weekly Report
NEJM: New England Journal of Medicine
Neph Dial Transpl: Nephrology Dialysis Transplantation
OFID: Open Forum Infectious Diseases
Ped Ann: Pediatric Annals
Peds: Pediatrics
Pharmacother: Pharmacotherapy
PIDJ: Pediatric Infectious Disease Journal
QJM: Quarterly Journal of Medicine
Scand J Inf Dis: Scandinavian Journal of Infectious Diseases
Sem Resp Inf: Seminars in Respiratory Infections
SGO: Surgery Gynecology and Obstetrics
SMJ: Southern Medical Journal
Surg Neurol: Surgical Neurology
Transpl Inf Dis: Transplant Infectious Diseases
Transpl: Transplantation
TRSM: Transactions of the Royal Society of Medicine

TABLE 1 – CLINICAL APPROACH TO INITIAL CHOICE OF ANTIMICROBIAL THERAPY*

Treatment based on presumed site or type of infection. In selected instances, treatment and prophylaxis based on identification of pathogens.
Regimens should be reevaluated based on pathogen isolated, antimicrobial susceptibility determination, and individual host characteristics. *(Abbreviations on 2)*

ANATOMIC SITE/DIAGNOSIS/ MODIFYING CIRCUMSTANCES	ETIOLOGIES (usual)	SUGGESTED REGIMENS*		ADJUNCT DIAGNOSTIC OR THERAPEUTIC MEASURES AND COMMENTS
		PRIMARY	ALTERNATIVE§	
ABDOMEN: *See Peritoneum, page 51; Gallbladder, page 18; and Pelvic Inflammatory Disease, page 28*				
BONE: Osteomyelitis. Microbiologic diagnosis is essential. If blood culture negative, need culture of bone *(Eur J Clin Microbiol Infect Dis 33:371, 2014)*. Culture of sinus tract drainage not predictive of bone culture.				
Hematogenous Osteomyelitis *(see IDSA guidelines for vertebral osteo: CID July 29, 2015)*				
Empiric therapy—Collect bone and blood cultures before empiric therapy				
Newborn (<4 mos.)	S. aureus, Gm-neg. bacilli, Group B strep, Kingella kingae in children	**MRSA possible: Vanco + (Ceftaz or CFP)**	**MRSA unlikely:** (**Nafcillin** or **Oxacillin** or **Cefazolin** 150 mg/kg/d div q8h) + (**Ceftaz or CFP**)	Severe allergy or toxicity: (**Linezolid**[NAI] 10 mg/kg IV/po q8h + **Aztreonam**).
Children (>4 mos.) — Adult: Osteo of extremity *(NEJM 370:352, 2014)*	S. aureus, Group A strep, Gm-neg. bacilli rare, Kingella kingae in children	**MRSA possible: Vanco** 30-60 mg/kg/d in 2-3 div doses, target AUC_{24} 400-600 µg/mL x h	**MRSA unlikely:** (**Nafcillin** or **Oxacillin**) 150 mg/kg/day div q6h (max 12 gm). **Cefazolin** 150 mg/kg/day div q8h in children equally effective	Severe allergy or toxicity: **Clinda** or **TMP-SMX** or **Linezolid**[NAI]. Early conversion to high dose oral therapy equally effective
		Add **Ceftaz or CFP** if Gm-neg. bacilli on Gram stain **Adult doses below.**		
Adult (>21 yrs) **Vertebral osteo ± epidural abscess** *(see IDSA guidelines for vertebral osteo: CID 61:859, 2015)* **Blood & bone cultures essential.**	S. aureus most common but variety other organisms. Brucella, M. tuberculosis, Coccidioides important in regions of high endemicity for the organisms	**Vanco** 30-60 mg/kg/d in 2-3 div doses, target AUC_{24} 400-600 µg/mL x h + (**Ceftriaxone** 2 gm q24h OR **CFP** 2 gm q8h OR **Levo** 750 mg q24h)	**Dapto** 8-10 mg/kg IV q24h OR **Linezolid** 600 mg q12h + (**Ceftriaxone** 2 gm q24h OR **CFP** 2 gm q8h OR **Levo** 750 mg q24h)	**Ceftriaxone** should not be used if pseudomonas suspected. **Piperacillin/Tazobactam** another option for pseudomonas or other Gram-negative coverage. **Dx: MRI diagnostic test of choice, indicated to rule out epidural abscess. Risk factors for recurrence:** end-stage renal disease, MRSA infection, undrained paravertebral or psoas abscess; pathogen-specific therapy for >8 wks recommended if any of these are present *(CID 62:1262, 2016)*; 6 wks of pathogen-specific therapy comparable to 12 wks for less complicated infection *(CID 62:1261, 2016 and Lancet 385:875, 2015)*. Whenever possible empirical therapy should be administered after cultures are obtained.

* **PRIMARY REGIMENS SUGGESTED are for adults (unless otherwise indicated) with clinically severe (often life-threatening) infections. Dosages also assume normal renal function, and not severe hepatic dysfunction.**
§ **ALTERNATIVE REGIMENS INCLUDE these considerations: allergy, pregnancy, pharmacology/pharmacokinetics, compliance, costs, local resistance profiles.**

TABLE 1 (2)

ANATOMIC SITE/DIAGNOSIS/ MODIFYING CIRCUMSTANCES	ETIOLOGIES (usual)	SUGGESTED REGIMENS*		ADJUNCT DIAGNOSTIC OR THERAPEUTIC MEASURES AND COMMENTS
		PRIMARY	ALTERNATIVE§	
BONE/Hematogenous Osteomyelitis *(continued)*				
Specific therapy—Culture and in vitro susceptibility results known. *See CID Jul 29, 2015 for IDSA Guidelines*				
	MSSA	**Nafcillin** or **Oxacillin** 2 gm IV q4h or **Cefazolin** 2 gm IV q8h	**Vanco** 30-60 mg/kg/d in 2-3 div doses, target AUC_{24} 400-600 µg/mL x h OR **Dapto** 8-10 mg/kg IV q24h OR **Linezolid** 600 mg IV/po q12h	In children, therapy can be completed with high dose oral therapy *(JAMA Pediatr 169:220,2015)*. **Other options if susceptible in vitro and allergy/toxicity issues *(see NEJM 362:11, 2010)*:** 1) **TMP-SMX** 8-10 mg/kg/d po/IV div q8h + **RIF** 300-450 mg bid: limited data, particularly for MRSA *(see AAC 53:2672, 2009)*; 2) **Levo** 750 mg po q24h) + **RIF** 600 mg po q24h; 3) **Fusidic acid**[NUS] 500 mg IV q8h + **RIF** 300 mg po bid. *(CID 42:394, 2006)*. Duration of therapy: 6 weeks, provided that epidural or paravertebral abscesses can be drained; consider longer course in those with extensive infection or abscess particularly if not amenable to drainage because of increased risk of treatment failure *(OFID Dec 5:1, 2014)*.
	MRSA—*See Table 6, page 88; IDSA Guidelines CID 52:e18-55, 2011; CID 52:285-92, 2011.* Combination therapy lessens relapse rate	**Vanco** 30-60 mg/kg/d in 2-3 div doses, target AUC_{24} 400-600 µg/mL x h ± **RIF** 300-450 mg bid.	**Linezolid** 600 mg q12h IV/po ± **RIF** 300 mg po/IV bid OR **Dapto** 8-10 mg/kg q24h IV ± **RIF** 300-450 mg po/IV bid	
Hemoglobinopathy: Sickle cell/thalassemia	Salmonella; other Gm-neg. bacilli	**CIP** 400 mg IV q12h OR **CIP** 750 mg po bid	**Levo** 750 mg IV/po q24h	Due to increasing levels of FQ resistance, consider adding a second agent (e.g., third generation cephalosporin) until susceptibility test results available. Alternative for salmonella is Ceftriaxone 2 gm IV q24h if nalidixic acid resistant which is predictive of fluoroquinolone resistance.
Contiguous Osteomyelitis Without Vascular Insufficiency				
Empiric therapy: Get cultures!				
Foot bone osteo due to nail through tennis shoe	P. aeruginosa	**CIP** 750 mg po bid or **Levo** 750 mg po q24h	**Ceftaz** 2 gm IV q8h or **CFP** 2 gm IV q8h	Empiric therapy not recommended: Get cultures. *S. aureus* and polymicrobial infections more common in diabetics *(J Am Podiatr Med Assoc. 2020 Nov 2;20-206)*. See also: *Skin—Nail puncture, page 63.* Need debridement to remove foreign body.
Long bone, post-internal fixation of fracture	S. aureus, Gm-neg. bacilli, P. aeruginosa	**Vanco** 30-60 mg/kg/d in 2-3 div doses, target AUC_{24} 400-600 µg/mL x h + [**Ceftaz** or **CFP**]. *See Comment*	**Linezolid** 600 mg IV/po bid[NAI] + (**Ceftaz** or **CFP**). *See Comment*	**Regimens listed are empiric.** Adjust after culture data available. If susceptible Gm-neg. bacillus, **CIP** 750 mg po bid or **Levo** 750 mg po q24h. For other *S. aureus* options: *See Hem. Osteo. Specific Therapy, page 6.*
Osteonecrosis of the jaw	Probably rare adverse reaction to bisphosphonates	Infection may be secondary to bone necrosis and loss of overlying mucosa. Treatment: minimal surgical debridement, chlorhexidine rinses, antibiotics (e.g., Amp-sulb). Evaluate for concomitant actinomycosis, for which specific long-term antibiotic treatment would be warranted.		
Prosthetic joint	*See prosthetic joint, page 36*			
Spinal implant infection	S. aureus, coag-neg staphylococci, gram-neg bacilli	Onset within 30 days: culture, treat for 3 mos.	Onset after 30 days remove implant, culture & treat	
Sternum, post-op	S. aureus, S. epidermidis, occasionally, gram-negative bacilli	**Vanco** 30-60 mg/kg/d in 2-3 div doses, target AUC_{24} 400-600 µg/mL x h recommended for serious infections.	**Linezolid** 600 mg po/IV[NAI] bid	Sternal debridement for cultures & removal of necrotic bone. If setting or gram stain suggests possibility of gram-negative bacilli, add appropriate coverage based on local antimicrobial susceptibility profiles (e.g., cefepime, Pip-tazo).

 **NOTE: All dosage recommendations are for adults (unless otherwise indicated) and assume normal renal function. § Alternatives consider allergy, PK, compliance, local resistance, cost.*

TABLE 1 (3)

ANATOMIC SITE/DIAGNOSIS/ MODIFYING CIRCUMSTANCES	ETIOLOGIES (usual)	SUGGESTED REGIMENS*		ADJUNCT DIAGNOSTIC OR THERAPEUTIC MEASURES AND COMMENTS
		PRIMARY	ALTERNATIVE§	
BONE *(continued)*				
Contiguous Osteomyelitis With Vascular Insufficiency.				
Most pts are **diabetics** with peripheral neuropathy & infected skin ulcers *(see Diabetic foot, page 17)*	Polymicrobic [Gm+ cocci (to include MRSA) (aerobic & anaerobic) and Gm-neg. bacilli (aerobic & anaerobic)]	Debride overlying ulcer & submit bone for histology & culture. Select antibiotic based on culture results. **No empiric therapy unless acutely ill.** If acutely ill, *see suggestions, Diabetic foot, page 17.*		**Diagnosis of osteo:** Culture bone biopsy (gold standard). Swab cultures unreliable. Sampling by needle puncture inferior to biopsy. Osteo likely if ulcer >2 cm², positive probe to bone, ESR >70 & abnormal plain x-ray. **Treatment:** (1) **Revascularize if possible;** (2) Culture bone; (3) Specific antimicrobial(s) based on culture results.
Chronic Osteomyelitis: Specific therapy By definition, implies presence of dead bone. **Need valid cultures**	S. aureus, Enterobacterales, P. aeruginosa	**Empiric rx not indicated.** Base systemic rx on results of culture, sensitivity testing. If acute exacerbation of chronic osteo, rx as acute hematogenous osteo. Surgical debridement important.		**Important adjuncts:** removal of orthopedic hardware, surgical debridement; vascularized muscle flaps, distraction osteogenesis (Ilizarov) techniques. Oral therapy equivalent to IV: *NEJM, 2019;380:425*
BREAST: Mastitis—*Obtain culture; need to know if MRSA present.*				
Postpartum mastitis *(Cochrane Review: Cochrane Database Syst Rev 2013 Feb 28;2:CD005458; see also CID 54:71, 2012)*				
Mastitis without abscess	S. aureus, strep, coag-neg. staph, other Gram-positives less common	**NO MRSA:** **Outpatient: Diclox** 500 mg po qid or **Cephalexin** 500 mg po qid. **Inpatient: Nafcillin/ Oxacillin** 2 gm IV q4-6h	**MRSA Possible:** **Outpatient: TMP-SMX-DS** tabs 1-2 po bid or, if suscepti-ble, **Clinda** 300 mg po tid **Inpatient: Vanco** 30-60 mg/ kg/d in 2-3 div doses, target AUC_{24} 400-600 µg/mL x h	If no abscess & controllable pain, ↑ freq of nursing may hasten response.
Mastitis with abscess				For painful abscess I&D is standard; needle aspiration reported successful. Resume breast feeding from affected breast as soon as pain allows. *(Breastfeed Med 9:239, 2014)*
Non-puerperal mastitis with abscess	S. aureus; less often Bacteroides sp., peptostreptococcus (Peptoniphilus sp.), & selected coagulase-neg. staphylococci	*See regimens for Postpartum mastitis, page 7.*		**If subareolar & odoriferous**, most likely anaerobes; **add Metro** 500 mg IV/po tid. Need pretreatment aerobic/anaerobic cultures. Surgical drainage for abscess. **I&D standard. Consider TB in chronic infections.**
Breast implant infection	Acute: S. aureus, S. pyogenes. TSS reported. Chronic: Look for rapidly growing Mycobacteria	Acute: **Vanco** 30-60 mg/kg/d in 2-3 div doses, target AUC_{24} 400-600 µg/mL x h	Chronic: Await culture results. *See Table 12A* for mycobacteria treatment.	Risk of complications higher with late-onset infection (>30 days post implantation). Antibiotics alone may be sufficient for minor infections; explantation often required for more serious infections. *Plast. Reconstr. Surg 139:20, 2017.*

**NOTE: All dosage recommendations are for adults (unless otherwise indicated) and assume normal renal function. § Alternatives consider allergy, PK, compliance, local resistance, cost.*

TABLE 1 (4)

ANATOMIC SITE/DIAGNOSIS/ MODIFYING CIRCUMSTANCES	ETIOLOGIES (usual)	SUGGESTED REGIMENS*		ADJUNCT DIAGNOSTIC OR THERAPEUTIC MEASURES AND COMMENTS
		PRIMARY	ALTERNATIVE§	
CENTRAL NERVOUS SYSTEM				
Brain abscess				
Primary or contiguous source Review: *NEJM 371:447, 2014.*	Streptococci (60–70%), bacteroides (20–40%), Enterobacterales (25-33%), S. aureus (10-15%), S. anginosus grp. Rare: Nocardia *(below)*, Listeria. *See S. aureus Comment*	(**Cefotaxime** 2 gm IV q4h or **Ceftriaxone** 2 gm IV q12h) + (**Metro** 7.5 mg/kg q6h or 15 mg/kg IV q12h)	**Pen G** 3-4 million units IV q4h + **Metro** 7.5 mg/kg q6h or 15 mg/kg IV q12h	If CT scan suggests cerebritis or abscesses <2.5 cm and pt neurologically stable and conscious, start antibiotics and observe. Otherwise, surgical drainage necessary. If blood cultures or other clinical data do not yield a likely etiologic agent, aspirate even small abscesses for diagnosis if this can be done safely. S. anginosus grp esp. prone to produce abscess. Ceph/metro does not cover listeria.
		Add **Vanco** 30-60 mg/kg/d in 2-3 div doses, target AUC_{24} 400-600 µg/mL x h or **Linezolid** 600 mg IV/po q12h to the regimen if S. aureus is a possibility. Duration of rx unclear; usually 4-6 wks or until resolution by neuro imaging (CT/MRI)		
Post-surgical, post-traumatic. Review: *NEJM 371:447, 2014.*	S. aureus, Enterobacterales	**For MSSA:** (**Nafcillin** or **Oxacillin**) 2 gm IV q4h + (**Ceftriaxone** or **Cefotaxime**)	**For MRSA: Vanco** 30-60 mg/kg/d in 2-3 div doses, target AUC_{24} 400-600 µg/mL x h + (**Ceftriaxone** or **Cefotaxime**)	Empiric coverage, de-escalated based on culture results. **Aspiration of abscess usually necessary for dx & rx. If P. aeruginosa suspected, substitute (Cefepime or Ceftazidime) for (Ceftriaxone or Cefotaxime).**
HIV-1 infected (AIDS)	Toxoplasma gondii	*See Table 13A, page 209*		
Nocardia: Haematogenous abscess	N. farcinica, N. asteroides & N. brasiliensis *See AAC 58:795, 2014* for other species.	**TMP-SMX:** 15 mg/kg/day of TMP & 75 mg/kg/day of SMX, IV/po div in 2-4 doses + **IMP** 500 mg q6h IV. If multiorgan involvement some add **Amikacin** 7.5 mg/kg q12h.	**Linezolid** 600 mg IV or po q12h + MER 2 gm q8h	Susceptibility testing should be performed to guide therapy. **TMP-SMX** remains a drug of choice for CNS nocardia infection. If sulfonamide resistant or sulfa-allergic, **Amikacin** plus one of: **IMP**, **MER**, **Ceftriaxone** or **Cefotaxime**. N. farcinica is resistant to third generation cephalosporins, which should not be used for treatment of infection caused by this species.
		After 3-6 wks of IV therapy, switch to po therapy. Immunocompetent pts: **TMP-SMX**, **minocycline** or **Amox-clav** x 3+ months. Immunocompromised pts: Treat with 2 drugs x 1 yr.		
Subdural empyema: In adults and children 60–90% is extension of sinusitis or otitis media. Rx same as primary brain abscess. Surgical emergency: must drain. Review in *LnID 7:62,* 2007.				
Encephalitis/encephalopathy *(For Herpes see Table 14A, page 227 and for rabies, Table 20B, page 328)*	H. simplex (42%), VZV (15%), M. TB (15%), Listeria (10%) *(CID 49:1838, 2009).* Other: arbovirus, West Nile, rabies, Lyme, Parvo B19, Cat-scratch, Mycoplasma, EBV and others.	Start IV **Acyclovir** while awaiting results of CSF PCR for H. simplex. For amebic encephalitis *see Table 13A.* Start **Doxy** 100 mg q12h if setting suggests R. rickettsii, Anaplasma, Ehrlichia or Mycoplasma. **Ceftriaxone** 2 gm IV q24h or **Doxy** 100 mg q12h x 14 days for Lyme encephalitis.		Increasing recognition of autoimmune antibody-mediated encephalitis, e.g., anti-N-methyl aspartate receptors & others. Dx: CSF antibody panel. Ref: *NEJM 2018,378:840.* Review of acute viral encephalitis *(NEJM 2018;379:557; Curr Opin Infect Dis. 2023; 36:177).*
Meningitis, "Aseptic": Pleocytosis of up to 100s of cells, CSF glucose normal, neg. culture for bacteria *(See Table 14A, page 224)*	Enteroviruses, HSV-2, LCM, HIV, VZV, other viruses, syphilis, drugs [NSAIDs, metronidazole, carbamazepine, lamotrigine TMP-SMX, IVIG, (e.g., detuximab, infliximab)], rarely leptospirosis, Lyme.	For all but leptospirosis, IV fluids and analgesics. D/C drugs that may be etiologic. For lepto (**Doxy** 100 mg IV/po q12h) or (**Pen G** 5 million units IV q6h) or (**AMP** 0.5–1 gm IV q6h). Repeat LP if suspect partially treated bacterial meningitis. **Acyclovir** 10 mg/kg IV q8h for HSV-2 meningitis.		If available, PCR of CSF for enterovirus. VZV, HSV-2: concurrent or history of prior genital lesions often absent. For lepto, positive epidemiologic history and concomitant hepatitis, conjunctivitis, dermatitis, nephritis. CNS Lyme: Varies – palsy, encephalitis, aseptic meningitis: *see page 65.* Etiologies: *Med 95:e2372, 2016.*

 **NOTE: All dosage recommendations are for adults (unless otherwise indicated) and assume normal renal function. § Alternatives consider allergy, PK, compliance, local resistance, cost.*

TABLE 1 (5)

ANATOMIC SITE/DIAGNOSIS/ MODIFYING CIRCUMSTANCES	ETIOLOGIES (usual)	SUGGESTED REGIMENS*		ADJUNCT DIAGNOSTIC OR THERAPEUTIC MEASURES AND COMMENTS
		PRIMARY	ALTERNATIVE§	
CENTRAL NERVOUS SYSTEM *(continued)*				
Meningitis, Bacterial, Acute: Goal is empiric therapy, then CSF exam within 30 min. If focal neurologic deficit, give empiric therapy, then head CT, then LP. If no focal deficit, empiric therapy, LP & then head CT *(CID 2018,66:321)*. Reviews: *JAMA 2022;328:2147* and *Neurol Clin. 2022; 40:77.*				
Empiric Therapy—CSF Gram stain is negative—immunocompetent				
Age: Preterm to <1 mo *LnID 10:32, 2010*	Group B strep 49%, E. coli 18%, listeria 7%, misc. Gm-neg. 10%, misc. Gm-pos. 10%	**AMP** 75-100 mg/kg IV q6h + **Cefotaxime** 75 mg/kg IV q6h + **Genta** 2.5 mg/kg IV q8h or 5-7 mg/kg IV q24h.	**AMP** 75-100 mg/kg IV q6h + **Cefotaxime** 75 mg/kg IV q6h OR **AMP** 75-100 mg/kg IV q6h + **Gent** 2.5 mg/kg IV q8h	Regimens active vs. Group B strep, most coliforms, & listeria. If premature infant with long nursery stay, S. aureus, enterococci, and resistant coliforms potential pathogens. **If high risk of MRSA,** use vanco + cefotaxime. Alter regimen after culture/ sensitivity data available. Cefepime is an option if Cefotaxime is unavailable
		Intraventricular treatment not recommended.		
Age: 1 mo– 50 yrs Recent review: *Lancet Infect Dis 16:339, 2016.*	S. pneumo, meningococci, H. influenzae now uncommon, **listeria unlikely if young adult & immunocompetent** (add **Ampicillin** if suspect listeria: 2 gm IV q4h)	Adult: [(**Cefotaxime** 2 gm IV q4–6h OR **Ceftriaxone** 2 gm IV q12h)] + **Dexamethasone** + **Vanco**	[(**MER** 2 gm IV q8h) (Peds: 40 mg/kg IV q8h)] + IV **Dexamethasone** + **Vanco**[1]	For patients with severe **β-lactam allergy,** *see below (Empiric Therapy—positive gram stain and Specific Therapy)* for alternative therapies. Dexamethasone shown to improve outcomes in children with *H. influenzae* but no data establishes role for *S. pneumoniae* in children.
		Dexamethasone: 0.15 mg/kg IV q6h x 2–4 days. **Give with, or just before, 1st dose of antibiotic** *(see Comment).*		
		See footnote[1] for Vanco Adult dosage and[2] for ped. dosage		
Age: >50 yrs or alcoholism or other **debilitating assoc diseases** or **impaired cellular immunity**	S. pneumo, listeria, meningococci, Gm-neg. bacilli	(**AMP** 2 gm IV q4h) + (**Ceftriaxone** 2 gm IV q12h or **Cefotaxime** 2 gm IV q4-6h) + **Vanco** + IV **Dexamethasone**	**MER** 2 gm IV q8h + **Vanco** + IV **Dexamethasone**. *For severe Pen allergy, see Comment*	For patients with severe **β-lactam allergy,** *see below (Empiric Therapy—positive gram stain and Specific Therapy)* for alternative agents that can be substituted to cover likely pathogens. LP without CT for patients with altered level of consciousness and non-focal neurological exam associated with earlier treatment and improved outcome *(CID 60:1162, 2015)*
		For Vanco dose, *see footnote[1]*. **Dexamethasone dose:** 0.15 mg/kg IV q6h x 2–4 days; 1st dose before, or concomitant with, 1st dose of antibiotic.		
Post-neurosurgery Ventriculostomy/lumbar catheter; ventriculoperitoneal (atrial) shunt or penetrating trauma w/o basilar skull fracture Shunt-related meningitis IDSA Guidelines: *CID 64:e34, 2017.*	S. epidermidis, S. aureus, Cutibacterium acnes. Facultative and aerobic gram-neg bacilli, including: P. aeruginosa & A. baumannii (may be multi-drug resistant)	**Vanco** 30-60 mg/kg/d in 2-3 div doses, target AUC_{24} 400-600 µg/mL x h + (**Cefepime** or **Ceftaz** 2 gm IV q8h)	**Vanco** + (**MER** 2 gm IV q8h)	• Remove infected shunt and place external ventricular catheter for drainage or pressure control. • Intraventricular therapy used if the shunt cannot be removed or cultures fail to clear with systemic therapy. • **Shunt reimplantation:** If coagulase-negative staphylococci, diphtheroids, or C. acnes: no CSF abnormalities, day 3 after externalization if CSF cultures are negative at 48h; CSF abnormalities present: 7-10 days after the last positive CSF culture. If S. aureus or Gram-negative organism: 10 days after last positive CSF culture.
		• **If severe Pen/Ceph allergy,** for possible gram-neg, substitute either: **Aztreonam** 2 gm IV q6-8h or **CIP** 400 mg IV q8h. **Intraventricular antibiotic dosing** (lower dose for slit ventricles, intermediate dose for normal size ventricles, higher dose for enlarged ventricles): **Amikacin** 30 mg, **Gent** 4-8 mg in adults, 1-2 mg in infants, children, **Polymyxin E** (Colistin) 10 mg, **Tobra** 5-20 mg, **Vanco** 5-20 mg, **Dapto** 5 mg. **Frequency of administration** depends on drainage output: < 50 ml/24h: every 3rd day, 50-100 ml/24h: every second day, 100-150 ml/day: once daily, 150-200 ml/24h: increase dose of vancomycin by 5 mg, gentamicin by 1 mg, 200-250 ml/24h: increase dose of vancomycin by 5 mg, gentamicin by 1 mg		

[1] **Vanco adult dose:** 30-60 mg/kg/d in 2-3 div doses, target AUC_{24} 400-600 µg/mL x h

[2] **Dosage of drugs used to treat children age ≥1 mo: Cefotaxime** 50 mg/kg per day IV q6h; **Ceftriaxone** 50 mg/kg IV q12h; **Vanco** 60-80 mg/kg/d in 3-4 doses, target AUC_{24} 400-600 µg/mL x h

Abbreviations on page 2. **NOTE: All dosage recommendations are for adults (unless otherwise indicated) and assume normal renal function. § Alternatives consider allergy, PK, compliance, local resistance, cost.*

TABLE 1 (6)

ANATOMIC SITE/DIAGNOSIS/ MODIFYING CIRCUMSTANCES	ETIOLOGIES (usual)	SUGGESTED REGIMENS* PRIMARY	SUGGESTED REGIMENS* ALTERNATIVE§	ADJUNCT DIAGNOSTIC OR THERAPEUTIC MEASURES AND COMMENTS
CENTRAL NERVOUS SYSTEM/Meningitis, Bacterial, Acute/Empiric Therapy—CSF Gram stain is negative—immunocompetent *(continued)*				
Trauma with basilar skull fracture	S. pneumoniae, H. influenzae, S. pyogenes	**Vanco** 30-60 mg/kg/d in 2-3 div doses, target AUC_{24} 400-600 μg/mL x h + (**Ceftriaxone** 2 gm IV q12h or **Cefotaxime** 2 gm IV q6h) + [**Dexamethasone** 0.15 mg/kg IV q6h x 2-4 d (1st dose with or before 1st antibiotic dose)].		
Empiric Therapy—Positive CSF Gram stain				
Gram-positive diplococci	S. pneumoniae	(**Ceftriaxone** 2 gm IV q12h or **Cefotaxime** 2 gm IV q4–6h) + **Vanco** 30-60 mg/kg/d in 2-3 div doses, target AUC_{24} 400-600 μg/mL x h + **Dexamethasone** 0.15 mg/kg IV q6h		**Alternative** if serious beta-lactam allergy: **MER** 2 gm IV q8h or **Moxi** 400 mg IV q24h + **Vanco**. First dose of dexamethasone given 15-20 minutes prior to first antibiotic dose, and then continued for 4 days for confirmed pneumococcal infection.
Gram-negative diplococci	N. meningitidis	(**Cefotaxime** 2 gm IV q4–6h or **Ceftriaxone** 2 gm IV q12h)		**Alternatives: Pen G** 4 mill. units IV q4h or **AMP** 2 gm q4h or **CIP** 400 mg IV q8h or **Chloro** 1 gm IV q6h (Chloro less effective than other alternatives: *see JAC 70:979, 2015*)
Gram-positive bacilli or coccobacilli	Listeria monocytogenes	**AMP** 2 gm IV q4h		If pen allergic use **TMP/SMX** 5 mg/kg (TMP component) q6-8h. Data showing beneficial effect of gentamicin combination therapy are inconclusive.
Gram-negative bacilli	H. influenzae, enterics, P. aeruginosa	(**Ceftazidime** or **Cefepime** 2 gm IV q8h)		**Alternatives: MER** 2 gm IV infused over 4h q8h (covers ESBLs); **Aztreonam** 2 gm IV q6-8h (safe in beta-lactam allergic patient). Dexamethasone, recommended only for suspected H. influenza infection, administered as stated above for S. pneumoniae.
Specific Therapy—Positive culture of CSF with in vitro susceptibility results available administered as stated above for *S. pneumoniae*.				
H. influenzae	β-lactamase positive	**Ceftriaxone** 2 gm IV q12h (adult), 50 mg/kg IV q12h (peds) + **Dexamethasone** 0.15 mg/kg IV q6h; first dose is given 15-20 minutes prior to first antibiotic dose, and then continued for 4 days in microbiologically confirmed cases.		**Pen. allergic: CIP** 400 mg IV q8h; **Aztreonam** 2 gm q6-8h.
Listeria monocytogenes		**AMP** 2 gm IV q4h		If pen allergic use **TMP/SMX** 5 mg/kg (TMP component) q6-8h. Data showing beneficial effect of gentamicin combination therapy are inconclusive.
N. meningitidis		**Pen G** (adult dose 4 million units q4h) x 7 days or **Ceftriaxone** 2 gm IV q12h x 7 days; if β-lactam allergic, **Aztreonam** 2 gm IV q6h.		Other alternatives: **MER** 2 gm IV q8h or **CIP** 400 mg IV q8h. FQ-resistant isolates encountered rarely. Increased risk of invasive meningococcal infection in recipients of eculizumab *(MMWR 66:734, 2017)*.

 **NOTE: All dosage recommendations are for adults (unless otherwise indicated) and assume normal renal function. § Alternatives consider allergy, PK, compliance, local resistance, cost.*

TABLE 1 (7)

ANATOMIC SITE/DIAGNOSIS/ MODIFYING CIRCUMSTANCES	ETIOLOGIES (usual)	SUGGESTED REGIMENS*		ADJUNCT DIAGNOSTIC OR THERAPEUTIC MEASURES AND COMMENTS
		PRIMARY	ALTERNATIVE§	
CENTRAL NERVOUS SYSTEM/Meningitis, Bacterial, Acute/Specific Therapy—Positive culture of CSF with in vitro susceptibility results available *(continued)*				
S. pneumoniae **Notes:** 1. Dexamethasone 0.15 mg/kg IV q6h; first dose 15-20 minutes prior to first antibiotic dose, and then continued for 4 days. 2. If MIC ≥1, repeat CSF exam after 24–48h. 3. Treat for 10–14 days	Pen G MIC <0.1 μg/mL	**Pen G** 4 million units IV q4h or **AMP** 2 gm IV q4h		**Alternatives: Ceftriaxone** 2 gm IV q12h
	Pen G MIC >0.1 / Ceftriax MIC ≤0.5	**Ceftriaxone** 2 gm IV q12h or **Cefotaxime** 2 gm IV q4–6h		**Alternatives: Cefepime** 2 gm IV q8h or **MER** 2 gm IV q8h, **Moxi** 400 mg IV q24h
	Pen G MIC ≥0.1 / Ceftriax MIC >0.5	**Vanco** 30-60 mg/kg/d in 2-3 div doses, target AUC_{24} 400-600 μg/mL x h + (**Ceftriaxone** or **Cefotaxime** as above)		**Alternatives: Vanco** + **Moxi** 400 mg IV q24h If MIC to Ceftriaxone ≥2 mcg/mL, add **RIF** 600 mg po/IV 1x/day or **Linezolid** 600 mg q12h
E. coli, other coliforms, or P. aeruginosa	**Consultation advised**— need susceptibility results	(**Ceftazidime** or **Cefepime** 2 gm IV q8h) + **Gent** 2 mg/kg IV x 1 dose, then 1.7 mg/kg IV q8h x 21 days.		**Alternatives: MER** 2 gm IV infused over 4h q8h; **CIP** 400 mg IV q8h (need to confirm susceptibility) **Reculture CSF after 4-5 days of therapy;** If culture is still positive, may need adjunctive intrathecal or intraventricular antibiotic therapy.
Prophylaxis for H. influenzae and N. meningitidis				
Haemophilus influenzae type B Household or close contact group defined as persons who reside with the patient or a nonresident who has spent 4 hours or more with the index patient for at least 5 of the 7 days preceding the day of hospitalization of the patient.		**RIF** 20 mg/kg (not to exceed 600 mg) once daily x 4 days for individuals ≥1 mo; 10 mg/mg once daily x 4 days for age <1 mo.		**Household or Close Contacts:** RIF chemoprophylaxis recommended for index patients (unless treated with Cefotaxime or Ceftriaxone) and all household contacts in households with members aged <4 years who are not fully vaccinated or members aged <18 years who are immunocompromised, regardless of their vaccination status. **Childcare Contacts:** RIF chemoprophylaxis recommended in childcare settings when two or more cases of invasive Hib disease have occurred within 60 days and unimmunized or underimmunized children attend the facility; when prophylaxis is indicated, it should be prescribed for all attendees, regardless of age or vaccine status, and for childcare providers.
Prophylaxis for Neisseria meningitidis exposure (close contact)		**RIF** 10 mg/kg (max dose 600 mg) q12h x 2 days (adult or child ≥1 mo); 5 mg/kg q12h x 2 dose child <1 mo OR **Ceftriaxone** single IM dose of 250 mg (adult) or 125 mg (child age <15 years) OR **CIP** single po 500 mg dose (age ≥18; not recommended in pregnant or lactating women, or if CIP resistant isolates circulating in the local community).		↑ risk if close contact for at least 4 hrs during wk before illness onset (e.g., housemates, day care contacts, cellmates) or exposure to pt's nasopharyngeal secretions (e.g., kissing, mouth-to-mouth resuscitation, intubation, nasotracheal suctioning).
Meningitis, chronic Defined as symptoms + CSF pleocytosis for ≥4 wks	MTB cryptococcosis, other fungal, neoplastic, Lyme, syphilis, Whipple's disease	Treatment depends on etiology. No urgent need for empiric therapy, but when TB suspected treatment should be expeditious.		Long list of possibilities: bacteria, parasites, fungi, viruses, neoplasms, vasculitis, and other miscellaneous. See *NEJM. 2021;385:930*
Meningitis, eosinophilic	Angiostrongyliasis, gnathostomiasis, baylisascaris	Corticosteroids	Anti-helminthic therapy probably not beneficial	1/3 lack peripheral eosinophilia. Need serology to confirm diagnosis.
Meningitis, HIV-1 infected (AIDS)	As in adults, >50 yrs: also consider cryptococci, M. tuberculosis, syphilis, HIV aseptic meningitis, Listeria monocytogenes	If etiology not identified: treat as adult >50 yrs + obtain CSF/serum cryptococcal antigen *(see Comments)*	For crypto rx, *see Table 11A, page 178*	C. neoformans most common etiology in AIDS patients. H. influenzae, pneumococci, listeria, TBc, syphilis, viral, histoplasma & coccidioides also need to be considered. Obtain blood cultures.

Abbreviations on page 2. **NOTE: All dosage recommendations are for adults (unless otherwise indicated) and assume normal renal function. § Alternatives consider allergy, PK, compliance, local resistance, cost.*

TABLE 1 (8)

ANATOMIC SITE/DIAGNOSIS/ MODIFYING CIRCUMSTANCES	ETIOLOGIES (usual)	SUGGESTED REGIMENS* PRIMARY	SUGGESTED REGIMENS* ALTERNATIVE§	ADJUNCT DIAGNOSTIC OR THERAPEUTIC MEASURES AND COMMENTS
EAR				
External otitis				
Acute external otitis: "Swimmer's ear", ear buds, headsets Ref: *JAMA 2018;320:1375*	*S. aureus, P. aeruginosa*	Ear drops: 1) **CIP** + (dexamethasone or hydrocortisone) bid x 7 days; 2) **Oflox** qd x 7 days; 3) **CIP** single dose. FQ eardrops assoc. with increased risk of tympanic membrane perforation *(CID 70:1103, 2020)*		Antiseptics, acidifying agents, glucocorticoids & topical antibiotics have similar outcomes *(Cochr Sys Rev 2010;1:CD004740)*. Topical antibiotic therapy favored with cure rates of 65-90%; all are expensive ($70-300).
Chronic	Usually 2° to seborrhea	Eardrops: [(**Polymyxin B** + **Neomycin** + **hydrocortisone** qid) + **selenium sulfide shampoo**]		Control seborrhea with dandruff shampoo containing selenium sulfide (Selsun) or [(ketoconazole shampoo) + (medium potency steroid solution, triamcinolone 0.1%)].
Fungal	Candida species	**Fluconazole** 200 mg po x 1 dose & then 100 mg po x 3-5 days.		
"Necrotizing (malignant) otitis externa" Risk groups: Diabetes mellitus, AIDS, chemotherapy. *See Am J Otolaryngol 37:425, 2016.*	Pseudomonas aeruginosa in >95% *(Otol & Neurotology 34:620, 2013)*	**CIP** Adult: 400 mg IV q8h; 750 mg po q8-12h only for early disease; Child: 20-30 mg/kg/day IV div q12h (max 800 mg/day)	**Pip-tazo** 4.5 gm IV over 30 minutes and then 4hrs later start 4.5 gm IV over 4hrs q8h + **Tobra** 5.1 mg/kg q24h	Very high ESRs are typical. Debridement usually required. R/O osteomyelitis: CT or MRI scans. If bone involved, treat for 6–8 wks. Other alternatives if P. aeruginosa is susceptible: **IMP** 0.5 gm q6h or **MER** 1 gm IV q8h or **CFP** 2 gm IV q12h or **Ceftaz** 2 gm IV q8h.
Perichondritis of the pinna Usually follows piercing through cartilage	Similar to malignant otitis	See malignant otitis, above		Unlike malignant otitis, surgery not always required for perichondritis.
Otitis media—infants, children, adults				
Acute				
Initial empiric therapy of acute otitis media (AOM) **NOTE: Treat children <2 yrs old**. If >2 yrs old, fever <39C, mild or no ear pain, neg./questionable exam— consider analgesic treatment without antimicrobials. Favorable results in mostly afebrile pts with waiting 48hrs before deciding on antibiotic use *(JAMA 296:1235, 1290, 2006)*	Overall detection in middle ear fluid: No pathogen 4% Virus 70% Bact. + virus 66% Bacteria 92% Bacterial pathogens from middle ear: S. pneumo 49%, H. influenzae 29%, M. catarrhalis 28%. Ref.: *CID 43:1417 & 1423, 2006.* Children 6 mos-3 yrs, 2 episodes AOM/yrs & 63% are virus positive *(CID 46:815 & 824, 2008).*	**If NO antibiotics in prior month:** **Amox** 80-90 mg/kg/d divided q8h or q12h (**preferred regimen**) OR **Amox-clav** 90/6.4 mg/kg/d divided bid Options for nonIgE PCN allergy: **Cefdinir** 14 mg/kg/d divided q12h or once q24h **Cefpodoxime proxetil** 10 mg/kg/d divided q12h or once q24h **Cefprozil** 15 mg/kg/d divided q12h **Cefuroxime axetil** 30 mg/kg/d divided q12h **All doses are pediatric** **Duration of rx:** <2 yrs old x 10 days; ≥2 yrs x 5–7 days. **For adult doses, *see Sinusitis, page 55, and Table 10A***	**Received antibiotics in prior month: Amox-clav** 90/6.4 mg/kg/d divided bid OR **Ceftriaxone** 50 mg/kg IV or IM once daily for 3 days **Levofloxacin** (Age < 5 yr: 10 mg/kg po bid x 10 days; age > 5 years 10 mg/g po qd for 10 days (max daily dose 750 mg). For adults also: **Levo** or **Moxi**	**Amoxicillin** remains first-line therapy with low rates of treatment failure and recurrence despite increase in frequency of *Moraxella* and non-typable H. flu *(J Pediatric Infect Dis Soc. 2024 Feb 5)*. **β-lactam allergy:** If history unclear or rash, oral ceph OK; avoid ceph if IgE-mediated allergy, e.g., anaphylaxis. **TMP-SMX:** high failure rate if etiology is DRSP or H. influenza. **Macrolides:** limited efficacy against S. pneumo and H. influenza, use only if β-lactam not an option. **Drug-resistant S. pneumo:** Uncommon risk ↑ if age <2 yrs, antibiotics last 3 mos, &/or daycare attendance. Selection of drug based on (1) effectiveness against β-lactamase producing H. influenzae & M. catarrhalis & (2) effectiveness against S. pneumo, inc. DRSP. Cefaclor, Loracarbef, & Ceftibuten less active vs. S. pneumo (Pen resistant) than other β-lactams. **Otitis media with effusion:** no benefit of antibiotics *(Cochrane Database Syst Rev. Sep 12:9:CD009163, 2012)*. **Persistent otorrhea with PE tubes:** Hydrocortisone/Bacitracin/Colistin eardrops[NUS] 5 drops tid x 7 d more effective than po Amox-clav *(NEJM:370:723, 2014)*. **Refractory or recurrent AOM, age 6 months to 5 years:** Levofloxacin 20 mg/kg/d in divided doses q12h if other options have failed. Tympanostomy tubes may prevent recurrent AOM.

 **NOTE: All dosage recommendations are for adults (unless otherwise indicated) and assume normal renal function. § Alternatives consider allergy, PK, compliance, local resistance, cost.*

TABLE 1 (9)

ANATOMIC SITE/DIAGNOSIS/ MODIFYING CIRCUMSTANCES	ETIOLOGIES (usual)	SUGGESTED REGIMENS*		ADJUNCT DIAGNOSTIC OR THERAPEUTIC MEASURES AND COMMENTS
		PRIMARY	ALTERNATIVE§	
EAR/Otitis media—infants, children, adults *(continued)*				
Treatment for clinical failure after 3 days	Drug-resistant S. pneumoniae main concern	**NO antibiotics in month prior to last 3 days:** **Amox-clav HD** or **Cefdinir** or **Cefpodoxime** or **Cefprozil** or **Cefuroxime Axetil** or IM **Ceftriaxone** x 3 days	**Antibiotics in month prior to last 3 days:** **Levofloxacin**: if Ceftriaxone is contraindicated or refractory infection Age < 5 years: 10 mg/kg po q12h x 10 days Age > 5 years: 10 mg/g po once daily for 10 days (max daily dose 750 mg)	**Levo** 20 mg/kg/d in divided doses q12h if other options have failed (not FDA approved).
		For dosage, see footnote[3] **All doses are pediatric** Duration of rx as above		
After >48 hrs of nasotracheal intubation	Pseudomonas sp., klebsiella, enterobacter	**Ceftazidime** or **CFP** or **IMP** or **MER** or (**Pip-tazo**) or **CIP**. *(For dosages, see Ear, Necrotizing (malignant) otitis externa, page 12)*		With nasotracheal intubation >48 hrs, about ½ pts will have otitis media with effusion.
Prophylaxis: acute otitis media	S. pneumo	**Antimicrobial prophylaxis is not recommended.**	**Use of antibiotics to prevent otitis media is a major contributor to emergence of antibiotic-resistant S. pneumo.**	
Mastoiditis: Complication of acute or chronic otitis media. If chronic, look for cholesteatoma (Keratoma)				
Acute				
Generally too ill for outpatient therapy	If complication of 1st episode of acute otitis media: S. pneumoniae (most common) S. pyogenes S. aureus If secondary to chronic otitis media: S. aureus P. aeruginosa	Child: 1st episode, uncomplicated disease. no prior antibiotics: **Amp-sulb** 200 mg/kg/d IV in 4 divided doses OR **Ceftriaxone** 50-100 mg/kg/d in 2 divided doses Adult: suspect complicated disease, treat for acute exacerbation of chronic infection	Acute exacerbation of chronic otitis media: Surgical debridement of auditory canal, then [**Vanco** 30-60 mg/kg/d in 2-3 div doses, target AUC24 400-600 µg/mL x h + **Pip-tazo** 4.5 gm IV q8h] OR [**Vanco** + **Cefepime** 2 gm IV q8h (Adult), 50 mg/kg IV q8h (Child) + **Metronidazole** 750 mg q8h (Adult), 22.5 mg/kg/d in 3 divided doses (Child)]	• Diagnosis: CT or MRI • Look for complication: osteomyelitis, suppurative lateral sinus thrombophlebitis, purulent meningitis, brain abscess • ENT consultation for possible mastoidectomy
Chronic				
Generally not ill enough for parenteral antibiotics	As per 1st episode and: S. aureus P. aeruginosa Anaerobes Fungi	Culture ear drainage. May need surgical debridement. Topical Fluoroquinolone ear drops. ENT consult.		• Diagnosis: CT or MRI

[3] **Drugs & peds dosage (all po unless specified) for acute otitis media: Amoxicillin UD (usual dose)** = 40 mg/kg per day div q12h or q8h. **Amoxicillin HD (high dose)** = 90 mg/kg per day div q12h or q8h. **AM-CL HD** = 90 mg/kg per day of amox component. **Extra-strength Amox-clav oral suspension** (Augmentin ES-600) available with 600 mg AM & 42.9 mg CL / 5 mL—dose: 90/6.4 mg/kg per day div bid. **Cefuroxime axetil** 30 mg/kg per day div q12h. **Ceftriaxone** 50 mg/kg IM x 3 days. **Clindamycin** 20–30 mg/kg per day div qid (may be effective vs. DRSP but no activity vs. H. influenzae). **Other drugs suitable for drug (e.g., Penicillin) - sensitive S. pneumo: TMP-SMX** 4 mg/kg of TMP q12h. **Erythro-sulfisoxazole** 50 mg/kg per day of erythro div q6–8h. **Clarithro** 15 mg/kg per day div q12h; **Azithro** 10 mg/kg per day x 1 & then 5 mg/kg q24h on days 2–5. Other FDA-approved regimens: 10 mg/kg q24h x 3 days & 30 mg/kg x 1. **Cefprozil** 15 mg/kg q12h; **Cefpodoxime proxetil** 10 mg/kg per day as single dose; **Cefaclor** 40 mg/kg per day div q8h. **Cefdinir** 7 mg/kg q12h or 14 mg/kg q24h.

Abbreviations on page 2. **NOTE: All dosage recommendations are for adults (unless otherwise indicated) and assume normal renal function. § Alternatives consider allergy, PK, compliance, local resistance, cost.*

TABLE 1 (10)

ANATOMIC SITE/DIAGNOSIS/ MODIFYING CIRCUMSTANCES	ETIOLOGIES (usual)	SUGGESTED REGIMENS* PRIMARY	SUGGESTED REGIMENS* ALTERNATIVE§	ADJUNCT DIAGNOSTIC OR THERAPEUTIC MEASURES AND COMMENTS
EYE				
Eyelid:				
Blepharitis	Etiol. unclear. Factors include Staph. aureus & Staph. epidermidis, seborrhea, rosacea, & dry eye	Lid margin care with baby shampoo & warm compresses q24h. Artificial tears if assoc. dry eye *(see Comment)*.		Topical ointments of uncertain benefit *(Cochrane Database Syst Rev. 2017 Feb 7;2:CD011965)*. If associated rosacea, add doxy 100 mg po bid for 2 wks and then q24h.
Hordeolum (Stye) Cochrane review of effectiveness of non-surgical interventions found no evidence for or against non-surgical interventions for treatment of acute internal hordeola *(Cochrane Database Syst Rev. 2017 Jan 9;1:CD00774)*.				
External (eyelash follicle)	Staph. aureus	Hot packs only. Will drain spontaneously		Infection of superficial sebaceous gland.
Internal (Meibomian glands): Can be acute, subacute or chronic.	Staph. aureus, MSSA	Oral **Diclox** + hot packs		Also called acute meibomianitis. Rarely drain spontaneously; may need I&D and culture. Role of fluoroquinolone eye drops is unclear. MRSA often resistant to lower conc.; may be susceptible to higher concentration of FQ in ophthalmologic solutions of gati, levo or moxi.
	Staph. aureus, MRSA	**TMP-SMX-DS**, tabs ii po bid		
	Staph. aureus, MRSA (MDR)	**Linezolid** 600 mg po bid		
Conjunctiva:				
Conjunctivitis of the newborn (ophthalmia neonatorum): by day of onset post-delivery—all dose pediatric				
Onset 1st day	Chemical due to silver nitrate prophylaxis	None		Usual prophylaxis is erythro ointment; hence, silver nitrate irritation rare.
Onset 2–4 days	N. gonorrhoeae	**Ceftriaxone** 25–50 mg/kg IV x 1 dose *(see Comment)*, not to exceed 125 mg		Treat mother and her sexual partners. Hyperpurulent. Topical rx inadequate. **Treat neonate for concomitant Chlamydia trachomatis.**
Onset 3–10 days	Chlamydia trachomatis	**Erythro base or ethylsuccinate syrup** 12.5 mg/kg q6h x 14 days. No topical rx needed.		Diagnosis by NAAT. Alternative: **Azithro suspension** 20 mg/kg po q24h x 3 days. Treat mother & sexual partner.
Onset 2–16 days	Herpes simplex types 1, 2	Topical anti-viral rx under direction of ophthalmologist.		Also give **Acyclovir** 60 mg/kg/day IV div 3 doses.
Ophthalmia neonatorum prophylaxis: **Erythro** 0.5% ointment x 1 or **Tetra** 1% ointment[NUS] x 1 application; effective vs. gonococcus but not C. trachomatis				
Pink eye (viral conjunctivitis) Usually unilateral	Adenovirus (types 3 & 7 in children, 8, 11 & 19 in adults)	No treatment. If symptomatic, artificial tears may help.		Highly contagious. Onset of ocular pain and photophobia in an adult suggests associated keratitis—rare.
Inclusion conjunctivitis (adult) Usually unilateral & concomitant genital infection	Chlamydia trachomatis	**Azithro** 1 gm once	**Doxy** 100 mg po bid x 7 days	Oculogenital disease. Diagnosis NAAT. Urine NAAT for both GC & chlamydia. Treat sexual partner. May need to repeat dose of azithro.
Trachoma —a chronic bacterial keratoconjunctivitis linked to poverty	Chlamydia trachomatis	**Azithro** 20 mg/kg po single dose—78% effective in children; Adults: 1 gm po.	**Doxy** 100 mg po bid x minimum of 21 days or **Tetracycline** 250 mg po qid x 14 days.	Starts in childhood and can persist for years with subsequent damage to cornea. Topical therapy of marginal benefit. Avoid doxy/tetracycline in young children. Mass treatment works.
Suppurative conjunctivitis, bacterial: Children and Adults (Eyedrops speed resolution of symptoms: *Cochrane Database Syst Rev. Sep 12;9:CD001211, 2012*)				
JAMA 310:1721, 2013	Staph. aureus, S. pneumoniae, H. influenzae, Viridans Strep., Moraxella sp.	FQ ophthalmic solns: **CIP** (generic); others expensive (**Levo, Moxi**) All 1-2 gtts q2h while awake 1st 2 days, then q4–8h up to 7 days.	**Polymyxin B + TMP** solution 1–2 gtts q3–6h x 7–10 days.	**FQs** best spectrum for empiric therapy. High concentrations ↑ likelihood of activity vs. S. aureus—even MRSA. **TMP** spectrum may include MRSA. Polymyxin B spectrum only Gm-neg. bacilli but no ophthal. prep of only **TMP**. Most S. pneumo resistant to Gent & Tobra.
Gonococcal (peds/adults)	N. gonorrhoeae	**Ceftriaxone** 25-50 mg/kg IV/IM (not to exceed 125 mg) as one dose in children; 1 gm IM/IV as one dose in adults		

Abbreviations on page 2. **NOTE: All dosage recommendations are for adults (unless otherwise indicated) and assume normal renal function. § Alternatives consider allergy, PK, compliance, local resistance, cost.*

TABLE 1 (11)

ANATOMIC SITE/DIAGNOSIS/ MODIFYING CIRCUMSTANCES	ETIOLOGIES (usual)	SUGGESTED REGIMENS*		ADJUNCT DIAGNOSTIC OR THERAPEUTIC MEASURES AND COMMENTS
		PRIMARY	ALTERNATIVE§	
EYE *(continued)*				
Cornea (keratitis): Usually serious and often sight-threatening. Prompt ophthalmologic consultation essential for diagnosis, antimicrobial and adjunctive therapy! Herpes simplex most common etiology in developed countries; bacterial and fungal infections more common in underdeveloped countries.				
Viral				
H. simplex	H. simplex, types 1 & 2	**Trifluridine** ophthalmic sol'n, one drop q2h up to 9 drops/ day until re-epithelialized, then one drop q4h up to 5x/ day, for total not to exceed 21 days. *See Comment*	**Ganciclovir** 0.15% ophthalmic gel: Indicated for acute herpetic keratitis. One drop 5 times per day while awake until corneal ulcer heals; then, one drop three times per day for 7 days.	**For severe infection or immunocompromised host**, consider adding **acyclovir** 400 mg po 5x daily or **valacyclovir** 1000 mg bid. Topical acyclovir 3% ointment 5x daily is a first-line treatment for HSV epithelial keratitis outside the United States. Approx 30% recurrence rate within one year; consider prophylaxis with acyclovir 400 mg bid for 12 months or valacyclovir 500 mg once daily to prevent recurrences.
Varicella-zoster ophthalmicus	Varicella-zoster virus	**Famciclovir** 500 mg po tid or **Valacyclovir** 1 gm po tid x 10 days	**Acyclovir** 3% ointment 5x/day is a first-line treatment outside the US **Acyclovir** 400 mg 5x/day or **Valacyclovir** 1000 mg bid	Clinical diagnosis most common: dendritic figures with fluorescein staining in patient with varicella-zoster of ophthalmic branch of trigeminal nerve.
Bacterial		**All treatment listed for bacterial, fungal, protozoan is topical unless otherwise indicated**		
Acute: No comorbidity	S. aureus Coagulase-negative staphylococci S. pyogenes P. aeruginosa Enterobacterales	Initial, empiric therapy for uncomplicated, community-acquired infection (**CIP** 3 mg/ml optic solution or **Levo** 15 mg/ml optic solution) 1 gtt hourly x 24–72 hrs then taper based on clinical response.	**Tobra** or **Gent** 3 mg/ml optic solution 1 gtt hourly x 24–72 hrs, then taper based on clinical response.	Regimens vary: some start rx by applying drops q5 min for 5 doses; some apply drops q15-30 min for several hours; some extend interval to q2h during sleep. **NOTE:** despite high concentrations, may fail vs. MRSA.
Contact lens users	P. aeruginosa	**CIP** 0.3% ophthalmic solution or **Levo** 0.5% ophthalmic solution 1-2 gtts hourly x24-72h, taper based on response.	**Gent** or **Tobra** 0.3% ophthalmic solution 1-2 gtts hourly x24h then taper based on clinical response.	Recommend alginate swab culture and susceptibility testing; refer to ophthalmologist. **Cornea abrasions:** treated with Tobra, Gent, or CIP gtts qid for 3-5 days; referral to ophthalmologist recommended cornea infiltrate or ulcer, visual loss, lack of improvement or worsening symptoms.
Dry cornea, diabetes, immunosuppression	Staph. aureus, S. epidermidis, S. pneumoniae, S. pyogenes, Enterobacterales, listeria	**CIP** 0.3% ophthalmic solution 1-2 gtts hourly x24–72 hrs, then taper based on clinical response.	**Vanco** (50 mg/mL) + **Ceftaz** (50 mg/mL) hourly for 24-72h, taper depending upon response. *See Comment.*	Specific therapy guided by results of alginate swab culture.
Fungal	Aspergillus, fusarium, candida and others.	**Natamycin** (5%): 1 drop q1-2h for several days; then q3-4h for several days; can reduce frequency depending upon response.	**Amphotericin B** (0.15%): 1 drop q1-2h for several days; can reduce frequency depending upon response.	Obtain specimens for fungal wet mount and cultures. Numerous other treatment options (**Itra** 1% topical x 6 wks, **Itra** 100 mg po bid x 3 wks, Vori 1% topical x 2 wks, **Miconazole** 1% topical 5x daily, **silver sulphadiazine** 0.5-1% topical 5x daily) appear to have similar efficacy.
Mycobacteria: Post-refractive eye surgery	*M. chelonae; M. abscessus; M. massiliense*	**Gati** or **Moxi** eye drops: 1 gtt qid in conjunction with other active antimicrobial eyedrops (**Amikacin** 50 mg/L and **Clarithro** 10 mg/L).		**Alternative:** systemic rx: **Doxy** 100 mg po bid + **Clarithro** 500 mg po bid *(PLoS One 10:doi16236, 2015).*

Abbreviations on page 2. **NOTE: All dosage recommendations are for adults (unless otherwise indicated) and assume normal renal function. § Alternatives consider allergy, PK, compliance, local resistance, cost.*

TABLE 1 (12)

ANATOMIC SITE/DIAGNOSIS/ MODIFYING CIRCUMSTANCES	ETIOLOGIES (usual)	SUGGESTED REGIMENS*		ADJUNCT DIAGNOSTIC OR THERAPEUTIC MEASURES AND COMMENTS
		PRIMARY	ALTERNATIVE§	
EYE/Cornea (keratitis) *(continued)*				
Protozoan Soft contact lens users. Uncommon. Trauma and soft contact lenses are risk factors.	Acanthamoeba castellanii Acanthamoeba polyphaga Other Acanthamoeba sp. Other free-living ameba species including Hartmannella and Vahlkampfiid amoebae are causative *(Cornea 36:785, 2017)*	Topical 0.02%-0.2% biguanide chlorhexidine or 0.02%-0.06% Polyhexamethylene biguanide (PHMB) in combination with propamidine (0.1 %) or hexamidine (0.1 %). Start with lower dose of PHMB and titrate to clinical response. **Alternate Rx:** Uncontrolled reports of amebic eradication with oral miltefosine but post-miltefosine inflammatory response leads to corneal thinning and possible perforation. Steroid coverage has been proposed. Cornea 2021 Sep 4 (online ahead of print). Also consider: voriconazole 1% solution *(Eye (Lond) 2020 Jul 27)*		Initially, drops should be applied up to hourly day and night for the first 48 hours then hourly during the daytime for the first week, then with subsequent taper over 3 - 4 weeks. Debridement may also be warranted.
Lacrimal apparatus				
Canaliculitis	Actinomyces Staph., Strep. Rarely, Arachnia, fusobacterium, nocardia, candida	Apply hot packs to punctal area 4x/day. Refer to ophthalmologist for removal of granules and local irrigation with an antibiotic solution.		Digital pressure produces exudate at punctum; Gram stain confirms diagnosis.
Dacryocystitis (lacrimal sac)	S. pneumo, S. aureus, H. influenzae, S. pyogenes, P. aeruginosa	Often consequence of obstruction of lacrimal duct. Empiric systemic antimicrobial therapy based on Gram stain of aspirate—*see Comment.*		Need ophthalmologic consultation. Surgery may be required. Can be acute or chronic. Culture to detect MRSA.
Endophthalmitis: Endogenous (secondary to bacteremia or fungemia) and exogenous (post-injection, post-operative) types. **Ophthalmologic consult imperative.**				
Bacterial: Haziness of vitreous key to diagnosis. Needle aspirate of both vitreous and aqueous humor for culture prior to therapy. Intravitreal administration of antimicrobials essential.				
Postocular surgery (cataracts)				
Early, acute onset (incidence 0.05%)	S. epidermidis 60%, Staph. aureus, streptococci, & enterococci each 5–10%, Gm-neg. bacilli 6%	**Immediate ophthal. consult.** If only light perception or worse, immediate vitrectomy + intravitreal vanco 1 mg & intravitreal ceftazidime 2.25 mg.		
Low grade, chronic	Cutibacterium acnes, S. epidermidis, S. aureus (rare) also fungal	Intraocular **Vanco**. Usually requires vitrectomy, lens removal.		
Post filtering blebs for glaucoma	Strep. species (viridans & others), H. influenzae	Referral to ophthalmologist for intravitreal **Vanco** 1 mg + **Ceftaz** 2.25 mg and a topical ophthalmic antimicrobial.		
Post-penetrating trauma	Bacillus sp., S. epiderm.	Referral to ophthalmologist for intravitreal **Vanco** 1 mg + (**Ceftaz** 2.25 mg or **Amikacin** 0.4 mg) + systemic **Vanco** 30-60 mg/kg/d in 2-3 div doses, target AUC_{24} 400-600 µg/mL x h + [**Ceftaz** 1 g IV q8h or **CIP** 400 mg IV/po q12h]. Vitrectomy may be required.		
Hematogenous	S. pneumoniae, N. meningitidis, Staph. aureus, Grp B Strep, K. pneumo	(**Cefotaxime** 2 gm IV q4h or **Ceftriaxone** 2 gm IV q24h or **Ceftazidime** 2 gm IV q8h) + **Vanco** 30-60 mg/kg/d in 2-3 div doses, target AUC_{24} 400-600 µg/mL x h pending cultures. Intravitreal antibiotics as with early postocular surgery. Urgent ophthalmological consultation.		
Mycotic (fungal): Broad-spectrum antibiotics, often corticosteroids, indwelling venous catheters	Candida sp., Aspergillus sp.	Intravitreal **Ampho B** 0.005–0.01 mg in 0.1 mL. *Also see Table 11A, page 177 for concomitant systemic therapy. See Comment*		Patients with *Candida* spp. chorioretinitis usually respond to systemically administered antifungals. Intravitreal ampho and/or vitrectomy may be necessary for those with vitritis or endophthalmitis. *(IDSA guidelines CID 62:409, 2016).*

 **NOTE: All dosage recommendations are for adults (unless otherwise indicated) and assume normal renal function. § Alternatives consider allergy, PK, compliance, local resistance, cost.*

TABLE 1 (13)

ANATOMIC SITE/DIAGNOSIS/ MODIFYING CIRCUMSTANCES	ETIOLOGIES (usual)	SUGGESTED REGIMENS* PRIMARY	ALTERNATIVE§	ADJUNCT DIAGNOSTIC OR THERAPEUTIC MEASURES AND COMMENTS
EYE *(continued)*				
Retinitis				
Acute retinal necrosis Review: *Clinical Ophthalmology 14:1931, 2020*	Varicella zoster virus (VZV), Herpes simplex	IV **Acyclovir** 10–12 mg/kg IV q8h x 5–7 days, then **Acyclovir** 800 mg po 5 x/day OR **Valacyclovir** 1000 mg po tid OR **Famciclovir** 500 mg po tid		Strong association of VZ virus with atypical necrotizing herpetic retinopathy. Ophthalmology consultation.
HIV+ (AIDS) CD4 usually <100/mm³	Cytomegalovirus	*See Table 14A, page 226*		Occurs in 5–10% of AIDS patients
Progressive outer retinal necrosis	VZV, H. simplex, CMV (rare)	**Acyclovir** 10-12 mg/kg IV q8h for 1-2 weeks, then (**Valacyclovir** 1000 mg po tid, or **Famciclovir** 500 mg po tid, or **Acyclovir** 800 mg po tid). Ophthalmology consultation imperative		Most patients are highly immunocompromised (HIV with low CD4 or transplantation). May be able to stop oral antivirals when CD4 recovers with ART *(Ocul Immunol Inflammation 15:425, 2007)*.
Retinochoroiditis (posterior uveitis)	Toxoplasma gondii	**Pyrimethamine** 200 mg po once on 1st day, then 50–75 mg q24h] + [**sulfadiazine** 1–1.5 gm po qid] + [**Leucovorin** (folinic acid) 5–20 mg 3x/week]. **TMP-SMX** 1 DS q12. Add Prednisone 1 mg/kg/day in 2 divided doses if threat of visual loss		The most common manifestation of toxoplasmosis in immunocompetent. Due to expense of pyrimethamine, can substitute TMP-SMX; Recurrent episodes can be treated with **TMP-SMX** 1 DS q12 x 45 days followed by 1 DS qod for 311 days *(Am J Ophth 213:195 2020)*.
Orbital cellulitis *(see page 60 for erysipelas, facial)*	S. pneumoniae, H. influenzae, M. catarrhalis, S. aureus, anaerobes, group A strep, occ. Gm-neg. bacilli post-trauma	**Vanco** 15-20 mg/kg IV q8-12h target AUC_{24} 400-600 µg/mL x h + ([**Ceftriaxone** 2 gm IV q24h + **Metro** 1 gm IV q12h] OR **Pip-tazo** 4.5 gm infused over 4h IV q8h OR **Ampicillin-sulbactam** 3 gm q6h IV)		**If Penicillin/Ceph allergy: Vanco** + **Moxi** 400 mg IV q24h. Problem is frequent inability to make microbiologic diagnosis. Image orbit (CT or MRI). Risk of cavernous sinus thrombosis. Options for MRSA: **Dapto** 6 mg/kg IV q24h or **Linezolid** 600 mg IV q12h.
FOOT				
"Diabetic foot" With extension into deeper tissues —Two thirds of patients have triad of neuropathy, deformity and pressure-induced trauma. IDSA Guidelines *CID 54:e132, 2012*.				
Ulcer without inflammation	Colonizing skin flora	No antibacterial therapy.		**General:** 1. Glucose control, eliminate pressure on ulcer 2. **Assess for peripheral vascular disease** 3. Caution in use of TMP-SMX in patients with diabetes, as many have risk factors for hyperkalemia (e.g., advanced age, reduced renal function, concomitant medications). 4. Improved outcomes in healing of diabetic foot ulcer with negative-pressure wound therapy (See *Curr Opin Infect Dis 29:145, 2016* for review). **Principles of empiric antibacterial therapy:** 1. For ulcer with superficial infection can use TMP-SMX as a single agent to cover MRSA or if no MRSA present, Amox-clav. 2. Obtain culture; cover for MRSA in moderate, more severe infections pending culture data. 3. Severe limb and/or life-threatening infections require initial parenteral therapy to cover. Gm-positive cocci including MRSA, coliforms & other aerobic Gm-neg. rods, & anaerobic Gm-neg. bacilli. 4. Risk of associated osteomyelitis is increased if ulcer area >2 cm², positive probe to bone *(CID 2016,63:944)*, ESR >70 and abnormal plain x-ray. MRI is best imaging modality.
Mild infection	*S. aureus (assume MRSA), S. agalactiae (Gp B), S. pyogenes predominate*	Oral therapy: (**Amox-clav** 875 mg/125 mg po bid + **TMP-SMX**-DS 1-2 tabs po bid) or [(**CIP** 750 mg po bid or **Levo** 750 mg po q24h or **Moxi** 400 mg po q24h) + (**Linezolid** 600 mg po bid)]		
Moderate infection. **Osteomyelitis** *See Comment.*	As above, plus coliforms possible	**Oral:** As above Parenteral therapy [based on prevailing susceptibilities]: (**Amp-sulb** 3 gm IV q6h or **Erta** 1 gm IV q24h) + **Vanco** 15-20 mg/kg IV q8-12h to achieve preferred target AUC_{24} 400-600 µg/mL x hr until MRSA is excluded. *Dosages in footnotes* [4]		
Extensive local inflammation plus systemic toxicity.	As above, plus anaerobic bacteria. Role of enterococci unclear.	**Parenteral therapy: Vanco** 15-20 mg/kg IV q8-12h to achieve preferred target AUC_{24} 400-600 µg/mL x hr + **Pip-tazo** 4.5 gm infused over 4h IV q8h OR **Vanco** as above + (**IMP** 0.5 gm IV q6h or **MER** 1 gm IV q8h) *Dosages in footnote* [4] **Assess for arterial insufficiency!**		

[4] **Vanco** 15-20 mg/kg IV q8-12h to achieve preferred target AUC_{24} level of 400-600 µg/mL x hr, **Parenteral β-lactam/β-lactamase inhibitors**; **Amp-sulb** 3 gm IV q6h, **Pip-tazo** 4.5 gm infused over 4h IV q8h; **carbapenems: Doripenem** 500 mg (1-hr infusion) q8h, **ERTA** 1 gm IV q24h, **IMP** 0.5 gm IV q6h, **MER** 1 gm IV q8h, **Dapto** 6 mg per kg IV q24h, **Linezolid** 600 mg IV q12h, **Aztreonam** 2 gm IV q8h. **CIP** 400 mg IV q12h, **Levo** 750 mg IV q24h, **Moxi** 400 mg IV q24h, **Metro** 1 gm IV loading dose & then 0.5 gm IV q6h or 1 gm IV q12h.

 **NOTE: All dosage recommendations are for adults (unless otherwise indicated) and assume normal renal function. § Alternatives consider allergy, PK, compliance, local resistance, cost.*

TABLE 1 (14)

ANATOMIC SITE/DIAGNOSIS/ MODIFYING CIRCUMSTANCES	ETIOLOGIES (usual)	SUGGESTED REGIMENS*		ADJUNCT DIAGNOSTIC OR THERAPEUTIC MEASURES AND COMMENTS
		PRIMARY	ALTERNATIVE§	
FOOT *(continued)*				
Onychomycosis: *See Table 11, page 180, fungal infections*				
Puncture wound *See J Am Podiatr Med Assoc. 2020 Nov 2;20-206.*	*P. aeruginosa, S. aureus, Strept*	Cleanse. Tetanus booster. Observe.		*See Osteomyelitis, page 5.* 1–2% evolves to osteo.
GALLBLADDER				
Cholecystitis, cholangitis, biliary sepsis, or common duct obstruction (partial: 2nd to tumor, stones, stricture).	Enterobacterales 68%, enterococci 14%, bacteroides 10%, Clostridium sp. 7%, rarely candida	(**Pip-tazo** or **ERTA**) If life-threatening: **IMP** or **MER** *Dosages in footnote* 4 * Add **Vanco** for empiric activity vs. enterococci	(**P Ceph 3*** + **Metro**) or (**Aztreonam*** + **Metro**) or (**CIP*** + **Metro**) or **Moxi**	• Establish adequate biliary drainage, surgical, percutaneous or ERCP-placed stent, in more severely ill patients. No benefit to continuation of antibiotics after surgery in pts with acute calculous cholecystitis *(JAMA 3312:145, 2014)*. • Increasing FQ resistant *E. coli* limits utility of FQ regimens for empiric therapy. Choice should be guided by local susceptibility profiles. • Avoid Amp-sulb due to high levels of resistance among *E. coli* isolates.
GASTROINTESTINAL				
Gastroenteritis—Empiric Therapy (laboratory studies not performed or culture, microscopy, toxin results NOT AVAILABLE) ***NEJM 370:16, 2014*****; IDSA Guideline (Diarrhea):** ***CID 2017,65:1963 & e45.***				
Premature infant with necrotizing enterocolitis	Associated with intestinal flora	Treatment should cover broad range of intestinal bacteria using drugs appropriate to age and local susceptibility patterns, e.g., **Pip-tazo** rationale as in diverticulitis/ peritonitis, *page 24.*		Pneumatosis intestinalis, if present on x-ray confirms diagnosis. Bacteremia-peritonitis in 30–50%. If Staph. epidermidis isolated, add vanco (IV). For review and general management, *see NEJM 364:255, 2011.*
Mild diarrhea 1-2 unformed stools per day	Bacterial *(see Severe, below)*, viral (norovirus), parasitic. Viral usually causes mild to moderate disease. For traveler's diarrhea, *see page 21*	Fluids only + lactose-free diet, avoid caffeine		**Rehydration: For po fluid replacement,** *see Cholera, page 20.* **Antimotility** (Do not use if fever, bloody stools, or suspicion of HUS): Loperamide (Imodium) 4 mg po, then 2 mg after each loose stool to max. of 16 mg per day. Bismuth subsalicylate (Pepto-Bismol) 2 tablets (262 mg) po qid. **Hemolytic uremic syndrome (HUS):** Risk in **children** infected with E. coli 0157:H7 is 8–10%. Early treatment with TMP-SMX or FQs ↑ risk of HUS. **Norovirus:** Etiology of over 90% of non-bacterial diarrhea (± nausea/ vomiting). Lasts 12-60 hrs. Hydrate. No effective antiviral. **Other potential etiologies (parasitic):** Cryptosporidia—no treatment in immunocompetent host. Cyclospora—usually chronic diarrhea, responds to TMP-SMX *(see Table 13A)*.
Moderate diarrhea 3-5 unformed stools per day		Antimotility agents *(see Comments)* + fluids		
Severe diarrhea (≥6 unformed stools/day, &/or temp ≥101°F, tenesmus, blood, or fecal leukocytes). **NOTE: Severe afebrile bloody diarrhea should ↑ suspicion of Shiga-toxin E. coli 0157:H7 & others**	Shigella, salmonella, C. jejuni, Shiga toxin + E. coli, toxin-positive C. difficile, Klebsiella oxytoca, E. histolytica, Vibrio sp. *For typhoid fever, see page 68*	(**CIP** 500 mg po q12h or **Levo** 500 mg q24h) x 3–5 days **Azithro** 1000 mg po once or 500 mg q 24h x 3 days preferred for Campylobacter and disease acquired in Southeast Asia. If *C. difficile* see **C. difficile toxin positive antibiotic-associated colitis** below for specific recommendations.	**TMP-SMX**-DS po bid x 3–5 days. Campylobacter resistance to TMP-SMX is common in the tropics. *C. diff* recommendations changed: See *CID 73:755, 2021 or Med Let 63:137, 2021*	
		If recent antibiotic therapy (C. difficile toxin colitis possible) promptly test stool for C. diff.		

Abbreviations on page 2. **NOTE: All dosage recommendations are for adults (unless otherwise indicated) and assume normal renal function. § Alternatives consider allergy, PK, compliance, local resistance, cost.*

TABLE 1 (15)

ANATOMIC SITE/DIAGNOSIS/ MODIFYING CIRCUMSTANCES	ETIOLOGIES (usual)	SUGGESTED REGIMENS*		ADJUNCT DIAGNOSTIC OR THERAPEUTIC MEASURES AND COMMENTS
		PRIMARY	ALTERNATIVE§	
GASTROINTESTINAL *(continued)*				
Gastroenteritis—Specific Therapy (results of culture, microscopy, toxin assay AVAILABLE) Ref.: *NEJM 370:1532, 2014*; IDSA infectious diarrhea guideline *(CID 2017,65:1963)*.				
If culture negative, probably **Norovirus (Norwalk)** other virus *(EID 17:1381, 2011) — see Norovirus, page 232* **NOTE**: WBC >15,000 suggestive of C. difficile in hospitalized patient. Campylobacter bacteremia: *CID 2022;75:702* (retrospective)	**Aeromonas/Plesiomonas**	**CIP** 750 mg po bid x 3 days.	**TMP-SMX DS** tab 1 po bid x 3 days	Aeromonas ref: *Eur J Clin Microbiol ID. 36:1393, 2017.*
	Amebiasis (Entamoeba histolytica, Cyclospora, Cryptosporidia and **Giardia)**, *see Table 13A*			
	Campylobacter jejuni History of fever in 53-83%. Self-limited diarrhea in normal host.	**Azithro** 500 mg po q24h x 3 days OR 1000 mg po one dose	**Erythro stearate** 500 mg po qid x 5 days or **CIP** 500 mg po bid (CIP resistance increasing) *(CID 2017;65:1624)*.	**Post-Campylobacter Guillain-Barré;** assoc. 15% of cases. **Reactive arthritis** another potential sequelae. *See Traveler's diarrhea, page 21.*
	Campylobacter fetus Diarrhea uncommon. More systemic disease in debilitated hosts. Don't treat immunocompetent.	**IMP** 500 mg IV q 6 or **MER** 1 gm IV q8	**AMP** 100 mg/kg/day IV div q6h or **Gent** 5 mg/kg IV q 24. **Erta** 1 gm q24	Draw blood cultures. In bacteremic pts, FQ resistance common in *C. fetus*. Meropenem inhibits C. fetus at low concentrations in vitro. Clinical review: *CID 58:1579, 2014*. Recommendations are for treatment of bacteremia or focal infections. Gastroenteritis is self-limiting and does not require antimicrobial therapy except for severe infection or immunocompromised host.
Differential diagnosis of toxin-producing diarrhea: • *C. difficile* • *Klebsiella oxytoca* • *S. aureus* • Shiga toxin producing *E. coli* (STEC) • Enterotoxigenic *B. fragilis* IDSA Guidelines *(C. diff)*: *CID 2018,66:987* Revised focused guidelines: *CID 73:755, 2021; Med Lett 63:137, 2021*	**C. difficile toxin positive antibiotic-associated colitis. Probiotics:** Cochrane review found moderate quality evidence the probiotics prevents C. diff. associated diarrhea *(Cochrane Database Syst Rev. 2017 Dec 19;12:CD006095)*.			
	po meds okay; WBC <15,000; no increase in serum creatinine.	**Fidaxomicin** 200 mg po bid x 10 days or **Vanco** 125 mg po qid x 10-14 days	*See Comment*	**D/C antibiotic if possible; avoid antimotility agents, hydration, enteric isolation.** Recent review suggests antimotility agents can be used cautiously in certain pts with mild disease who are receiving rx *(CID 48: 598, 2009)*. **Relapse in 10-20%.** Note: **Metro 500 mg tid no longer recommended as first-line therapy.**
	po meds okay; Sicker; WBC >15,000; ≥50% increase in baseline creatinine	**Fidaxomicin** 200 mg po bid x 10 days or **Vanco** 125 mg po qid x 10 days. For oral use of IV Vanco, *see Table 10A, page 156.*	**Fidaxomicin** 200 mg po bid x 10 days	**Vanco superior to metro in sicker pts.** Relapse in 10-20%. Fidaxomicin had lower rate of recurrence than Vanco for diarrhea with non-NAP1 strains *(N Engl J Med 364:422, 2011)*. Bezlotoxumab 1 dose IV + standard rx reduced relapse rate 11-14% *(NEJM 2017, 376:305)*.
	Post-treatment relapse. Ideally use a regimen not used previously.	**Fidaxomicin** 200 mg po bid x 10 days or **Vanco** 125 mg po qid x 10-14 days, then immediately start taper *(See Comments)*	**Fidaxomicin** 200 mg po bid x 10 days then 200 mg po qod x 20 days	**Vanco taper** (all doses 125 mg po): week 1 – tid, week 2 – bid week 3 – q24h week 4 – q48h, week 5 – q72h. Ref: *CID 2017;65:1624*. Prevention of recurrent CDI (age >18 yrs) following antibiotic treatment: Fecal microbiota regimen with either of 2 FDA-approved products: **Rebyota** or **Vowst**. **Bezlotoxumab**, anti C. diff toxin B approved and recommended in 2021 IDSA focused guidelines, decreases recurrence 10% but very expensive *CID 68:699, 2019*. If **Metro** used for initial therapy can use standard 10-day course of **Vanco**.
(Continued on next page)	Post-op ileus; severe disease with toxic megacolon *(CID 61:934, 2015)*.	**Metro** 500 mg IV q8h + **Vanco** 500 mg q6h via nasogastric tube (or naso-small bowel tube) ± vanco 500 mg q6h retention enema. *See comment* for dosage. No data on efficacy of **Fidaxomicin** in severe life-threatening disease.		For vanco instillation into bowel, add 500 mg vanco to 500 mL of saline. **NOTE: IV vanco not effective.**

Abbreviations on page 2. **NOTE: All dosage recommendations are for adults (unless otherwise indicated) and assume normal renal function. § Alternatives consider allergy, PK, compliance, local resistance, cost.*

TABLE 1 (16)

ANATOMIC SITE/DIAGNOSIS/ MODIFYING CIRCUMSTANCES	ETIOLOGIES (usual)	SUGGESTED REGIMENS* PRIMARY	ALTERNATIVE§	ADJUNCT DIAGNOSTIC OR THERAPEUTIC MEASURES AND COMMENTS
GASTROINTESTINAL/Gastroenteritis—Specific Therapy (results of culture, microscopy, toxin assay AVAILABLE) *(continued)*				
Differential diagnosis of toxin-producing diarrhea *(Continued from previous page)*	**Shiga-toxin producing E. coli** [formerly **Enterohemorrhagic E. coli (EHEC)]:** 0157:H7 & 0104:H4 & others. Hemolytic uremic syndrome complicates 6-9% *(see Comment)*	Treatment: 1. If afebrile, bloody diarrhea: a. Hydration b. Avoid antiperistaltic drugs c. No antibiotics 2. If febrile, bloody diarrhea, risk of bacteremia: **Azithro** 500 mg IV/po once daily x 3 d		**Risk of antibiotic therapy is HUS due to Shiga toxin production.** HUS = renal failure, hemolytic anemia, thrombocytopenia. Restrict antibiotics to patients with increased risk of, or documentation of, bacteremia due to EHEC. Ref: *CID 62:1251 & 1259, 2016*. Pro and con of antibiotic use *(Curr Opin Gastroenterol 2022;38:30)*.
	Klebsiella oxytoca— antibiotic-associated diarrhea	Responds to stopping antibiotic		Suggested that stopping NSAIDs helps.
	Listeria monocytogenes	Usually self-limited. Value of oral antibiotics (e.g., AMP or TMP-SMX) unknown, but their use might be reasonable in populations at risk for serious listeria infections.		Cause of food-associated febrile gastroenteritis. Not detected in standard stool cultures. Populations at ↑ risk of severe systemic disease: pregnant women, neonates, the elderly, and immunocompromised hosts.
	Salmonella, non-typhi— For typhoid (enteric) fever, *see page 68* Fever in 71–91%, history of bloody stools in 34%	**If asymptomatic or illness mild, antimicrobial therapy not indicated. Treat if:** age <1 yr or >50 yrs, immunocompromised, vascular grafts or prosthetic joints, bacteremic, hemoglobinopathy, or hospitalized with fever and severe diarrhea *(see typhoid fever, page 68)*.		
		(**CIP** 500 mg bid) or (**Levo** 500 mg q24h) x 7-10 days (14 days if immunocompromised). **If infection acquired in Asia**, avoid FQ and treat with **Azithro** or **Ceftriaxone**.	**Azithro** 500 mg po once daily x 7 days (14 days if immunocompromised).	↑ resistance to TMP-SMX and chloro. Ceftriaxone, cefotaxime usually active if IV therapy required *(see footnote⁷ on page 28, for dosage)*. CIP: susceptible strains, MIC ≤0.06 µg/mL. **Primary treatment of enteritis is fluid and electrolyte replacement.**
	Shigella	**CIP** 750 mg po q12-24h or **Levo** 500 mg q24h x 3 days **Pockets of resistance** ***(see Comment)*** **Peds doses: Azithro** 10 mg/kg/day once daily x 3 days. For severe disease, **Ceftriaxone** 50–75 mg/kg per day x 2–5 days. **CIP** suspension 10 mg/kg bid x 5 days.	**Azithro** 500 mg po once daily x 3 days	**Immunocompromised children & adults: Treat for 7–10 days.** Avoid FQ if CIP MIC ≥0.12 µg/mL. Pockets of resistance reported, especially to FQ in Asia. Resistance more common in international travelers and immunocompromised; clusters of resistance to FQ, Azithro, Ceftriaxone in MSM. For most individuals, treatment not necessary. May be associated with traveler's diarrhea, where one dose of treatment may be sufficient.
	Spirochetosis (Brachyspira pilosicoli)	Benefit of treatment unclear. Susceptible to **Metro**, **Ceftriaxone**, and **Moxi**.		Anaerobic intestinal spirochete that colonizes colon of domestic & wild animals plus humans. Called enigmatic disease due to uncertain status *(Digest Dis & Sci 58:202, 2013)*.
(Continued on next page)	**Vibrio cholerae (toxigenic - 01 & 039)** Treatment decreases duration of disease, volume losses, & duration of excretion	**Primary therapy is rehydration.** Select antibiotics based on susceptibility of locally prevailing isolates. Options include: **Doxy** 300 mg po single dose, **Azithro** 1 gm po single dose, **Tetra** 500 mg po qid x 3 days, **Erythro** 500 mg po qid x 3 days.	**Pregnancy: Azithro** 1 gm po single dose **OR Erythro** 500 mg po qid x 3 days **Peds: Azithro** 20 mg/kg po as single dose; for other age-specific alternatives, *see CDC website http://www.cdc.gov/haiticholera/hcp_goingtohaiti.htm*	**Antimicrobial therapy shortens duration of illness, but rehydration is paramount.** When IV hydration is needed, use Ringer's lactate. Switch to po repletion with Oral Rehydration Salts (ORS) as soon as able to take oral fluids. ORS are commercially available for reconstitution in potable water. If not available, WHO suggests a substitute can be made by dissolving ½ teaspoon salt and 6 level teaspoons of sugar per liter of potable water *(http://www.who.int/cholera/technical/en/)*.

 **NOTE: All dosage recommendations are for adults (unless otherwise indicated) and assume normal renal function. § Alternatives consider allergy, PK, compliance, local resistance, cost.*

TABLE 1 (17)

ANATOMIC SITE/DIAGNOSIS/ MODIFYING CIRCUMSTANCES	ETIOLOGIES (usual)	SUGGESTED REGIMENS*		ADJUNCT DIAGNOSTIC OR THERAPEUTIC MEASURES AND COMMENTS
		PRIMARY	ALTERNATIVE§	
GASTROINTESTINAL/Gastroenteritis—Specific Therapy (results of culture, microscopy, toxin assay AVAILABLE) *(continued)*				
Differential diagnosis of toxin-producing diarrhea	**Vibrio parahaemolyticus, V. mimicus, V. fluvialis**	**Antimicrobial rx does not shorten course. Hydration.**		Shellfish exposure common. Treat severe disease: **FQ, Doxy, 3rd gen Ceph**
(Continued from previous page)	**Vibrio vulnificus** Usual presentation is skin lesions & bacteremia; life-threatening	Adult: (**Doxy** or **Minocycline** 100 mg IV/po bid) + (**Ceftriaxone** 2 gm IV once daily or **Ceftaz** 1 gm IV q8h). Peds: **Doxy** 4.4 mg/kg/day div bid (max 200 mg/day). Alternatives: **Levo** or **CIP**.		
	Yersinia enterocolitica Fever in 68%, bloody stools in 26%	**No treatment unless severe.** If severe, **Doxy** 100 mg IV bid + (**Tobra** or **Gent** 5 mg/kg per day once q24h). **TMP-SMX** or **FQs** are alternatives.		Mesenteric adenitis pain can mimic acute appendicitis. Lab diagnosis difficult: requires "cold enrichment" and/or yersinia selective agar. Desferrioxamine therapy increases severity, discontinue if pt on it. Iron overload states predispose to yersinia.
Gastroenteritis—Specific Risk Groups–Empiric Therapy				
Anoreceptive intercourse				
Proctitis (distal 15 cm only)	Herpes viruses, gonococci, chlamydia, syphilis. *See Genital Tract, page 25*			
Colitis	Shigella, salmonella, campylobacter, E. histolytica *(see Table 13A)*			*See specific GI pathogens, Gastroenteritis, above.*
HIV-1 infected (AIDS): >10 days diarrhea	G. lamblia Acid fast: Cryptosporidium parvum or hominis, Cyclospora cayetanensis Other: Cystoisospora belli, microsporidia (Enterocytozoon bieneusi, Septata intestinalis)			*See Table 13A*
Neutropenic enterocolitis or "typhlitis" *(CID 56:711, 2013) (World J Gastroenterol 23: 42, 2017)*	Mucosal invasion by **Clostridium septicum** and others. Occasionally caused by C. sordellii or P. aeruginosa	Bowel rest and **Pip-tazo** 4.5 gm infused over 4h IV q8h or **IMP** 500 mg IV q6h or **MER** 2 gm IV q8h	**Cefepime** 2 gm IV q8h + **Metro** 500 mg IV q8h	Need surgical consult. Surgical resection controversial but may be necessary. **NOTE:** Resistance of clostridia to clindamycin reported. Pip-tazo, IMP, MER, DORI should cover most pathogens.
Traveler's diarrhea, self-medication. Patient often afebrile Single dose **Azithro** rec therapy and usually sufficient, can continue for 3 days if not resolved	**Acute**: 60% due to diarrheagenic E. coli; shigella, salmonella, or campylobacter. C. difficile, amebiasis *(see Table 13A)*. **If chronic**: cyclospora, cryptosporidia, giardia, isospora	**Adult: Azithro** 1000 mg po once or 500 mg po q24h for 3 days **CIP** 500 mg po bid x 3 days **OR** **Levo** 500 mg po q24h for 1-3 days **OR** **Oflox** 300 mg po bid for 3 days **OR** **Rifaximin** 200 mg po tid for 3 days **OR** **Rifamycin SV** 2 tabs bid x 3 days **Peds: Azithro** 10 mg/kg/day as a single dose for 3 days or **Ceftriaxone** 50 mg/kg/day as single dose for 3 days. Avoid FQs. **Pregnancy:** Use Azithro. Avoid FQs. **For loperamide**, *see Comment*.		**Antimotility agent:** For non-pregnant adults with no fever or blood in stool, add **loperamide** 4 mg po x 1, then 2 mg po after each loose stool to a maximum of 16 mg per day. **Rifaximin** approved only for ages 12 and older. Works only for diarrhea due to non-invasive E. coli; do not use if fever or bloody stool. **Rifamycin SB**: adult only; for E. coli. Do not use if fever or bloody diarrhea. **Ref:** *Clin Micro Inf 21:744, 2015.* **NOTE:** Self-treatment with FQs associated with acquisition of resistant Gm-neg bacilli *(CID 60:837, 847, 872, 2015)*. Increasing resistance of Campylobacter to FQ, particularly in Asia. Azithro now first line choice.
Prevention of Traveler's diarrhea	Preventative treatment of traveler's diarrhea is **not routinely indicated**. Preferred approach in the current recommendation is **Azithro** 1000 mg once + Imodium with first loose stool. Consider **CIP** 500 mg po daily for short trips with vital missions that cannot be disrupted and in immunocompromised patients and those with HIV and CD4 <200. As an alternative during the first 3 weeks (if activities are essential): **Rifaximin** 200 mg po bid.			

 **NOTE: All dosage recommendations are for adults (unless otherwise indicated) and assume normal renal function. § Alternatives consider allergy, PK, compliance, local resistance, cost.*

TABLE 1 (18)

ANATOMIC SITE/DIAGNOSIS/ MODIFYING CIRCUMSTANCES	ETIOLOGIES (usual)	SUGGESTED REGIMENS*		ADJUNCT DIAGNOSTIC OR THERAPEUTIC MEASURES AND COMMENTS
		PRIMARY	ALTERNATIVE§	
GASTROINTESTINAL *(continued)*				
Gastrointestinal Infections by Anatomic Site: Esophagus to Rectum				
Esophagitis	Candida albicans, HSV, CMV	*See Table 11A and Table 14A.*		
Duodenal/Gastric ulcer; gastric cancer, MALT lymphomas (not secondary NSAIDs)	**Helicobacter pylori** Prevalence of pre-treatment resistance increasing, especially clarithro. Ask about previous antibiotics and try to avoid prior antibiotic given. Where available treatment should be guided by susceptibility testing; all H. pylori + should be treated. Test & treat without EGD if age <45 yrs.	**Quadruple therapy:** (**Bismuth subsalicylate** 2 tabs qid + **Tetra** 500 mg qid + **Metro** 500 mg tid + **PPI**) x 14 days. Also can be administered as Pylera (fixed dose quad combination) 3 capsules qid For doses, *see footnote*[5] *& Comments*	**Rifabutin based triple therapy** (**Rifabutin** 150 bid + **Amox** 1 gm tid + **Esomeprazole** or **Rabeprazole** 40 mg bid); also can be administered as **Talicia** (fixed combination, 4 capsules tid). **Triple therapy if susceptibility known:** **Clarithro** 500 bid + **Amox** 1 gm bid + PPI or **Metro** 500 bid + **Amox** 1 gm bid + PPI or **Levo** 500 qd + **Amox** 1 gm bid + **PPI** Newer combination treatments: **Talicia** and **Pylera** In Japan: combination of **Vonoprazan** + **Clarithro** *(Inter Med 59:153, 2020)*	**Comment:** Any one of these **proton pump inhibitors (PPI)** may be used: omeprazole 20 mg bid, Lansoprazole 30 mg bid, esomeprazole 20 mg bid, pantoprazole 40 mg bid, rabeprazole 20 mg bid. High failure rates with previously recommended *triple* regimens **(PPI + Amox + Clarithro)**. Exercise caution regarding potential interactions with other drugs, contraindications in pregnancy and warnings for other special populations. **Dx: Stool antigen**—Monoclonal EIA >90% sens. & 92% specific. Other tests: if endoscoped, rapid urease &/or histology &/or culture; serology less sens & spec; urea breath test, but some office-based tests underperform. Testing ref: *BMJ 344:44, 2012.* **Test of cure:** Repeat stool antigen and/or urea breath test >8 wks post-treatment. **Treatment outcome:** Failure rate of triple therapy >20% due to clarithro resistance.
Small intestine: Whipple's disease *See Infective endocarditis, culture-negative, page 32.*	Tropheryma whipplei	(**Doxy** 100 mg po bid + **Hydroxychloroquine** 200 mg po tid) x 1 year, then **Doxy** 100 mg po bid for life (Peds dose, *see Comment*) Immune reconstitution inflammatory response (IRIS) reactions occur.		In vitro resistance to TMP-SMX plus frequent clinical failures & relapses. Frequent in vitro resistance to carbapenems. Ceftriaxone demonstrates high MICs against intracellular organisms in vitro.

[5] **Bismuth preparations:** (1) In U.S., **bismuth subsalicylate (Pepto-Bismol)** 262 mg tabs; adult dose for helicobacter is 2 tabs (524 mg) qid. (2) Outside U.S., **colloidal bismuth subcitrate** (De-Nol) 120 mg chewable tablets; dose is 1 tablet qid. In the U.S., bismuth subcitrate is available in combination cap only (Pylera: each cap contains bismuth subcitrate 140 mg + Metro 125 mg + Tetracycline 125 mg), given as 3 caps po 4x daily for 10 days **together with** a twice daily PPI.

 **NOTE: All dosage recommendations are for adults (unless otherwise indicated) and assume normal renal function. § Alternatives consider allergy, PK, compliance, local resistance, cost.*

TABLE 1 (19)

ANATOMIC SITE/DIAGNOSIS/ MODIFYING CIRCUMSTANCES	ETIOLOGIES (usual)	SUGGESTED REGIMENS*		ADJUNCT DIAGNOSTIC OR THERAPEUTIC MEASURES AND COMMENTS
		PRIMARY	ALTERNATIVE§	
GASTROINTESTINAL/Gastrointestinal Infections by Anatomic Site: Esophagus to Rectum *(continued)*				
Appendicitis, acute	Aerobic & anaerobic gram-negative bacilli	**Uncomplicated, no apparent perforation**		
		If decision is not to perform appendectomy but treat with antibiotics. CT scan shows no evidence of appendicolith, perforation or abscess. Suggested antibacterial therapy: Adult: **Erta** 1 gm IV q24h Pediatric: **Erta** 15 mg/kg IV bid (max daily 1 gm)	**Surgery:** Adult: **Ceftriaxone** 2 gm IV q24h + **Metro** 500 mg IV q8h Pediatric: **Ceftriaxone** 75 mg/kg IV q24h (max daily 2 gm) + **Metro** 10 mg/kg IV q8h (max dose 500 mg; max 1500 mg/day). With this approach, most patients were able to be discharged with no antibiotic therapy within a mean (±SD) of 23.5 (20) hrs *(J Ped Surgery 2015;50:1566)*. Can further streamline: **Ceftriaxone** 50 mg/kg/dose every 24hrs (max 2 gm/day) + **Metro** 30 mg/kg/ dose q24h (max 1500 mg/dose if ≥ to 80 kg or max of 1000 mg/dose if < 80 kg). Efficacious and cost-saving *(J Ped Infect Dis 2017;6:57-64)*. PK/PD justification of once daily metronidazole; studies in human volunteers: *Antimicrob Agents Chemother 2004;48:4597*	Goal: Activity vs. both aerobic & anaerobic bacteria. Active vs; anaerobes: Metro. Active vs. aerobic gram neg bacilli: AG, P Ceph 2/3/4, Aztreonam, Cip, Levo, Ceftaz-avi. Active vs. both: Pip-tazo, Amox-clav, carbapenems, eravacycline, Moxi, Delaflox. Refs: Non-operative rx of uncomplicated appendicitis *(J Trauma Acute Care Surg 86:722, 2019; JAMA 32:1245 & 1259, 2018)*. Note: No firm guidance on dose for Metro: range 500 mg q6-8h to 30 mg/kg IV once daily (max 1500 mg). Note: Amox-clav may reduce FQ harm without impacting efficacy *(Ann Intern Med 174:737, 2021)*
		Perforation, peritonitis, shock *Emergency surgery:* **MER** 1 gm IV q8h or CIP 400 mg IV q8h + Metro 500 mg IV q8h *(See Comments for other options)*		

Abbreviations on page 2. **NOTE: All dosage recommendations are for adults (unless otherwise indicated) and assume normal renal function. § Alternatives consider allergy, PK, compliance, local resistance, cost.*

TABLE 1 (20)

ANATOMIC SITE/DIAGNOSIS/ MODIFYING CIRCUMSTANCES	ETIOLOGIES (usual)	SUGGESTED REGIMENS*		ADJUNCT DIAGNOSTIC OR THERAPEUTIC MEASURES AND COMMENTS
		PRIMARY	ALTERNATIVE§	
GASTROINTESTINAL/Gastrointestinal Infections by Anatomic Site: Esophagus to Rectum *(continued)*				
Diverticulitis, perirectal abscess, peritonitis *Also see Peritonitis, page 51* *NEJM 2018;379:1635*	Enterobacterales, occasionally P. aeruginosa, Bacteroides sp., enterococci	**Outpatient rx—mild diverticulitis, drained perirectal abscess:**		Must "cover" both Gm-neg. aerobic & Gm-neg. anaerobic bacteria. **Drugs active only vs. anaerobic Gm-neg. bacilli:** clinda, metro. **Drugs active only vs. aerobic Gm-neg. bacilli:** APAG[6], P Ceph 2/3/4 *(see Table 10A, page 150)*, aztreonam, CIP, Levo. **Drugs active vs. both aerobic/anaerobic Gm-neg. bacteria:** cefoxitin, cefotetan, TC-CL, Pip-tazo, Amp-sulb, ERTA, DORI, IMP, MER, Moxi, & tigecycline. **Resistance (B. fragilis):** Metro, Pip-tazo rare. Resistance to FQ increased in enteric bacteria, particularly if any FQ used recently. **Concomitant surgical management important**, esp. with moderate-severe disease. **Tigecycline: Black Box Warning:** All cause mortality higher in pts treated with tigecycline (2.5%) than comparators (1.8%) in meta-analysis of clinical trials. Note: Amox-clav may reduce FQ harm without impacting efficacy *(Ann Intern Med 174:737, 2021)*
		Amox-clav 875/125 mg po bid If beta-lactam allergic or intolerant: [(**TMP-SMX**-DS tab po bid) or (**CIP** 750 mg po bid or **Levo** 750 mg po q24h)] + **Metro** 500 mg q6h. Duration of treatment varies based on clinical response. Usually Treat for 7-10 days. Can customize duration by trending serum procalcitonin serum levels. Treat until PCT level is <0.5 ng/ml	**Moxi** 400 mg po q24h Duration varies with clinical response. Usually 7-10 days	
		Inpatient, mild-moderate disease		
		Surgical consultation advisable **Pip-tazo** 4.5 gm IV over 30 min as a loading dose. Then, 4 hrs later, start 3.375 gm IV infused over 4 hrs. Repeat 4 hr infusion q8h **Erta** 1 gm IV q24h **Moxi** 400 mg IV q24h (resistance of Bacteroides group maybe increasing)	[(**CIP** 400 mg IV q12h) or (**Levo** 750 mg IV q24h)] + (**Metro** 500 mg IV q6h or 1 gm IV q12h) **Moxi** 400 mg IV q24h **Cefepime** 2 gm IV q12h + **Metro** 1 gm IV q12h **Amox-clav** 1000 mg-200 mg IV q8h (non-US)	
		Severe life-threatening disease, ICU patient:		
		IMP 500 mg IV q6h **or MER** 1 gm IV q8h **or Dori** 500 mg q8h (1-hr infusion). For **Ceftolo-tazo** & **Ceftaz-avi** dosing, *see Peritonitis, page 51.*	**AMP** + **Metro** + (**CIP** 400 mg IV q12h or **Levo** 750 mg IV q24h) **OR** [**AMP** 2 gm IV q6h + **Metro** 500 mg IV q6h + **Aminoglycoside**[6] *(see Table 10C, page 166)*]	
		Severe penicillin/cephalosporin allergy: (**Aztreonam** 2 gm IV q6h to q8h) + [**Metro** (500 mg IV q6h) or (1 gm IV q12h)] **OR** [(**CIP** 400 mg IV q12h) or (**Levo** 750 mg IV q24h) + **Metro**].		

[6] **Aminoglycoside = antipseudomonal aminoglycosidic aminoglycoside, e.g., Amikacin, Gentamicin, Tobramycin, Plazomicin**

Abbreviations on page 2. **NOTE: All dosage recommendations are for adults (unless otherwise indicated) and assume normal renal function. § Alternatives consider allergy, PK, compliance, local resistance, cost.*

TABLE 1 (21)

ANATOMIC SITE/DIAGNOSIS/ MODIFYING CIRCUMSTANCES	ETIOLOGIES (usual)	SUGGESTED REGIMENS*		ADJUNCT DIAGNOSTIC OR THERAPEUTIC MEASURES AND COMMENTS
		PRIMARY	ALTERNATIVE§	
GENITAL TRACT: Mixture of empiric & specific treatment. Divided by sex of the patient. For sexual assault (rape), *see Table 15A, page 261.* ***See CDC Guidelines for Sexually Transmitted Diseases:*** *MMWR 70:1, 2021.* ***CDC now recommends Doxy PEP for MSM and TGW 200 mg 24-72 h after sex for those with STI in past 12 mo:*** *MMWR 73:1, 2024*				
Both Women & Men:				
Chancroid *(Curr Op Inf Dis 29:52, 2016)* Ulcer is painful.	H. ducreyi	**Ceftriaxone** 250 mg IM single dose OR **Azithro** 1 gm po single dose	**CIP** 500 mg bid po x 3 days OR **Erythro base** 500 mg po tid x 7 days.	In HIV+ pts, failures reported with single dose azithro *(CID 21:409, 1995)*. Evaluate after 7 days, ulcer should objectively improve. All patients treated for chancroid should be tested for HIV and syphilis. All sex partners of pts with chancroid should be examined and treated if they have evidence of disease or have had sex with index pt within the last 10 days.
Non-gonococcal or post-gonococcal urethritis, cervicitis **NOTE: Assume concomitant N. gonorrhoeae** (Chlamydia conjunctivitis, *see page 14*)	Chlamydia 50%, Mycoplasma genitalium (30%). Other known etiologies (10–15%): trichomonas, herpes simplex virus.	(**Doxy** 100 mg po bid x 7 days) or (**Azithro** 1 gm po as single dose). Evaluate & treat sex partner	(**Erythro base** 500 mg po qid x 7 days) or (**Oflox** 300 mg q12h po x 7 days) or (**Levo** 500 mg q24h x 7 days)	**Diagnosis:** NAAT for C. trachomatis & N. gonorrhoeae on urine or cervix or urethra specimens. Test all urethritis/cervicitis pts for HIV & syphilis. **Evaluate & treat sex partners.** Re-test for cure in pregnancy.
		Pregnancy: Azithro 1 gm po single dose OR **Amox** 500 mg po tid x 7 days.	**In pregnancy: Erythro** base 500 mg po qid for 7 days **Doxy & FQs contraindicated**	
Non-gonococcal urethritis: **Mycoplasma genitalium**	Mycoplasma genitalium. If macrolide resistance testing available, treatment guided by testing.	**If *macrolide sensitive*: Doxy** 100 mg po bid x 7 days, followed by **Azithro** 1 gm po x1 then 500 mg x 3 days	**If macrolide resistant or unknown: Doxy** 100 mg po bid x 7 days followed by **Moxi** 400 mg po x 7 days **Pristinamycin** 1 gm qid x 10 days (where available)	Diagnosis by NAAT, but often not available. Beta-lactams ineffective. Cure with single dose Azithro only 67% *(CID 61:1389, 2015)*. Emerging resistance with no good alternatives *(Em Inf Dis 23:809, 2017)*.
Recurrent/persistent urethritis	**C. trachomatis** (43%), **M. genitalium** (30%), **T. vaginalis** (13%) *(CID 52:163, 2011)*.	**Metro** 2 gm po x 1 dose + or **Tinidazole** 2 gm po x1 then treat for macrolide resistant *M. genitalium* with **Doxy** 100 bid x 7 d followed by **Moxi** 400 po qd x 7 days	No good alternatives	
Rectal, proctitis MSM and increasingly in women	C. trachomatis, M. genitalium, N. gonorrhoeae, syphilis, HSV	If NAAT not available, treat for GC and chlamydia; **Doxy** 100 mg po bid x 7 days	If LGV suspected treat **Doxy** 100 mg po bid x 21 days	**Proctitis:** Doxy x 7 days.
Gonorrhea. FQs no longer recommended for treatment of gonococcal infections *(See CDC Guidelines MMWR 69:1911, 2020; MMWR 70:1, 2021)*: **Dual therapy with Ceftriaxone and Azithro no longer recommended. If Chlamydia suspected Doxy 100 mg po bid x 7 days.**				
Conjunctivitis (adult)	N. gonorrhoeae	**Ceftriaxone** 1 gm IM or IV single dose		Consider one-time saline lavage of eye.
Disseminated gonococcal infection (DGI, dermatitis-arthritis syndrome)	N. gonorrhoeae	**Ceftriaxone** 1 gm IV q24h	(**Cefotaxime** 1 gm q8h IV or **Ceftizoxime** 1 gm q8h IV)	**Treat for 7 days.** Owing to high-level resistance to oral cephalosporins and fluoroquinolones in the community, "Step-down" therapy should be avoided unless susceptibilities are known.
Endocarditis	N. gonorrhoeae	**Ceftriaxone** 1-2 gm IV q12-24 hours x 4 weeks		Severe valve destruction may occur. Ceftriaxone resistance in *N. gonorrhoeae* has been reported; determine susceptibility of any isolate recovered.
Pharyngitis Dx: NAAT	N. gonorrhoeae	**Ceftriaxone** 500 mg IM x 1	Due to resistance concerns, **do not use FQs.**	Pharyngeal GC more difficult to eradicate. **Repeat NAAT 14 days post-rx. Spectinomycin[NUS], cefixime, cefpodoxime & cefuroxime not effective**

Abbreviations on page 2. **NOTE: All dosage recommendations are for adults (unless otherwise indicated) and assume normal renal function. § Alternatives consider allergy, PK, compliance, local resistance, cost.*

TABLE 1 (22)

ANATOMIC SITE/DIAGNOSIS/ MODIFYING CIRCUMSTANCES	ETIOLOGIES (usual)	SUGGESTED REGIMENS* PRIMARY	SUGGESTED REGIMENS* ALTERNATIVE§	ADJUNCT DIAGNOSTIC OR THERAPEUTIC MEASURES AND COMMENTS
GENITAL TRACT/Both Women & Men/Gonorrhea *(continued)*				
Urethritis, cervicitis, proctitis (uncomplicated) 2020 CDC Guidelines: *MMWR 69:1911.* **Diagnosis:** Nucleic acid amplification test (NAAT) on vaginal swab, urine or urethral *swab.*	N. gonorrhoeae (50% of pts with urethritis, cervicitis have concomitant C. trachomatis — **treat for both unless NAAT indicates single pathogen**).	**Ceftriaxone** 500 mg IM x 1 **Rx failure: Ceftriaxone** 1 gm IM x 1; treat partner; NAAT for test of cure 1 wk post-treatment **Severe Pen/Ceph allergy**: (**Gent** 240 mg IM + **Azithro** 2 gm po x 1 dose) OR (**Gemi** 320 mg + **Azithro** 2 gm po x 1 dose) (nausea in >20%)		Screen for syphilis. **Other alternatives for GC (Test of Cure recommended one week after Rx for ALL of these approaches listed below):** • **Oral cephalosporin use is no longer recommended** as primary therapy owing to emergence of resistance. • Other single-dose cephalosporins: ceftizoxime 500 mg IM, cefotaxime 500 mg IM, cefoxitin 2 gm IM + probenecid 1 gm po.
Pregnancy		**Ceftriaxone** 500 mg IM x1; if Chlamydia not excluded **Azithro** 1 gm po x1		
Granuloma inguinale (Donovanosis)	Klebsiella (formerly Calymmatobacterium) granulomatis	**Azithro** 1 gm po q wk x 3 wks	**TMP-SMX** one DS tablet bid x 3 wks **OR Erythro** 500 mg po qid x 3 wks OR **CIP** 750 mg po bid x 3 wks OR **Doxy** 100 mg po bid x 3 wks	Clinical response usually seen in 1 wk. **Rx until all lesions healed,** may take 4 wks. Treatment failures & recurrence seen with Doxy & TMP-SMX. Relapse can occur 6-18 months after apparently effective Rx. If improvement not evidence in first few days, some experts add Gent 1 mg/kg IV q8h.
Herpes simplex virus	*See Table 14A, page 227*			
Human papilloma virus (HPV)	*See Table 14A, page 232*			
Lymphogranuloma venereum Ref: *CID 61:S865, 2015*	Chlamydia trachomatis, serovars. L1, L2, L3	**Doxy** 100 mg po bid x 21 days	**Erythro** 500 mg po qid x 21 days or **Azithro** 1000 mg po q wk x 3 wks (clinical data lacking)	Dx based on serology; biopsy contraindicated because sinus tracts develop. Nucleic acid ampli tests for *C. trachomatis* will be positive. In MSM, presents as fever, rectal ulcer, anal discharge.
Phthirus pubis **(pubic lice, "crabs")** & scabies	Phthirus pubis & Sarcoptes scabiei	*See Table 13A, page 217*		
Syphilis *CDC 2021 STI guidelines MMWR 70:1, 2021.* Diagnosis: *CID 71 (Suppl 1):S1, 2020*; treatment: *JAMA 312:1905, 2014;* management: *CID 61:S818, 2015.* Overview: *Lancet 389: 1550, 2017.*				
Early: primary, secondary, or latent <1 yr **Chancre is painless.**	T. pallidum **NOTE:** Test all pts with syphilis for HIV; test all HIV patients for latent syphilis. Screen MSM and/or HIV pts every 3-12 mos Pregnancy: screen all *(JAMA 2018;320:911)*	**Benzathine pen G (Bicillin L-A)** 2.4 million units IM x 1 *(See Comment for other alternatives if unavailable due to shortages)*	(**Doxy** 100 mg po bid x 14 days) or (**Tetra** 500 mg po qid x 14 days) or (**Ceftriaxone** 1 gm IM/IV q24h x 10–14 days). Follow-up mandatory. Ceftriaxone efficacy *(CID 2017;65:1683).*	If early or congenital syphilis, **quantitative VDRL at 0**, 3, 6, 12 & 24 mos after rx. If 1° or 2° syphilis, VDRL should ↓ 2 tubes at 6 mos, 3 tubes 12 mos, & 4 tubes 24 mos. If titers fail to fall, examine CSF; if CSF (+), treat as neurosyphilis; if CSF is negative, retreat with benzathine Pen G 2.4 mu IM weekly x 3 wks. **NOTE:** Use of **benzathine procaine penicillin** is inappropriate!! **Benzathine Pen G (Bicillin) now often scarce.** Small RCT in HIV+ compared **Amox** 1 gm tid + **Probenecid** 250 mg tid vs Amox 500 mg tid; 97.9% vs 93.5% serological response in 12 mo for early syphilis. Treated 14d for early or 28d for late *(CID 77:779 2023).*

Abbreviations on page 2. **NOTE: All dosage recommendations are for adults (unless otherwise indicated) and assume normal renal function. § Alternatives consider allergy, PK, compliance, local resistance, cost.*

TABLE 1 (23)

ANATOMIC SITE/DIAGNOSIS/ MODIFYING CIRCUMSTANCES	ETIOLOGIES (usual)	SUGGESTED REGIMENS*		ADJUNCT DIAGNOSTIC OR THERAPEUTIC MEASURES AND COMMENTS
		PRIMARY	ALTERNATIVE§	
GENITAL TRACT/Both Women & Men/Syphilis *(continued)*				
More than 1 yr's duration (latent of indeterminate duration, cardiovascular, late benign gumma)	For penicillin desensitization method, *see Table 7, page 89*	**Benzathine Pen G (Bicillin L-A)** 2.4 million units IM q week x 3 = 7.2 million units total. *(See Comments for alternative if unavailable due to shortages)*	**Doxy** 100 mg po bid x 28 days or **Tetra** 500 mg po qid x 28 days; **Ceftriaxone** 1 gm IV or IM daily for 10-14 days MAY be an alternative; consult an ID specialist	**Indications for LP (CDC): neurologic symptoms, treatment failure, any eye or ear involvement, other evidence of active syphilis (aortitis, gumma, iritis).** Neurosyphilis *(NEJM 381:1358, 2019)*. Small RCT for Amox +/- probenecid *(CID 77:779 2023)*. Serological cure: 90.6% for Amox 500 mg tid vs 94.4% for Amox 1 gm tid / Probenecid 250 tid. If alternative regimen used, need serological follow-up.
Neurosyphilis—Very difficult to treat. Includes ocular (retro-bulbar neuritis) syphilis		**Pen G** 18-24 million units per day either as continuous infusion or as 3–4 million units IV q4h x 10–14 days.	(**Procaine Pen G** 2.4 million units IM q24h + **probenecid** 0.5 gm po qid) both x 10–14 days *(CID 71:267, 2020)*	**Ceftriaxone** 2 gm (IV or IM) q24h x 14 days *(Lancet Inf Dis 21:1441, 2021)*. For penicillin allergy: either desensitize to penicillin or obtain infectious diseases consultation. **Serologic criteria for response to rx: 4-fold or greater ↓ in VDRL titer over 6–12 mos.**
HIV infection (AIDS) CDC STD guidelines: *MMWR 70:1, 2021*		Treatment same as HIV uninfected with closer follow-up. Treat early neurosyphilis for 10-14 days regardless of CD4 count.		*See https://www.cdc.gov/std/treatment-guidelines/syphilis.htm* for recent guidelines. Treat for neurosyphilis if CSF VDRL negative but >20 CSF WBCs; 5-20 WBC in HIV+, lower specificity.
Pregnancy and syphilis		Same as for non-pregnant, some recommend 2nd dose (2.4 million units) **Benzathine Pen G** 1 wk after initial dose esp. in 3rd trimester or with 2° syphilis	Skin test for penicillin allergy. Desensitize if necessary, as parenteral pen G is only therapy with documented efficacy!	Monthly quantitative VDRL or equivalent. If 4-fold ↑, re-treat. Doxy, tetracycline contraindicated. Erythro not recommended because of high risk of failure to cure fetus.
Congenital syphilis		**Aqueous crystalline Pen G** 50,000 units/kg per dose IV q12h x 7 days, then q8h for 10 days total.	**Procaine Pen G** 50,000 units/kg IM q24h for 10 days	Another alternative: **Ceftriaxone** ≤30 days old, 75 mg/kg IV/IM q24h (use with caution in infants with jaundice) or >30 days old 100 mg/kg IV/IM q24h. Treat 10–14 days. If symptomatic, ophthalmologic exam indicated. If more than 1 day of rx missed, restart entire course. **Need serologic follow-up!**
Warts, anogenital	*See Table 14A, page 232*			
Women:				
Amnionitis, septic abortion	Bacteroides, esp. Prevotella bivia; Group B, A streptococci; Enterobacterales; C. trachomatis. Rarely U. urealyticum, Mycoplasma sp.	**Pip-tazo** 4.5 gm infused over 4h IV q8h If critically ill: **MER** 1-2 gm IV loading dose, then 0.5-1 gm IV q8h	Other potential empiric regimens: **IMP** 0.5 gm IV q6h or **Erta** 1 gm IV q24h **Amp-sulb** 3 gm IV q6h (up to 50% of *E. coli* are now resistant in some locations) Clindamycin 900 mg IV q8h + Ceftriaxone 2 gm IV q24h. NOTE: one-third of Group B streptococci are resistant to Clindamycin	D&C of uterus. **In septic abortion,** Clostridium perfringens may cause fulminant intravascular hemolysis. **In postpartum patients** with enigmatic fever and/or pulmonary emboli, **consider septic pelvic vein thrombophlebitis** *(see Vascular septic pelvic vein thrombophlebitis, page 74)*. Add doxy for C. trachomatis, Ureaplasma or Mycoplasma. Review: *Frontiers Pharm 8:97, 2017.* NOTE: in US and Europe, 1/3 of Grp B Strep resistant to clindamycin.

**NOTE: All dosage recommendations are for adults (unless otherwise indicated) and assume normal renal function. § Alternatives consider allergy, PK, compliance, local resistance, cost.*

TABLE 1 (24)

ANATOMIC SITE/DIAGNOSIS/ MODIFYING CIRCUMSTANCES	ETIOLOGIES (usual)	SUGGESTED REGIMENS*		ADJUNCT DIAGNOSTIC OR THERAPEUTIC MEASURES AND COMMENTS
		PRIMARY	ALTERNATIVE§	
GENITAL TRACT/Women *(continued)* Updated CDC Guidelines: *MMWR 70:1, 2021*				
Cervicitis, mucopurulent Treatment based on results of nucleic acid amplification test	N. gonorrhoeae	Treat for Gonorrhea, *page 26*		Criteria for diagnosis: 1) (muco) purulent endocervical exudate and/or 2) sustained endocervical bleeding after passage of cotton swab. >10 WBC/hpf of vaginal fluid is suggestive. Intracellular gram-neg diplococci are specific but insensitive. If in doubt, send swab or urine for culture, EIA or nucleic acid amplification test and treat for both.
	Chlamydia trachomatis	Treat for non-gonococcal urethritis, *page 25*. If due to *Mycoplasma genitalium*, less likely to respond to doxy and emerging resistance to both azithro and FQ.		
Endomyometritis/septic pelvic phlebitis				
Early postpartum (1st 48 hrs) (usually after C-section)	Bacteroides, esp. Prevotella bivia; Group B, A streptococci; Enterobacterales; C. trachomatis	Severe: **Pip-tazo** or **MER** Strep TSS: **Ceftriaxone** + **Clinda** Mild: **Amox-clav** 875/125 po bid Associated C. trachomatis: add **Doxy** *Dosage: see footnote*[7]		*See Comments under Amnionitis, septic abortion, above*
Late postpartum (48 hrs to 6 wks) (usually after vaginal delivery)	Chlamydia trachomatis, M. hominis	**Doxy** 100 mg IV or po q12h times 14 days		Tetracyclines not recommended in nursing mothers; discontinue nursing. M. hominis sensitive to tetra, clinda, not erythro.
Fitzhugh-Curtis syndrome	C. trachomatis, N. gonorrhoeae	Treat as for pelvic inflammatory disease immediately below.		Perihepatitis (violin-string adhesions). Sudden onset of RUQ pain. Associated with salpingitis. Transaminases elevated in <30% of cases.
Pelvic actinomycosis; usually tubo-ovarian abscess	A. Israelii most common	**AMP** 200 mg/kg/day in 3-4 divided doses x 4-6 wks then Pen VK 2-4 gm/day in 4 divided doses x 6-12 mo	**Doxy** or **Ceftriaxone** or **Clinda**	Complication of intrauterine device (IUD). Remove IUD. Can use **Pen G** 10-20 million units/day IV instead of **AMP** x 4-6 wks.
Pelvic Inflammatory Disease (PID), salpingitis, tubo-ovarian abscess				
Outpatient rx: limit to pts with temp <38°C, WBC <11,000 per mm³, minimal evidence of peritonitis, active bowel sounds & able to tolerate oral nourishment	N. gonorrhoeae, chlamydia, bacteroides, Enterobacterales, streptococci, especially S. agalactiae Less commonly: G. vaginalis, Haemophilus influenzae, cytomegalovirus (CMV), M. genitalium, U. urealyticum	**Outpatient rx: Ceftriaxone** 500 mg IM or IV x 1 + **Metro** 500 mg po bid x 14 days + **Doxy** 100 mg po bid **OR** (**Cefoxitin** 2 gm IM with **Probenecid** 1 gm po both as single dose) plus (**Doxy** 100 mg po bid with **Metro** 500 mg bid—both times 14 days)	**Inpatient regimens:** [(**Cefotetan** 2 gm IV q12h or **Cefoxitin** 2 gm IV q6h) + (**Doxy** 100 mg IV/po q12h)] (**Clinda** 900 mg IV q8h) + (**Gent** 2 mg/kg loading dose, then 1.5 mg/kg q8h or 4.5 mg/kg once per day), then **Doxy** 100 mg po bid x 14 days	**Another alternative parenteral regimen:** **Amp-sulb** 3 gm IV q6h + **Doxy** 100 mg IV/po q12h. Recommended treatments don't cover M. genitalium so if no response after 7-10 days consider M. genitalium NAAT and treat with **Moxi** 400 mg/day 14 days. Remember: Evaluate and treat sex partner. FQs not recommended due to increasing resistance. Suggest initial inpatient evaluation/therapy for pts with tubo-ovarian abscess. For inpatient regimens, continue treatment until satisfactory response for ≥ 24-hr before switching to outpatient regimen.

[7] **P Ceph 2** (**Cefoxitin** 2 gm IV q6–8h, **Cefotetan** 2 gm IV q12h, Cefuroxime 750 mg IV q8h); **Amp-sulb** 3 gm IV q6h; **Pip-tazo** 4.5 gm infused over 4h IV q8h; **Doxy** 100 mg IV/po q12h; **Clinda** 450–900 mg IV q8h; **Aminoglycoside** (**Gent**, *see Table 10C, page 166*); **P Ceph 3** (**Cefotaxime** 2 gm IV q8h, **Ceftriaxone** 2 gm IV q24h); **Dori** 500 mg IV q8h (1-hr infusion); **Erta** 1 gm IV q24h; **IMP** 0.5 gm IV q6h; **MER** 1-2 gm IV q8h; **Azithro** 500 mg IV q24h; **Linezolid** 600 mg IV/po q12h; **Vanco** 30-60 mg/kg/d in 2-3 div doses, target AUC_{24} 400-600 µg/mL x h.

Abbreviations on page 2. **NOTE: All dosage recommendations are for adults (unless otherwise indicated) and assume normal renal function. § Alternatives consider allergy, PK, compliance, local resistance, cost.*

TABLE 1 (25)

ANATOMIC SITE/DIAGNOSIS/ MODIFYING CIRCUMSTANCES	ETIOLOGIES (usual)	SUGGESTED REGIMENS*		ADJUNCT DIAGNOSTIC OR THERAPEUTIC MEASURES AND COMMENTS
		PRIMARY	ALTERNATIVE§	
GENITAL TRACT/Women *(continued)*				
Vaginitis *(MMWR 70:1, 2021)*				
Candidiasis Pruritus, thick cheesy discharge, pH <4.5 *See Table 11A, page 176*	Candida albicans 80–90%. C. glabrata, C. tropicalis may be increasing—they are less susceptible to azoles	**Oral azoles: Fluconazole** 150 mg po x 1; **Itraconazole** 200 mg po bid x 1 day. For milder cases, Topical Therapy with non-prescription agent usually is successful (e.g., clotrimazole, butoconazole, miconazole, or tioconazole) as creams or vaginal suppositories.	**Butoconazole, Clotrimazole, Miconazole, Tioconazole** or **Terconazole** (all intravaginal): variety of strengths - from 1 dose to 7–14 days *(See Table 11A, page 176)*	Nystatin vag. tabs times 14 days less effective. Other rx for azole-resistant strains: gentian violet, boric acid. If recurrent candidiasis (4 or more episodes per yr): 6 mos. suppression with: fluconazole 150 mg po q week or itraconazole 100 mg po q24h or clotrimazole vag. suppositories 500 mg q week.
Trichomoniasis Copious foamy discharge, pH >4.5 Treat sexual partners—*see Comment*	Trichomonas vaginalis **Dx:** NAAT & PCR available & most sensitive; wet mount not sensitive.	**Metro** 500 mg po bid x 7 days for women OR 2 gm single dose for men. 7 days more effective in RCT, If HIV+ always give 7-day course OR **Tinidazole** 2 gm po single dose or **Secnidazole** 2 g packet x1 **Pregnancy:** *See Comment*	**For rx failure:** Re-treat with metro 500 mg po bid x 7 days; if 2nd failure: metro 2 gm po q24h x 3–5 days. If still failure, **Tinidazole** 2 gm po q24h x 5 days	**Treat male sexual partners: Metro** 2 gm x 1 dose or **Secnidazole** Nearly 20% men with NGU are infected with trichomonas *(JID 188:465, 2003)*. For alternative option in refractory cases, *see CID 33:1341, 2001.* **Pregnancy:** No data indicating metro teratogenic or mutagenic. For discussion of treating trichomonas, including issues in pregnancy, *see MMWR 70:1, 2021 (CDC Guidelines)*.
Bacterial vaginosis (BV) Malodorous vaginal discharge, pH >4.5 No rec to screen during pregnancy *(JAMA 2020,323:1286)*	Etiology unclear: associated with Gardnerella vaginalis, mobiluncus, Mycoplasma hominis, Prevotella sp., & Atopobium vaginae et al.	**Metro** 0.5 gm po bid x 7 days or **Metro vaginal gel**[8] (1 applicator intravaginally) 1x/day x 5 days OR 2% **Clinda vaginal cream** 5 gm intravaginally at bedtime x 7 days	**Clinda** 0.3 gm bid po x 7 days or **Clinda ovules** 100 mg intravaginally at bedtime x 3 days. **Secnidazole** 2 gm packet (granules on applesauce, yogurt, pudding) x 1 dose over 30 min.	**Treatment of male sex partner not indicated unless balanitis present.** **Pregnancy:** Oral **Metro** or oral **Clinda** 7-day regimens. If recurrent BV, can try adding **boric acid** to suppressive regimen: Metro 0.5 gm po bid x 7 days, then vaginal boric acid gelatin capsule 600 mg hs x 21 days, followed by Metro vaginal gel 2x/week x 16 weeks *(Sex Trans Dis 36:732, 2009)*. **Post gel rx, Lactin-V (probiotic) reduced recurrence rate (p 0.01)** *(NEJM 382:1906, 2020)*.
Men:				
Balanitis	Candida 40%, Group B strep, gardnerella	**Metro** 2 gm po x 1 dose OR **Fluconazole** 150 mg po x 1 dose OR **Itra** 200 mg po bid x 1 day.		Exclude circinate balanitis (Reiter's syndrome); (non-infectious) responds to hydrocortisone cream.
Epididymo-orchitis *(MMWR 70:1, 2021)*				
Age <35 years	N. gonorrhoeae, Chlamydia trachomatis	(**Ceftriaxone** 500 mg IM x 1 + **Doxy** 100 mg po bid x 10 days) + bed rest, scrotal elevation, analgesics.		Enterobacterales occasionally encountered. Test all pts age <35 yrs for HIV and syphilis.
Age >35 years or MSM (insertive partners in anal intercourse)	Enterobacterales	**Levo** 500-750 mg IV/po once daily for 10-14 days. If STI unlikely, low local resistance, **TMP-SMX** 1 DS bid x 10-14 days. **Amp-sulb**, **P Ceph 3**, **Pip-tazo** *(Dosage: see footnote[7] on page 28)* for MSM can be mixed GC/chlamydia with enterics so treat with FQ AND Ceftriaxone 500 mg IM x1) Also: bed rest, scrotal elevation, analgesics		Midstream pyuria and scrotal pain and edema. **NOTE:** Do urine NAAT (nucleic acid amplification test) to ensure absence of N. gonorrhoeae with concomitant risk of FQ-resistant gonorrhoeae or of chlamydia if using agents without reliable activity. Other causes include: mumps, brucella, TB, intravesicular BCG, B. pseudomallei, coccidioides, Behcet's disease.
Non-gonococcal urethritis	*See page 25* *(MMWR 70:1, 2021)*			

[8] 1 applicator contains 5 gm of gel with 37.5 mg metronidazole

Abbreviations on page 2. **NOTE: All dosage recommendations are for adults (unless otherwise indicated) and assume normal renal function. § Alternatives consider allergy, PK, compliance, local resistance, cost.*

TABLE 1 (26)

ANATOMIC SITE/DIAGNOSIS/ MODIFYING CIRCUMSTANCES	ETIOLOGIES (usual)	SUGGESTED REGIMENS*		ADJUNCT DIAGNOSTIC OR THERAPEUTIC MEASURES AND COMMENTS
		PRIMARY	ALTERNATIVE§	
GENITAL TRACT/Men *(continued)*				
Prostatitis—Review: *CID 50:1641, 2010. See Guidelines 2015 http://onlinelibrary.wiley.com/doi/10.1111/bju.13101/epdf*				
Acute Uncomplicated (with risk of STD; age <35 yrs)	N. gonorrhoeae, C. trachomatis	**Ceftriaxone** 500 mg IM x 1 dose or **Cefixime** 400 mg po x 1 dose; then **Doxy** 100 mg po bid x 10 days		FQs no longer recommended for gonococcal infections. Test for HIV. In AIDS pts, prostate may be focus of Cryptococcus neoformans.
Uncomplicated with low risk of STD	Enterobacterales	**FQ** *(dosage: see Epididymo-orchitis, >35 yrs, above)* or **TMP-SMX** 1 DS tablet (160 mg TMP) po bid x 10–14 days (minimum). Some recommend 3-6 weeks.		Treat as acute urinary infection, 14 days (not single dose regimen). If uncertain, do NAAT for C. trachomatis and N. gonorrhoeae.
Chronic bacterial	Enterobacterales 80%, enterococci 15%, P. aeruginosa	**CIP** 500-750 mg po bid x 4 wks OR **Levo** 750 mg po q24h x 4 wks.	**TMP-SMX-DS** 1 tab po bid x 1–3 mos (Fosfomycin: *see Comment*)	**With treatment failures** consider infected prostatic calculi. Fosfomycin penetrates prostate; case report of success with 3 gm po q24h x 12-16 wks *(CID 61:1141, 2015)* or 3 gm q3d x 6 wks *(AAC 60:1854, 2016).*
Chronic prostatitis/chronic pain syndrome	The most common prostatitis syndrome. Etiology is unknown.	α-adrenergic blocking agents are controversial.		Pt has sx of prostatitis but negative cultures and no cells in prostatic secretions.
HAND *(Bites: See Skin)*				
Paronychia				
Nail biting, manicuring	Staph. aureus (MSSA or MRSA)	Incision & drainage; culture	**Cephalexin** 500 tid while waiting for culture result. **TMP-SMX-DS** 1-2 tabs po bid	*See Table 6 for alternatives*. Occasionally--candida, gram-negative rods.
Contact with saliva— dentists, anesthesiologists, wrestlers	Herpes simplex (Whitlow)	**Acyclovir** 400 mg tid po x 10 days	**Famciclovir** or **Valacyclovir**, *see Comment*	Gram stain and routine culture negative. Famciclovir/valacyclovir for primary genital herpes; *see Table 14A, page 227*
Fungal/Chronic Paronychia *(see Comments)*, e.g., Dishwasher (prolonged water immersion)	Candida sp.	**Clotrimazole** (topical)	Topical **Ampho B**, **Clotrimazole**, **Econazole**, **Miconazole**, or **Nystatin** tid/qid x 7–14 days **Ketoconazole** 400 mg po qd or **Itraconazole** 200 mg po qd x 14 days **Ciclopirox olamine** 1% cream/lotion; apply topically bid x 7–14 days	Avoid immersion of hands in water as much as possible.
HEART Duke Criteria for Infective Endocarditis: *CID 2023;77:518 & 527*				
Infective endocarditis—Native valve—empirical rx awaiting cultures—No IV illicit drugs	**Diagnostic criteria** include evidence of continuous bacteremia (multiple positive blood cultures), new murmur (worsening of old murmur) of valvular insufficiency, definite emboli, and echocardiographic (transthoracic or transesophageal) evidence of valvular vegetations. Refs.: *Circulation 132:1435, 2015.* For antimicrobial prophylaxis, *see Table 15C, page 266.*			
Valvular or congenital heart disease but no modifying circumstances *See Table 15C, page 266 for prophylaxis*	Viridans strep 30–40%, "other" strep 15–25%, enterococci 5–18%, staphylococci 20-35% (including coag-neg staphylococci- *CID 46:232, 2008).*	**Vanco** 30-60 mg/kg/d in 2-3 div doses, target AUC_{24} 400-600 μg/mL x h + **Ceftriaxone** 2g q24h OR **Vanco** 30-60 mg/kg/d	Substitute **Dapto** 10 mg/kg IV q24h (or q48h for CrCl <30 mL/min) for **Vanco**	If serious beta-lactam allergy can substitute Gent 1 mg/kg IV/IM q8h for Ceftriaxone; even low-dose Gent for only a few days carries risk of nephrotoxicity. Modify therapy based on identification of specific pathogen as soon as possible to obtain best coverage and to avoid toxicity.

 **NOTE: All dosage recommendations are for adults (unless otherwise indicated) and assume normal renal function. § Alternatives consider allergy, PK, compliance, local resistance, cost.*

ANATOMIC SITE/DIAGNOSIS/ MODIFYING CIRCUMSTANCES	ETIOLOGIES (usual)	SUGGESTED REGIMENS*		ADJUNCT DIAGNOSTIC OR THERAPEUTIC MEASURES AND COMMENTS
		PRIMARY	ALTERNATIVE§	
HEART *(continued)*				
Infective endocarditis—Native valve—culture positive Ref: *Circulation 132:1435, 2015.*				
Viridans strep, S. bovis *(S. gallolyticus)* with **pen G MIC ≤0.12 mcg/mL.** IV rx is gold standard. Insufficient evidence for po step down.	**Viridans strep, S. bovis (S. gallolyticus subsp. gallolyticus)**	(**Pen G** 12-18 million units/ day IV, divided - q4h x 4 wks) **OR** (**Ceftriaxone** 2 gm IV q24h x 4 wks)	[(**Pen G or Ceftriaxone** 2 gm IV q24h) + **Gent** 3 mg per kg IV q24h] x 2 wks.	4-wks regimen preferred for most patients. Avoid 2-wks regimen for patients age >65 years, those with cardiac or extracardiac abscess, creatinine clearance of <50 mL/min, impaired eighth cranial nerve function, or Abiotrophia, Granulicatella, or Gemella spp infection. Vanco 15-20 mg/kg q12h x 4 wks, target AUC24 400-600 µg/mL x h or trough 10-15 µg/mL an option for patients allergic to or intolerant of Pen or Ceftriaxone.
Viridans strep, S. bovis (S. gallolyticus) with **pen G MIC >0.12 to <0.5 mcg/mL**	**Viridans strep, S. bovis (S. gallolyticus subsp. gallolyticus)**	**Ceftriaxone** 2 gm IV q24h x 4 weeks if Ceftriaxone MIC ≤0.5 mcg/mL	**Vanco** 15-20 mg/kg q12h x 4 wks, target AUC_{24} 400-600 µg/mL x h	**Pen G** 24 million units/day IV (divided q4h) x 4 wks + **Gent** 3 mg/kg IV q24h x 2 wk an option if ceftriaxone or vancomycin is not an option.
For viridans strep or S. bovis with pen MIC ≥0.5 mcg/mL or gram-positive cocci. **NOTE:** Inf. Dis. consultation suggested	**Viridans strep, S. bovis, Gram-positive cocci** (new names are: Abiotrophia sp. & Granulicatella sp.). Also Gemella sp.	[(**Pen G** 24 million units per 24h IV, divided q4h x 4 wks) + (**Gent** 3 mg/kg/d in 2-3 divided doses x 4 wks)] OR (**AMP** 12 gm/day IV, divided q4h + **Gent** as above x 4 wks)	**Vanco** 15-20 mg/kg q12h x 4 wks, target AUC_{24} 400-600 µg/mL x h	For streptococci with Ceftriaxone MIC ≤0.5 µg/mL, Ceftriaxone 2 gm q24h can be substituted for ampicillin or penicillin. For gentamicin given 1 mg/kg q8h target peak serum concentration of 3-4 µg/mL and trough serum concentration of <1 µg/mL.
Enterococci, penicillin and aminoglycoside susceptible	E. faecalis E. faecium *(see Comments)*	Pen sensitive and synergy with Gent positive: (**Amp** 12 gm/day IV divided q4h + **Ceftriaxone** 2 gm IV q12h) x 6 weeks **Pen G** 24 million units/day IV divided q4h + **Gent** 1 mg/kg q8h IV x 4-6 weeks (6-week course for patients with > 3 months of symptoms or for prosthetic valve infection) **Amp** 12 gm/day IV, divided q4h + **Gent** 1 mg/kg q8h IV x 4-6 weeks (6-weeks for patients with > 3 months of symptoms or for prosthetic valve infection)	(**AMP** 2 gm IV q4h + **Ceftriaxone** 2 gm IV q12h) x 6 wks Penicillin-intolerant patient only: (**Vanco** 30 mg/kg/d IV in 2 divided doses + **Gent** 1 mg/kg IV q8h) x 6 wks	**Native valve:** 4 wks Pen or AMP + Gent if symptoms <3 mo; 6 wks if symptoms >3 mo; **prosthetic valve:** 6 wks. **Vanco** target AUC_{24} 400-600 µg/mL x h. Adjust dose of Gent to achieve peak serum conc. of 3-4 µg/mL and trough of <1 µg/mL. Limited data suggest that efficacy of amp-gent combination therapy for 2 weeks followed by amp alone for 4 to 6 weeks is similar to that of the standard combination regimen for 4 to 6 weeks and is less toxic *(NEJM 2020; 383:567).* **AMP + Ceftriaxone** preferred for patients with creatinine clearance <50 mL/min or who develop such on gent regimen. Unproven efficacy versus E. faecium; **AMP or Pen + Gent** recommended. Vanco + Gent toxic: consider pen desensitization.
Enterococci, Penicillin susceptible, Gentamicin resistant (MIC >500 µg/mL), streptomycin susceptible (MIC <1500 µg/mL)	E. faecalis E. faecium *(see Comments)*	(**AMP** 2 gm IV q4h + **Ceftriaxone** 2 gm IV q12h) x 6 wks	[(**AMP** 2 gm IV q4h or **Pen G** 24 million units) + **streptomycin** 15 mg/kg IV q24h] x 4-6 wks	Must confirm streptomycin MIC for synergy if strep combo used. **AMP + Ceftriaxone** regimen preferred, if creatinine clearance <50 mL/min, concern for impaired eighth nerve function. Unproven efficacy versus E. faecium; ID consultation recommended.
Enterococci, Penicillin, aminoglycoside, Vancomycin resistant	E. faecalis E. faecium	**Dapto** 8-12 mg/kg IV q24h + **AMP** 2 gm IV q4h	**Linezolid** 600 mg IV/po q12h	Duration of therapy ≥8 weeks, expert consultation strongly advised. Valve replacement often required for cure.

TABLE 1 (28)

ANATOMIC SITE/DIAGNOSIS/ MODIFYING CIRCUMSTANCES	ETIOLOGIES (usual)	SUGGESTED REGIMENS*		ADJUNCT DIAGNOSTIC OR THERAPEUTIC MEASURES AND COMMENTS
		PRIMARY	ALTERNATIVE§	
HEART/Infective endocarditis—Native valve—culture positive *(continued)*				
Infective endocarditis, Gram-negative bacilli	Enterobacterales or P. aeruginosa	Optimal therapy unknown, infectious diseases consult recommended: an aminoglycoside (**Tobra** if P. aeruginosa) + (**Cefepime** or **MER**) is a reasonable option.		Choice of agents based on in vitro susceptibilities, fluoroquinolone an option instead of aminoglycoside, but few data.
Infective endocarditis, fungal	Candida sp. Aspergillus	Optimal therapy unknown, infectious diseases consultation recommended; an azole or echinocandin is a reasonable empirical choice. High failure rate with medical therapy alone, consider early surgery		
Staphylococcal endocarditis Aortic &/or mitral valve infection—MSSA Surgery indications: *see Comment page 30.*	**Staph. aureus, methicillin-sensitive**	**Nafcillin/Oxacillin** 2 gm IV q4h x 6 wks	[(**Cefazolin** 2 gm IV q8h x 6 wks) OR **Vanco** 30-60 mg/kg/d in 2-3 div doses, target AUC_{24} 400-600 µg/mL x h x 6 wks	If IgE-mediated penicillin allergy, 10% cross-reactivity to cephalosporins. **Cefazolin** and **Nafcillin** probably similar in efficacy and Cefazolin better tolerated. Vanco only for patients unable to tolerate a beta-lactam; dapto 8-12 mg/kg once daily also an option in this circumstance.
Aortic and/or mitral valve—MRSA	**Staph. aureus, methicillin-resistant**	**Vanco** 30-60 mg/kg/d in 2-3 div doses, target AUC_{24} 400-600 µg/mL x h	**Dapto** 8-12 mg/kg q24h IV	For other alternatives, *see Table 6, page 88.*
Tricuspid valve infection (usually IVDUs): MSSA, uncomplicated	**Staph. aureus, methicillin-sensitive**	**Nafcillin/Oxacillin** 2 gm IV q4h x 4 wks	**If penicillin allergy: Vanco** 30-60 mg/kg/d in 2-3 div doses, target AUC_{24} 400-600 µg/mL x h x 4 wks OR **Dapto** 8-12 mg/kg IV q24h x 4 wks OR **Cefazolin** 2 gm IV q8h x 4 wks	**Dapto** resistance can occur de novo, after or during vanco, or after/during dapto therapy. *See Comments on MSSA above.*
Tricuspid valve--MRSA	**Staph. aureus, methicillin-resistant**	**Vanco** 30-60 mg/kg/d in 2-3 div doses, target AUC_{24} 400-600 µg/mL x h recommended for serious infections x 6 wks	**Dapto** 8-12 mg/kg IV q24h x 6 wks	
Slow-growing fastidious Gm-neg. bacilli--any valve	**HACEK group** *(see Comments).*	**Ceftriaxone** 2 gm IV q24h x 4 wks OR **CIP** 400 mg IV q12h x 4 wks	**Amp-sulb** 3 gm IV q6h x 4 wks OR **Levo** 750 mg po/IV q24h x 4 wks OR **Moxi** 400 mg po/IV q24h x 4 wks	**HACEK** (acronym for Haemophilus parainfluenza, Aggregatibacter, Actinobacillus, Cardiobacterium, Eikenella, Kingella). **AMP** 2 gm IV q4h an option if growth of isolate in vitro is sufficient for reliable determination of ampicillin susceptibility.
Bartonella species--any valve	B. henselae, B. quintana	**Doxy** 100 mg IV/po bid x 6 weeks + **Gent** 3 mg/kg/day IV divided in 3 equal doses x 2 wks, then continue doxy for an additional 3 months unless valve resected, then 6 wks	**Doxy** 100 mg IV/po bid x 6 wks + **RIF** 300 mg IV/po bid x 2 wks, then continue doxy for an additional 3 months unless valve resected, then 6 wks	**Dx:** Immunofluorescent antibody titer ≥1:800. Note, at low titers, cross-reactivity with C. burnetii & Brucella sp. blood cultures only occ. positive, or PCR of tissue from surgery *(J Clin Micro 2021;59:e02217).* B. quintana transmitted by body lice among homeless.
Infective endocarditis— "culture negative"				
Fever, valvular disease, and ECHO vegetations ± emboli and neg. cultures.		Etiology in 348 cases studied by serology, culture, histopath, & molecular detection: C. burnetii 48%, Bartonella sp. 28%, and rarely (Abiotrophia elegans (nutritionally variant strep), Mycoplasma hominis, Legionella pneumophila, Tropheryma whipplei—together 1%), & rest without etiology identified (most on antibiotic).		

 **NOTE: All dosage recommendations are for adults (unless otherwise indicated) and assume normal renal function. § Alternatives consider allergy, PK, compliance, local resistance, cost.*

TABLE 1 (29)

ANATOMIC SITE/DIAGNOSIS/ MODIFYING CIRCUMSTANCES	ETIOLOGIES (usual)	SUGGESTED REGIMENS* PRIMARY	ALTERNATIVE§	ADJUNCT DIAGNOSTIC OR THERAPEUTIC MEASURES AND COMMENTS
HEART *(continued)*				
Infective endocarditis—<u>Prosthetic valve—empiric therapy (cultures pending)</u> *(Medicine. 2005; 84:162)*				
Early (<2 mos post-op)	S. epidermidis, S. aureus. Rarely, Enterobacterales, diphtheroids, fungi	**Vanco** 30-60 mg/kg/d in 2-3 div doses, target AUC_{24} 400-600 µg/mL x h + **Gent** 1 mg/kg IV q8h + **RIF** 600 mg po q24h		Early surgical consultation advised especially if etiology is S. aureus, evidence of heart failure, presence of diabetes and/or renal failure, or concern for valve ring abscess.
Late (>2 mos post-op)	S. epidermidis, viridans strep, enterococci, S. aureus			
Infective endocarditis— <u>Prosthetic valve—positive blood cultures</u> **Surgical consultation advised:** Indications for surgery: severe heart failure, S. aureus infection, prosthetic dehiscence, resistant organism, emboli due to large vegetation *(See AHA guidelines; Circulation 132:1435, 2015).*	Staph. epidermidis	(**Vanco** 30-60 mg/kg/d in 2-3 div doses, target AUC_{24} 400-600 µg/mL x h + **RIF** 300 mg po q8h) x 6 wks + **Gent** 1 mg/kg IV q8h x 14 days.		If S. epidermidis is susceptible to nafcillin/oxacillin in vitro, then substitute nafcillin (or oxacillin) for vanco. Some clinicians prefer to wait 2-3 days after starting vanco/ gent before starting RIF, to decrease bacterial density and thus minimize risk of selecting rifampin-resistant subpopulations.
	Staph. aureus	Methicillin sensitive: (**Nafcillin/Oxacillin** 2 gm IV q4h + **RIF** 300 mg po q8h) x 6 wks + **Gent** 1 mg per kg IV q8h x 2 wks. Methicillin resistant: (**Vanco** 30-60 mg/kg/d in 2-3 div doses, target AUC_{24} 400-600 µg/mL x h + **RIF** 300 mg po q8h) x 6 wks + **Gent** 1 mg per kg IV q8h x 2 wks.		
	Viridans strep, enterococci	*See infective endocarditis, native valve, culture positive, page 30.* Treat for 6 weeks.		
	Enterobacterales or P. aeruginosa	[(**Cefepime** 2 gm IV q8h or **MER** 1 gm IV q8h) or (**Pip-tazo** 4.5 gm infused over 4h IV q8h) + **Tobra** 1.5-2 mg/kg IV q8h]		In theory, could substitute CIP for aminoglycoside, but no clinical data and resistance is common. Select definitive regimen based on susceptibility results.
	Candida, aspergillus	*Table 11, page 174*		High mortality. Valve replacement plus antifungal therapy standard therapy but some success with antifungal therapy alone.
Infective endocarditis—Q fever *CID 2021;73:1476*	Coxiella burnetii Dx: serologic. Chronic illness, phase i antibody ≥1:800	**Doxy** 100 mg po bid + **hydroxychloroquine** 600 mg/day for at least 18 mos *(Mayo Clin Proc 83:574, 2008). Pregnancy: Need long term* **TMP-SMX** *(see CID 45:548, 2007).*		**Dx:** IFA > 800 phase I IgG plus evidence of endocarditis or vasculopathy or signs of chronic Q fever **OR** positive Coxiella burnetii PCR of blood or tissue. Possible chronic Q fever = IFA > 800 phase I IgG. Treatment duration: 18 mos for native valve, 24 mos for prosthetic valve. Monitor serologically for 5 yrs.
Pacemaker/defibrillator infections	S. aureus (40%), S. epidermidis (40%), Gram-negative bacilli (5%), fungi (5%).	MRSA/MRSE: **Device removal + Vanco** 30-60 mg/kg/d in 2-3 div doses, target AUC_{24} 400-600 µg/mL x h. MSSA/MSSE: **Nafcillin/ Oxacillin** 2 gm IV q4h OR **Cefazolin** 2 gm IV q8h	MRSA/MRSE: **Device removal** + **Dapto** 8-10 mg per kg IV q24h[NAI]	**Duration of rx after device removal:** For "pocket" or subcutaneous infection, 10–14 days; if lead-assoc. endocarditis, 4–6 wks depending on organism. Device removal and absence of valvular vegetation assoc. with significantly higher survival at 1 yr *(JAMA 307:1727, 2012).* British guidelines: *JAC 70:325, 2015.* Prophylaxis: Antibiotic eluting envelope (Tyrx) reduced infection of implantable devices *(NEJM 380:1895, 2019).*
Pericarditis, bacterial	Staph. aureus, Strep. pneumoniae, Group A strep, Enterobacterales	[**Vanco** 30-60 mg/kg/d in 2-3 div doses, target AUC_{24} 400-600 µg/mL x h + (**Ceftriaxone** 2 gm q24h OR **Cefepime** 2 gm IV q8h)] *(Dosage, see footnote[9])*	**Vanco + CIP** 400 mg q12h *(see footnote[9])*	Drainage required if signs of tamponade. Adjust regimen based on results of organism ID and susceptibility. Use Nafcillin, Oxacillin, or Cefazolin for confirmed MSSA infection.

[9] **Aminoglycosides** *(see Table 10C, page 166)*, **IMP** 0.5 gm IV q6h, **MER** 1 gm IV q8h, **Nafcillin** or **Oxacillin** 2 gm IV q4h, **Pip-Tazo** 4.5 gm infused over 4h IV q8h, **Amp-sulb** 3 gm IV q6h, **P Ceph** 1 (**cephalothin** 2 gm IV q4h or **cefazolin** 2 gm IV q8h), **CIP** 750 mg po bid or 400 mg IV bid, **Vanco** 30-60 mg/kg/d in 2-3 div doses, target AUC_{24} 400-600 µg/mL x h, **RIF** 600 mg po q24h, **Aztreonam** 2 gm IV q8h, **Cefepime** 2 gm IV q12h

TABLE 1 (30)

ANATOMIC SITE/DIAGNOSIS/ MODIFYING CIRCUMSTANCES	ETIOLOGIES (usual)	SUGGESTED REGIMENS*		ADJUNCT DIAGNOSTIC OR THERAPEUTIC MEASURES AND COMMENTS
		PRIMARY	ALTERNATIVE§	
HEART *(continued)*				
Rheumatic fever with carditis Ref.: *Ln 366:155, 2005*	Post-infectious sequelae of Group A strep infection (usually pharyngitis)	ASA, and usually prednisone 2 mg/kg po q24h for symptomatic treatment of fever, arthritis, arthralgia. May not influence carditis.		Clinical features: Carditis, polyarthritis, chorea, subcutaneous nodules, erythema marginatum. Prophylaxis: *see page 68.* ASA dose: 80-100 mg/kg/day (pediatric), 4-8 gm/day (adult). Eradication of group A streptococcus also recommended: Child, Penicillin V, 250 mg po tid x 10 days; adult, Penicillin V 500 mg po tid x 10 days.
Ventricular assist device-related infection *Clin. Transplant. 2019;33:e13552; OFID. 2020 Nov 16;8(1):ofaa532*	S. aureus, S. epidermidis, aerobic gm-neg bacilli, Candida sp. (rare)	After culture of blood, wounds, drive line, device pocket and maybe pump: **Vanco** 30-60 mg/kg/d in 2-3 div doses, target AUC_{24} 400-600 µg/mL x h + **Cefepime** 2 gm IV q12h.		Can substitute **Daptomycin** 10 mg/kg/d[NAI] for **Vanco,** (**CIP** 400 mg IV q12h or **Levo** 750 mg IV q24h) for **Cefepime**.
JOINT—*Also see Lyme Disease, page 65*				
Reactive arthritis				
Reiter's syndrome *(See Comment for definition)*	Occurs wks after infection with C. trachomatis, Campylobacter jejuni, Yersinia enterocolitica, Shigella/Salmonella sp.	Only treatment is non-steroidal anti-inflammatory drugs		**Definition:** Urethritis, conjunctivitis, arthritis, and sometimes uveitis and rash. **Arthritis:** asymmetrical oligoarthritis of ankles, knees, feet, sacroiliitis. **Rash:** palms and soles—keratoderma blennorrhagica; circinate balanitis of glans penis. HLA-B27 positive predisposes to Reiter's.
Poststreptococcal reactive arthritis *(See Rheumatic fever, above)*	Immune reaction after strep pharyngitis: (1) arthritis onset in <10 days, (2) lasts months, (3) unresponsive to ASA	Treat strep pharyngitis and then NSAIDs (prednisone needed in some pts)		A reactive arthritis after a β-hemolytic strep infection in absence of sufficient Jones criteria for acute rheumatic fever. Ref.: *Pediatr Emerg Care 28:1185, 2012.*
Septic arthritis: Treatment requires both adequate drainage of purulent joint fluid and appropriate antimicrobial therapy. **There is no need to inject antimicrobials into joints.** Empiric therapy after collection of blood and joint fluid for culture; review Gram stain of joint fluid. 2 wk of oral step-down after surgical drainage and 1-2 days of IV therapy non-inferior to 4 wk for septic arthritis, principally hand or wrist, in adults *(Ann Rheum Dis 2019; 78:1114)*.				
Infants <3 mos (neonate)	Staph. aureus, Enterobacterales, Group B strep	**If MRSA not a concern:** (**Nafcillin** OR **Cefazolin**) + **Cefotaxime**	**If MRSA a concern:** **Vanco + Cefotaxime**	Blood cultures frequently positive. Adjacent bone involved in 2/3 pts. Group B strep and gonococci most common community-acquired etiologies. Kingella kingae suscept. to ceftriaxone *(Ped Infect Dis J 2016, 35:340)*.
Children (3 mos–14 yrs) *K. kingella* most common for age 6-48 mos. *(Peds 2019;144:e20191509)*	S. aureus 27%, S. pyogenes & S. pneumo 14%, H. influ 3%, Gm-neg. bacilli 6%, other (GC, N. mening) 14%, unk 36%	MRSA prevalence high: **Vanco** + **Cefotaxime** MRSA prevalence low: **Cefazolin**		Marked ↓ in H. influenzae since use of conjugate vaccine. **Usual duration is 3 weeks for S. aureus, 2-3 weeks others.** High dose oral therapy appropriate after initial response *(J Pediatr Infect Dis Soc 2024 Jan 29;13(1):1)*.
Adults *(review Gram stain): See page 65 for Lyme Disease and page 65 for gonococcal arthritis*				
Acute monoarticular				
At risk for sexually-transmitted disease	**N. gonorrhoeae** *(see page 25)*, S. aureus, streptococci, rarely aerobic Gm-neg. bacilli	**Gram stain negative:** **Ceftriaxone** 1 gm IV q24h	If Gram stain shows Gm+ cocci in clusters: **Vanco** 30-60 mg/kg/d in 2-3 div doses, target AUC_{24} 400-600 µg/mL x h	Suspected gonococcal infections (GC): culture urethra, cervix, anal canal, throat, blood, joint fluid. For treatment comments, *see Disseminated GC, page 25.* Nucleic acid amplification tests now available for diagnosis of gonococcal infection in a variety of specimens, including endocervical and vaginal swabs and urine for women, urethral swabs and urine for men, and rectal swabs and pharyngeal swabs for men and women.

TABLE 1 (31)

ANATOMIC SITE/DIAGNOSIS/ MODIFYING CIRCUMSTANCES	ETIOLOGIES (usual)	SUGGESTED REGIMENS*		ADJUNCT DIAGNOSTIC OR THERAPEUTIC MEASURES AND COMMENTS
		PRIMARY	ALTERNATIVE§	
JOINT/Septic arthritis/Adults/Acute monoarticular *(continued)*				
Not at risk for sexually-transmitted disease	S. aureus, streptococci, Gm-neg. bacilli	Gram stain shows Gram-pos. cocci: **Vanco** 30-60 mg/kg/d in 2-3 div doses, target AUC_{24} 400-600 μg/mL x h Gram stain shows Gram-neg bacilli: **Cefepime** 2 gm q8h IV OR **IMP** 0.5 gm IV q6h Gram stain neg: **Vanco** 30-60 mg/kg/d in 2-3 div doses, target AUC_{24} 400-600 μg/mL x h + [**Ceftriaxone** 1 gm IV q24h OR **Cefepime** 2 gm q8h IV q8h (preferred for possible healthcare-associated infection)] *For treatment duration, see Table 3, page 75*		Differential includes gout and chondrocalcinosis (pseudogout). **Look for crystals in joint fluid.** Adjust regimen based on culture and susceptibility. **NOTE:** *See Table 6* for MRSA treatment.
Chronic monoarticular	Brucella, nocardia, mycobacteria, fungi	*See specific bacterial organism and/or mycobacteria (Table 12)*		*See Brucellosis, page 67*
Polyarticular, usually acute	**Gonococci,** B. burgdorferi (Lyme), acute rheumatic fever; viruses, e.g., hepatitis B, rubella vaccine, parvo B19, staph and strep may also cause polyarticular infections	Gram stain usually negative for GC. If sexually active, culture urethra, cervix, anal canal, throat, blood, joint fluid, and then: **Ceftriaxone** 1 gm IV q24h. No STD risk, Gram stain negative: **Vanco** + **Ceftriaxone** OR **Cefepime**.		GC may be associated with pustular/hemorrhagic skin lesions and tenosynovitis; treat with **Ceftriaxone** for **7 days**, ideally. Consider Lyme disease if exposure areas known to harbor infected ticks *(see page 65)*; usually large joint. Vanco+ CIP or Levo also an option if low STD risk. Expanded differential includes gout, pseudogout, reactive arthritis (HLA-B27 pos.).
Septic arthritis, post intra-articular injection	MSSE/MRSE 40%, MSSA/ MRSA 20%, P. aeruginosa, Cutibacterium, AFB	**NO empiric therapy.** Arthroscopy for culture/sensitivity, crystals, washout		**Treat based on culture results x 14 days** (assumes no foreign body present).

Abbreviations on page 2. **NOTE: All dosage recommendations are for adults (unless otherwise indicated) and assume normal renal function. § Alternatives consider allergy, PK, compliance, local resistance, cost.*

TABLE 1 (32)

ANATOMIC SITE/DIAGNOSIS/ MODIFYING CIRCUMSTANCES	ETIOLOGIES (usual)	SUGGESTED REGIMENS*		ADJUNCT DIAGNOSTIC OR THERAPEUTIC MEASURES AND COMMENTS
		PRIMARY	ALTERNATIVE§	
JOINT *(continued)*				
Infected prosthetic joint (PJI) • Suspect infection if sinus tract or wound drainage; acutely painful prosthesis; chronically painful prosthesis; or high ESR/CRP assoc. w/painful prosthesis. • **Empiric therapy is NOT recommended.** Treat based on culture and sensitivity results. • **3 surgical options:** 1) debridement and prosthesis retention (if sx <3 wks or implantation <30 days); 2) 1 stage, direct exchange; 3) 2 stage: debridement, removal, reimplantation • **IDSA Guidelines:** *CID 56:e1, 2013.* **Mgmt Review:** *NEJM 2023;388:251* See also: *CID 2023:77:939*	MSSA/MSSE	**Debridement/Retention**: (**Nafcillin/Oxacillin** 2 gm IV q4h + **RIF** 300 mg po bid) OR (**Cefazolin** 2 gm IV q8h + **RIF** 300 mg po bid) x 2-6 wks followed by [(**CIP** 750 mg po bid OR **Levo** 750 mg po q24h) + **RIF** 300 mg po bid] for 3-6 months (shorter duration for total hip arthroplasty) **1-stage exchange:** IV/po regimen as above for 3 mos **2-stage exchange:** regimen as above for 6 wks	(**Dapto** 8-10 mg/kg IV q24h OR **Linezolid** 600 mg po/IV bid) ± **RIF** 300 mg po bid	• **Confirm isolate susceptibility to fluoroquinolone and rifampin:** for fluoroquinolone-resistant isolate consider using other active highly bioavailable agent, e.g., TMP-SMX, Doxy, Minocycline, Amoxicillin-Clavulanate, Clindamycin, or Linezolid. • Enterococcal infection: addition of aminoglycoside optional. • *P. aeruginosa* infection: consider adding aminoglycoside if isolate is susceptible, (but if this improves outcome unclear). • Prosthesis retention most important risk factor for treatment failure. (Linezolid 600 mg + Rifampin 300 mg) may be effective as salvage therapy if device removal not possible. • If prosthesis is retained, consider long-term, suppressive therapy, particularly for staphylococcal infections: depending on in vitro susceptibility options include TMP-SMX, Doxycycline, Minocycline, Amoxicillin, Ciprofloxacin, Cephalexin. • Culture yield may be increased by sonication of prosthesis. • Other treatment consideration: Rifampin is bactericidal vs. biofilm-producing bacteria. **Never use Rifampin alone due to rapid development of resistance.** • Watch for toxicity if Linezolid is used for more than 2 weeks of therapy. • Role of longer durations of therapy or chronic suppressive therapy in Gram-negative or Pseudomonas PJI not established. • Alpha-defensin immunoassay (Synovasure) with a sensitivity ~0.8-0.9 and specificity ~0.9-0.95 may be a useful biomarker for diagnosis of PJI. • Observational study of 156 pts, 35.6% given FQ vs. 3% given non-FQ treatment required cessation of the FQ due to AEs *(CID 73:850 & 857, 2021).*
	MRSA/MRSE	**Debridement/Retention:** (**Vanco** 30-60 mg/kg/d in 2-3 div doses, target AUC_{24} 400-600 µg/mL x h + **RIF** 300 mg po bid) x 2-6 weeks *followed by* [(**CIP** 750 mg po bid OR **Levo** 750 mg po q24h) + **RIF** 300 mg po bid] for 3-6 months (shorter duration for total hip arthroplasty) **1-stage exchange:** IV/po regimen as above for 3-6 mos (shorter duration for hip) **2-stage exchange:** regimen as above for 4-6 wks	(**Dapto** 8-10 mg/kg IV q24h OR **Linezolid** 600 mg po/IV bid) ± **RIF** 300 mg po bid	
(Continued on next page)	Streptococci (Grps A, B, C, D, viridans, other)	**Debridement/Retention** (Poorer outcomes with retention compared with removal and exchange, *CID 64:1742, 2017*): **Pen G** 20 million units IV continuous infusion q24h or in 6 divided doses OR **Ceftriaxone** 2 gm IV q24h x 4-6 wks **1 or 2 stage exchange:** regimen as above for 4-6 wks	**Vanco** 15 mg/kg IV q12h	*(Continued on next page)*

 **NOTE: All dosage recommendations are for adults (unless otherwise indicated) and assume normal renal function. § Alternatives consider allergy, PK, compliance, local resistance, cost.*

ANATOMIC SITE/DIAGNOSIS/ MODIFYING CIRCUMSTANCES	ETIOLOGIES (usual)	SUGGESTED REGIMENS*		ADJUNCT DIAGNOSTIC OR THERAPEUTIC MEASURES AND COMMENTS
		PRIMARY	ALTERNATIVE§	
JOINT/Infected prosthetic joint (PJI) *(continued)*				
(Continued from previous page)	Enterococci	**Debridement/Retention:** **Pen-susceptible:** (**AMP** 200 mg/kg/day IV in divided doses q6h or **Pen G** 20 million units/day IV by continuous infusion or in 6 divided doses) x 4-6 wks **Pen-resistant: Vanco** 15 mg/kg IV q12h x 4-6 wks **1 or 2 stage exchange:** regimen as above for 4-6 wks	**Dapto** 8-10 mg/kg IV q24h OR **Linezolid** 600 mg po/IV bid	*(Continued from previous page)*
	Cutibacterium acnes (Hold broth cultures, especially in infections of the shoulder, for 10 days with blind subculture to maximize recovery of C. acnes *(Clin Infect Dis 2018;66:54; J Clin Microbiol 54:3043, 2016)*).	**Debridement/Retention:** **Pen G** 20 million units IV continuous infusion or in 6 divided doses OR **Ceftriaxone** 2 gm IV q24h x 4-6 wks **1 or 2 stage exchange:** regimen as above for 4-6 wks	**Vanco** 15 mg/kg IV q12h OR **Clinda** 300-450 mg po qid	
	Gm-neg enteric bacilli	**Debridement/Retention:** **Erta** 1 gm q24h IV OR other beta-lactam (e.g., **Ceftriaxone** 2 gm IV q24h OR **Cefepime** 2 gm IV q12h, based on susceptibility) x 4-6 wks **1 or 2 stage exchange:** regimen as above for 4-6 wks	**CIP** 750 mg po bid	
	P. aeruginosa	**Debridement/Retention:** **Cefepime** 2 gm IV q12h OR **MER** 1 gm IV q8h + **Tobra** 5.1 mg/kg once daily IV x 4-6 wks **1 or 2 stage exchange:** regimen as above for 4-6 wks	**CIP** 750 mg po bid or 400 mg IV q8h	
Rheumatoid arthritis	**TNF inhibitors** (adalimumab, certolizumab, etanercept, golimumab, infliximab) and other anti-inflammatory biologics (tofacitinib, rituximab, tocilizumab, abatacept) ↑ risk of TBc, fungal infection, legionella, listeria, and malignancy. Hep B flare may be fatal. *See Med Lett 55:1, 2013 for full listing.*			
Septic bursitis: Olecranon bursitis; prepatellar bursitis	Staph. aureus >80%, M. tuberculosis (rare), M. marinum (rare)	(**Nafcillin/Oxacillin** 2 gm IV q4h or **Cefazolin** 2 gm IV q8h if **MSSA**. Oral step-down: **Diclox** 500 mg po qid	(**Vanco** 30-60 mg/kg/d in 2-3 div doses, target AUC_{24} 400-600 µg/mL x h or **Linezolid** 600 mg po bid) if **MRSA**. Another option: **Dapto** 6 mg/kg IV q24h	Empiric MRSA coverage recommended if risk factors are present and in high prevalence areas. Immunosuppression, not duration of therapy, is a risk factor for recurrence; 7 days of therapy may be sufficient for immunocompetent patients undergoing one-stage bursectomy *(JAC 65:1008, 2010)*.

 **NOTE: All dosage recommendations are for adults (unless otherwise indicated) and assume normal renal function. § Alternatives consider allergy, PK, compliance, local resistance, cost.*

TABLE 1 (34)

ANATOMIC SITE/DIAGNOSIS/ MODIFYING CIRCUMSTANCES	ETIOLOGIES (usual)	SUGGESTED REGIMENS*		ADJUNCT DIAGNOSTIC OR THERAPEUTIC MEASURES AND COMMENTS
		PRIMARY	ALTERNATIVE§	
KIDNEY & BLADDER *(Reviewed in Nature Rev 13:269, 2015; IDSA Guidelines CID 52: e103, 2011)*				
Acute Uncomplicated Cystitis & Pyelonephritis in Women				
Cystitis Diagnosis: dysuria, frequency, urgency, suprapubic pain & no vaginal symptoms	E. coli (75-95%) P. mirabilis K. pneumoniae S. saprophyticus Presence of enterococci, Grp B streptococcus, other S. epidermidis suggests contamination Often no need for culture if uncomplicated	**Nitrofurantoin (Macrobid)** 100 mg po bid x 5 d OR **TMP-SMX DS** 1 tab po bid x 3 days (Avoid TMP-SMX if 20% or more local E. coli are resistant)	**CIP** 250 mg bid or extended release 500 mg q24h x 3 days **Levo** 250 mg q24h x 3 days **Amox-clav** 875/125 mg bid x 5-7 days **Cephalexin** 500 mg bid x 5-7 days **Cefdinir** 300 mg bid x 3-7 days **Pivmecillinam** 400 mg bid x 3-7 days **Fosfomycin** 3 gm po x 1 dose	**Pyridium** (phenazopyridine) may hasten resolution of dysuria. Beta lactams are less effective. Nitrofurantoin & Fosfomycin active vs. ESBLs; however, if pyelonephritis avoid these drugs due to low renal concentrations. Outpatient therapy of UTIs due to MDR bacteria: - Fosfomycin & nitrofurantoin usually active. - Increasing TMP-SMX & FQ resistance. - Beta-lactams least efficacious.
Pyelonephritis Diagnosis: fever, CVA, pain, nausea/vomiting	Same as for Cystitis, above. Need urine culture & sensitivity testing	*LOW RISK for resistant bacteria:* (**CIP** 500 mg po bid OR **CIP-ER** 1000 mg po once daily OR **Levo** 750 mg po once daily) x 5-7 days OR **Ceftriaxone** 1 gm IV qd x 10 days (can transition to po FQ or TMP-SMX 1 DS bid if suscept) *HIGH RISK for MDR bacteria* consider **Erta** 1 gm IV qd or, if critically ill and/or had recent Pseudomonas infection, **MER** 1 gm IV q8h	*Low risk for resistant bacteria:* **Erta** 1 gm IV q24. When transitioning to po, if FQ or TMP-SMX not an option, consider oral B-lactams to complete 14 days (may be less effective): **Cefixime** 400 mg po qd **Amox-clav** 875 mg/125 mg po bid	When tolerating po fluids, can transition to oral therapy; drug choice based on culture/sens results. Consider imaging (US / CT) if critical illness, new renal failure, history of nephrolithiasis, ureteral colic, obstructive uropathy, urine pH ≥ 7.0, or failure to respond to appropriate therapy. **HIGH-RISK for resistant bacteria include prior highly resistant bacteria in urine, recent inpatient health-care facility stay, obstructive uropathy, recent fluoroquinolone or B-lactam exposure, recent travel to Asia, Middle East or Africa in past 3 months).** Review of pyelonephritis *(N Engl J Med 2018;378:48).*
Pregnancy: Asymptomatic bacteriuria & cystitis Drug choice based on culture / sensitivity results; do follow-up culture one week after last dose of antibiotic	E. coli (70%) Klebsiella sp. Enterobacter sp. Proteus sp. Grp B Streptococcus	**Nitrofurantoin (Macrobid)** (but not in 3rd trimester) 100 mg po q12h x 5-7 days OR **Amox-clav** 500 mg po q8h x 3-7 days OR **Cephalexin** 500 mg po bid x 3-7 days	**TMP-SMX DS** (but not in 1st trimester or at term) 1 tab po q12h x 3 days OR **Cefpodoxime** 100 mg po q12h x 3-7 days	Treatment recommended to avoid progression to cystitis or pyelonephritis. Untreated bacteriuria associated with increased risk of low birth wt, preterm birth & increased perinatal mortality. If post-treatment culture positive, re-treat with different drug of longer course of same drug. Avoid nitrofurantoin in 3rd trimester due to risk of hemolytic anemia in newborn.
Pregnancy: Acute pyelonephritis Diagnosis: CVA pain, fever, nausea/vomiting in 2nd/3rd trimester. *See Comment*	Same as for Cystitis, above Regimens are empiric therapy *(see Comment)*	**Moderately ill**: **Ceftriaxone** 1 gm IV q24h OR **Cefepime** 1 gm IV q12h. If Pen-allergic, **Aztreonam** 1 gm IV q8h (no activity vs. Gram-pos cocci)	**Severely ill**: **Pip-Tazo** 4.5 gm infused over 4h IV q8h OR **MER** 500 mg IV q8h OR **Erta** 1 gm IV q24h	Try to avoid FQs and AGs during pregnancy. Switch to po therapy after afebrile x 48 hrs. **Treat for 10-14 days.** If pyelo recurs, re-treat. Once asymptomatic continue suppressive therapy for duration of pregnancy: Nitrofurantoin 50-100 mg po qhs OR Cephalexin 250-500 mg po qhs.

 **NOTE: All dosage recommendations are for adults (unless otherwise indicated) and assume normal renal function. § Alternatives consider allergy, PK, compliance, local resistance, cost.*

TABLE 1 (35)

ANATOMIC SITE/DIAGNOSIS/ MODIFYING CIRCUMSTANCES	ETIOLOGIES (usual)	SUGGESTED REGIMENS*		ADJUNCT DIAGNOSTIC OR THERAPEUTIC MEASURES AND COMMENTS
		PRIMARY	ALTERNATIVE§	
KIDNEY & BLADDER/Acute Uncomplicated Cystitis & Pyelonephritis in Women *(continued)*				
Recurrent UTIs in Women (2 or more infections in 6 mos/ 3 or more infections in 1 yr) Risk factors: family history, spermicide use, presence of cystocele, elevated post-void residual urine volume	Same as for Cystitis, above Regimens are options for antimicrobial prophylaxis	Preventive strategies include avoid spermicide, increase fluid intake (additional 1.5 L/ day), Methenamine hippurate 1 gm PO BID, post-coital antibiotics (**Nitrofurantoin** 100 mg OR TMP-SMX 80 mg/400 mg OR TMP 100 mg OR **Cephalexin** 250 mg immediately after intercourse . *See Comment regarding post-menopause.*	When primary options fail, consider daily abx prophylaxis based on susceptibilities of pathogen. Can include **TMP-SMX SS**, **cephalexin** 250 mg, or **nitrofurantoin** 50-100 mg daily)	No strong evidence to support use of cranberry juice. Studies have not shown benefit of oral probiotics but intravaginal probiotics are likely beneficial but not yet FDA approved. In DBRPCT of women age >65 yrs in nursing home, cranberry capsules resulted in no difference in bacteriuria/pyuria *(JAMA 2016,316:1873 & 1879)*. Primary Regimens: In post-menopausal women use Intravaginal estrogen: 0.5 mg Estriol cream intravaginal daily x 2 weeks and then twice weekly as maintenance. Post-menopausal person (not woman) - add methenamine hippurate 1g po bid. Intravaginal probiotics have show promise in several studies but are not yet FDA approved.
Asymptomatic Bacteriuria in Women Defined: 2 consecutive clean catch urine cultures with ≥105 CFU/mL of same organism	Same as for Cystitis, above	**Treatment indicated:** pregnancy, urologic procedure causing bleeding from mucosa	**No treatment indicated:** premenopausal, nonpregnant women, diabetic women, older persons living in the community, elderly, institutionalized subjects, persons with spinal cord injury, catheterized patients while the catheter remains in situ, patients > 2 months post kidney transplant	Asymptomatic bacteriuria & pyuria are discordant. 60% of pts with pyuria have no bacteriuria and pyuria commonly accompanies asymptomatic bacteriuria. In DBRPCT of women in nursing homes, compared cranberry capsules vs. placebo; no difference in bacteriuria/pyuria *(JAMA 2016;316:1873 (ed) & 1879)*.
Acute Uncomplicated Cystitis & Pyelonephritis in Men. Risk of uncomplicated UTI increased with history of BPH, insertive anal sex & lack of circumcision. *See also, Complicated UTIs in Men & Women, below*				
Cystitis	E. coli (75-95%) Rarely other Enterobacterales	**TMP-SMX DS** 1 tab po bid x 7 days OR (**CIP** 500 mg po bid OR **CIP-ER** 1000 mg po once daily OR **Levo** 750 mg po once daily) x 7 days also **Nitrofurantoin** (Macrobid) 100 mg po bid x 7 days.	**Amox-clav** 875/125 mg bid x 5-7 days, **Cephalexin** 500 mg bid x 5-7 days	If recurrent, evaluate for prostatitis. Studies have revealed that for men with UTI without fever that 7 days of treatment is adequate *(JAMA Intern Med 2013; 173:1153)*. But if fever with UTI, 14 days is superior to 7 days *(Clin Infect Dis 2023; 26: 2154)*. Cystitis plus symptoms of bladder outlet obstruction suggests concomitant acute bacterial prostatitis. Consider presence of STDs. Recommend NAAT for C. trachomatis & N. gonorrhoeae. If any hint of obstructive uropathy, image collecting system asap.
Pyelonephritis	Pockets of FQ-resistant ESBL producing E. coli *(EID 2016,22:1594)*	*Low risk of MDR-GNB:* (**CIP** 400 mg IV q12h OR **Levo** 750 mg IV once daily) x 7-14 days	*High risk of MDR GNB:* **MER** 0.5-1 gm IV q8h x 7-14 days OR **Erta** 1 gm IV q12. If critically illness or recent Pseudomonas infection use **MER** 1 gm IV q8h.	

 **NOTE: All dosage recommendations are for adults (unless otherwise indicated) and assume normal renal function. § Alternatives consider allergy, PK, compliance, local resistance, cost.*

TABLE 1 (36)

ANATOMIC SITE/DIAGNOSIS/ MODIFYING CIRCUMSTANCES	ETIOLOGIES (usual)	SUGGESTED REGIMENS*		ADJUNCT DIAGNOSTIC OR THERAPEUTIC MEASURES AND COMMENTS
		PRIMARY	ALTERNATIVE§	
KIDNEY & BLADDER *(continued)*				
Acute Complicated UTIs in Men & Women				
Defined: UTI plus co-morbid condition that increases infection severity & risk of failure, e.g., diabetes, pregnancy, late diagnosis, chronic foley catheter, suprapubic tube, obstruction secondary to stone, anatomic abnormalities, immunosuppression	E. coli or Other Enterobacterales plus: P. aeruginosa Enterococci S. aureus Candida sp.	Prior to empiric therapy: urine culture & sensitivity. If hypotensive: blood cultures. If obstructive uropathy suspected, need imaging of urinary tract asap. *See Comments*		Due to high incidence of resistance and infection severity, Nitrofurantoin, Fosfomycin & TMP-SMX should not be used for empiric therapy. If enterococci cultured, need to adjust therapy based on in vitro susceptibility. Duration of treatment varies with status of co-morbid conditions, need for urologic procedures & individualized pt clinical response. Pip-Tazo inferior to MER vs. ceftriaxone-resistant E. coli/K. pneumo *(JAMA 2018;320:979 & 984).* Men with afebrile UTIs can be treated for 7 days while men who are febrile UTIs benefit from 14 days of treatment *(Clin Infect Dis 2023; 26: 2154).*
		Low risk of MDR GNB: **Levo** 750 mg IV once daily OR **Ceftriaxone** 1 gm IV once daily OR **Cefepime** 1 gm IV q12h OR **Pip-Tazo** 4.5 gm infused over 4h IV q8h OR **Gent** 5 mg/kg IV Once daily. If **Pen-allergic: Aztreonam** 2 gm IV q8h	*Risk of MDR GNB ≥20%:* **MER** 0.5-1 gm IV q8h OR **Ceftolo-tazo** 1.5 gm IV q8h OR **Ceftaz-avi** 2.5 gm IV q8h **MER-vabor** 4 gm IV q8h, *see Comment*	
LIVER *(for Primary (Spontaneous) Bacterial Peritonitis (SBP), see page 51)*				
Cholangitis		*See Gallbladder, page 18*		
Cirrhosis & variceal bleeding	Esophageal flora	**CIP** 400 mg IV q12h x max. of 7 days	**Ceftriaxone** 1 gm IV once daily for max. of 7 days	Short term prophylactic antibiotics in cirrhotics with G-I hemorr, with or without ascites, decreases rate of bacterial infection & ↑ survival *(J Hepatol 60:1310, 2014).*
Hepatic abscess	Enterobacterales (esp. Klebsiella sp.), bacteroides, enterococci, Entamoeba histolytica, Yersinia entero-colitica (rare), Fusobacterium necrophorum *(Lemierre's).*	**Metro** + (**Ceftriaxone** OR **Pip-Tazo** OR **CIP** OR **Levo**)	**Metro** (for amoeba) + either **IMP**, **MER** OR **Dori**	**Serological tests for amebiasis should be done on all patients;** if neg., surgical drainage or percutaneous aspiration. In pyogenic abscess, ½ have identifiable GI source or underlying biliary tract disease. If amoeba serology positive, treat with **Metro** alone without surgery. Empiric **Metro** included for both E. histolytica & bacteroides. **Hemochromatosis** associated with Yersinia enterocolitica liver abscess; regimens listed are effective for yersinia. Klebsiella pneumonia genotype K1 associated ocular & CNS Klebsiella infections.
Hepatic encephalopathy	Urease-producing gut bacteria	**Rifaximin** 550 mg po bid (take with lactulose)		Ref: *NEJM 375:1660, 2016.*
Leptospirosis	Leptospirosis, *see page 67*			
Peliosis hepatis in AIDS pts	Bartonella henselae and B. quintana	*See page 64*		
Post-transplant infected "biloma"	Enterococci (incl. VRE), candida, Gm-neg. bacilli (P. aeruginosa 8%), anaerobes 5%	**Linezolid** 600 mg IV bid + **Pip-Tazo** 4.5 gm infused over 4h IV q8h + **Fluconazole** 400 mg IV q24h	**Levo** 750 m IV q24h + **Dapto** 10 mg/kg IV once daily + **Micafungin** 100 mg IV q24h	Suspect if fever & abdominal pain post-transplant. Exclude hepatic artery thrombosis. Presence of candida and/or VRE bad prognosticators.
Viral hepatitis	Hepatitis A, B, C, D, E, G	*See Table 14E and Table 14F*		

 **NOTE: All dosage recommendations are for adults (unless otherwise indicated) and assume normal renal function. § Alternatives consider allergy, PK, compliance, local resistance, cost.*

TABLE 1 (37)

ANATOMIC SITE/DIAGNOSIS/ MODIFYING CIRCUMSTANCES	ETIOLOGIES (usual)	SUGGESTED REGIMENS*		ADJUNCT DIAGNOSTIC OR THERAPEUTIC MEASURES AND COMMENTS
		PRIMARY	ALTERNATIVE§	
LUNG/Bronchi				
Bronchiolitis/wheezy bronchitis (expiratory wheezing)				
Infants/children (≤ age 5) *See RSV, Table 14A page 233* Ref: *Ln 368:312, 2006*	**Respiratory syncytial virus** (RSV) 50%, parainfluenza 25%, human metapneumovirus	Antibiotics not useful, mainstay of therapy is oxygen and hydration. Ribavirin not recommended for bronchiolitis except HSCT and perhaps other transplant pts		RSV most important. For prevention a humanized mouse monoclonal antibody, **palivizumab**. *See Table 14A, page 233.* Guidance from the American Academy of Pediatrics recommends use of Palivizumab only in newborn infants born at 29 weeks gestation (or earlier) and in special populations (e.g., those infants with significant heart disease). *(Pediatrics 2014;134:415–420)*
Bronchitis				
Infants/children (≤ age 5) Bronchiolitis is characterized by wheezing and crackles, most often in children <2 yrs	<Age 2: Adenovirus; age 2–5: Respiratory syncytial virus, influenza, parainfluenza 3 virus, human metapneumovirus		Antibiotics not indicated for bronchitis or bronchiolitis.	
Adolescents and adults with acute tracheobronchitis (Acute bronchitis)	Usually viral. M. pneumoniae 5%; C. pneumoniae 5%. *See Persistent cough (Pertussis)*	**Antibiotics not indicated.** Antitussive ± inhaled bronchodilators. Throat swab PCR available for Dx of mycoplasma or chlamydia.		Purulent sputum alone not an indication for antibiotic therapy. Expect cough to last 2 weeks. If fever/rigors, get chest x-ray. **If mycoplasma documented, prefer doxy over macrolides due to increasing macrolide resistance.**
Persistent cough (>14 days), afebrile during community outbreak: Pertussis (whooping cough) 10–20% adults with cough >14 days have pertussis	Bordetella pertussis & occ. Bordetella parapertussis. Also consider asthma, gastro-esophageal reflux, post-nasal drip, mycoplasma and also chlamydia.	**Peds doses: Azithro/ Clarithro** OR **TMP-SMX** *(doses in footnote[10])*	**Adult doses: Azithro** po 500 mg day 1, 250 mg q24h days 2–5 OR **TMP-SMX-DS** 1 tab po bid times 14 days OR (**Clarithro** 500 mg po bid or 1 gm **extended release** q24h x 7 days)	**3 stages of illness:** catarrhal (1–2 wks), paroxysmal coughing (2–4 wks), and convalescence (1–2 wks). Treatment may abort or eliminate pertussis in catarrhal stage, but does not shorten paroxysmal stage. **Diagnosis:** PCR on nasopharyngeal secretions or ↑ pertussis-toxin antibody. **Rx aimed at eradication of NP carriage.**
Pertussis: Prophylaxis of household contacts	Drugs and doses as per treatment immediately above. Vaccination of newborn contacts: *CID 58:830, 2014.*			Recommended by Am. Acad. Ped. Red Book 2006 for all household or close contacts; community-wide prophylaxis not recommended.

[10] **ADULT DOSAGE: Amox-clav** 875/125 mg po bid or 500/125 mg po q8h or 2000/125 mg po bid; **Azithro** 500 mg po x 1 dose, then 250 mg q24h x 4 days or 500 mg po q24h x 3 days; *Oral cephalosporins:* **Cefaclor** 500 mg po q8h or 500 mg extended release q12h; **Cefdinir** 300 mg po q12h or 600 mg po q24h; **Cefditoren** 200 mg tabs—2 tabs bid; **Cefixime** 400 mg po q24h; **Cefpodoxime proxetil** 200 mg po q12h; **Cefprozil** 500 mg po q12h; **Ceftibuten** 400 mg po q24h; **Cefuroxime axetil** 250 or 500 mg q12h; **Loracarbef** 400 mg po q12h; **Clarithro** extended release 1000 mg po q24h; **Doxy** 100 mg po bid; **Erythro base** 40 mg/kg/day po div q6h; **Erythro estolate** 40 mg/kg/day po div qid; FQs: **CIP** 750 mg po q12h; **Levo** 500 mg po q24h; **Moxi** 400 mg po q24h; **Prulifloxacin** 600 mg po q24h (where available); **TMP-SMX** 1 DS tab po bid.

PEDS DOSAGE: Azithro 10 mg/kg/day po on day 1, then 5 mg/kg po q24h x 4 days; **Clarithro** 7.5 mg/kg po q12h; **Erythro base** 40 mg/kg/day div q6h; **Erythro estolate** 40 mg/kg/day div q8-12h; **TMP-SMX** (>6 mos. of age) 8 mg/kg/day (TMP component) div bid.

 **NOTE: All dosage recommendations are for adults (unless otherwise indicated) and assume normal renal function. § Alternatives consider allergy, PK, compliance, local resistance, cost.*

TABLE 1 (38)

ANATOMIC SITE/DIAGNOSIS/ MODIFYING CIRCUMSTANCES	ETIOLOGIES (usual)	SUGGESTED REGIMENS* PRIMARY	SUGGESTED REGIMENS* ALTERNATIVE§	ADJUNCT DIAGNOSTIC OR THERAPEUTIC MEASURES AND COMMENTS
LUNG/Bronchi/Bronchitis *(continued)*				
Acute bacterial exacerbation of chronic bronchitis (ABECB), adults (almost always smokers with COPD) Ref: *NEJM 359:2355, 2008.* Severe ABECB = ↑ dyspnea, ↑ sputum viscosity/purulence, ↑ sputum volume. For severe ABECB: (1) consider chest x-ray, esp. if febrile &/or low O2 sat.; (2) inhaled anticholinergic bronchodilator; (3) oral corticosteroid for just 5 days; (4) D/C tobacco use; (5) non-invasive positive pressure ventilation.	Viruses 20–50%, C. pneumoniae 5%, M. pneumoniae <1%; role of S. pneumo, H. influenzae & M. catarrhalis controversial. Tobacco use, air pollution contribute.	**Role of antimicrobial therapy is debated even for severe disease. For mild or moderate disease, no antimicrobial treatment** or maybe **Amox**, **Doxy**, **TMP-SMX**, or **O Ceph.** **For severe disease:** **Amox-clav** 875/125 mg po bid **Azithro** 500 mg po x 1 dose, then 250 mg q24h x 4 days or 500 mg po q24h x 3 days **Clarithro** extended release 1000 mg po q24h **Levo** 750 mg po q24h or **Moxi** 400 mg po q24h **Hospitalized patients, severe disease:** *High risk for pseudomonas* (confirm with culture): **Levo** 750 mg IV/po q24h **Cefepime** 2 gm q8h **Pip-tazo** 4.5 gm infused over 4h IV q8h *Low risk for pseudomonas:* **Levo** 750 mg IV/po q24h or **Moxi** 400 mg IV/po q24h **Ceftriaxone** 2 gm q24h *Drugs & doses in footnote.* Guidelines suggest duration of 5 days *(Ann Intern Med 174:822, 2021)*		
Bronchiectasis *NEJM. 2022;387:533* Acute exacerbation	H. influ., P. aeruginosa, and rarely S. pneumo.	**Levo**, or **Moxi** x 10-14 days. *Dosage in footnote*[10].		Many potential etiologies: obstruction, ↓ immune globulins, cystic fibrosis, dyskinetic cilia, tobacco, prior severe or recurrent necrotizing bronchitis: e.g., pertussis. Choice of therapy based on pre-treatment cultures.
Prevention of exacerbation	Not applicable	**Azithro** 250 mg q24h for 6-12 months		**Caveats:** higher rates of macrolide resistance in oropharyngeal flora; potential for increased risk of a) cardiovascular deaths from macrolide-induced QTc prolongation, b) liver toxicity, or c) hearing loss *(see JAMA 309:1295, 2013).* **Pre-treatment screening:** baseline liver function tests, electrocardiogram; assess hearing; sputum culture to exclude mycobacterial disease.
Specific organisms	Aspergillus *(see Table 11)* MAI *(Table 12)* and P. aeruginosa *(Table 5B).*			
Pneumonia:				
Neonatal: Birth to 1 month	**Viruses:** CMV, rubella, H. simplex **Bacteria:** Group B strep, listeria, S. aureus, P. aeruginosa, Enterobacterales **Other:** Chlamydia trachomatis, syphilis, ureaplasma urealyticum, Mycoplasma hominis	For term infants with normal bilirubin **Ceftriaxone** or **AMP** + **Gent** ± **Cefotaxime**. Add **Vanco** if MRSA is a concern. For chlamydia therapy, **Erythro** 12.5 mg per kg po or IV qid times 14 days.		Blood cultures indicated. Consider C. trachomatis if afebrile pneumonia, staccato cough, IgM >1:8; therapy with erythro or sulfisoxazole. If MRSA documented, **Vanco**, **Clinda**, & **Linezolid** alternatives. **Linezolid** dosage from birth to age 11 yrs is 10 mg per kg q8h.

 **NOTE: All dosage recommendations are for adults (unless otherwise indicated) and assume normal renal function. § Alternatives consider allergy, PK, compliance, local resistance, cost.*

ANATOMIC SITE/DIAGNOSIS/ MODIFYING CIRCUMSTANCES	ETIOLOGIES (usual)	SUGGESTED REGIMENS*		ADJUNCT DIAGNOSTIC OR THERAPEUTIC MEASURES AND COMMENTS
		PRIMARY	ALTERNATIVE§	
LUNG/Bronchi/Pneumonia *(continued)*				
Age 1–3 months				
Pneumonitis syndrome. Usually afebrile	C. trachomatis, RSV, parainfluenza virus 3, human metapneumovirus, Bordetella, S. pneumoniae, S. aureus (rare)	**Outpatient: po** **Amox** 90-100 mg/kg/d x 10-14 days OR **Azithro** 10 mg/kg x 1 dose then 5 mg/kg once daily x 4 days	**Inpatient:** • **If afebrile: Erythro** 10 mg/kg IV q6h or **Azithro** 2.5 mg/kg IV q12h *(see Comment).* • **If febrile: Cefotaxime** 200 mg/kg per day div q8h OR **Ceftriaxone** 75-100 mg/kg q24h	Pneumonitis syndrome: Cough, tachypnea, dyspnea, diffuse infiltrates, afebrile. Usually requires hospital care. Reports of hypertrophic pyloric stenosis after erythro under age 6 wks; not sure about azithro; bid azithro dosing theoretically might ↓ risk of hypertrophic pyloric stenosis. If lobar pneumonia, give AMP 200–300 mg per kg per day for S. pneumoniae. No empiric coverage for S. aureus, as it is rare etiology.
		For **RSV**, *see Bronchiolitis, page 41*		
Infants and Children, age >3 months to 18 yrs (IDSA Treatment Guidelines: *CID 53:617, 2011*).				
Outpatient Consider influenza virus, RSV (respiratory syncytial virus), human metapneumovirus, parainfluenza virus, adenovirus, SARS-CoV-2.	RSV, human metapneumovirus, rhinovirus, influenza virus, adenovirus, parainfluenza virus, Mycoplasma, H. influenzae, S. pneumoniae, S. aureus (rare)	**Amox** 90 mg/kg in 2 divided doses x 5 days	**Azithro** 10 mg/kg x 1 dose (max 500 mg), then 5 mg/kg (max 250 mg) x 4 days OR **Amox-clav** 90 mg/kg (Amox comp) in 2 divided doses x 5 days	Antimicrobial therapy may not be necessary for preschool-aged children with CAP as most infections are viral etiologies. 2011 Guidelines recommend 10-14 days but shorter duration (5 days) superior in recent trial: *JAMA Pediatr 2022;176:253.*
Inpatient (3 mos - 18 yrs) Influenza testing recommended for all hospitalized children in winter season.	As above	Fully immunized: **AMP** 200 mg/kg/day IV q6h Not fully immunized: **Cefotaxime** 150 mg/kg IV divided q8h or **Ceftriaxone** 75-100 mg/kg/day	*See Comments* If influenza is diagnosed or strongly suspected: **Oseltamivir**	If atypical infection suspected, add **Azithro** 10 mg/kg x 1 dose (max 500 mg), then 5 mg/kg (max 250 mg) x 4 days. If community MRSA suspected, add **Vanco** 30-60 mg/kg/d in 2-3 div doses, target AUC_{24} 400-600 µg/mL x h OR **Clinda** 40 mg/kg/day divided q6-8h x 10-14d; may switch to oral agents as early as 2-3 days if good clinical response.
Adults (over age 18) — IDSA/ATS Guideline for CAP in adults: *Am J Crit Care Med 2019, 200:e45.*				
Community-acquired, empiric therapy for outpatient CAP patients with Pneumonia Severity Index (PSI) ≤90 (level I, II, or III) are candidates for out-patient therapy	S. pneumo, atypicals and mycoplasma in particular, Hemophilus, Moraxella, viral pathogens: up to 30% of cases	**No co-morbidity**: **Amox** 1 gm po tid OR **Doxy** 100 mg po bid **Co-morbidity present**: [(**Amox-clav** 875 mg/125 mg po bid x 5-7d + (**Azithro** 500 mg po x1, then 250 mg daily x 4d OR **Levo** 750 mg po q24h x 5d	**No co-morbidity**: if local rates of macrolide resistant S. pneumo < 25%: **Azithro** 500 mg po x 1 dose then 250 mg po q24h x 4 days OR **Clarithro** 500 mg po bid x 7 days **Co-morbidity present**: **Amox-clav + Doxy**	Levo substitutes: **Moxi** 400 mg po q24h or **Gemi** 320 mg po q24h Amox-clav substitutes: **Cefpodoxime** 200 mg po bid or **Cefuroxime** 500 mg po bid. **Treat for 5-7 days**

Abbreviations on page 2. **NOTE: All dosage recommendations are for adults (unless otherwise indicated) and assume normal renal function. § Alternatives consider allergy, PK, compliance, local resistance, cost.*

TABLE 1 (40)

ANATOMIC SITE/DIAGNOSIS/ MODIFYING CIRCUMSTANCES	ETIOLOGIES (usual)	SUGGESTED REGIMENS* PRIMARY	ALTERNATIVE§	ADJUNCT DIAGNOSTIC OR THERAPEUTIC MEASURES AND COMMENTS
LUNG/Bronchi/Pneumonia *(continued)*				
Community-acquired, empiric therapy for patient admitted to hospital	As above plus *S. aureus* in IVDU or influenza-associated CAP; legionella. No pathogen detected in majority of patients, virus > bacteria *(NEJM 373:415, 2015)*	(**Ceftriaxone** 1-2 gm IV q24h or **Ceftaroline** 600 mg IV q12h) + **Azithro** 500 mg IV q24h OR **Levo** 750 mg IV/po q24h **(not recommended as monotherapy for severe CAP)** For severe CAP use beta-lactam + macrolide	(**Ceftriaxone** 1-2 gm IV q24h or **Ceftaroline** 600 mg IV q12h) + **Doxy** 100 mg IV/po q12h OR **Moxi** 400 mg IV/po q24h For severe CAP beta-lactam + respiratory fluoroquinolone	Sputum and blood cultures recommended for in-patients, especially for severe CAP. Coverage for MRSA or *P. aeruginosa* not routinely recommended in absence of risk factors (e.g., prior isolation of the pathogen or hospitalization AND treatment with parenteral antibiotics within prior 90 days; additional risk factors for MRSA include IVDU and influenza-associated CAP. if empirical coverage is used obtain cultures/nasal PCR to allow de-escalation (cultures negative) or confirmation for need of continued therapy (cultures positive). **Treat for 5-7 days**. Safe to discontinue antibiotics with normalization of procalcitonin to 0.1-0.2 mcg/mL.
Hospital-acquired or Ventilator-associated pneumonia IDSA guidelines: *CID 63:e61, 2016*	As above + MDR Gram-negatives. In 39 of 174 pts with non-ventilator HAP, respiratory virus detected *(Resp Med 2017,122:76)*	**Cefepime** 2 gm IV q12h OR **Pip-tazo** 4.5 gm infused over 4h IV q8h Note: no supportive evidence for use of nebulized/inhaled antibiotics *(CCM 47: 890 & e470, 2019); Lancet ID 20:330, 2020.* Suscept. testing may identify other active agents, e.g., **Ceftaz-avibactam, MER-vabor, Cefiderocol**. Duration: 8 days treatment as effective as 15 days *(PLoS 7:e41290, 2012)*	**MER** 1 gm IV q8h OR **Levo** 750 mg IV/po q24h	Add **Vanco** or **Linezolid** if unit or hospital MRSA prevalence >10-20%, prior IV antibiotic use within 90 days, acute renal replacement therapy prior to VAP onset, septic shock or high risk of mortality, ARDS preceding VAP, unknown MRSA prevalence or presence of MRSA risk factors (e.g., IVDU, prior MRSA infection or colonization). For suspected pseudomonas or high risk of mortality add **CIP** 400 mg IV q8h or **Levo** 750 mg IV q24h or **Tobra** 5 mg/kg IV q24h or **AMK** 15 mg/kg IV q24h. **Aztreonam** 2 gm IV q8h can substitute for other beta-lactams if there is beta-lactam hypersensitivity, but lacks coverage for S. aureus. Colistin if carbapenem-resistant Gram-negative is suspected.
Pneumonia —Selected specific therapy after culture results (sputum, blood, pleural fluid, etc.) available.				
Acinetobacter baumannii complex (ABC)	Patients with VAP; long ICU stay with repeated antibiotic exposure	**Empiric rx:** positive culture, no in vitro suscept results, prevalence of resistance < 15%: **Cefepime**, **Ceftazidime**, **Amp-sulb, Mero** *(Doses in footnote[11])*.	**Specific rx:** culture & suscept results known, susceptible organism: **Cefepime**, **Ceftazidime**, **Amp-sulb, Mero** or **FQ**. For carbapenem-resistant strain: **Cefiderocol** 2 gm IV, 3h infusion, q8h OR **Sulbactam-durlobactam + IMP** *(see Comments)*.	*See Table 5E for treatment of MDR infections* (Sulbactam 1 g IV + Durlobatam 1 g IV) q6h + IMP 1 gm IV q6h background therapy compared to Colistin 2.5 mg/kg + IMP background therapy in a RCT *(Lancet ID 2023; 23:1072)* of serious ABC infections, including pneumonia, was significantly less nephrotoxic than the Colistin regimen and was associated with a numerically lower mortality in laboratory-confirmed cases of ABC, 12 (19%) of 63 in the Sulbactam-Durlobactam group and 20 (32%) of 62 in the colistin group, a difference of –13.2% (95% CI, – 30.0 to 3.5).
Actinomycosis	A. Israelii and rarely others	**AMP** 200 mg/kg/day in 3-4 divided doses x 4-6 wks then **Pen** VK 2-4 gm/day in 4 divided doses x 6-12 mo	**Doxy** or **Ceftriaxone** OR **Clinda** IV x 4-6 wks, then po x 6-12 mo	Can use **Pen G** instead of AMP: 10-20 million units/day IV x 4-6 wks, then **Pen VK** 2-4 g/d in four divided doses or Amoxicillin 2 gm po bid x 6-12 months.

[11] Doses of antibiotics used to treat pneumonia due to Acinetobacter sp., Klebsiella sp. and Pseudomonas sp. *Penicillins:* **Pip-Tazo** 4.5 gm infused over 4h IV q8h; **Amp-sulb** 3 gm IV q6h or HD 9 gm IV q8h over 4 hrs. *Cephalosporins:* **Ceftazidime** 2 gm IV q8h; **Ceftaz-avi** 2.5 gm IV q8h over 3 hrs; **Ceftolo-tazo** 3 gm IV q8h over 3 hrs; **IMP-relebactam** 1.25 gm IV over 30 min; **Aztreonam** 2 gm IV q8h. *FQs:* **CIP** 400 mg IV q8h (septic shock: may need 600 mg q8h); **Levo** 750 mg IV q24h. *Carbapenems:* **MER** 1-2 gm IV q8h; **MER-vabor** 4 gm IV over 3 hrs q8h; **IMP** 0.5-1 gm q8h. *Aminoglycosides:* **Gent/Tobra** 7 mg/kg IV x 1, then 5 mg/kg IV q8h. **Polymyxin B** 2.5 mg/kg IV over 2 hrs, then 12 hrs later, 1.5 mg/kg over 1 hr & repeat q12h. **Minocycline** 200 mg IV x 1, then 100 mg IV q12h

Abbreviations on page 2. **NOTE: All dosage recommendations are for adults (unless otherwise indicated) and assume normal renal function. § Alternatives consider allergy, PK, compliance, local resistance, cost.*

ANATOMIC SITE/DIAGNOSIS/ MODIFYING CIRCUMSTANCES	ETIOLOGIES (usual)	SUGGESTED REGIMENS*		ADJUNCT DIAGNOSTIC OR THERAPEUTIC MEASURES AND COMMENTS
		PRIMARY	ALTERNATIVE§	
LUNG/Bronchi/Pneumonia/Selected specific therapy after culture results (sputum, blood, pleural fluid, etc.) available. *(continued)*				
Anthrax, systemic (includes oral, gastrointestinal, inhalational) **Treatment** consists of antibacterial regimen + antitoxin	*B. anthracis*	Primary: Adult, including pregnancy: **CIP** 400 mg IV q8h + **MER** 2 gm q8h + **Doxy** 200 mg IV x1 then 100 mg IV q12h + antitoxin (Raxibacumab or Obiltoxaximab or Anthrax immune globulin intravenous (see package insert for dosing) Primary: Child, age ≥ 1 mo. to < 18 yr: **CIP** 10 mg/kg (max dose 400 mg) IV q8h + **MER** 40 mg/kg (max dose 2 gm) IV q8h + **Doxy** 4.4 mg/kg (max dose 200 mg) IV x1 then 2.2 mg/kg (max dose 100 mg) IV q12h + antitoxin (as above) **See *MMWR/Nov. 17, 2023/72 (6):1-47* for complete CDC guidelines and use of alternative agents**		1. Duration of therapy 2 weeks or longer depending on clinical response. 2. Prolonged therapy no longer recommended for aerosol exposure for immunocompetent patients who will have developed natural immunity. 3. Immunocompromised patients with aerosol exposure should be transitioned to an oral post-exposure prophylaxis regimen to complete 42-60 days of therapy.
Anthrax, prophylaxis Empiric regimens for post-exposure prophylaxis if an aerosol exposure might have occurred.	*B. anthracis*	Adult, including pregnancy: **CIP** 500 mg po q12h or **Doxy** 100 mg po q12h Child, age ≥ 1 mo. to < 18 yr.: **CIP** 15 mg/kg (max dose 500 mg) po q12h or **Doxy** 2.2 mg/kg (max dose 100 mg) po q12h Immunocompetent unvaccinated persons age 18-65, who have been exposed or potentially exposed to aerosolized *B. anthracis* should receive Anthrax Vaccine Adsorbed (Cyfendus; Emergent Biosolutions) 2 doses: 2 doses at 0, 14 days plus concurrent prophylactic antimicrobial therapy x 42 days.		1. 60 days of therapy if antimicrobial therapy is administered without post-exposure vaccination. 2. Duration of therapy and vaccination in other groups guided by data available at the time of an anthrax event. **See *MMWR/Nov. 17, 2023/72 (6):1-47* for complete CDC guidelines and use of alternative agents.**
Burkholderia (Pseudomonas) pseudomallei (etiology of melioidosis) Can cause primary or secondary skin infection *See NEJM 367:1035, 2012*	Gram-negative	**Initial parenteral rx:** **Ceftaz** 30–50 mg per kg IV q8h or **MER** 1 gm IV q8h. Rx minimum of 14 days, longer in those with more severe or extensive disease, then transition to oral eradication therapy.	**Eradication therapy:** **TMP-SMX** 5 mg/kg (TMP component) bid (adults and children) x 3 mos.	Eradication therapy in pregnancy and children <8 yrs intolerant of TMP/SMX: **AM-CL** 20 mg/5 mg po tid x 3 mos. **Doxy** 100 mg bid x 3 mos also an option but TMP-SMX preferred because of lower failure rate. Extend duration of therapy to 6 mos for bony or CNS infection.
Chlamydia pneumoniae	Chlamydophila pneumoniae	**Azithro** 500 mg on day one then 250 mg qd x 4 days OR **Levo** 750 mg x 5 days	**Doxy** 100 mg q12h x 5 days OR **Clarithro** 500 mg bid x 5 days	Clinical diagnosis, rarely confirmed microbiologically.
Haemophilus influenzae	β-lactamase negative	**AMP** IV, **Amox** po, **TMP-SMX**, **Azithro/Clarithro**, **Doxy.**		25–35% strains β-lactamase positive. ↑ resistance to both TMP-SMX and doxy. *See Table 10A, page 150 for dosages.*
	β-lactamase positive	**Amox-clav**, **O Ceph 2/3**, **P Ceph 3**, **FQ.** Dosage: *Table 10A*		
Influenza virus	See *Table 14A, page 231*. Ref: *IDSA Guidelines, CID 68:895, 2019.*			
Klebsiella sp.—ESBL pos. & other coliforms *(see Table 5C)*	β-lactamase positive	**Ceftolo-tazo**, **IMP** or **MER**; if resistant: **Ceftaz-avi**, **MER-vabor** or **IMP-relebactam** *(See footnote[11] for dosing)*		ESBL inactivates all cephalosporins, co-resistance to all FQs & often aminoglycosides. Failure of Pip-tazo vs. ESBLs *(JAMA 2018;320:979 & 984)*.

 **NOTE: All dosage recommendations are for adults (unless otherwise indicated) and assume normal renal function. § Alternatives consider allergy, PK, compliance, local resistance, cost.*

TABLE 1 (42)

ANATOMIC SITE/DIAGNOSIS/ MODIFYING CIRCUMSTANCES	ETIOLOGIES (usual)	SUGGESTED REGIMENS*		ADJUNCT DIAGNOSTIC OR THERAPEUTIC MEASURES AND COMMENTS
		PRIMARY	ALTERNATIVE§	
LUNG/Bronchi/Pneumonia/Selected specific therapy after culture results (sputum, blood, pleural fluid, etc.) available. *(continued)*				
Legionella pneumonia	Legionella pneumophila, other legionella species	(**Levo** 750 mg po/IV or **Moxi** 400 mg po/IV) x 7-10 days	**Azithro** 500 mg IV/po x 7-10 days	If immunocompromised or severe disease, treat for 14-21 days. FQs and Azithro equally efficacious *(CID 72:1979, 1990, 2021)*.
Moraxella catarrhalis	93% β-lactamase positive	**Amox-clav**, **O Ceph 2/3**, **P Ceph 2/3**, **Macrolide**[12], **FQ**, **TMP-SMX**. **Doxy** another option. *See Table 10A, page 150 for dosages*		
Mycoplasma pneumoniae	M. pneumoniae	**Doxy** 100 mg q12h x 7-10 days; Peds: Doxy safe regardless of age for rx ≤ 21 days *(AAP Redbook 2018)*.	**Azithro** 500 mg po on day 1 and then 250 mg po once daily for 4 days *(see Comments)* OR **Levo** 750 mg po/IV x 5 days	If Doxy not available, Mino 200 g po/IV x 1 dose, then 100 mg po/IV bid. Increasing macrolide resistance *(Infect Dis Clin N Amer 33:1087, 2019)* so Doxy then Levo are preferred for documented mycoplasma infection. For cold agglutinin complications, see *JAMA 319:1377, 2018*.
Nocardia pneumonia Expert Help: Wallace Lab (+1) 903-877-7680; CDC (+1) 404-639-3158 Ref: *Medicine 88:250, 2009*.	Nocardia spp.	**TMP-SMX** 15 mg/kg/day IV/po in 2-4 divided doses + **Imipenem** 500 mg IV q6h for first 3-4 weeks then **TMP-SMX** 10 mg/kg/day in 2-4 divided doses x 3-6 mos.	**IMP** 500 mg IV q6h + **Amikacin** 7.5 mg/kg IV q12h x 3-4 wks & then po **TMP-SMX**	**Duration:** 3 mos. if immunocompetent; 6 mos. if immunocompromised. **Linezolid:** active in vitro. Important to send for susceptibility testing.
Pseudomonas aeruginosa (For resistant strains, see *Table 5D*) *(CID 2022;75:187)*	Risk factors: cystic fibrosis, neutropenia, mechanical ventilation, tracheostomy	*Mild, low risk of MDR: Monotherapy:* [**Pip-Tazo**, **Ceftazidime**, **Cefepime**, **IMP**, **MER** or **Aztreonam**] or [**CIP** or **Levo**] *(Dosing in footnote*[11]*)*	*Septic ± high risk for MDR: Combination rx:* **Ceftolozane-tazobactam** 3 gm IV over 1h q8h or a Primary agent + **Tobra** 7 mg/kg IV x 1, then 5 mg/kg IV q8h	*Known ESBL producer:* MER or **Ceftolo-tazo*** or **Ceftaz-avi*** or **MER-vabor***. *Known KPC producer:* **Ceftaz-avi*** or **MER-vabor** or **IMP-rela**. *Known metallo-type (NDM) carbapenemase producer:* (**Ceftaz-avi*** + **Aztreonam**) *(CID 72:1871, 2021)*. **Cefiderocol**, if susceptible. * not FDA-approved indication
Q Fever Acute atypical pneumonia.	Coxiella burnetii Dx: PCR and/or Phase II antibody (IgG≥1:200 or IgM≥50	No valvular heart disease: **Doxy** 100 mg po bid x 14 days Doxy safe regardless of age for rx ≤21 days *(AAP Redbook 2018)*	Valvular heart disease: (**Doxy** 100 mg po bid + **hydroxychloroquine** 200 mg tid) x 12 months *See Comment*	In pregnancy: **TMP-SMX DS** 1 tab po bid throughout pregnancy. Even in absence of valvular heart disease, 1% of pts develop endocarditis *(CID 62:537, 2016)*. If hydroxychloroquine intolerant, Doxy + FQ is alternative *(CID 2018,66:719)*.
Staphylococcus aureus Duration of treatment: 2-3 wks if just pneumonia; 6-8 wks if concomitant endocarditis and/or osteomyelitis.	Nafcillin/oxacillin susceptible	**Nafcillin/oxacillin** 2 gm IV q4h	**Vanco** 30-60 mg/kg/d in 2-3 div doses, target AUC_{24} 400-600 µg/mL x h or **Linezolid** 600 mg IV q12h	**Telavancin** 10 mg/kg IV x 60 min q24h another option. Value of negative nasal S. aureus PCR *(CID 67:1, 2018)*. Linezolid should not be used in cases of endocarditis.
	MRSA (see *Table 6*)	**Vanco** 30-60 mg/kg/d in 2-3 div doses, target AUC_{24} 400-600 µg/mL x h or **Linezolid** 600 mg IV/po q12h	**Dapto** not an option; pneumonia developed during dapto rx *(CID 49:1286, 2009)*. **Ceftaroline** 600 mg IV q8h	
Stenotrophomonas maltophilia (see *Table 5E*) *(CID 2022;74:2089)*		**TMP-SMX** 8-12 mg/kg/d (dosed based on TMP component) IV/po divided q8h or q12h + **Mino** 200 mg IV/po q12h	Combo therapy with two of the following agents: **TMP-SMX** (8-12 mg/kg/d IV/po divided q8h or q12h), **Levo** (750 mg Iv/po q24h), **Mino** (200 mg IV/po q12h), **Tigecycline** (200 mg IV x1, then 100 mg IV q12h)	Can step down to oral monotherapy with TMP-SMX or Mino once patient has improved. Rarely may need to use polymyxin combination therapy. **Cefiderocol** also an option.

[12] **Macrolide** = Azithromycin, Clarithromycin and Erythromycin.

 **NOTE: All dosage recommendations are for adults (unless otherwise indicated) and assume normal renal function. § Alternatives consider allergy, PK, compliance, local resistance, cost.*

TABLE 1 (43)

ANATOMIC SITE/DIAGNOSIS/ MODIFYING CIRCUMSTANCES	ETIOLOGIES (usual)	SUGGESTED REGIMENS*		ADJUNCT DIAGNOSTIC OR THERAPEUTIC MEASURES AND COMMENTS
		PRIMARY	ALTERNATIVE§	
LUNG/Bronchi/Pneumonia/Selected specific therapy after culture results (sputum, blood, pleural fluid, etc.) available. *(continued)*				
Streptococcus pneumoniae	Pen-susceptible	**AMP** 2 gm IV q6h, **Amox** 1 gm po tid, **Pen G** IV[13], **Doxy**, **O Ceph 2**, **P Ceph 2/3;** may add **Azithro** 500 mg IV/po qd *(JAC 69:1441, 2014). See Table 10A, page 150 for other dosages.* Treat until afebrile, (min. of 5 days) and/or until serum procalcitonin normal.		
	Pen-resistant, high level	**FQs** with enhanced activity: **Gemi**, **Levo**, **Moxi**; **P Ceph 3** (resistance rare); high-dose IV **AMP**; **Vanco** IV—*see Table 5A, page 85 for more data.* If all options not possible (e.g., allergy), **Linezolid** active: 600 mg IV or po q12h. *Dosages Table 10A.* Treat until afebrile, 3-5 days (min. of 5 days). In CAP trial, **Ceftaroline** 600 mg IV q12h superior to Ceftriaxone *(CID 51:641, 2010).*		
Tularemia **Inhalational tularemia** *CID 2024. 78(Suppl1):S1-S71*	Francisella tularemia **Treatment**	**Doxy** 100 mg IV or po bid times 14-21 days or **CIP** 400 mg IV (or 750 mg po) bid times 14-21 days	(**Streptomycin** 15 mg per kg IV bid) or (**Gent** 5 mg per kg IV qd) times 10 days	Pregnancy: *as for non-pregnant adults.* **Tobramycin** should work. **Streptomycin** and **gentamicin** have been preferred agents historically for severe disease but **fluoroquinolones** and **doxycycline** also appear to be effective *(CID 2024; 78(Suppl 1): S38).*
	Postexposure prophylaxis	**Doxy** 100 mg po bid times 14 days	**CIP** 500 mg po bid times 14 days	Pregnancy: *As for non-pregnant adults*
Viral (interstitial) pneumonia suspected *See Influenza, Table 14A, page 231.*	**Rule out: COVID-19/SARS CoV-2 and RSV** Consider: **Influenza**, adenovirus, coronavirus (MERS/SARS), hantavirus, metapneumovirus, parainfluenza virus, respiratory syncytial virus	**For influenza: Oseltamivir** 75 mg po bid for 5 days or **Zanamivir** two 5 mg inhalations twice a day for 5 days. **COVID-19:** see *https://web.sanfordguide.com/* for free access to continual COVID-19 updates.		No known efficacious drugs for adenovirus, coronavirus, hantavirus, metapneumovirus, parainfluenza.
Yersinia pestis (Plague) *MMWR 2021;70(RR-3):1*	Y. pestis If aerosolized, suspect bioterror.	(**Gent** 5 mg/kg IV q24h or **Streptomycin** 30 mg/kg/day in 2 div doses) x 10 days	(**CIP** 500 mg po bid or 400 mg IV q12h or **Levo** 500 mg IV/po) x 10 d or **Moxi** 400 mg po/IV once daily x 10 d	**Doxy** 200 mg IV q12h x 1 day, then 100 mg po bid x 7-10 days. **Chloro** also effective but potentially toxic. Consider if evidence of plague meningitis.
LUNG—Other Specific Infections				
Aspiration pneumonia/Anaerobic lung infection/lung abscess	Anaerobes and viridans group streptococci predominate.	**Parenteral regimens** **Ceftriaxone** 1-2 gm IV q24h + **Metro** (500 mg IV q6h or 1 gm IV q12h) **Amp-sulb** 3 gm IV q6h **Oral regimens** **Clinda** 300-450 mg po tid **Moxi** 400 mg po once daily	**Parenteral regimens** **Pip-tazo** 3.375 gm IV q6h or 4-hr infusion of 4.5 gm initial dose then 3.375 gm q8h (q12h for CrCl < 20 ml/min) **Erta** 1 gm IV q24h **Oral regimens** **Amox-clav** 875/125 mg po bid	Typically anaerobic infection of the lung: aspiration pneumonitis, necrotizing pneumonia, lung abscess and empyema *(NEJM 380:651, 2019).* Routine coverage for anaerobes not recommended unless lung abscess or empyema is suspected (ATS/IDSA Guidelines: *Am J Respir Crit Care Med. 2019; 200:e45-e67).* Note: Different from chemical pneumonitis after aspiration of sterile gastric acid *(CID 2018;67:513).*
Chronic pneumonia with fever, night sweats and weight loss	M. tuberculosis, coccidioidomycosis, histoplasmosis	*See Table 11 and Table 12.* For risk associated with TNF inhibitors, *see CID 41(Suppl 3):S187, 2005.*		Risk factors: HIV+, nationality, alcoholism, contact with TB, travel into developing countries
COVID-19	Coronavirus: SARS CoV-2	See *Table 14A* and *http://web.sanfordguide.com* for updated information, treatment recommendations and prevention measures.		
RSV	Respiratory syncitial virus			

[13] **IV Pen G dosage:** no meningitis, 2 million units IV q4h. If concomitant meningitis, 4 million units IV q4h.

Abbreviations on page 2. **NOTE: All dosage recommendations are for adults (unless otherwise indicated) and assume normal renal function. § Alternatives consider allergy, PK, compliance, local resistance, cost.*

TABLE 1 (44)

ANATOMIC SITE/DIAGNOSIS/ MODIFYING CIRCUMSTANCES	ETIOLOGIES (usual)	SUGGESTED REGIMENS* PRIMARY	SUGGESTED REGIMENS* ALTERNATIVE§	ADJUNCT DIAGNOSTIC OR THERAPEUTIC MEASURES AND COMMENTS
LUNG—Other Specific Infections *(continued)*				
Cystic fibrosis **Acute exacerbation of pulmonary symptoms** *BMC Medicine 9:32, 2011* Choice of therapy should be based on results of respiratory cultures.	S. aureus or H. influenzae early in disease; P. aeruginosa later in disease Nontuberculous mycobacteria emerging as an important pathogen *(Semin Respir Crit Care Med 34:124, 2013)*	**For P. aeruginosa:** (Peds doses) **Tobra** 3.3 mg/kg q8h or 12 mg/kg IV q24h. Combine tobra with **Pip-Tazo** 4.5 gm infused over 4h IV q8h **or** **Ceftaz** 50 mg/kg IV q8h to max of 6 gm per day. If resistant to above, **CIP/ Levo** used if P. aeruginosa susceptible. *See footnote[14] & Comment*	**For S. aureus: (1) MSSA—Oxacillin/Nafcillin** 2 gm IV q4h. **(2) MRSA—Vanco** 30-60 mg/kg/d in 2-3 div doses, target AUC_{24} 400-600 µg/mL x h	**Cystic Fibrosis Foundation Guidelines:** 1. Combination therapy for P. aeruginosa infection. 2. Once-daily dosing for aminoglycosides. 3. Routine use of steroid not recommended. **Inhalation options** (P. aeruginosa suppression): 1) Nebulized tobra 300 mg bid x 28 days, no rx for 28 days, repeat; 2) Inhaled tobra powder-hand held: 4-28 mg cap bid x 28 days, no rx for 28 days, repeat; Nebulized aztreonam (Cayston): 75 mg tid after pre-dose bronchodilator. Ref: *Med Lett 56:51, 2014.*
	Burkholderia (Pseudomonas) cepacia	**TMP-SMX** 5 mg per kg (TMP) IV q6h	**Chloro** 15–20 mg per kg IV/po q6h	Patients develop progressive respiratory failure, 62% mortality at 1 yr. **Fail to respond to aminoglycosides,** anti-pseudomonal beta-lactams. Patients with B. cepacia should be isolated from other CF patients.
		Need culture & sens results to guide rx.		
Empyema. *IDSA Treatment Guidelines for Children, CID 53:617, 2011*; exudative pleural effusion criteria *(JAMA 311:2422, 2014)*.				
Neonatal	Staph. aureus	*See Pneumonia, neonatal, page 42*		Drainage indicated.
Infants/children (1 month–5 yrs)	Staph. aureus, Strep. pneumoniae, H. influenzae	*See Pneumonia, age 1 month–5 years, page 42*		Drainage indicated.
Child >5 yrs to Adult—Diagnostic thoracentesis; chest tube for empyemas				
Acute, usually parapneumonic *For dosage, see footnote on page 28*	Strep. pneumoniae, Group A strep	**Cefotaxime** or **Ceftriaxone** *(Dosage, see footnote[7] page 28)*	**Vanco**	Tissue Plasminogen Activator (10 mg) + DNase (5 mg) bid x 3 days via chest tube. In adults but not children addition of DNase improves outcome *(NEJM 365:518, 2011)*.
	Staph. aureus: Check for MRSA	**Nafcillin/Oxacillin** if MSSA	**Vanco** or **Linezolid** if MRSA.	Usually complication of S. aureus pneumonia &/or bacteremia.
	H. influenzae	**Ceftriaxone**	**TMP-SMX** or **Amp-sulb**	Pleomorphic Gm-neg. bacilli. ↑ resistance to TMP-SMX.
Subacute/chronic	Anaerobic strep, Strep. milleri, Bacteroides sp., Enterobacterales, M. tuberculosis	**Clinda** 450–900 mg IV q8h + **Ceftriaxone**	**Cefoxitin** or **IMP** or **Pip-tazo** or **Amp-sulb** *(Dosage, see footnote[7] page 28)*	Intrapleural tissue plasminogen activator (t-PA) 10 mg + DNase 5 mg via chest tube twice daily for 3 days improved fluid drainage, reduced frequency of surgery, and reduced duration of the hospital stay; neither agent effective alone *(N Engl J Med 365:518, 2011)*.
Human immunodeficiency virus infection (HIV+):				
CD4 T-lymphocytes <200 per mm³ or clinical AIDS Dry cough, progressive dyspnea, & diffuse infiltrate **Prednisone first if suspect pneumocystis** *(see Comment)*	Pneumocystis jirovecii (PJP or PCP) most likely; also MTB, fungi, Kaposi's sarcoma, & lymphoma **NOTE:** AIDS pts may develop pneumonia due to DRSP or other pathogens--*see below*	*Rx listed here is for* **severe** *pneumocystis; see Table 11A, page 183 for po regimens for* **mild** *disease.* **Prednisone 1st** *(see Comment),* **then:** **TMP-SMX** [IV: 15 mg per kg per day div q8h (TMP component) or po: 2 DS tabs q8h], total of 21 days	(**Clinda** 600 mg IV q8h + **Primaquine** 30 mg po q24h) or (**pentamidine isethionate** 4 mg per kg per day IV) times 21 days.	**Diagnosis (induced sputum or bronchial wash) for:** histology or monoclonal antibody strains or PCR. **Prednisone 40 mg bid po times 5 days then 40 mg q24h po times 5 days then 20 mg q24h po times 11 days is indicated with PCP should be given at initiation of anti-PCP rx; don't wait until pt's condition deteriorates.** If PCP studies negative, consider bacterial pneumonia, TBc, cocci, histo, crypto, Kaposi's sarcoma or lymphoma.

[14] Other options: (**Tobra** + **Aztreonam** 50 mg per kg IV q8h); (**IMP** 15–25 mg per kg IV q6h + **Tobra**); **CIP commonly used in children**, e.g., **CIP** IV/po + **Ceftaz** IV *(LnID 3:537, 2003)*.

Abbreviations on page 2. **NOTE: All dosage recommendations are for adults (unless otherwise indicated) and assume normal renal function. § Alternatives consider allergy, PK, compliance, local resistance, cost.*

TABLE 1 (45)

ANATOMIC SITE/DIAGNOSIS/ MODIFYING CIRCUMSTANCES	ETIOLOGIES (usual)	SUGGESTED REGIMENS*		ADJUNCT DIAGNOSTIC OR THERAPEUTIC MEASURES AND COMMENTS
		PRIMARY	ALTERNATIVE§	
LUNG—Human immunodeficiency virus infection (HIV+) *(continued)*				
CD4 T-lymphocytes normal Acute onset, purulent sputum & pulmonary infiltrates ± pleuritic pain. **Isolate pt until TBc excluded: Adults**	Strep. pneumoniae, H. influenzae, aerobic Gm-neg. bacilli (including P. aeruginosa), Legionella rare, MTB.	**Ceftriaxone** 1 gm IV q24h (over age 65 1 gm IV q24h) + **Azithro**. Could use **Levo,** or **Moxi** IV as alternative *(see Comment)*		For suspected bacterial pneumonia, other regimens for CAP also are options.
LYMPH NODES (approaches below apply to lymphadenitis without an obvious primary source)				
Lymphadenitis, acute				
Generalized	Etiologies: EBV, early HIV infection, syphilis, toxoplasma, tularemia, Lyme disease, sarcoid, lymphoma, systemic lupus erythematosus, **Kikuchi-Fujimoto** disease and others. For differential diagnosis of fever and lymphadenopathy *see NEJM 369:2333, 2013.*			
By Region:				
Cervical—*see cat-scratch disease (CSD)*	CSD (B. henselae), Grp A strep, Staph. aureus, anaerobes, MTB (scrofula), M. avium, M. scrofulaceum, M. malmoense, toxo, tularemia		History & physical exam directs evaluation. If nodes fluctuant, aspirate and base rx on Gram & acid-fast stains. **Kikuchi-Fujimoto** disease causes fever and benign self-limited adenopathy; the etiology is unknown *(Blood 129:917, 2017).*	
Inguinal				
Sexually transmitted	HSV, chancroid, syphilis, LGV			
Not sexually transmitted	GAS, SA, tularemia, CSD, Y. pestis (plague)		Consider bubonic plague & glandular tularemia.	
Axillary	GAS, SA, CSD, tularemia, Y. pestis, sporotrichosis		Consider bubonic plague & glandular tularemia.	
Extremity, with associated nodular lymphangitis	Sporotrichosis, leishmania, Nocardia brasiliensis, Mycobacterium marinum, Mycobacterium chelonae, tularemia		Treatment varies with specific etiology	A distinctive form of lymphangitis characterized by subcutaneous swellings along inflamed lymphatic channels. Primary site of skin invasion usually present; regional adenopathy variable.
Nocardia lymphadenitis & skin abscesses	Nocardia sp.	**TMP-SMX** 5-10 mg/kg/day based on TMP IV/po div in 2-4 doses	**Minocycline** 100-200 mg po bid	**Duration:** 3 mos. if immunocompetent; 6 mos. if immunocompromised. **Linezolid:** active in vitro *(Clin Microbiol Infect. 2021;27:550).*
By Pathogen:				
Cat-scratch disease—immunocompetent patient Axillary/epitrochlear nodes 46%, neck 26%, inguinal 17%.	Bartonella henselae	Adult: **Azithro** 500 mg po x 1, then 250 mg/day x 4 days. **Peds** (<45.5 kg): **Azithro** sol'n 10 mg/kg x 1, then 5 mg/kg per day x 4 days	Adult: **Clarithro** 500 mg po bid or **RIF** 300 mg po bid or **TMP-SMX** DS 1 tab po bid or **CIP** 500 mg po bid (duration at least 10 days)	**Dx:** Antibody titer; PCR increasingly available. **Hepatosplenic, CNS or Retinal infection:** (**Doxy** 100 mg po bid + **RIF** 300 mg po bid) x 4-6 wks. Needle drainage of suppurative node(s) provides patient comfort.
Bubonic plague *(See MMWR/Vol.70/No. 3, July 16, 2021)*	Yersinia pestis	**CIP** 400 mg IV q8h or 750 mg po q12h OR **Levo** 750 mg IV/po once daily OR **Moxi** 400 mg IV/po q24h	**Streptomycin** 30 mg/kg/day IV in 2 div doses OR **Gentamicin** 5 mg/kg/day IV single dose	Duration of therapy 10-14 days. **Doxy** 200 mg IV/po x 1, then 100 mg IV/po bid x 10-14 days another option. Doxy acceptable at any age for up to 21 days *(AAP Red Book 2018).*

 **NOTE: All dosage recommendations are for adults (unless otherwise indicated) and assume normal renal function. § Alternatives consider allergy, PK, compliance, local resistance, cost.*

TABLE 1 (46)

ANATOMIC SITE/DIAGNOSIS/ MODIFYING CIRCUMSTANCES	ETIOLOGIES (usual)	SUGGESTED REGIMENS*		ADJUNCT DIAGNOSTIC OR THERAPEUTIC MEASURES AND COMMENTS
		PRIMARY	ALTERNATIVE§	
MOUTH				
Aphthous stomatitis, recurrent	Etiology unknown	Topical steroids (Kenalog in Orabase) may ↓ pain and swelling		
Actinomycosis: "Lumpy jaw" after dental or jaw trauma	Actinomyces israelii	**AMP** 200 mg/kg/day in 3-4 divided doses x 2-6 wks then **Pen VK** 2-4 gm/day in 4 divided doses x 6-12 mo	(**Ceftriaxone** 2 gm IV q24h or **Clinda** 600-900 mg IV q8h or **Doxy** 100 mg IV/po bid) x 4-6 wks, then **Pen VK** 2-4 gm/d x 6-12 mos	**NOTE:** Metro not active. Recommendations for a 2-6 week run-in IV therapy prior to oral therapy are traditional and empirical. There are case reports of successful treatment with oral therapy preceded by much shorter durations of IV therapy, as little as 3 days, or no IV therapy at all, particularly for less severe disease. Durations shorter than 3 months may also be effective in less bulky disease.
Buccal cellulitis Children <5 yrs	H. influenzae	**Ceftriaxone** 50 mg/kg IV q24h	**Amox-clav** 45-90 mg/kg po div bid or **TMP-SMX** 8-12 mg/kg (TMP comp) IV/po div bid	With Hib immunization, invasive H. influenzae infections have ↓ by 95%. Now occurring in infants prior to immunization.
Candida Stomatitis ("Thrush")	C. albicans	**Fluconazole**	Echinocandin	*See Table 11, page 174.*
Dental (Tooth) abscess	Aerobic & anaerobic Strep sp.	Mild: **Amox-clav** 875/125 mg po bid	Severe: **Pip-tazo** 4.5 gm infused over 4h IV q8h	Surgical drainage / debridement. If Pen-allergic: **Clinda** 600 mg IV q6-8h
Herpetic stomatitis	Herpes simplex virus 1 & 2	*See Table 14A*		
Submandibular space infection, bilateral (Ludwig's angina)	Oral anaerobes, facultative streptococci, S. aureus (rare)	**Pip-tazo** or (**Pen G** IV + **Metro** IV)	**Clinda** 600 mg IV q6-8h (for Pen-allergic pt)	**Ensure adequate airway** and early surgical debridement. Add Vanco IV if gram-positive cocci on gram stain. Look for dental infection.
Ulcerative gingivitis (Vincent's angina or Trench mouth)	Oral anaerobes + vitamin deficiency	**Pen G** 4 million units IV q4h or **Metro** 500 mg IV q6h	**Clinda** 600 mg IV q8h	Replete vitamins (A-D). Can mimic scurvy. Severe form is NOMA (Cancrum oris)
MUSCLE				
"Gas gangrene" Contaminated traumatic wound. Can be spontaneous without trauma.	C. perfringens, other histotoxic Clostridium sp.	(**Clinda** 900 mg IV q8h) + (**Pen G** 24 million units/day div. q4–6h IV)		Susceptibility of C. tertium to penicillins and metronidazole is variable; resistance to clindamycin and 3GCs is common, so vanco or metro (500 mg q8h) recommended. IMP or MER expected to have activity in vitro against Clostridium spp.
Pyomyositis	Staph. aureus, Group A strep, (rarely Gm-neg. bacilli), variety of anaerobic organisms	(**Nafcillin** or **Oxacillin** 2 gm IV q4h) or **Cefazolin** 2 gm IV q8h if **MSSA**	**Vanco** 30-60 mg/kg/d in 2-3 div doses, target AUC_{24} 400-600 µg/mL x h if **MRSA**	In immunocompromised or if otherwise suspected, add gram-negative and/or anaerobic coverage. Evaluate for drainage of abscesses.
PANCREAS				
Acute alcoholic (without necrosis) (idiopathic) **pancreatitis**	Not bacterial	None No necrosis on CT	1–9% become infected but prospective studies show no advantage of prophylactic antimicrobials. Observe for pancreatic abscesses or necrosis which require therapy.	
Post-necrotizing pancreatitis; infected pseudocyst; pancreatic abscess	Enterobacterales, enterococci, S. aureus, S. epidermidis, anaerobes, candida	Need culture of abscess/infected pseudocyst to direct therapy; **Pip-tazo** is reasonable empiric therapy		Can often get specimen by fine-needle aspiration. **Moxi**, **MER**, **IMP**, **ERTA** are all options *(Gastroenterol 158:67, 2020)*.
Antimicrobial prophylaxis, necrotizing pancreatitis	As above	Patients with necrotizing pancreatitis who develop gas in the area of necrosis, rising inflammatory markers or persistent fever are candidates for antibiotic therapy. Meta-analysis: initiation of antibiotics within 72 hrs of sx onset reduced infected pancreatic necrosis *(J Hepatobil Pancreat Sci 2015;22:316)*.		

 **NOTE: All dosage recommendations are for adults (unless otherwise indicated) and assume normal renal function. § Alternatives consider allergy, PK, compliance, local resistance, cost.*

ANATOMIC SITE/DIAGNOSIS/ MODIFYING CIRCUMSTANCES	ETIOLOGIES (usual)	SUGGESTED REGIMENS*		ADJUNCT DIAGNOSTIC OR THERAPEUTIC MEASURES AND COMMENTS
		PRIMARY	ALTERNATIVE§	
PAROTID GLAND				
"Hot" tender parotid swelling	S. aureus, S. pyogenes, oral flora, & aerobic Gm-neg. bacilli (rare), mumps, rarely enteroviruses/ influenza; parainfluenza: **Amp-sulb** 3 gm IV q6h OR **Ceftriaxone** 1 gm IV q24h + (**Metro** or **Clinda**); if MRSA is a concern add **Vanco** to one of the above regimens *(Am Fam Physician. 2024; 109:550)*			Oral therapies, if appropriate **Amox-clav** OR **Moxi**, if MRSA is a concern add **Linezolid** 600 mg po bid. Predisposing factors: stone(s) in Stensen's duct, dehydration. Therapy depends on ID of specific etiologic organism.
"Cold" non-tender parotid swelling	Granulomatous disease (e.g., mycobacteria, fungi, sarcoidosis, Sjögren's syndrome), drugs (iodides, et al.), diabetes, cirrhosis, tumors			History/lab results may narrow differential; may need biopsy for diagnosis.
PERITONEUM/PERITONITIS:				
Primary (Spontaneous) Bacterial Peritonitis (SBP) Dx: Pos culture & ≥250 PMN/mcL of ascites fluid Ref: *Aliment Pharmacol Ther 2015,41:1116*	E. coli 33% Other Enterobacterales 11% P. aeruginosa 1% Gm+ cocci 40% Strept sp 15% Staph sp 18% Enterococci 9%	**Community-acquired: low risk of MDR GNB, VRE:** **Cefotaxime** 2 gm IV q8h (q4h if life-threatening) OR **Pip-tazo** 4.5 gm infused over 4h IV q8h OR **Ceftriaxone** 2 gm IV q24h OR **Erta** 1 gm IV q24h OR **CIP** 400 mg IV q12h	**Nosocomial: high risk of MDR GNB, VRE:** **MER** 1 gm IV q8h + **Dapto** 6 mg/kg IV q24h **Note:** In RCT, combination superior to Ceftaz alone	VRE, may need higher doses of Dapto, eg 8-10 mg/kg per day. **Secondary prophylaxis:** Norfloxacin 400 mg po daily or CIP 500 mg po daily until transplantation or liver function improves to compensated state. In RCT, CIP 750 mg po once weekly as effective as Norflox 400 mg po daily *(Am J Gastroenterol 2018;113:1167)*.
		• Average duration of rx 5 days but varies with severity of infection • To protect renal function: on day 1 & day 3 give IV albumin 1.5 gm/kg		
Prophylaxis after UGI (Variceal) bleeding		Hospitalized pts: **Ceftriaxone** 1 gm, IV once daily x 7 days or **Norfloxacin** 400 mg po bid x 7 days or **CIP** 500 mg po bid x 7 days		
Prevention of SBP: Cirrhosis & ascites *For prevention after UGI bleeding, see Liver, page 40*		**CIP** 500 mg/day		

Abbreviations on page 2. *NOTE: All dosage recommendations are for adults (unless otherwise indicated) and assume normal renal function. § Alternatives consider allergy, PK, compliance, local resistance, cost.

TABLE 1 (48)

ANATOMIC SITE/DIAGNOSIS/ MODIFYING CIRCUMSTANCES	ETIOLOGIES (usual)	SUGGESTED REGIMENS*		ADJUNCT DIAGNOSTIC OR THERAPEUTIC MEASURES AND COMMENTS
		PRIMARY	ALTERNATIVE§	
PERITONEUM/PERITONITIS *(continued)*				
Secondary (bowel perforation, ruptured appendix, ruptured diverticula) Ref: *CID 50:133, 2010 (IDSA Guidelines)* **Antifungal rx?** No need if successful uncomplicated 1st surgery for viscus perforation. Treat for candida if: pure culture from abdomen or blood. In controlled study, no benefit from preemptive rx to prevent invasive candidiasis *(CID 61:1671, 2015)*. **Pediatric appendicitis.** In retrospective review, **Ceftriaxone** 50 mg/kg (max 2 gm) once daily + **Metro** 30 mg/kg (max 1500 mg) once daily as effective as **Erta** *(JPIDS 2017,6:57)* PK/PD basis for once daily Metro	Enterobacterales, Bacteroides sp., enterococci, P. aeruginosa (3-15%). C. albicans *(see Comment)* If VRE documented, dapto may work *(Int J Antimicrob Agents 32:369, 2008)*. *See Table 5A* for other options for treatment of VRE.	**Mild-moderate disease—Inpatient—parenteral rx:** (e.g., focal periappendiceal peritonitis, peridiverticular abscess). **Usually need surgery for source control**. *See Comment*		Must "cover" both Gm-neg. aerobic & Gm-neg. anaerobic bacteria. Empiric coverage of MRSA, enterococci and candida not necessary unless culture indicates infection. Cover enterococci if valvular heart disease. **Drugs active only vs. anaerobic Gm-neg. bacilli:** Metro. **Drugs active only vs. aerobic Gm-neg. bacilli:** aminoglycosides, P Ceph 2/3/4, Aztreonam, AP Pen, CIP, Levo, Ceftolozane-tazo, Ceftaz-avibactam. **Drugs active vs. both aerobic/anaerobic Gm-neg. bacteria:** Pip-tazo, DORI, IMP, MER, tigecycline, eravacycline. **Ertapenem** not active vs. P. aeruginosa/Acinetobacter species. If absence of ongoing fecal contamination, **aerobic/anaerobic culture** of peritoneal exudate/abscess may be of help in guiding specific therapy. Less need for aminoglycosides. **With severe pen allergy,** can "cover" Gm-neg. aerobes with **CIP** or **Aztreonam.** IMP dose increased to 1 gm q6h if suspect P. aeruginosa and pt. is critically ill. Resistance to Moxi increasing. *See CID 59:698, 2014* (suscept. of anaerobic bacteria). Recent data suggest that short course antibiotic Rx (approx 4 days) may be sufficient where there is adequate source control of complicated intra-abdominal infections *(NEJM 372:21, 2015)*. **Appendicitis:** Randomized trial of antibiotics vs. appendectomy with similar 30 day outcome; if no initial surgery by day 90, 30% of antibiotics only group required appendectomy *(NEJM 383:907, 2020; NEJM 385:1116, 2021)*.
		Pip-tazo 4.5 gm infused over 4h IV q8h OR **Erta** 1 gm IV q24h OR **Moxi** 400 mg IV q24h	[(**CIP** 400 mg IV q12h or **Levo** 750 mg IV q24h) + (**Metro** 1 gm IV q12h)] or (**CFP** 2 gm q12h + **Metro**) **NOTE:** avoid tigecycline unless no other alternative due to increased mortality risk (FDA warning)	
		Severe life-threatening disease—ICU patient: Surgery for source control +		
		IMP 500 mg IV q6h or **MER** 1 gm IV q8h or **Dori** 500 mg IV q8h (1-hr infusion) or (**Ceftolo-tazo** 1.5 gm IV q8h + **Metro** 500 mg q8h) or (**Ceftaz-avi** 2.5 gm IV over 2 hrs q8h + **Metro** 500 mg q8h)	[**AMP** + **Metro** + (**CIP** 400 mg IV q8h or **Levo** 750 mg IV q24h)]	
		Concomitant surgical management important.		
Abdominal actinomycosis	A. Israelii and rarely others	**AMP** 200 mg/kg/day in 3-4 divided doses x 4-6 wks then **Pen VK** 2-4 gm/day in 4 divided doses x 6-12 mo	**Doxy** or **Ceftriaxone** or **Clinda**	Presents as mass +/- fistula tract after abdominal surgery, e.g., for ruptured appendix. Can use IV Pen G instead of AMP: 10-20 million units/day IV x 4-6 wks.
Associated with chronic ambulatory peritoneal dialysis (Abdominal pain, cloudy dialysate, dialysate WBC >100 cell/μL with >50% neutrophils; normal = <8 cells/μL.	Gm+ 45%, Gm- 15%, Multiple 1%, Fungi 2%, MTB 0.1% *General review: NEJM 385:1786, 2021.*	**Empiric therapy:** Need activity vs. MRSA **(Vanco)** & aerobic gram-negative bacilli (**Ceftaz**, **CFP**, **Carbapenem**, **CIP**, **Aztreonam**, **Gent**). Add **Fluconazole** if gram stain shows yeast. Use intraperitoneal dosing, unless bacteremia (rare). For bacteremia, IV dosing. For dosing detail, *see Table 19, page 325.*		A positive Gram stain will guide initial therapy. If culture shows Staph. epidermidis and no S. aureus, good chance of "saving" dialysis catheter; **if multiple Gm-neg. bacilli cultured, consider catheter-induced bowel perforation and need for catheter removal.** Other indications for catheter removal: relapsing/refractory peritonitis, fungal peritonitis, catheter tunnel infection.

 **NOTE: All dosage recommendations are for adults (unless otherwise indicated) and assume normal renal function. § Alternatives consider allergy, PK, compliance, local resistance, cost.*

ANATOMIC SITE/DIAGNOSIS/ MODIFYING CIRCUMSTANCES	ETIOLOGIES (usual)	SUGGESTED REGIMENS*		ADJUNCT DIAGNOSTIC OR THERAPEUTIC MEASURES AND COMMENTS
		PRIMARY	ALTERNATIVE§	
PHARYNX				
Pharyngitis/Tonsillitis: "Strept throat" Reviews: Known, emerging, reemerging pharyngitis pathogens *(JID 2024, 230 (Suppl 3):S173)*; Laboratory and point of care diagnostic testing *(JID 2024, 230 (Suppl 3):S182)*.				
Exudative or Diffuse Erythema				
Associated cough, rhinorrhea, hoarseness and/or oral ulcers suggest viral etiology. Pros & cons of diagnostics *(JCM 2016,54:2413)* Even with rapid detection of S. pyogenes, probably still need back3-up culture if rapid test is negative *(AJM 2016,54:2413)*.	Group A, C, G Strep.; EBV; Primary HIV; *N. gonorrhea*; Respiratory viruses. F. necrophorum	Strep. pharyngitis - no allergy: **Pen V** or **Amox**. Mild Pen allergy: **Cephalexin** or **Cefpodoxime** or **Cefdinir**. F. necrophorum: **Amox-clav** or **Clinda** *Doses in footnote*[15].	Strep. pharyngitis - anaphylaxis after **Pen**: **Azithro** or **Clarithro** or **Clinda**. Resistance around 30% *Doses in footnote*[15].	**Dx: Rapid Strep test**. If rapid test neg., do culture *(CID 59:643, 2014)*. No need for post-treatment rapid strep test or culture. **Complications of Strep pharyngitis:** 1. Acute rheumatic fever – follows Grp A *S. pyogenes* infection, rare after Grp C/G infection. *See footnote*[16]. For prevention, start treatment within 9 days of onset of symptoms. 2. Children age <7 yrs at risk for post-streptococcal glomerulonephritis. 3. Pediatric autoimmune neuropsychiatric disorder associated with Grp A Strep (PANDAS) infection. 4. Peritonsillar abscess and suppurative phlebitis are potential complications.
		FQs, tetracyclines & TMP-SMX not recommended due to resistance, clinical failures *(JCM 2012;50:4067)*		
2 POC PCR (NAAT) assays for GpA strep: COBAS Strept A, Alere Strept A. Superior to antigen detection *(JCM 2018;56:e01310)*.	Gonococcal pharyngitis	**Ceftriaxone** 500 mg IM x 1 dose (1 gm for wt >150kg)	FQs not recommended due to resistance	Not effective for pharyngeal GC: spectinomycin, cefixime, cefpodoxime and cefuroxime. Always have test of cure for pharyngeal GC. Always perform a test of cure for pharyngeal GC.
	Proven *S. pyogenes* recurrence or documented relapse	**Cefdinir** OR **Cefpodoxime**	**Amox-clav** OR **Clinda**	*Doses in footnote*[15]. Prospective study favors Amox-clav *(JAC 1989,24:227)*
	Grp A infections: more than 7/yr	Tonsillectomy guideline *(Oto Head Neck Surg 160:187, 2019)*		Hard to distinguish true Grp A Strep infection from chronic Grp A Strep carriage and/or repeat viral infections.
Peritonsillar abscess – Sometimes a serious complication of exudative pharyngitis ("Quinsy")	**F. necrophorum** (44%) Grp A Strep (33%) Grp C/G Strep (9%) S. anginosus grp	**Surgical drainage plus**		**Avoid macrolides: Fusobacterium is resistant.** *See jugular vein suppurative phlebitis, page 54.* Culture results may allow de-escalation to **Amp-sulb** 3 gm IV q6h.
		Amp-sulb 3 gm iv q6h	**Metro** 500 mg iv q6-8h or 1 g IV q 12h + **Ceftriaxone** 2 gm IV once daily Pen allergic: **Clinda** 600-900 mg IV q6-8h	
Other complications	*See parapharyngeal space infection and jugular vein suppurative phlebitis (see next page)*			

[15] **Treatment of Group A, C & G strep: Treatment durations are from approved package inserts. Subsequent studies indicate efficacy of shorter treatment courses. All po unless otherwise indicated.**

PEDS DOSAGE; Benzathine penicillin 25,000 units per kg IM to max. 1.2 million units; **Pen V** 250 mg bid or tid x 10d (wt < 27 kg); **Amox** 50 mg/kg po once daily (max 1000 mg) x 10 days; **Amox-clav** 45 mg per kg per day div. q12h x 10 days; **Cephalexin** 20 mg/kg/dose bid (max 500 mg/dose) x 10 days; **Cefuroxime axetil** 20 mg per kg per day div. bid x 5 days; **Cefpodoxime proxetil** 10 mg per kg div. bid x 5 days; **Cefdinir** 7 mg per kg q12h x 5 days or 14 mg per kg q24h x 10 days; **Cefprozil** 15 mg per kg per day div. bid x 10 days; **Cefadroxil** 30 mg/kg once daily (max 1 gm/day) x 10 days; **Clarithro** 15 mg per kg per day div. bid or 250 mg qid x 10 days; **Azithro** 12 mg per kg once daily x 5 days; clinda 20–30 mg per kg per day div. q8h x 10 days.

ADULT DOSAGE; Benzathine penicillin 1.2 million units IM x 1; **Pen V** 500 mg po bid x 10 days; **Cefditoren** 200 mg bid x 10 days; **Cefuroxime axetil** 250 mg bid x 4 days; **Cefpodoxime proxetil** 100 mg bid x 5 days; **Cefdinir** 300 mg q12h x 5 days or 600 mg q24h x 5 days; **Cefditoren** 200 mg bid; **Cefprozil** 500 mg q24h x 10 days; **NOTE:** All **O Ceph 2** drugs approved for 10-day rx of strep pharyngitis; increasing number of studies show efficacy of 4–6 days; **Clarithro** 250 mg bid x 10 days; **Azithro** 500 mg x 1 and then 250 mg q24h x 4 days or 500 mg q24h x 3 days; Clinda 300 mg po tid x 10 days.

[16] Primary rationale for therapy is eradication of Group A strep (GAS) and prevention of acute rheumatic fever (ARF). Benzathine penicillin G has been shown in clinical trials to ↓ rate of ARF from 2.8 to 0.2%. This was associated with clearance of GAS on pharyngeal cultures (CID 19:1110, 1994). Subsequent studies have been based on cultures, not actual prevention of ARF. Treatment decreases duration of symptoms.

TABLE 1 (50)

ANATOMIC SITE/DIAGNOSIS/ MODIFYING CIRCUMSTANCES	ETIOLOGIES (usual)	SUGGESTED REGIMENS*		ADJUNCT DIAGNOSTIC OR THERAPEUTIC MEASURES AND COMMENTS
		PRIMARY	ALTERNATIVE§	
PHARYNX/Pharyngitis/Tonsillitis *(continued)*				
Membranous pharyngitis: due to **Diphtheria** Respiratory isolation, nasal & pharyngeal cultures (special media), obtain antitoxin. **Place pt in respiratory droplet isolation**.	*C. diphtheriae* (human to human), *C. ulcerans* and *C. pseudotuberculosis* (animal to human) (rare)	Adult: **Azithro** 500 mg IV/po once daily or **Aqueous Pen G** 25,000 units/kg IV q12h. Switch to **Pen VK** 500 mg po qid when tolerated. Treat for 14 days	Child: **Azithro** 10-12 mg/kg IV once daily; switch to po when tolerated or **Aqueous Pen G** 300,000 units/kg/day IV divided q6h. Treat for 14 days	Diphtheria equine antitoxin: In US obtain from CDC (1-404-639-2880 or -1231)
Vesicular, ulcerative pharyngitis (viral)	Coxsackie A9, B1-5, ECHO (multiple types), Enterovirus 71, Herpes simplex 1,2	Antibacterial agents not indicated. For HSV-1, 2: **acyclovir** 400 mg tid po x 10 days.	HSV: **Famciclovir** 250 mg po tid x 7-10 days or **Valacyclovir** 1000 mg po bid x 7-10 days	Small vesicles posterior pharynx suggests enterovirus. Viruses are most common etiology of acute pharyngitis. **Suspect viral if concurrent conjunctivitis, coryza, cough, skin rash, hoarseness.**
Epiglottitis (Supraglottis): Concern in life-threatening obstruction of the airway				
Children	H. influenzae (rare), S. pyogenes, S. pneumoniae, S. aureus (includes MRSA), viruses	**Peds dosage:** (**Cefotaxime** 50 mg per kg IV q8h or **Ceftriaxone** 50 mg per kg IV q24h) + **Vanco**	**Peds dosage: Levo** 10 mg/kg IV q24h + **Clinda** 7.5 mg/kg IV q6h	Have tracheostomy set "at bedside". **Levo** use in children is justified as emergency empiric therapy in pts with severe beta-lactam allergy. *Ref: Ped Clin No Amer 53:215, 2006.* Use of steroids is controversial; do not recommend.
Adults	Group A strep, H. influenzae (rare) & many others	Same regimens as for children. **Adult dosage:** *See footnote*[17]		
Parapharyngeal space infection [Spaces include: sublingual, submandibular (Ludwig's angina) *(see page 50)* lateral pharyngeal, retropharyngeal, pretracheal & descending mediastinitis]				
Poor dental hygiene, dental extractions, foreign bodies (e.g., toothpicks, fish bones)	Polymicrobic: S. aureus, Strep sp., anaerobes, Eikenella corrodens. Anaerobes outnumber aerobes 10:1.	**Ceftriaxone** 2 gm IV q24h + **Metro** 500 mg IV q8h	**Pip-tazo** 4.5 gm infused over 4h IV q8h or **Amp-sulb** 3 gm IV q6h	Close observation of airway, 1/3 require intubation. MRI or CT to identify abscess; **surgical drainage. Metro** may be given 1 gm IV q12h. Complications: infection of carotid (rupture possible) & jugular vein phlebitis. Dx: FDG PET CT.
Jugular vein suppurative phlebitis (Lemierre's syndrome)	Fusobacterium necrophorum in vast majority *(JCM 2018;56:e00487-18)*	**Pip-tazo** 4.5 gm infused over 4h IV q8h or **IMP** 500 mg IV q6h or another carbapenem or (**Metro** 500 mg po/IV q8h + **Ceftriaxone** 2 gm IV q24h	**Clinda** 600–900 mg IV q8h. **Avoid macrolides: fusobacterium is resistant**	Emboli: pulmonary and systemic common. Erosion into carotid artery can occur. Other anaerobes & Gm-positive cocci are less common etiologies of suppurative phlebitis post-pharyngitis. Add **vanco** to cover MRSA if the phlebitis is related to and infected catheter.
Laryngitis (hoarseness)	Viral (90%)	Not indicated		

[17] Parapharyngeal space infection: **Ceftriaxone** 2 gm IV q24h; **Cefotaxime** 2 gm IV q4–8h; **Pip-tazo** 4.5 gm infused over 4h IV q8h; **TMP-SMX** 8–10 mg per kg per day (based on TMP component) div q6h, q8h, or q12h; **Clinda** 600-900 mg IV q6-8h; **Levo** 750 mg IV q24h; **Vanco** 30-60 mg/kg/d in 2-3 div doses, target AUC_{24} 400-600 µg/mL x h.

Abbreviations on page 2. **NOTE: All dosage recommendations are for adults (unless otherwise indicated) and assume normal renal function. § Alternatives consider allergy, PK, compliance, local resistance, cost.*

TABLE 1 (51)

ANATOMIC SITE/DIAGNOSIS/ MODIFYING CIRCUMSTANCES	ETIOLOGIES (usual)	SUGGESTED REGIMENS*		ADJUNCT DIAGNOSTIC OR THERAPEUTIC MEASURES AND COMMENTS
		PRIMARY	ALTERNATIVE§	
SINUSES, PARANASAL				
Sinusitis, acute *Guidelines: Pediatrics 132:e262 & 284, 2013 (American Academy of Pediatrics); Otolaryngol Head Neck Surg 2015,152 (Suppl 2):S1; JAMA 314:926, 2015*				
Treatment goals: • Speed resolution • Prevent bacterial complications *(see Comment)* • Prevent chronic sinusitis • Avoid unnecessary use of antibiotics Discussion of when to start antibacterial rx *(AnIM 2017,166:201)*	S. pneumonia 33% H. influenza 32% M. catarrhalis 9% Anaerobes 6% Grp A strep 2% Viruses 15-18% S. aureus 10% *(see Comment)*	Most common: obstruction of sinus ostia by inflammation from virus or allergy. Treatment: Saline irrigation **Antibiotics for bacterial sinusitis if:** 1) fever, pain, purulent nasal discharge; 2) still symptomatic after 10 days with no antibiotic; 3) clinical failure despite antibiotic therapy		**Treatment:** • Clinda: Haemophilus & Moraxella sp. are resistant; may need 2nd drug • Duration of rx: 5-7 days *(IDSA Guidelines)*, 10-14 days *(Amer Acad Ped Guidelines)* • Adjunctive rx: 1) do not use topical decongestant for >3 days; 2) no definite benefit from nasal steroids & antihistamines; 3) saline irrigation may help • Avoid macrolides & TMP-SMX due to resistance • Empiric rx does not target S. aureus: incidence same in pts & controls *(CID 45:e121, 2007)* Potential complications: transient hyposmia, orbital infection, epidural abscess, brain abscess, meningitis, cavernous sinus thrombosis.
		No penicillin allergy **Peds: Amox** 90 mg/kg/day divided q12h or **Amox-clav** suspension 90 mg/kg/day (Amox comp) divided q12h. Treat for 10-14 days **Adult: Amox-clav** 875/125 mg po bid x 5-7 days	*Empiric penicillin allergy* **Peds (if anaphylaxis): Clinda** 30-40 mg/kg/day divided tid or qid x 10-14 days *(see Comment)* **Peds (no anaphylaxis): Cefpodoxime** 10 mg/kg/day po div q12h **Adult (if anaphylaxis): Levo** 750 mg q24h or **Doxy** 100 mg bid. **Adult (no anaphylaxis): Cefpodoxime** 200 mg po bid	
Clinical failure after 3 days of empiric antibiotics (pain, discharge, fever)	Possibilities: resistant bacteria, ostia obstruction, non-infectious disease, e.g., granulomatosis with poly angiitis	Adjustment of empiric therapy pending results of culture & sensitivity *Child failing Amoxicillin:* **Amox-clav** 90 mg/kg/d div q12h or **Clinda** 30-40 mg/kg/d div q8h + oral cephalosporin: **Cefuroxime** axetil 30 mg/kg/d div q12h or **Cefdinir** 14 mg/kg/d div q12h or **Cefpodoxime** 10 mg/kg/d div q12h *Adult outpatient:* **Amox-clav** 1000/62.5 mg tab 2 po bid or **Levofloxacin** 750 mg po once daily *Inpatient:* **Ceftriaxone** 1-2 gm IV q24h or **Amp-sulb** 3 gm IV q6h or **Levofloxacin** 750 mg IV q24h *Treat 5-10 days.*		**Collect sinus exudate for culture & sensitivity.** If no response within 24 hrs, CT scan of sinuses and surgical consult.
Diabetes mellitus with acute ketoacidosis; neutropenia; deferoxamine rx: Mucormycosis	Rhizopus sp., (mucor), aspergillus	*See Table 11, pages 173 & 182.*		
Hospitalized + nasotracheal nasogastric intubation	Gm-neg. bacilli (pseudomonas, acinetobacter, E. coli common) 47%, Gm+ (S. aureus) 35%, yeasts 18%. Polymicrobial in 80%	**Remove nasotracheal tube:** if fever persists and ENT available, recommend sinus aspiration for C/S & S. aureus PCR prior to empiric therapy		Fluid in sinus common for nasogastric or nasotracheal intubation > 1 wk; bacterial sinusitis is uncommon. Postulated role in development of HAP/VAP *(J Intens Care Med 34:844, 2019)*.
		IMP 0.5 gm IV q6h or **MER** 1 gm IV q8h. Add **Vanco** for MRSA if Gram stain suggestive.	(**Ceftaz** 2 gm IV q8h + **vanco**) or (**CFP** 2 gm IV q12h + **Vanco**).	

Abbreviations on page 2. **NOTE: All dosage recommendations are for adults (unless otherwise indicated) and assume normal renal function. § Alternatives consider allergy, PK, compliance, local resistance, cost.*

TABLE 1 (52)

ANATOMIC SITE/DIAGNOSIS/ MODIFYING CIRCUMSTANCES	ETIOLOGIES (usual)	SUGGESTED REGIMENS*		ADJUNCT DIAGNOSTIC OR THERAPEUTIC MEASURES AND COMMENTS
		PRIMARY	ALTERNATIVE§	
SINUSES, PARANASAL *(continued)*				
Sinusitis, chronic Adults **Defined:** Inflammatory disease of sinuses lasting 12+ wks despite medical management	Some combination of allergy, obstruction (polyps); antibiotics only indicated for acute exacerbation of chronic sinusitis due to mix of aerobic/anaerobic bacteria	Oral therapy is usually adequate: **Amox-clav** 875 mg po bid IF PCR detects MRSA: add **Doxy** 100 mg po bid If immunocompromised and worried about P. aeruginosa: **Levo** 750 mg po once daily + **Metro** 500 mg po tid Duration is usually 7-10 days but is adjusted for clinical response; there are no clinical trials for guidance	**Moxi** 400 mg po once daily If MRSA: **TMP/SMX** 160/800 mg po bid + **Metro** 500 mg po tid Oral cephalosporin (**Cefdinir** or **Cefuroxime axetil** or **Cefpodoxime proxetil**) + **Metro** 500 mg po tid	Coordinate culture from sinuses or sinus ostia. Treatment duration: 7-10 days. Topical antibacterials of no value. Antibiotic use, see *Cochrane Database Sys Rev 4:CD011994, 2016.*
SKIN				
Anthrax, cutaneous	*B. anthracis* Spores introduced to skin by contact with infected animals/ animal product *See Anthrax, systemic, page 45.*	Primary: Adult, including pregnancy: **CIP** 500 mg po q12h or **Doxy** 100 mg po q12h Child, age ≥ 1 mo to < 18 yr: **CIP** 15 mg/kg (max dose 500 mg) po q12h or **Doxy** 2.2 mg/kg (max dose 100 mg po q12h Alternatives: **Levo**, **Clinda**, **Minocycline**; **Amox** or **Pen VK** for pen-susceptible strains only **See *MMWR/Nov. 17, 2023/72 (6):1-47* for complete CDC guidelines and use of alternative agents.**		Duration of therapy 7-10 days unless an aerosol exposure may have occurred in which case transition to a post-exposure prophylaxis regimen *(see page 45)* to complete 60 days of treatment.
Bacillary angiomatosis: For other Bartonella infections, see *Cat-scratch disease lymphadenitis, page 49, and Bartonella systemic infections, page 64*				
In immunocompromised (HIV-1, bone marrow transplant) patients	Bartonella henselae and quintana	**Clarithro** 500 mg po bid or ext. release 1 gm po q24h or **Azithro** 500 mg po q24h *(see Comment)*	**Erythro** 500 mg po qid or **Doxy** 100 mg po bid or (**Doxy** 100 mg po bid + **RIF** 300 mg po bid)	For AIDS pts, continue suppressive therapy until HIV treated and CD >200 cells/μL for 6 mos. **Drugs to avoid:** TMP-SMX, CIP, Pen, cephalosporins.

 **NOTE: All dosage recommendations are for adults (unless otherwise indicated) and assume normal renal function. § Alternatives consider allergy, PK, compliance, local resistance, cost.*

ANATOMIC SITE/DIAGNOSIS/ MODIFYING CIRCUMSTANCES	ETIOLOGIES (usual)	SUGGESTED REGIMENS*		ADJUNCT DIAGNOSTIC OR THERAPEUTIC MEASURES AND COMMENTS
		PRIMARY	ALTERNATIVE§	
SKIN *(continued)*				
Bite: Remember tetanus prophylaxis— *See Table 20B, page 328 for rabies prophylaxis.* Review: *CMR 24:231, 2011.* **Avoid primary wound closure.**				
Alligator *(Alligator mississippiensis)*	Gram negatives including Aeromonas hydrophila, Clostridia sp.	Severe wound: Surgical debridement. (**CIP** 400 mg IV or 750 mg po bid or **Levo** 750 mg IV once daily) + **Metro** 500 mg IV/po q8h OR **Pip-tazo** 4.5 gm infused over 4h IV q8h	Severe wound: Surgical debridement. (**TMP-SMX** 8-10 mg/kg /day IV divided q6h or q8h or **Cefepime** 2 gm IV q8h) + **Metro** 500 mg IV or po q8h	Oral flora of American alligator isolated: Aeromonas hydrophila and other gram-negatives, and anaerobes including Clostridium spp *(S Med J 82:262, 1989).*
Bat, raccoon, skunk	Strep & staph from skin; rabies	**Amox-clav** 875/125 mg po bid or 500/125 mg po tid	**Doxy** 100 mg po bid	In Americas, **anti-rabies rx indicated:** rabies immune globulin + vaccine. *(See Table 20B, page 328)*
Bear	S. aureus, coagulase-negative staph, viridans streptococci, Enterobacterales, Aeromonas, B. cereus, Neisseria spp, E. durans *(Clin Microbiol Rev 24: 231, 2011)*	**Pip-tazo** 4.5 gm infused over 4h IV q8h	**Vanco** 30-60 mg/kg/d in 2-3 div doses, target AUC_{24} 400-600 µg/mL x h + [**Cefepime** 2 gm IV OR **CIP** 400 mg IV q8-12h] + **Metro** 500 mg q8h OR **Amox-clav** 875 mg po bid + **CIP** 500-750 mg po bid.	Injuries often result in hospital level care. Infection with Mycobacterium fortuitum reported *(J Clin Micro 43: 1009, 2005).* Rabies occurs in bears *(MMWR 48: 761, 1999).*
Camel	S. aureus, Streptococcus spp, P. aeruginosa, Other Gm-neg bacilli	**Pip-tazo** 4.5 gm infused over 4h IV q8h	**Cephalexin** 500 mg po qid + **CIP** 750 mg po bid	*See EJCMID 18:918, 1999.* Rabies can occur in camels *(PLoS Negl Trop Dis. 2016; 10(9): e0004890).*
Cat: 80% get infected, culture & treat empirically. Cat-scratch disease: *page 49*	**Pasteurella multocida**, Streptococci, Staph. aureus, Neisseria, Moraxella, Capnocytophaga spp., B. henselae, oral anaerobes	**Amox-clav** 875/125 mg po bid 1000/62.5 mg 2 tabs po bid	**Cefuroxime axetil** 0.5 gm po q12h or **Doxy** 100 mg po bid. **Do not use cephalexin.** Sens. to FQs in vitro.	**P. multocida resistant to dicloxacillin, cephalexin, clinda; many strains resistant to erythro** (most sensitive to azithro but no clinical data). P. multocida infection develops within 24 hrs. Observe for osteomyelitis. If culture + for only P. multocida, can switch to pen G IV or pen VK po. *See Dog Bite*
Catfish sting	Toxins (pain may respond to immersion in hot water as tolerated). Evaluate for retained foreign body (spine). May become secondarily infected	**Doxy** 100 mg po bid + **Amox-clav** 875/125 mg po bid		Toxin injury presents as immediate pain, erythema, edema; resembles strep cellulitis. May become infected with marine organisms or staphylococci
Dog: Only 5% get infected; treat only if bite severe or bad co-morbidity (e.g., diabetes).	**Pasteurella canis**, S. aureus, Streptococci, Fusobacterium sp., Capnocytophaga canimorsus	**Amox-clav** 875/125 mg po bid or 1000/62.5 mg 2 tabs po bid	Adult: **Clinda** 300 mg po q6h + **FQ** Child: **Clinda** + **TMP-SMX**	Consider anti-rabies prophylaxis: rabies immune globulin + vaccine *(see Table 20B).* Capnocytophaga in splenectomized pts may cause local eschar, sepsis with DIC. **P. canis resistant to diclox, cephalexin, clinda and erythro;** sensitive to Ceftriaxone, cefuroxime, cefpodoxime and FQs.
Horse	Actinobacillus, Pasteurella, Enteric Gram negative bacilli, S aureus, streptococci, anaerobes, Neisseria spp. Prevotella spp, B. fragilis, Campylobacter ureolyticus, Yersinia spp.	**Amox-clav** 875/125 mg po bid	**Doxy** 100 mg po bid	Debridement often needed. IV antibiotics may be needed for severe wounds.

 **NOTE: All dosage recommendations are for adults (unless otherwise indicated) and assume normal renal function. § Alternatives consider allergy, PK, compliance, local resistance, cost.*

TABLE 1 (54)

ANATOMIC SITE/DIAGNOSIS/ MODIFYING CIRCUMSTANCES	ETIOLOGIES (usual)	SUGGESTED REGIMENS*		ADJUNCT DIAGNOSTIC OR THERAPEUTIC MEASURES AND COMMENTS
		PRIMARY	ALTERNATIVE§	
SKIN/Bite *(continued)*				
Human For bacteriology, *see CID 37:1481, 2003*	Viridans strep 100%, Staph epidermidis 53%, corynebacterium 41%, **Staph. aureus 29%, eikenella 15%,** bacteroides 82%, peptostrep (Peptoniphilus) 26%	Serious infection until MRSA ruled out, add **Vanco** standard dose or **Dapto** 6 mg/kg IV q24h; alternate if pen allergic: **Clinda** + **CIP** or **Levo** or **Moxi**; **Amox-clav** 1000-200 IV q8h (non-US). **Early** (not yet infected): **Amox-clav** 875/125 mg po bid times 5 days. **Later:** Signs of infection (usually in 3–24 hrs): (**Amp-sulb** 1.5 gm IV q6h or **Cefoxitin** 2 gm IV q8h) or (**Pip-tazo** 4.5 gm infused over 4h IV q8h).		**Cleaning, irrigation and debridement most important.** For clenched fist injuries, x-rays should be obtained. Bites inflicted by hospitalized pts, consider aerobic Gm-neg. bacilli. **Eikenella resistant to clinda, nafcillin/ oxacillin, metro, P Ceph 1, and erythro; susceptible to FQs and TMP-SMX.**
Komodo dragon	Staphylococcus spp, Bacillus spp, Aeromonas, Pseudomonas spp, Enterobacterales, Burkholderia, anaerobes	**Amox-clav** 875/125 mg po bid plus **CIP** 750 po bid	**Pip-tazo** 4.5 gm infused over 4h IV q8h	
Leech (Medicinal) *(Ln 381:1686, 2013)*	Aeromonas hydrophila	**CIP** 750 or 400 bid or parenteral cephalosporin 3rd gen; alternative: **TMP-SMX** DS 1 tab bid	**TMP-SMX DS** 1 tab po bid	Aeromonas in GI tract of leeches. Some use prophylactic antibiotics when leeches used medicinally.
Pig (swine)	Polymicrobic: Gm+ cocci, Gm-neg. bacilli, anaerobes, Pasteurella sp., Actinobacillus suis	**Amox-clav** 875/125 mg po bid	**P Ceph 3** or **Amp-sulb** or **IMP**	Information limited but infection is common and serious *(Ln 348:888, 1996)*. Pigs may be colonized with MRSA *(Clin Microbiol Rev 24: 231, 2011)*. Potential pathogens include Streptococcus suis leading to meningitis.
Prairie dog	Monkeypox	*See Table 14A, page 232.* No rx recommended		Tularemia and bubonic plague reported after prairie dog bites.
Primate, Monkey, non-human *See Table 14A, Herpes simiae.*	Herpesvirus simiae. *See Comments*	**Valacyclovir** (PEP) or **Acyclovir** or **Ganciclovir**		From macaques, risk of infection with herpes B virus; rare but potentially fatal encephalitis/myelitis. Potential risk of rabies. Etiologies: Bacteria similar to human bites; for deep bites, can use antibiotics as for human bites.
Rat	Spirillum minus & Streptobacillus moniliformis	Prophylaxis: **Amox-clav** 875/125 mg po bid x 3 days Rat bite fever: **Pen G** 2 million units IV q4h or **Doxy** 100 mg po bid x 10-14 days	**Doxy** 100 mg po bid	Anti-rabies rx not indicated. Causes rat bite fever (Streptobacillus moniliformis): Pen G or doxy, alternatively erythro or clinda.
Seal	Marine mycoplasma	**Tetracycline** or **Doxy** for 2-4 wks		Can take weeks to appear after bite. Disseminated disease reported *(CID 62:491, 2016)*. Differential includes sealpox, resembling Orf *(Br J Derm 152: 791, 2005)* and other bacteria: Bisgaardia hudsonensis *(J Infect 63: 86, 2011)* and Streptococcus halichoeri *(J Clin Microbiol 54: 739, 2016)*.
Snake: pit viper (Ref.: *NEJM 386:68, 2022*)	Pseudomonas sp., Enterobacterales, Staph. aureus and epidermidis, Clostridium sp.		**Primary therapy is antivenom.** Tetanus prophylaxis indicated. No need for antibiotic prophylaxis *(Am J Med 2018;131:1367)*. **Pip/Tazo** for empirical therapy of infected wound. Adjust per culture results *(Emerg Clin N Amer 35: 339, 2017)*.	
Spider bite: Most necrotic ulcers attributed to spiders are probably due to another cause, e.g., cutaneous anthrax *(Ln 364:549, 2004)* or **MRSA infection** (spider bite painful; anthrax not painful.)				
Widow (Latrodectus)	Not infectious	None	May be confused with "acute abdomen". Diazepam or calcium gluconate helpful to control pain, muscle spasm. Tetanus prophylaxis.	
Brown recluse (Loxosceles)	Not infectious. Overdiagnosed! Spider distribution limited to S. Central & desert SW of US	Bite usually self-limited & self-healing. No therapy of proven efficacy.	**Dapsone** 50 mg po q24h often used despite marginal supportive data	Dapsone causes hemolysis (check for G6PD deficiency). Can cause hepatitis; baseline & weekly liver panels suggested.

 **NOTE: All dosage recommendations are for adults (unless otherwise indicated) and assume normal renal function. § Alternatives consider allergy, PK, compliance, local resistance, cost.*

ANATOMIC SITE/DIAGNOSIS/ MODIFYING CIRCUMSTANCES	ETIOLOGIES (usual)	SUGGESTED REGIMENS* PRIMARY	ALTERNATIVE§	ADJUNCT DIAGNOSTIC OR THERAPEUTIC MEASURES AND COMMENTS
SKIN/Bite *(continued)*				
Swan	P aeruginosa	**CIP** 750 mg po bid		Case report of P aeruginosa infection *(Lancet 350: 340, 1997)*. However, other aquatic organisms or host skin organisms have potential to cause infection.
Tasmanian devil	Pasteurella multocida *(CID 14: 1266, 1992)*	Treat as cat bite		15% of P multocida from devils were TMP-SMX resistant *(Lett Appl Microbiol 62: 237, 2016)*
Boils—Furunculosis				
Active lesions *See Table 6, page 88*	Staph. aureus, both MSSA & MRSA	Oral therapy, outpatient, empiric therapy *(see Comments)* Low suspicion, low prevalence of MRSA: Incision and drainage + **Diclox** 500 mg po tid-qid OR **Cephalexin** 500 mg po tid-qid Moderate or high suspicion, moderate or high prevalence of MRSA: Incision and drainage + **TMP-SMX** 160/800 (1 DS tab; 2 DS tabs in obese patient, BMI > 40) po bid or **Clinda** 300-450 mg (higher dose in obese patient, BMI > 40) po tid If no response after 2-3 days, look for undrained abscess Inpatients: Incision and drainage: culture abscess and blood + Empiric antibiotic therapy (in absence of specific culture and sensitivity data select an agent with activity against MRSA) **Vanco** 15-20 mg/kg IV q8-12h to achieve preferred target AUC24 400-600 µg/mL x hr Definitive therapy once culture results are available: MSSA: **Nafcillin** or **Oxacillin** 1 gm IV q4h or **Cefazolin** 1 gm IV q8h MRSA: **Vancomycin** 15-20 mg/kg IV q8-12h to achieve preferred target AUC24 400-600 µg/mL x hr		Incision and Drainage mainstay of therapy! Other options: **Doxy** 100 mg po bid or **Minocycline** 100 mg po bid for 5-10 days; **Cephalexin** 500 mg po tid-qid or **Dicloxacillin** 500 mg po tid-qid, only in low prevalence setting for MRSA. Also: **Dalbavancin** 1.5 gm IV x 1 or **Oritavancin** 1200 mg IV x 1. If dx uncertainty or for assessing adequacy of I&D, ultrasound is helpful. **NOTE: needle aspiration is inadequate.**
To lessen number of furuncle recurrences --decolonization *For surgical prophylaxis, see Table 15B, page 262.*	MSSA & MRSA.	(4% **Chlorhexidine** shower/bath daily + 0.12% **Chlorhexidine** mouthwash 2x daily + 2% nasal **Mupirocin** 2x daily) x 5 days, twice monthly for 6 months		Only proven effective regimen in a high quality RCT of hospitalized patients colonized with MRSA: MRSA infection rate reduced by 32% with decolonization with 44% reduction in those fully adherent *(NEJM 2019;380:638)*.
Burns. Overall management: ISBI Practice Guideline (Burns): *Burns 2016,42:953.*				
Initial wound care Use burn unit, if available	**Not infected** Prophylaxis for potential pathogens: Gm-pos cocci, Gm-neg bacilli, Candida	Early excision & wound closure. Variety of skin grafts/substitutes. Shower hydrotherapy. Topical antimicrobials	**Silver sulfadiazine** cream 1% applied 1-2 x daily. Minimal pain. Transient reversible neutropenia due to margination in burn – not marrow toxicity	Mafenide acetate cream is an alternative but painful to apply. Anti-tetanus prophylaxis indicated.
Burn wound sepsis	Strep. pyogenes, Enterobacter sp., S. aureus, S. epidermidis, E. faecalis, E. coli, P. aeruginosa. Fungi (rare). Herpesvirus (rare).	**Vanco** 30-60 mg/kg/d in 2-3 div doses, target AUC_{24} 400-600 µg/mL x h + (**MER** 1 gm IV q8h or **Cefepime** 2 gm IV q8h) + **Fluconazole** 6 mg/kg IV qd (if Candida suspected) *See Comments for alternatives*		Vanco allergic/intolerant: **Dapto** 8-10 mg/kg IV qd IgE mediated allergy to beta lactams: **Aztreonam** 2 gm IV q6h. ESBL pos: use a carbapenem; carbapenemase-producer: **Ceftaz-avi or MER-vabor** *(See Table 5B)*

 **NOTE: All dosage recommendations are for adults (unless otherwise indicated) and assume normal renal function. § Alternatives consider allergy, PK, compliance, local resistance, cost.*

TABLE 1 (56)

ANATOMIC SITE/DIAGNOSIS/ MODIFYING CIRCUMSTANCES	ETIOLOGIES (usual)	SUGGESTED REGIMENS*		ADJUNCT DIAGNOSTIC OR THERAPEUTIC MEASURES AND COMMENTS
		PRIMARY	ALTERNATIVE§	
SKIN *(continued)*				
Cellulitis, erysipelas: NOTE: Consider diseases that masquerade as cellulitis, e.g., stasis dermatitis *(Clev Clin J Med 79:547, 2012)*				
Extremities, non-diabetic *For diabetes, see below.* Practice guidelines: *CID 59:147, 2014.* **NOTE:** stasis dermatitis can masquerade as erysipelas	Streptococcus sp., Groups A, B, C & G. Staph. aureus, including MRSA (but rare). Strept sp: No purulence Staph sp: Purulence. Etiologic study *(OFID, doi 10.1093 OFID/OFV181)*	**Inpatients: Elevate legs. Pen G** 2-4 million units IV q4-6h or **Cefazolin** 1 gm IV q8h. If **Pen allergic** (if not IgE-mediated): **Cefazolin**. If IgE mediated: **Vanco** 15 mg/kg IV q12h to achieve target AUC_{24} of 400-600 mcg/mL x hr. When afebrile: **Pen VK** 500 mg po qid ac & hs. Total therapy: 10 days	**Outpatient: Elevate legs. Pen VK** 500 mg po qid ac & hs or **Cephalexin** 500 mg qid. **Pen-allergic: Azithro** 500 mg po x 1 dose, then 250 mg po once daily. Rarely, **Linezolid** 600 mg po bid or **Tedizolid** 200 mg po q24h or **Delaflox** 450 mg po q12h. Treat for 5-6 days *(Ann IM 174:822, 2021)*(ACP Guidelines)	• Erysipelas: elevation, IV antibiotic, treat T. pedis if present, if no purulence, no need for culture. • If unsure as to presence of deep abscess, bedside ultrasound can help. If present: furunculosis (boils) • **TMP-SMX** 1 DS bid OR **Clinda** 300 mg tid effective for uncomplicated cellulitis in non-diabetic outpatients *(NEJM 372:2460, 2015)* • **Oritavancin** 1200 mg IV x1 OR **Dalbavancin** 1.5 gm IV x 1 also effective for outpatient therapy of more severe infections in patients who might otherwise be admitted to the hospital. • No benefit of adding TMP-SMX to Cephalexin for MRSA coverage *(JAMA 317:2088, 2017).*
Facial, adult (erysipelas)	Strep. sp. (Grp A, B, C & G), Staph. aureus (to include MRSA), S. pneumo	**Vanco** 30-60 mg/kg/d in 2-3 div doses, target AUC_{24} 400-600 µg/mL x h x 7-10 days	**Dapto** 4 mg/kg IV q 24h or **Linezolid** 600 mg IV q 12h. Treat 7-10 days if not bacteremic	**Choice of empiric therapy must have activity vs. S. aureus**. S. aureus erysipelas of face can mimic streptococcal erysipelas of an extremity. Forced to treat empirically for MRSA until in vitro susceptibilities available.
Diabetes mellitus and erysipelas *(See Foot, "Diabetic", page 17)*	Strep. sp. (Grp A, B, C & G), Staph. aureus, Enterobacterales; Anaerobes	**Early mild: TMP-SMX-DS** 1-2 tabs po bid + (**Pen VK** 500 mg po qid or **Cephalexin** 500 mg po qid). **For severe disease: IMP**, **MER**, **Erta** or **Dori** IV + (**Linezolid** 600 mg IV/po bid or **vanco** IV or **dapto** 4 mg/kg IV q 24h). *Dosage, page 17, Diabetic foot*	**Early mild: Omadacycline** 200 mg IV (over 60 min) loading dose and then 100 mg (over 30 min) q24 h OR 100 mg IV over 30 min bid on day one and then 100 mg iv over 30 min q24h OR 450 mg po q24h on days 1 and 2 and then 300 mg po q24h. Do not use an older tetracycline for reason of resistance and/or clinical failures. For hospitalized severe disease, forced to use broad spectrum therapy that targets both Staph. aureus and Enterobacterales: (**IMP** 0.5 gm IV q6h) + either **Vanco** 15-20 mg/kg IV q8-12h to achieve preferred target AUC24 400-600 µg/mL x hr or Dapto 4 mg/kg IV q24h or Linezolid 600 mg IV/po bid Can substitute for IMP: **Erta** 1 gm IV q24h or **Dori** 500 mg IV q8h or **MER** 1 gm IV q8h	Prompt surgical debridement indicated to rule out necrotizing fasciitis and to obtain cultures. If septic, consider x-ray of extremity to demonstrate gas. **Prognosis dependent on blood supply: assess arteries.** *See diabetic foot, page 17.* For severe disease, use regimen that targets both aerobic gram-neg bacilli & MRSA. Caution re hyperkalemia with TMP-SMX in those with reduced renal function or concomitant drugs causing hyperkalemia.

 **NOTE: All dosage recommendations are for adults (unless otherwise indicated) and assume normal renal function. § Alternatives consider allergy, PK, compliance, local resistance, cost.*

ANATOMIC SITE/DIAGNOSIS/ MODIFYING CIRCUMSTANCES	ETIOLOGIES (usual)	SUGGESTED REGIMENS*		ADJUNCT DIAGNOSTIC OR THERAPEUTIC MEASURES AND COMMENTS
		PRIMARY	ALTERNATIVE§	
SKIN/Cellulitis, erysipelas *(continued)*				
Erysipelas 2° to lymphedema (congenital = Milroy's disease); post-breast surgery with lymph node dissection	Streptococcus sp., Groups A, C, G	**Benzathine pen G** 1.2 million units IM q4 wks or **Pen VK** 500 mg po bid or **Azithro** 250 mg po qd		Indicated only if pt is having frequent episodes of cellulitis. Compression rx reduced recurrent cellulitis in random trial *(NEJM 383:630, 2020)*.
Erythema multiforme	H. simplex type 1, mycoplasma, Strep. pyogenes, drugs (sulfonamides, phenytoin, penicillins)			Treat underlying disorder / Remove offending drug; symptomatic Rx.
Erythema nodosum	Sarcoidosis, inflammatory bowel disease, MTB, coccidioidomycosis, yersinia, sulfonamides, Whipple's disease.			**Rx: NSAIDs; glucocorticoids** if refractory. Identify and treat precipitant disease if possible.
Erythrasma	Corynebacterium minutissimum	Localized infection: **Topical Clinda** 2-3 x daily x 7-14 days	Widespread infection: **Clarithro** 500 mg po bid or **Erythro** 250 mg po bid) x 14 days	Dx: Coral red fluorescence with Wood's lamp. If infection recurs, prophylactic bathing with anti-bacterial soap or wash with benzyl peroxide. **Clarithro** 1 gm po x 1 reported to be effective. Mupirocin 2% ointment x 2-4 weeks also effective.
Folliculitis	S. aureus, candida, P. aeruginosa common	Usually self-limited, no Rx needed. Could use topical mupirocin for Staph and topical antifungal for Candida.		
Furunculosis	Staph. aureus	*See Boils, page 59*		
Hemorrhagic bullous lesions				
Hx of sea water-contaminated abrasion or eating raw seafood in cirrhotic pt.	**Vibrio vulnificus**	Severe disease: (**Ceftaz** 1 gm IV q8h or **Ceftriaxone** 2 gm IV q24h) + **CIP** 750 mg po bid or 400 mg IV q12h or **Doxy** 100 mg IV or po bid	**CIP** 750 mg po bid or 400 mg IV bid OR **Levo** 750 mg IV/po 750 mg once daily	Wound infection in healthy hosts, but bacteremia mostly in cirrhotics or use of TNF-inhibitors. Pathogenesis: Exposure to contaminated seawater. Can cause necrotizing fasciitis. Surgical debridement needed.
Herpes zoster (shingles): *See Table 14A*				
Impetigo				
"Honey-crust" lesions (non-bullous). Ecthyma is closely related. Causes "punched out" skin lesions.	**Group A strep impetigo** (rarely Strept. sp. Groups B, C or G); crusted lesions can be Staph. aureus + streptococci. Staph. aureus may be secondary colonizer.	Few lesions: (**Mupirocin** ointment 2% tid or **fusidic acid** cream[NUS] 2%, OR **retapamulin** ointment, 1% bid. Treat for 5 days	Numerous lesions: **Pen VK** 250-500 mg po q6h x 5 days or **Benzathine Pen** 600,000 units IM x 1 or **TMP-SMX** po x 3-5 days	Topical rx: OTC ointments (bacitracin, neomycin, polymyxin B not as effective as prescription ointments. For mild disease, topical rx as good as po antibiotics *(Cochrane Database Syst Rev CD003261, 2012)*. **Ecthyma:** Infection deeper into epidermis than impetigo. May need parenteral penicillin. Military outbreaks reported.
Bullous (if ruptured, thin "varnish-like" crust)	**Staph. aureus** MSSA & MRSA: strains that produce exfoliative toxin A.	**For MSSA:** po therapy with **Diclox, Oxacillin, Cephalexin, Amox-clav, Clinda, TMP-SMX-DS**, OR **Mupirocin** ointment OR **Retapamulin** ointment	**For MRSA: Mupirocin** ointment OR po therapy with, **TMP-SMX-DS, Minocycline, Doxy, Clinda.** Treat for 7 days	
		For dosages, see Table 10A		

Abbreviations on page 2. *NOTE: All dosage recommendations are for adults (unless otherwise indicated) and assume normal renal function. § Alternatives consider allergy, PK, compliance, local resistance, cost.

TABLE 1 (58)

ANATOMIC SITE/DIAGNOSIS/ MODIFYING CIRCUMSTANCES	ETIOLOGIES (usual)	SUGGESTED REGIMENS*		ADJUNCT DIAGNOSTIC OR THERAPEUTIC MEASURES AND COMMENTS
		PRIMARY	ALTERNATIVE§	
SKIN *(continued)*				
Infected wound, extremity —Post-trauma *(for bites, see page 57; for post-operative, see below)*— **Gram stain negative**				
Uncomplicated: Mild to moderate Debride wound, if necessary	Polymicrobic: S. aureus (MSSA & MRSA), aerobic & anaerobic strep, Enterobacterales, C. perfringens, C. tetani; if water exposure, Pseudomonas sp., Aeromonas sp.	**TMP-SMX** DS 1-2 tab po bid or **Clinda** 300-450 mg po tid + (if GNB suspected) **Amox-clav** 875/125 po bid or **FQ**	**Minocycline** 100 mg po bid or **linezolid** 600 mg po bid or **Omadacycline**	**Culture & sensitivity, check Gram stain. Tetanus toxoid if indicated.** **Mild infection:** Suggested drugs focus on S. aureus & Strep species. If suspect Gm-neg. bacilli, add **Amox-clav-ER** 1000/62.5 two tabs po bid. If MRSA is erythro-resistant, may have inducible resistance to clinda. **Fever—sepsis:** Another alternative is **Linezolid** 600 mg IV/po q12h. If Gm-neg. bacilli & severe pen allergy, **CIP or Levo. Do not use an older tetracycline for reason of resistance and/or clinical failures.**
Complicated, severe: Febrile with sepsis—hospitalized Debride wound, if necessary		[**Pip-tazo** or **IMP** or **MER** or **Erta** *(Dosage, page 28)*] + **Vanco** 30-60 mg/kg/d in 2-3 div doses, target AUC_{24} 400-600 µg/mL x h	(**Vanco** 30-60 mg/kg/d in 2-3 div doses, target AUC_{24} 400-600 µg/mL x h OR **Dapto** 6 mg/kg IV q 24h OR **Telavancin** 10 mg/kg IV q24h) + (**CIP** 400 mg IV q12h (q8h if P. aeruginosa) OR **Levo** 750 mg IV q24h)	
Infected wound, post-operative—Gram stain negative: for Gram stain positive cocci – ***see below***				
Surgery not involving GI or female genital tract				
Without sepsis (mild, afebrile)	Staph. aureus, Group A, B, C or G strep sp.	**Clinda** 300–450 mg po tid		Check Gram stain of exudate. If Gm-neg. bacilli, **add** β-lactam/β-lactamase inhibitor: **Amox-clav-ER** po or (**ERTA** or **Pip-tazo**) IV. *Dosage on page 28.*
With sepsis (severe, febrile)		**Vanco** 30-60 mg/kg/d in 2-3 div doses, target AUC_{24} 400-600 µg/mL x h	**Dapto** 8-10 mg per kg IV q24h or **Telavancin** 10 mg/kg IV q24h	
Surgery involving GI tract (includes oropharynx, esophagus) or female genital tract—fever, neutrophilia	MSSA/MRSA, coliforms, bacteroides & other anaerobes	[**Pip-tazo** or (**P Ceph 3** + **Metro**) or **Dori** or **Erta** or **IMP** or **MER**] + (**Vanco** 30-60 mg/kg/d in 2-3 div doses, target AUC_{24} 400-600 µg/mL x h or **Dapto** 6 mg/kg IV q 24h) **if severely ill.** **Mild infection: Amox-clav** 875/125 mg po bid + **TMP-SMX-DS** 1-2 tabs po bid if Gm+ cocci on Gram stain.		For all treatment options, *see Peritonitis, page 51.* Most important: Drain wound & get cultures. Can sub **Linezolid** for vanco. Can sub **CIP or Levo** for β-lactams if local susceptibility permits.
Infected wound, post-op, febrile patient— Positive gram stain: Gram-positive cocci in clusters	S. aureus, possibly MRSA	**Do culture & sensitivity; open & drain wound** **Oral: TMP-SMX-DS** 1 tab po bid or **Clinda** 300–450 mg po tid *(see Comment)*	**IV: Vanco** 30-60 mg/kg/d in 2-3 div doses, target AUC_{24} 400-600 µg/mL x h or **Dapto** 4-6 mg/kg IV q24h or **Ceftaroline** 600 mg IV q12h	Need culture & sensitivity to verify MRSA. Oral options for CA-MRSA include **minocycline** 100 mg po q12h or **Doxy** 100 mg po bid or **linezolid** 600 mg po q12h. If MRSA clinda-sensitive but erythro-resistant, watch out for inducible clinda resistance. **Dalbavancin** and **oritavancin** recently FDA approved for acute bacterial skin and skin structure infections; single dose options for parenteral out-patient therapy.

 **NOTE: All dosage recommendations are for adults (unless otherwise indicated) and assume normal renal function. § Alternatives consider allergy, PK, compliance, local resistance, cost.*

TABLE 1 (59)

ANATOMIC SITE/DIAGNOSIS/ MODIFYING CIRCUMSTANCES	ETIOLOGIES (usual)	SUGGESTED REGIMENS*		ADJUNCT DIAGNOSTIC OR THERAPEUTIC MEASURES AND COMMENTS
		PRIMARY	ALTERNATIVE§	
SKIN *(continued)*				
Necrotizing fasciitis ("flesh-eating bacteria") Reviews: *Infect Dis Clin N Amer 2017;31:497; NEJM 2017,377:2253.*				
Post-surgery, trauma, or strepto-coccal skin infections *See Gas gangrene, page 50*	**5 types:** (1) Strep sp., Grp A, C, G; (2) Clostridia sp.; (3) polymicrobic: aerobic + anaerobic (if S. aureus + anaerobic strep = Meleney's synergistic gangrene); (4) MRSA; (5) *V. vulnificus*; (6) Klebsiella sp.; (7) Aeromonas sp.	*For treatment of clostridia, see Muscle, gas gangrene, page 50.* The terminology of **polymicrobic** wound infections is not precise: Meleney's synergistic gangrene, Fournier's gangrene, necrotizing fasciitis have common pathophysiology. **All require prompt surgical debridement** + antibiotics. Dx of necrotizing fasciitis req incision & probing of fascial plane. **Need Gram stain/culture** to determine if etiology is strep, clostridia, polymicrobial, or S. aureus. Empiric Treatment: **Pip-tazo**, **IMP** or **MER** + **vanco** or **dapto**; add **clindamycin** 900 mg IV if streptococcal infection is a possibility. **If strep necrotizing fasciitis**, treat with **penicillin** & **clinda** (900 mg IV q6h); **if clostridia ± gas gangrene**, add clinda to penicillin *(see page 50)*. ***See toxic shock syndrome, streptococcal,*** *page 71.* IVIG not recommended except for group A strep infection: 0.5 gm/kg day 1, then 25 gm days 2 and 3 *(CID 71:1772, 2020).*		
Puncture wound	*P. aeruginosa*, *S. aureus*, mixed infection	Local debridement to remove foreign body & tetanus prophylaxis; no antibiotic therapy.		Osteomyelitis evolves in only 1–2% of plantar puncture wounds. Consider x-ray if chance of radio-opaque foreign body.
Staphylococcal scalded skin syndrome	Toxin-producing S. aureus	**Nafcillin/Oxacillin** 2 gm IV q4h (children: 150 mg/kg/ day div. q6h) x 5–7 days for MSSA; **Vanco** 30-60 mg/kg/d in 2-3 div doses, target AUC_{24} 400-600 µg/mL x h) for MRSA		Toxin causes **intraepidermal split** and positive Nikolsky sign. Biopsy differentiates: drugs cause epidermal/dermal split, **called toxic epidermal necrolysis**—more serious.
Ulcerated skin lesions: Differential Dx	Consider: anthrax, diphtheria, tularemia, P. aeruginosa (ecthyma gangrenosum), plague, blastomycosis, spider (rarely), mucormycosis, mycobacteria, leishmania, YAWS, arterial insufficiency, venous stasis, and others.			
Ulcerated skin: venous/arterial insufficiency; pressure with secondary infection (infected decubiti)	Polymicrobic: Streptococcus sp. (Groups A, C, G), enterococci, anaerobic strep, Enterobacterales, Pseudomonas sp., Bacteroides sp., Staph. aureus	Severe local or possible bacteremia: **MER** 1 gm IV q8h or **Pip-tazo** 4.5 gm infused over 4h IV q8h. If Gm-pos cocci on gram stain, add **Vanco** 1 gm q12h. **Surgery: debridement, deep cultures & wound coverage. Sacral osteo** *(CID 68:338, 2019)*	(**Levo** 750 mg po/IV + **Metro** 500 mg po/IV) q8h or **CFP** 1-2 gm IV q8-12h. If Gm-pos cocci on gram stain, add **Vanco** 1 gm q12h.	• If ulcer clinically inflamed, treat IV. If not clinically inflamed, consider debridement, removal of foreign body, lessening direct pressure for weight-bearing limbs & leg elevation (if no arterial insufficiency). • Society of Vascular Surgery guidelines recommend against routine use of topical antimicrobials. • Silver sulfadiazine 1% cream: insufficient evidence. • **Chlorhexidine & povidone iodine may harm "granulation tissue"–Avoid.** If not inflamed, healing improved on air bed, protein supplement, radiant heat, electrical stimulation.
Whirlpool: (Hot Tub) folliculitis	Pseudomonas aeruginosa	Usually self-limited, treatment not indicated		Decontaminate hot tub: drain and chlorinate. Also associated with exfoliative beauty aids (loofah sponges).
Whirlpool: Nail Salon, soft tissue infection	Mycobacterium (fortuitum or chelonae)	**Minocycline**, **Doxy** or **CIP**		For more serious or progressive infection see recommendations for M. fortuitum.
SPLEEN. For post-splenectomy prophylaxis, *see Table 15A, page 260; for Septic Shock Post-Splenectomy, see Table 1, page 71. Vaccines: CID 58:309, 2014.*				
Splenic abscess				
Endocarditis, bacteremia	Staph. aureus, streptococci	**Vanco** 30-60 mg/kg/d in 2-3 div doses, target AUC24 400-600 µg/mL x h	**Nafcillin/Oxacillin** 2 gm IV q4h or **Cefazolin** 2 gm IV q8h if MSSA	Burkholderia (Pseudomonas) pseudomallei is common cause of splenic abscess in SE Asia. Presents with fever and LUQ pain. Usual treatment is antimicrobial therapy and splenectomy.
Contiguous from intra-abdominal site	Polymicrobic	*Treat as Peritonitis, secondary, page 51*		
Immunocompromised	Candida sp.	Lipid based **Ampho B** 3-5 mg/kg IV daily or **Fluconazole** or **Caspo/Micafungin**		*See Candida, Table 11*

Abbreviations on page 2. **NOTE: All dosage recommendations are for adults (unless otherwise indicated) and assume normal renal function. § Alternatives consider allergy, PK, compliance, local resistance, cost.*

TABLE 1 (60)

ANATOMIC SITE/DIAGNOSIS/ MODIFYING CIRCUMSTANCES	ETIOLOGIES (usual)	SUGGESTED REGIMENS* PRIMARY	ALTERNATIVE§	ADJUNCT DIAGNOSTIC OR THERAPEUTIC MEASURES AND COMMENTS
SYSTEMIC SYNDROMES (FEBRILE/NON-FEBRILE) Spread by infected TICK, FLEA, or LICE				
Epidemiologic history crucial. **Babesiosis, Lyme disease, & Anaplasma (Ehrlichiosis)** have same reservoir & tick vector.				
Babesiosis: Do not treat if asymptomatic, young, has spleen, and immunocompetent; can be fatal in lymphoma pts.	Etiol.: B. microti et al. Vector: Usually Ixodes ticks Host: White-footed mouse & others	[(**Atovaquone** 750 mg po q12h) + (**Azithro** 600 mg po day 1, then 500-1000 mg per day) times 7-10 days]. If severe infection [**Clinda** 1.2 gm IV bid or 600 mg po tid times 7 days + **Quinine** 650 mg po tid times 7 days. **Ped. dosage: Clinda** 20–40 mg per kg per day and **quinine** 25 mg per kg per day]. **Exchange transfusion**–*See Comment*		**Seven diseases where pathogen visible in peripheral blood smear:** African/ American trypanosomiasis; babesia; bartonellosis; filariasis; malaria; relapsing fever. **Dx:** Giemsa-stained blood smear; antibody test available. PCR if available. **Rx: Exchange transfusions successful adjunct if used early, in severe disease.** May need treatment for 6 or more wks if immunocompromised. Look for Lyme and/or Anaplasma co-infection.
Bartonella infections				
Bacteremia, asymptomatic	B. quintana, B. henselae	**Doxy** 100 mg po/IV bid x 4 wks + **Gent** 1 mg/kg qhs x 1st 2 wks		Rule out endocarditis. Found in homeless, alcoholics, esp. if lice/leg pain. Often missed since asymptomatic.
Cat-scratch disease	B. henselae	**Azithro** 500 mg po x 1 dose, then 250 mg/day po x 4 days. For symptomatic only--*see Lymphadenitis, page 49:* usually lymphadenitis, hepatitis, splenitis, FUO, neuroretinitis, transverse myelitis, oculoglandular syndrome.		
Bacillary angiomatosis; Peliosis hepatis—AIDS	B. henselae, B. quintana	**Uncomplicated:** **Erythro** 500 mg po qid, **Azithro** 500 mg po qd or **Doxy** 100 mg po bid x 3 months or longer.	**Complicated (CNS involvement):** **Doxy** 100 mg IV/po bid + **RIF** 300 mg po bid	**Do not use:** TMP-SMX, CIP, Pen, Ceph. **Manifestations of Bartonella infections:** **HIV/AIDS:** Bacillary angiomatosis; Bacillary peliosis; Bacteremia/endocarditis/FUO **Immunocompetent:** Bacteremia/endocarditis/FUO/ encephalitis; Cat scratch disease; Vertebral osteo; Trench fever; Parinaud's oculoglandular syndrome
		Regardless of CD4 count, DC therapy after 3-4 mos. & observe. If no relapse, no suppressive rx. If relapse, **Doxy**, **Azithro** or **Erythro** x 3 mos. Stop when CD4 >200 x 6 mos.		
Endocarditis *(see page 30)*	B. henselae, B. quintana	Surgical removal of infected valve		**Gentamicin toxicity:** If Gent toxicity, substitute Rifampin 300 mg IV/po bid x 14 days. Presents as SBE. Diagnosis: ECHO, serology & PCR of resected heart valve. **Note:** Empiric Ceftriaxone for possible endocarditis due to Strept. sp. while awaiting results of microbiology.
		If suspect endocarditis: **Ceftriaxone** 2 gm IV once daily x 6 weeks + **Gent** 1 mg/ kg IV q8h x 14 days + **Doxy** 100 mg IV/po bid x 6 wks	*If proven endocarditis:* **Doxy** 100 mg IV/po bid x 6 wks + **Gent** 1 mg/kg IV q8h or **Rifampin** 300 mg po/IV bid x 14 days, then doxycycline for another 3 months (6 wk if valve resected)	
Oroya fever (acute) & Verruga peruana (chronic) (South American Bartonellosis)	B. bacilliformis; *AAC 48:192, 2014; Pediatrics 128:e1034, 2011*	**Oroya fever:** (Adult) (**CIP** 500 mg po bid + **Ceftriaxone** 1 gm IV once daily) x 14 days OR (**Chloro** 50-75 mg/kg/day IV/po in 4 div doses + **Ceftriaxone** 1 gm IV once daily) x 14 days	**Verruga peruana:** (Adult) **Azithro** 500 mg po once daily x 7 days OR **CIP** 500 mg po bid x 7-10 days	**Oroya fever** (Pregnancy): **Amox-clav** 875/125 mg po bid. Oroya fever, severe infection (Child): (**CIP** or **Chloro**) + **Ceftriaxone** **Verruga peruana** (Child): **Azithro** 10 mg/kg po once daily x 7 days or **CIP** 20 mg/kg po in 2 div doses x 14 days
Trench fever (FUO)	B. quintana	No endocarditis: **Doxy** 100 mg po bid x 4 wks + **Gent** 3 mg/kg once daily for 1st 2 wks of therapy *(AAC 48:1921, 2004)*.		Vector is body louse. If endocarditis, need longer rx.

 **NOTE: All dosage recommendations are for adults (unless otherwise indicated) and assume normal renal function. § Alternatives consider allergy, PK, compliance, local resistance, cost.*

TABLE 1 (61)

ANATOMIC SITE/DIAGNOSIS/ MODIFYING CIRCUMSTANCES	ETIOLOGIES (usual)	SUGGESTED REGIMENS*		ADJUNCT DIAGNOSTIC OR THERAPEUTIC MEASURES AND COMMENTS
		PRIMARY	ALTERNATIVE§	
SYSTEMIC SYNDROMES (FEBRILE/NON-FEBRILE)/Spread by infected TICK, FLEA, or LICE *(continued)*				
Ehrlichiosis[18]. CDC def. is one of: (1) 4x ↑ IFA antibody, (2) detection of Ehrlichia DNA in blood or CSF by PCR, (3) visible morulae in WBC and IFA ≥1:64. New species in WI, MN *(NEJM 365:422, 2011)*.				
Human monocytic ehrlichiosis (HME)	Ehrlichia chaffeensis (Lone Star tick is vector)	**Doxy** 100 mg po/IV bid x 7–10 days *(Peds, see footnote[19])*	**Tetracycline** 500 mg po qid x 7–10 days. No current rec. for children or pregnancy	30 states: mostly SE of line from NJ to Ill. to Missouri to Oklahoma to Texas. History of outdoor activity and tick exposure. April-Sept. Fever, rash (36%), leukopenia and thrombocytopenia. Blood smears no help. PCR for early dx.
Human Anaplasmosis (formerly known as Human granulocytic ehrlichiosis)	Anaplasma (Ehrlichia) phagocytophilum (Ixodes sp. ticks are vector). Dog variant is Ehrlichia ewingii	**Doxy** 100 mg bid po or IV x 7–14 days *(Peds, see footnote[19])*	**Tetracycline** 500 mg po qid x 7–14 days. Not in children or pregnancy. **Chloro** is an alternative.	Upper Midwest, NE, West Coast & Europe. H/O tick exposure. April-Sept. Febrile flu-like illness after outdoor activity. No rash. Leukopenia/ thrombocytopenia common. **Dx:** PCR best; blood smear insensitive *(Am J Trop Med Hyg 93:66, 2015)*. **Rx:** Minocycline should work if doxy not available.
Lyme Disease NOTE: Think about concomitant tick-borne disease—e.g., babesiosis, anaplasmosis and ehrlichiosis. **Clinical Practice Guidelines:** *CID 72:1-48, 2021*				
Bite by ixodes-infected tick in an endemic area -- **Postexposure prophylaxis**	Borrelia burgdorferi Rarely, Borrelia mayonii	**If endemic area,** if nymphal partially engorged deer tick: **Doxy** 200 mg po x 1 dose with food *(Peds, see footnote[19])*	**If not endemic area,** not engorged, not deer tick: No treatment	Prophylaxis study in endemic area: erythema migrans developed in 3% of the control group and 0.4% doxy group *(NEJM 345:79 & 133, 2001)*. Can substitute **Minocycline** for Doxy, if Doxy is unavailable.
Early (erythema migrans) Serologic tests negative	**Two-tier testing for Dx** - First Tier: FDA-approved Enzyme-linked immunoassay (EIA or ELISA) or immunofluorescence assay (IFA). If the test is equivocal or positive a confirmatory, second tier test should be done. - Second Tier: Western immunoblot	**Doxy** 100 mg po bid x 10 days or **Amoxicillin** 500 mg po tid or **cefuroxime axetil** 500 mg po bid x 14 days (10 days as effective as 20: *AnIM 138:697, 2003*). **Azithro** 500 mg per day x 7-10 days. *(Peds dosing, see Comments and footnote[19])*		High rate of clinical failure with azithro & erythro *(Drugs 57:157, 1999)*. **Peds** (all po for 14–21 days): **Amox** 50 mg per kg per day in 3 div. doses or **Cefuroxime axetil** 30 mg per kg per day in 2 div. doses or **Azithro** 10 mg/kg (max 500 mg) per day for 7-10 days. Lesions usually homogenous--not target-like *(AnIM 136:423, 2002)*.
Carditis *See Comment*		(**Ceftriaxone** 2 gm IV q24h) or (**Cefotaxime** 2 gm IV q4h) or (**Pen G** 3 million units IV q4h) x 14–21 days	**Doxy** *(see Comments)* 100 mg po bid x *(Peds, see footnote[19])* 14–21 days or **Amoxicillin** 500 mg po tid x 14–21 days.	First degree AV block: Oral regimen. Generally self-limited. High degree AV block (PR >0.3 sec.): IV therapy—permanent pacemaker not necessary, but temporary pacing in 39% *(CID 59:996, 2014)*.
Facial nerve paralysis (isolated finding, early)	Food and Drug Administration (FDA) has cleared several Lyme disease serologic assays	(**Doxy** 100 mg po bid) *(Peds, see footnote[19])* or (**Amoxicillin** 500 mg po) tid x 14–21 days	**Ceftriaxone** 2 gm IV q24h x 14–21 days	LP suggested excluding central neurologic disease. If LP neg., oral regimen OK. If abnormal or not done, suggest parenteral Ceftriaxone.
Meningitis, encephalitis *For encephalopathy, See Comment*	allowing for an EIA rather than western immunoblot assay as the second test in a Lyme disease testing algorithm.	**Ceftriaxone** 2 gm IV q24h x 14–28 days	(**Pen G** 20 million units IV q24h in div. dose) or (**Cefotaxime** 2 gm IV q8h) x 14–28 days	Encephalopathy: memory difficulty, depression, somnolence, or headache, CSF abnormalities. 89% had objective CSF abnormalities. No compelling evidence that prolonged treatment has any benefit in post-Lyme syndrome.
Arthritis	*See Updated CDC Recommendation for Serologic Diagnosis of Lyme Disease*	(**Doxy** 100 mg po bid) *(Peds, see footnote[19])* or (**Amoxicillin** 500 mg po tid) x 28 days	(**Ceftriaxone** 2 gm IV q24h) or (**Pen G** 20–24 million units per day IV) x 14–28 days	Start with 1 mo of therapy; if only partial response, treat for a second mo.
Pregnancy		**Amoxicillin** 500 mg po tid x 21 days.	**If pen. allergic:** (**Azithro** 500 mg po q24h x 7–10 days) or (**Erythro** 500 mg po qid x 14–21 days). Choice should not include doxy.	
Post-Lyme Disease Syndromes		None indicated		No benefit from rx

[18] In endemic area (New York), high % of both adult ticks and nymphs were jointly infected with both Anaplasma (HGE) and B. burgdorferi *(NEJM 337:49, 1997)*.
[19] Important Note: Use of **Doxycycline** in children is considered safe regardless of age for treatment duration of ≤21 days. Pediatric dose: 4.4 mg/kg/day divided bid *(AAP Redbook 2018)*.

Abbreviations on page 2. **NOTE: All dosage recommendations are for adults (unless otherwise indicated) and assume normal renal function. § Alternatives consider allergy, PK, compliance, local resistance, cost.*

TABLE 1 (62)

ANATOMIC SITE/DIAGNOSIS/ MODIFYING CIRCUMSTANCES	ETIOLOGIES (usual)	SUGGESTED REGIMENS*		ADJUNCT DIAGNOSTIC OR THERAPEUTIC MEASURES AND COMMENTS
		PRIMARY	ALTERNATIVE§	
SYSTEMIC SYNDROMES (FEBRILE/NON-FEBRILE)/Spread by infected TICK, FLEA, or LICE *(continued)*				
Plague, bacteremic *(See MMWR/Vol.70/No. 3, July 16, 2021)*	Yersinia pestis	**CIP** 400 mg IV q8h or 750 mg po q12h OR **Levo** 750 mg IV/po q24h OR **Moxi** 400 mg IV/po q24h	**Streptomycin** 30 mg/kg/day IV in 2 div doses OR **Gentamicin** 5 mg/kg/day IV single dose	Duration of therapy 10-14 days. **Doxy** 200 mg IV/po x 1, then 100 mg IV/po bid x 10-14 days another option. Doxy acceptable at any age for up to 21 days *(AAP Red Book 2018)*.
Relapsing fever				
Louse-borne (LBRF)	*Borrelia recurrentis* Reservoir: human Vector: Louse pediculus humanus	**Tetracycline** 500 mg IV/po x 1 dose or **Doxy** 100 mg IV/po x 1 dose *(Peds, see footnote[19])*	**Erythro** 500 mg IV/po x 1 dose	Jarisch-Herxheimer (fever, ↑ pulse, ↑ resp., ↓ blood pressure) in most patients (occurs in ~2 hrs). Not prevented by prior steroids. **Dx: Examine peripheral blood smear during fever for spirochetes.** Can relapse up to 10 times.
Tick-borne (TBRF)	No Amer: *B. hermsii, B. turicata;* Africa: *B. hispanica, B. crocidurae, B. duttonii;* Russia: *B. miyamotoi* *(see Comment)*	**Doxy** 100 mg po bid x 7-10 days *(Peds, see footnote[19])* **Prophylaxis: Doxy** 100 mg single dose within 72 hrs of exposure is effective *(CID 71:1768, 2020)*	**Erythro** 500 mg po qid x 7-10 days	Jarisch-Herxheimer reaction may occur. Postexposure **Doxy** pre-emptive therapy highly effective *(NEJM 355:148, 2006)*. B. miyamotoi: Dx by ref lab serum PCR. Fever, headache, thrombocytopenia & tick exposure (NE USA). Seems to respond to Doxy, Azithro, Ceftriaxone *(AnIM 163:91 & 141, 2015; NEJM 373:468, 2015)*. Resistant to Amox *(Am J Med 132:136, 2019)*.
Rickettsial diseases				
Spotted fevers (NOTE: Rickettsial pox not included)				
Rocky Mountain spotted fever (RMSF) *CID 71:188, 2020*	R. rickettsii (Dermacentor tick vector)	**Doxy** 100 mg po/IV bid x 7 days or x 2 days after temp. normal. For critical illness some suggest a loading dose of 200 mg IV/po q2h x 3 days, then 100 mg po/IV bid	**Pregnancy: Doxy**	Fever, rash (88%), petechiae 40–50%. **Rash spreads from distal extremities to trunk.** Rash in <50% pts in 1st 72 hrs. Dx: Immunohistology on skin biopsy; confirmation with antibody titers. Highest incidence in SE and South Central states; also seen in Oklahoma, S. Dakota, Montana. Cases reported from 42 U.S. states. **NOTE: Only 3–18% of pts present with fever, rash, and hx of tick exposure; many early deaths in children & empiric doxy reasonable**. Chloro is less effective alternative ro Doxy.
NOTE: Can mimic ehrlichiosis. Pattern of rash important—*see Comment*				
Other spotted fevers, e.g., Rickettsial pox, African tick bite fever, R. parkeri	At least 8 species on 6 continents *(CID 45 (Suppl 1) S39, 2007)*.	**Doxy** 100 mg po bid x 7 days *(Peds, see footnote[19])*	**Chloro** 500 mg po/IV qid x 7 days Children age < 8 yrs: **Azithro** or **Clarithro** *(if mild disease)*	Clinical diagnosis suggested by: 1) fever, intense myalgia, headache; 2) exposure to mites or ticks; 3) localized eschar (tache noire) or rash. Definitive Dx: PCR of blood, skin biopsy or sequential antibody tests.
Typhus group—Consider in returning travelers with fever				
Louse-borne: epidemic typhus	R. prowazekii (vector is body or head louse)	**Doxy** 100 mg IV/po bid x 7 days; single 200 mg dose 95% effective. *(Peds, see footnote[19])*	**Chloro** 500 mg IV/po qid x 5 days	Truncal rash (64%) spreads centrifugally—opposite of RMSF. Louse borne typhus is a winter disease. Diagnosis by serology.
Murine typhus (cat flea typhus):	R. typhi (rat reservoir and flea vector)	**Doxy** 100 mg IV/po bid x 7 days *(Peds, see footnote[19])*	**Chloro** 500 mg IV/po qid x 5 days	Rash in 20-54%, not diagnostic. Without treatment most pts recover in 2 wks. Faster recovery with treatment. Dx based on suspicion; confirmed serologically. Azithro failure *(CID 68:738, 2019)*.
Scrub typhus	O. tsutsugamushi [rodent reservoir; vector is larval stage of mites (chiggers)]	**Doxy** 200 mg IV bid on day 1, then 100 mg bid x 6 days + **Azithro** 500 mg IV bid on day 1, then 500 mg once daily x 6 days		Regimen based on prospective DB RCT: *NEJM 2023;388:792*.

Abbreviations on page 2. **NOTE: All dosage recommendations are for adults (unless otherwise indicated) and assume normal renal function. § Alternatives consider allergy, PK, compliance, local resistance, cost.*

ANATOMIC SITE/DIAGNOSIS/ MODIFYING CIRCUMSTANCES	ETIOLOGIES (usual)	SUGGESTED REGIMENS*		ADJUNCT DIAGNOSTIC OR THERAPEUTIC MEASURES AND COMMENTS
		PRIMARY	ALTERNATIVE§	
SYSTEMIC SYNDROMES (FEBRILE/NON-FEBRILE)/Spread by infected TICK, FLEA, or LICE *(continued)*				
Tularemia, typhoidal type	Francisella tularensis. (Vector depends on geography: ticks, biting flies, mosquitoes identified). Direct inoculation of wounds.	Moderate/severe: [(**Gent** or **Tobra** 5 mg per kg per day div. q8h IV) or (**Streptomycin** 10 mg/kg IV/IM q12h)] x 10 days	Mild: [**CIP** 400 mg IV (or 750 mg po) bid or **Doxy** 100 mg IV/po bid] x 14-21 days *(Peds, see footnote[19])*	Diagnosis: Culture on cysteine-enriched media & serology. Dangerous in the lab. Hematogenous meningitis is a complication: treatment is **Streptomycin** + **Chloro** 50-100 mg/kg/day IV in 4 divided doses.
Other Zoonotic Systemic Bacterial Febrile Illnesses (not spread by fleas, lice or ticks): Obtain careful epidemiologic history				
Brucellosis				
MMWR 61:461, 2012; details of diagnostic testing: Clin Micro Rev 33:e0073-19, 2020.	B. abortus–cattle B. suis–swine B. melitensis–goats B. canis–dogs	**Non focal disease:** [**Doxy** 100 mg po bid x 6 wks + **Gent** 5 mg/kg once daily for 1st 7 days	(**Doxy** 100 mg po bid + **RIF** 600-900 mg po once daily) x 6 wks. Less optimal: **CIP** 500 mg po bid + (**Doxy** or **RIF**) x 6 wks	Bone involvement, esp. sacroiliitis in 20-30%. **Neurobrucellosis:** Usually meningitis. 1% of all pts with brucellosis. Role of corticosteroids unclear; not recommended. **Endocarditis:** Rare but most common cause of death. Need surgery + antimicrobials. **Pregnancy:** TMP-SMX + RIF x 6 wks. Note: TMP-SMX may cause kernicterus if given during last week of pregnancy. **Children (age < 8 yrs):** TMP-SMX x 6 wks + Gent x 2 wks.
		Spondylitis, Sacroiliitis: [**Doxy** + **Gent** (as above) + **RIF**] x min 3 mos	(**CIP** 750 mg po bid + **RIF** 600-900 mg po once daily) x min 3 mos	
		Neurobrucellosis: [**Doxy** + **RIF** (as above) + **Ceftriaxone** 2 gm IV q12h until CSF returned to normal *(AAC 56:1523, 2012)*		
		Endocarditis: Surgery + **[(RIF** + **Doxy** + **TMP-SMX)** x 45 days to 6 mos + **Gent** for 2-4 wks		
		Pregnancy: Not much data. **RIF** 900 mg po once daily x 6 wks	**RIF** 900 mg po once daily + **TMP-SMX** 5 mg/kg (TMP comp) po bid x 4 wks	
Leptospirosis	Leptospira—in urine of domestic livestock, dogs, small rodents	**Severe illness: Pen G** 1.5 million units IV q6h or **Ceftriaxone** 2 gm q24h. Duration: 7 days	**Mild illness: Doxy** 100 mg IV/po q12h *(Peds, see footnote[19])* or **Amox** 500 mg po tid x 7 days or **Azithro** 1 gm po x 1, then 500 mg po once daily x 2 days	**Severity varies**. Varies from mild anicteric illness to severe icteric disease (Weil's disease) with renal failure and myocarditis. AST/ALT do not exceed 5x normal. Jarisch-Herxheimer reaction can occur post-Pen therapy.
Salmonella bacteremia other than S. typhi–non-typhoidal)	Salmonella enteritidis— a variety of serotypes from animal sources	If NOT acquired in Asia: (**CIP** 400 mg IV q12h or **Levo** 750 mg po once daily) x 14 days *(See Comment)*	If acquired in Asia: **Ceftriaxone** 2 gm IV q24h or **Azithro** 1 gm po x 1 dose, then 500 mg po once daily x 5-7 days. Do NOT use FQs until susceptibility determined. *(See Comment)*	In vitro resistance to nalidixic acid indicates relative resistance to FQs. Bacteremia can infect any organ/tissue: look for infection of atherosclerotic aorta, osteomyelitis in sickle cell pts. Rx duration range 14 days (immunocompetent) to ≥6 wks if mycotic aneurysm or endocarditis. Alternative, if susceptible: **TMP-SMX** 8-10 mg/kg/day (TMP comp) divided q8h. If highly resistant use **MER, IMP, or Erta**. CLSI has established new interpretive breakpoints for susceptibility to Ciprofloxacin: susceptible strains, MIC <0.06 µg/mL.

 **NOTE: All dosage recommendations are for adults (unless otherwise indicated) and assume normal renal function. § Alternatives consider allergy, PK, compliance, local resistance, cost.*

TABLE 1 (64)

ANATOMIC SITE/DIAGNOSIS/ MODIFYING CIRCUMSTANCES	ETIOLOGIES (usual)	SUGGESTED REGIMENS*		ADJUNCT DIAGNOSTIC OR THERAPEUTIC MEASURES AND COMMENTS
		PRIMARY	ALTERNATIVE§	
SYSTEMIC SYNDROMES (FEBRILE/NON-FEBRILE) *(continued)*				
Miscellaneous Systemic Febrile Syndromes				
Fever in Returning Travelers Etiology by geographic exposure & clinical syndrome	Dengue (Flavivirus)	Supportive care; *see Table 14A, page 223*		Average incubation period 4 days; serodiagnosis.
	Malaria (Plasmodia sp)	Diagnosis: peripheral blood smear		*See Table 13A, page 204*
	Typhoid (Salmonella sp)	See Typhoidal syndrome; More resistant than non-Typhi, treat with **Azithro** or **MER/IMP/Erta** until sensitivities known: wide FQ resistance		Average incubation 7-14 days; diarrhea in 45%.
Rheumatic Fever, acute	Post-Group A strep pharyngitis (not Group B, C, or G)	(1) Symptom relief: **ASA** 80–100 mg per kg per day in children; 4–8 gm per day in adults. (2) Eradicate Group A strep: **Pen** times 10 days *(see Pharyngitis, page 53)*. (3) Start prophylaxis: *see below*		
Prophylaxis				
Primary prophylaxis (treatment of initial episode to eradicated S. pyogenes)	Child: **Benzathine pen G** 600,000 units (<27 kg) OR 1.2 million units(≥27 kg) IM x1 OR **Cephalexin** 25-50 mg/kg/day in 2-4 divided doses x 10 days OR **Azithro** 10 mg/kg (max 500 mg) x1 then 5 mg/kg (max 250 mg) days 2-5 Adult: **Benzathine pen G** 1.2 million units(≥27 kg) IM x1 OR **Cephalexin** 500 mg po bid x 10 days OR **Azithro** 500 mg x1 then 250 mg days 2-5			
Secondary prophylaxis (previous documented rheumatic fever, prevention of recurrence)	**Benzathine Penicillin G:** weight <27 kg, 600,000 units IM q3-4 weeks; weight >27 kg: 1.2 million units IM q3-4 weeks OR **Penicillin V** 250 mg po bid (preferred oral regimen) OR **Azithromycin** (preferred regimen for penicillin allergy): weight <27 kg: 5 mg/kg (up to 250 mg) po once daily; weight >27 kg: 250 mg po once daily		**Duration?** No carditis: 5 yrs or until age 21, whichever is longer; carditis without residual heart disease: 10 since last attack; carditis with residual valvular disease: 10 yrs since last episode or until age 40 whichever is longer.	
Typhoidal syndrome (typhoid fever, enteric fever) Widespread FQ resistance	Salmonella typhi, S. paratyphi A, B, C & S. choleraesuis. **NOTE: In vitro resistance to nalidixic acid predicts clinical failure of CIP (FQs).** Do not use empiric FQs. Need susceptibility results.	**If NOT acquired in Pakistan or Iraq:** (**Ceftriaxone** 2 gm IV daily x 7-14 d) or (**Azithro** 1 gm po x 1 dose, then 500 mg po daily x 7 days) *(See Comment)* **Peds: Azithro** 10 mg/kg once daily x 7 days	**If acquired in Pakistan or Iraq or Typhi in the US with no international travel: MER** 1-2 gm IV q8h (or other carbapenem); for severe infections can use MER + Azithro *(See Comment)*	**Dexamethasone: Use in severely ill pts: 1st dose just prior to antibiotic, 3 mg/kg IV, then 1 mg/kg q6h x 8 doses.** **Complications:** perforation of terminal ileum &/or cecum, osteo, septic arthritis, **mycotic aneurysm**, meningitis, hematogenous pneumonia. Failure of MER in pt with *S. enterica* strain producing ESBLs and resistant to FQs & azithro responded to addition of fosfomycin IV *(CID 2017;65:1754)*

 **NOTE: All dosage recommendations are for adults (unless otherwise indicated) and assume normal renal function. § Alternatives consider allergy, PK, compliance, local resistance, cost.*

ANATOMIC SITE/DIAGNOSIS/ MODIFYING CIRCUMSTANCES	ETIOLOGIES (usual)	SUGGESTED REGIMENS*		ADJUNCT DIAGNOSTIC OR THERAPEUTIC MEASURES AND COMMENTS
		PRIMARY	ALTERNATIVE§	
SYSTEMIC SYNDROMES (FEBRILE/NON-FEBRILE)/Miscellaneous Systemic Febrile Syndromes *(continued)*				
Sepsis: Following suggested **empiric** therapy assumes pt is bacteremic; mimicked by viral, fungal, rickettsial infections and pancreatitis *(Intensive Care Med. 2017;43:304)*.				
Neonatal—early onset Age <7 days	Group B strep, E. coli, klebsiella, enterobacter, Staph. aureus (uncommon), listeria (rare in U.S.)	**AMP** 150 mg/kg/day IV div q8h + **Cefotaxime** 100 mg/kg/day div q12h ± **Gent** 5 mg/kg q 24 h or 2.5 mg/kg q8h IV or IM (if meningitis, consider increasing to **AMP** 200 mg/kg/day IV div q6h and **Cefotaxime** 150 mg/kg/day div q8h)		Blood cultures are key but only 5–10% of febrile infants have bacterial infection. Discontinue antibiotics after 72 hrs if cultures and course do not support diagnosis. In Spain, Listeria more common; in S. America, salmonella.
Neonatal—late onset Age >7 days	As above + H. influenzae & S. epidermidis	**AMP** 200-300 mg/kg/day IV q6h + **Cefotaxime** 75 mg/kg q8h ± **Gent** 5 mg/kg q24h IV or IM	(**AMP** 200 mg/kg/day IV div q6h + **Ceftriaxone** 75-100 mg/kg IV q24h) or **AMP** 200 mg/kg/day IV div q6 + **Gent** 5 mg/kg/day div once daily or q8h IV or IM.	**If MRSA is a concern**, add **Vanco** 30 mg/kg/d in 2 div doses, target AUC_{24} 400-600 µg/mL x h (Wt < 2000 gm). *See also Comment (early onset).*
Child; not neutropenic	Strep. pneumoniae, meningococci, Staph. aureus (MSSA & MRSA), H. influenzae now rare	(**Cefotaxime** 50 mg/kg IV q8h or **Ceftriaxone** 100 mg/kg IV q24h) + **Vanco** 60-80 mg/kg/d in 3-4 div doses, target AUC_{24} 400-600 µg/mL x h	**Aztreonam** 7.5 mg/kg IV q6h + **Linezolid**	Major concerns are S. pneumoniae, MSSA, and community-associated MRSA. Coverage for Gm-neg. bacilli included but H. influenzae infection now rare. Meningococcemia mortality remains high *(Ln 356:961, 2000)*.
Adult Sepsis; not neutropenic; NO HYPOTENSION but LIFE-THREATENING!—*For Septic shock, see page 71*				Overview: *Med Clin N Amer 104:573, 2021.* For patients in septic shock unresponsive to volume resuscitation, requiring on-going vasopressor therapy to maintain systolic BP > 90 mm Hg or MAP > 65 mm Hg consider hydrocortisone 50 mg IV q6h + fludrocortisone 50 mcg once daily via NG tube *(NEJM 2018; 378:797, 809, 860 [editorial])*. **Note: Pip-tazo inferior to MER vs. ceftriaxone-resistant ESBL-producing E. coli/K. pneumo** *(JAMA 2018;320:979 & 984)*. Surviving Sepsis Guideline: *Crit Care Med 2021;49:1974; JAMA 2023;329:535.*
Source unclear—consider primary bacteremia, intra-abdominal or skin source. May be **Life-threatening.** Ref: *CCM 2024; 52:1138; CID 2024; 78:505*	Aerobic Gm-neg. bacilli; S. aureus; streptococci; others	[(**IMP** or **MER**) + **Vanco**] OR (**Pip-tazo + Vanco**) If ESBL and/or carbapenemase-producing GNB. Empiric options pending clarification of clinical syndrome and culture results: **Low prevalence of resistance: Vanco + Pip-tazo** **If high prevalence of resistance,** *see Table 5B, page 85* for treatment options *Dosages in footnote*[20]	(**Dapto** 8-12 mg/kg IV q24h) + (**Cefepime** or **Pip-tazo**)	
If suspect biliary source *(See Gallbladder page 18)*	Enterococci + aerobic Gm-neg. bacilli	**Pip-tazo** (Do not use if ESBL producer)	**Ceftriaxone** + **Metro** or [(**CIP** or **Levo**) + **Metro**] *Dosages–footnote*[20]	If enterococci a concern, add ampicillin or vanco to ceftriaxone or FQ regimen
If community-acquired pneumonia with severe sepsis or septic shock *(see page 43 and following pages)*	**S. pneumoniae; MRSA, Legionella, Gm-neg. bacillus, others**	(**Levo** or **Moxi**) + (**Pip-tazo**) + **Vanco**	**Aztreonam** + (**Levo** or **Moxi**) + **Linezolid**	Many categories of CAP, *see material beginning at page 43*. Suggestions based on most severe CAP, e.g., MRSA after influenza or Klebsiella pneumonia in an alcoholic.

[20] **P Ceph 3** (**Cefotaxime** 2 gm IV q8h, use q4h if life-threatening; **Ceftizoxime** 2 gm IV q4h; **Ceftriaxone** 2 gm IV q12h), **Pip-tazo** 4.5 gm infused over 4h IV q8h, **Aminoglycosides** *(see Table 10C, page 166)*, **AMP** 200 mg/kg/day divided q6h, **Clinda** 900 mg IV q8h, **IMP** 0.5 gm IV q6h, **MER** 1-2 gm IV q8h, **Erta** 1 gm IV q24h, **Dori** 500 mg IV q8h (1-hr infusion), **Nafcillin/Oxacillin** 2 gm IV q4h, **Aztreonam** 2 gm IV q8h, **Metro** 1 gm loading dose then 0.5 gm q6h or 1 gm IV q12h, **Vanco** 30-60 mg/kg/d in 2-3 div doses, target AUC_{24} 400-600 µg/mL x h (dose in obese pt, *see Table 17C, page 321*), **Ceftazidime** 2 gm IV q8h, [Cefepime 2 gm IV q12h (q8h if neutropenic), **Cefpirome**[NUS] 2 gm IV q12h], **CIP** 400 mg IV q12h, **Levo** 750 mg IV q24h, **Linezolid** 600 mg IV q12h, **Dapto** 8-12 mg/kg IV q24h.

Abbreviations on page 2. **NOTE: All dosage recommendations are for adults (unless otherwise indicated) and assume normal renal function. § Alternatives consider allergy, PK, compliance, local resistance, cost.*

TABLE 1 (66)

ANATOMIC SITE/DIAGNOSIS/ MODIFYING CIRCUMSTANCES	ETIOLOGIES (usual)	SUGGESTED REGIMENS*		ADJUNCT DIAGNOSTIC OR THERAPEUTIC MEASURES AND COMMENTS
		PRIMARY	ALTERNATIVE§	
SYSTEMIC SYNDROMES (FEBRILE/NON-FEBRILE)/Miscellaneous Systemic Febrile Syndromes *(continued)*				
Persons who inject drugs	S. aureus (MSSA, MRSA)	**Vanco** to cover MRSA.	**Dapto**	
If suspect intra-abdominal source	Mixture aerobic & anaerobic Gm-neg. bacilli	*See secondary peritonitis, page 52.*		
If petechial rash	Meningococcemia	**Ceftriaxone** 2 gm IV q12h (until sure no meningitis); consider Rocky Mountain spotted fever—*see page 66*. If RMSF: **Doxy**.		
If suspect urinary source, e.g., pyelonephritis	Aerobic Gm-neg. bacilli & enterococci	*See pyelonephritis, page 38*. Prefer a carbapenem for patients with severe sepsis or septic shock to cover ESBL producers.		
Neutropenia: Child or Adult (absolute PMN count <500 per mm³) in cancer and transplant patients. Guidelines *(Inpatients: CID 2011,52:427; Outpatients: J Clin Oncol doi:10.1200/JCO.2017.77.6211)*				
Prophylaxis *(J Clin Oncol 31:794, 2013; Pediatric Guidelines: CID 71:226, 2020)*				
Post-chemotherapy—impending neutropenia	Pneumocystis (PCP), Viridans strep	In patients expected to have PMN <100 for >7 days consider Levo 500-750 mg po q24h. Acute leukemia undergoing intensive induction consider addition of Fluc 400 mg q24h. In patients with AML or MDS who have prolonged neutropenia, consider Posa instead at 200 mg TID *(N Engl J Med 356:348, 2007)*. Safe & effective during induction rx for acute lymphoblastic leukemia (ALL) *(CID 2017,65:1790)*		
Post allogeneic stem cell transplant	Aerobic Gm-neg bacilli, ↑ risk pneumocystis, herpes viruses, candida aspergillus	**TMP-SMX** (vs. PCP) + **Acyclovir** (vs. HSV/VZV)+ **pre-emptive** monitoring for **CMV** + **Posaconazole** (vs. mold)		In autologous HCT, not active prophylaxis nor CMV screening is recommended. Fluc OK with TMP-SMX and acyclovir.
Empiric therapy—febrile neutropenia (≥38.3°C for >1 hr or sustained >38°C and absolute neutrophil count <500 cells/μL) (IDSA Guidelines: *CID 52:427, 2012*). *(Outpatients: J Oncol Prac 14:250, 2018)*				
Low-risk adults Anticipate <7 days neutropenia, no co-morb, can take po meds	Aerobic Gm-neg bacilli, Viridans strep	**CIP** 750 mg po bid + **Amox-clav** 875 /125 mg po bid. Treat until absolute neutrophil count >1000 cells/μL	Treat as outpatients with 24/7 access to inpatient care if: no focal findings, no hypotension, no COPD, no fungal infection, no dehydration, age range 16-60 yrs; motivated and compliant pts & family. If pen allergy: can substitute **Clinda** 300 mg po qid for Amox-clav	
High-risk adults and children (Anticipate >7 days profound neutropenia, active co-morbidities)	**Aerobic Gm-neg. bacilli; to include P. aeruginosa; cephalosporin-resistant viridans strep; MRSA**	**Empiric therapy:** **CFP**, **IMP**, **MER**, **Dori**, or **Pip-tazo**. Consider addition of **Vanco** as below. *Dosages: See footnote on page 69* **Include empiric Vanco if:** Suspected CLABSI, severe mucositis, SSTI, PNA, or hypotension	**Combination therapy:** If pt has severe sepsis/shock, consider add **Tobra** + **Vanco** + **Echinocandin**	Increasing resistance of viridans streptococci to penicillins, cephalosporins & FQs *(CID 34:1469 & 1524, 2002)*. **What if severe IgE-mediated β-lactam allergy?** Aztreonam plus Tobra. Work-up should include blood, urine, CXR with additional testing based on symptoms. Low threshold for CT scan. If cultures remain neg, but pt afebrile, treat until absolute neutrophil count ≥500 cells/μL. **Note**: Pip-tazo inferior to MER vs. ceftriaxone-resistant E. coli/K. pneumo *(JAMA 2018;320:979 & 984)*.
Persistent fever and neutropenia after 5 days of empiric antibacterial therapy—*see CID 52:427, 2011.*				
	Candida species, aspergillus, VRE, resistant GNB	Add either (**Caspofungin** 70 mg IV day 1, then 50 mg IV q24h or **Micafungin** 100 mg IV q24h or **Anidulafungin** 200 mg IV x 1 dose, then 100 mg IV q24h) **OR Voriconazole** 6 mg per kg IV q12h times 2 doses, then 4 mg per kg IV q12h		Conventional **Ampho B** causes more fever & nephrotoxicity & lower efficacy than lipid-based ampho B; both **Caspofungin** & **Voriconazole** better tolerated & perhaps more efficacious than lipid-based Ampho B *(NEJM 346:225, 2002 & 351:1391 & 1445, 2005)*.

 **NOTE: All dosage recommendations are for adults (unless otherwise indicated) and assume normal renal function. § Alternatives consider allergy, PK, compliance, local resistance, cost.*

TABLE 1 (67)

ANATOMIC SITE/DIAGNOSIS/ MODIFYING CIRCUMSTANCES	ETIOLOGIES (usual)	SUGGESTED REGIMENS*		ADJUNCT DIAGNOSTIC OR THERAPEUTIC MEASURES AND COMMENTS
		PRIMARY	ALTERNATIVE§	
SYSTEMIC SYNDROMES (FEBRILE/NON-FEBRILE) *(continued)*				
Shock syndromes				
Septic Shock, Bacteremic Shock, endotoxin Shock Surviving Sepsis Guideline: antibiotic treatment within 1 hr of dx of septic shock. Ref: *CCM 2024;52:1138; CID 2024; 78:505.* Excellent general ref on septic shock: *NEJM 2024, 391:2133*	Bacteremia due to aerobic GNB or GPC. Other possibilities include toxic shock syndrome and cytokine storm due to immunotherapy *(NEJM 383:1907, 2020).* Consider concomitant causes of shock: e.g., pulmonary embolis, congestive heart failure, etc.	**Management Bundle** *(NEJM 376:2235 & 2282, 2017)* 1. Two blood cultures, other pertinent cultures, nasal NAAT for S. aureus 2. Serum lactate 3. Baseline procalcitonin (if available); if < 0.25 ng/mL, repeat in 4-6 hrs 4. Empiric antibiotics: - *if low prevalence of MDR-GNB*, **Pip-tazo** or **CFP** + **Vanco** (add **Metro** if intra-abdominal source) - *if high prevalence of MDR-GNB*, (**MER** or **IMP**) + **Vanco** 5. IV crystalloid 20-40 mL/kg *(JAMA 326:818, 2021).* - *if persistent low BP*, start norepinephrine 6. Vigorous attempt to identify and correct source of bacteremia 7. Monitor adequacy of perfusion with lactate levels and central venous O2 saturation (target ≥ 70%)		- If persistent systolic BP < 90 mmHg or MAP < 65 mmHg, do random serum cortisol, then hydrocortisone 50 μg po once daily + fludrocortisone 50 μg via ng tube once daily. - Insulin to maintain serum glucose between 140-280 mg/dL. - Prognosis: survival correlates with rapid source control and effective antibiotic therapy. - Active debate as to the value of the elements of the standard bundle; latter used as a quality-of-care measure by Medicare: "Septic shock early management (SEP-1) sepsis quality measure". Refs: *CID 72:541, 2021* (IDSA opinion); *CID 72:553, 2021* (Medicare & Critical Care opinion). - Note: combination of Vit C, hydrocortisone & Thiamine failed to reduce septic shock severity score in prospective multi-center PCRCT *(JAMA 324:642, 2020).* - Hydrocortisone + fludrocortisone Phase 3 RT *(Lancet Respir Med 2024; 12:366).*
Septic shock: post-splenectomy or functional asplenia Asplenic pt care: *Chest 2016, 150:1394*	S. pneumoniae, N. meningitidis, H. influenzae, Capnocytophaga (DF-2)	No dog bite: **Ceftriaxone** 2 gm IV q24h (↑ to 2 gm q12h if meningitis) Post-dog bite: (**Pip-tazo** 4.5 gm IV (over 4h) q8h OR **MER** 1 gm IV q8h) OR **Clinda** 900 mg IV q8h	No dog bite: (**Levo** 750 mg or **Moxi** 400 mg) once IV q24h	Howell-Jolly bodies in peripheral blood smear confirm absence of functional spleen. Often results in **symmetrical peripheral gangrene of digits** due to severe DIC. For prophylaxis, *see Table 15A, page 260.* Vaccines: *CID 58:309, 2014.*
Toxic shock syndrome, Clostridium sordellii				
Clinical picture: shock, capillary leak, hemoconcentration, leukemoid reaction, afebrile	Clostridium sordellii-hemorrhagic & lethal toxins	Fluids, aq. **Pen G** 18–20 million units per day div. q4–6h + **Clinda** 900 mg IV q8h. **Surgical debridement is key.**	Occurs in variety of settings that produce anaerobic tissue, e.g., illicit drug use, post-partum. Several deaths reported after use of abortifacient regimen of mifepristone (RU486) & misoprostol.	
Toxic shock syndrome, staphylococcal				
Colonization by toxin-producing Staph. aureus of: vagina (tampon-assoc.), surgical/traumatic wounds, endometrium, burns	Staph. aureus (toxic shock toxin-mediated)	(**Nafcillin/Oxacillin** 2 gm IV q4h) or (if MRSA, **Vanco** 30-60 mg/kg/d in 2-3 div doses, target AUC_{24} 400-600 μg/mL x h) + **Clinda** 600-900 mg IV q8h	(**Cefazolin** 1–2 gm IV q8h) or (if MRSA, **Vanco** 30-60 mg/kg/d in 2-3 div doses, target AUC_{24} 400-600 μg/mL x h OR **Dapto** 10 mg/kg IV q24h) + **Clinda** 900 mg IV q8h	Rationale for Clinda is inhibition of toxin production; Linezolid also an option to inhibit toxin production. Can consider adding IVIG 1 gm/kg on day 1, then 0.5 gm/kg on days 2, 3.
Toxic shock syndrome, streptococcal. NOTE: For Necrotizing fasciitis without toxic shock, *see page 63.* Ref: *NEJM 2017,377:2253.*				
Associated with **invasive disease**, i.e., erysipelas, necrotizing fasciitis; secondary strep infection of varicella. Secondary household contact TSS cases reported.	Group A, B, C, & G Strep. pyogenes, Group B strep ref: *EID 15:223, 2009.*	(**Pen G** 24 million units per day IV in div. doses) + (**Clinda** 900 mg IV q8h) Prospective observational study *(CID 59:358, 366 & 851, 2014)* indicates: • Clinda decreases mortality • High incidence of secondary cases in household contacts	**Ceftriaxone** 2 gm IV q24h + **Clinda** 900 mg IV q8h	**Definition:** Isolation of Group A strep, hypotension and ≥2 of: renal impairment, coagulopathy, liver involvement, ARDS, generalized rash, soft tissue necrosis. Associated with invasive disease. **Surgery usually required.** Clinda added to decrease toxin production. **Adjunctive IVIG** 1 gm/kg day 1, then 0.5 gm/kg days 2 & 3 *(CID 2020;71:1772)*

Abbreviations on page 2. **NOTE: All dosage recommendations are for adults (unless otherwise indicated) and assume normal renal function. § Alternatives consider allergy, PK, compliance, local resistance, cost.*

TABLE 1 (68)

ANATOMIC SITE/DIAGNOSIS/ MODIFYING CIRCUMSTANCES	ETIOLOGIES (usual)	SUGGESTED REGIMENS*		ADJUNCT DIAGNOSTIC OR THERAPEUTIC MEASURES AND COMMENTS
		PRIMARY	ALTERNATIVE§	
SYSTEMIC SYNDROMES (FEBRILE/NON-FEBRILE) *(continued)*				
Toxin-Mediated Syndromes—no fever unless complicated				
Botulism *(Review: MMWR 2021 (RR-2):1). As **biologic weapon:** https://www.cdc.gov/botulism/index.html)*				
	Clostridium botulinum	For all types: Follow vital capacity; other supportive care		**Equine antitoxin:** Contact the local or state health department (1-800-222-1222) or CDC (1-770-488-7100) or for infant botulism 1-510-231-7600. **Antimicrobials:** May make infant botulism worse. Untested in wound botulism. When used, pen G 10–20 million units per day usual dose. If complications (pneumonia, UTI) occur, avoid antimicrobials with assoc. neuromuscular blockade, i.e., aminoglycosides, tetracycline, polymyxins. **Differential dx:** Guillain-Barré, myasthenia gravis, tick paralysis, organo-phosphate toxicity, West Nile virus. EMG can help.
Food-borne Dyspnea at presentation bad sign	Less common: C. baratii, C. butyricum	If no ileus, purge GI tract	Heptavalent equine serum antitoxin—CDC *(see Comment)*	
Infant	Submit blood, wound tissue, and/or implicated food (as pertinent) for mouse toxin bioassay.	Age < 1 year: Human botulinum immunoglobulin. Age > 1 year: Equine serum heptavalent botulinum antitoxin. **DO NOT WAIT FOR LAB CONFIRMATION TO TREAT SUSPECTED CASES**	**No antibiotics;** may lyse C. botulinum in gut and ↑ load of toxin	
Wound		Debridement & anaerobic cultures. No proven value of local antitoxin. Role of antibiotics untested.	Trivalent equine antitoxin	Wound botulism associated with injection drug use. Mouse bioassay failed to detect toxin in 1/3 of patients.
Tetanus: Trismus, generalized muscle rigidity, muscle spasm Ref: *AnIM 154:329, 2011.*	C. tetani–production of tetanospasmin toxin	**Six treatment steps:** 1. Urgent endotracheal intubation to protect the airway. Laryngeal spasm is common. Early tracheostomy. 2. Eliminate reflex spasms with diazepam, 20 mg/kg/day IV or midazolam. Reports of benefit combining diazepam with magnesium sulfate *(Ln 368:1436, 2006)*. Worst cases: need neuromuscular blockade with vecuronium. 3. Neutralize toxin: Human hyperimmune globulin IM; start tetanus immunization–no immunity from clinical tetanus. 4. Surgically debride infected source tissue. Start antibiotic: (**Pen G** 3 million units IV q4h or **Doxy** 100 mg IV q12h or **Metro** 1000 mg IV q12h) x 7-10 days. 5. Avoid light as may precipitate muscle spasms. 6. Use beta blockers, e.g., short acting esmolol, to control sympathetic hyperactivity.		

 **NOTE: All dosage recommendations are for adults (unless otherwise indicated) and assume normal renal function. § Alternatives consider allergy, PK, compliance, local resistance, cost.*

ANATOMIC SITE/DIAGNOSIS/ MODIFYING CIRCUMSTANCES	ETIOLOGIES (usual)	SUGGESTED REGIMENS* PRIMARY	ALTERNATIVE§	ADJUNCT DIAGNOSTIC OR THERAPEUTIC MEASURES AND COMMENTS
VASCULAR				
Catheter Related Blood Stream Infections (CRBSI). Ref: *Infect Dis Clin No Amer 2018 Dec;32(4):765-787*				
Tunneled & non-tunneled central venous catheters (CVC), including peripherally inserted central catheters (PICC). For management of peripheral IV, midline, arterial & hemodialysis catheters, see *Infect Dis Clin No Amer 2018 Dec;32(4):765-787.* **Diagnosis:** concomitant blood cultures from CVC & peripheral vein. A differential time to positive (DTP) of ≥2 hr favors infection of the CVC.	If suspect Gm+ bacteria: empiric rx for MSSA, MRSA, MRSE	**Vanco**	**Dapto**	Recommend in all clinical settings due to high prevalence of MSSA, MRSA & MRSE
	If suspect Gm-neg bacteria, e.g., femoral line, neutropenic	Not critically ill: **Cefepime** or **Pip-tazo** Critically ill: **MER** or **IMP**		
	Empiric rx if high risk of candidemia, e.g., prolonged antibiotic therapy, post-transplant neutropenia, hyperalimentation	**Micafungin** or **Caspofungin**	**Isavuconazole**	
	S. epidermidis in blood: MSSE or MRSE (most often)	IF no attempt to salvage catheter; remove catheter. For MRSE: **Vanco** or **Dapto** For MSSE: **Cefazolin** IF attempt to salvage catheter. Antibiotic as above + antibiotic lock therapy (ALT) x 10-14 days. *(See Comment)*		Antibiotic lock therapy (ALT) not FDA approved. Several options, but prefer sol'n of Minocycline 5 mg + EDTA 30 mg/mL in 25% alcohol. See *AAC 2016;60:3426*. Catheter "dwell" time of a minimum 2-4 hrs/day.
	S. aureus or S. lugdunensis in blood; attempts at salvage therapy not recommended	Remove catheter. For MSSA: (**Nafcillin/Oxacillin**) or **Cefazolin** x 2-6 wks For MRSA: **Vanco** or **Dapto** x 2-6 wks		If bacteremia for >72 hrs after catheter removal, TEE 5-7 days after diagnosis of bacteremia. New CVC: after removal of infected CVC, new blood cultures for 48-72 hrs.
	Enterococcus sp. In blood.	Specific antibiotic rx based on culture ID & susceptibility testing If short term CVC: remove & treat for 7-14 days. If long term CVC: can attempt salvage with combination IV antibiotic + ALT x 10-14 days		TEE if bacteremia persists longer than 72 hrs after start of antibiotic therapy or patient has a prosthetic heart valve.
	Aerobic Gm-neg bacilli (GNB) in blood *(See Comment)*	Mono- or combination therapy for *P. aeruginosa* (or other MDR bacteria). Remove catheter. Can attempt to salvage catheter with systemic antibiotic + ALT x 10-14 days		If gram positive bacilli (GPB) in blood, maybe Leuconostoc sp. or Lactobacillus sp. Both are Vanco resistant but sensitive to **Pen G**, **AMP** or **Clinda**.
	Candida sp. In blood	Remove CVC. **Micafungin**	Remove CVC. **Fluconazole** unless *C. krusei*, then **Isavuconazole**	
Mycotic aneurysm	S. aureus (28-71%), S. epidermidis, Salmonella sp. (15-24%), M.TBc, S. pneumonia, many others	**Vanco** 30-60 mg/kg/d in 2-3 div doses, target AUC_{24} 400-600 µg/mL x h + (**Ceftriaxone** or **Pip-tazo** or **CIP**) **Treatment is combination of antibiotic + surgical resection with revascularization.**	**Dapto** could be substituted for Vanco. For GNB: **Cefepime** or **Carbapenems**	Best diagnostic imaging: CT angiogram. Blood cultures positive in 50-85%. **De-escalate to specific therapy when culture results known.** Treatment duration varies but usually 6 wks from date of definitive surgery.

Abbreviations on page 2. **NOTE: All dosage recommendations are for adults (unless otherwise indicated) and assume normal renal function. § Alternatives consider allergy, PK, compliance, local resistance, cost.*

TABLE 1 (70)

ANATOMIC SITE/DIAGNOSIS/ MODIFYING CIRCUMSTANCES	ETIOLOGIES (usual)	SUGGESTED REGIMENS*		ADJUNCT DIAGNOSTIC OR THERAPEUTIC MEASURES AND COMMENTS
		PRIMARY	ALTERNATIVE§	
VASCULAR *(continued)*				
Suppurative (Septic) Thrombophlebitis				
Cranial dural sinus:				
Cavernous Sinus CN III, IV, V (branches V1/V2), VI at risk (Note: V1 and V2, numbers are subscript)	S. aureus (70%) Streptococcus sp. Anaerobes (rare) Mucormycosis (diabetes) *(See Table 11A)*	[**Vanco** 30-60 mg/kg/d in 2-3 div doses, target AUC_{24} 400-600 µg/mL x h + **Ceftriaxone** 2 gm IV q12h], add **Metro** 500 mg IV q8h if dental/sinus source	Can substitute **Dapto** 8-12 mg/kg IV q24h OR **Linezolid** 600 mg IV q12h for **Vanco**.	• Diagnosis: CT or MRI • Treatment: 1) obtain specimen for culture; 2) empiric antibiotics; 3) may need adjunctive surgery; 4) heparin until afebrile, then coumadin for several weeks
Lateral Sinus: Complication of otitis media/mastoiditis (pathogens similar to otitis media)	Polymicrobial (often) Aerobes, e.g., Proteus sp, E. coli S. aureus P. aeruginosa B. fragilis Other GNB	**Cefepime** 2 gm IV q8h + **Metro** 500 mg IV q8h + **Vanco** (30-60 mg/kg/d in 2-3 div doses, target AUC_{24} 400-600 µg/mL x h conc of 15-20 µg/mL)	**MER** 2 gm IV q8h + **Linezolid** 600 mg IV q12h	• Diagnosis: CT or MRI • Treatment: 1) consider radical mastoidectomy; 2) obtain cultures; 3) antibiotics; 4) anticoagulation controversial • Prognosis: favorable
Superior Sagittal Sinus: Complication of bacterial meningitis or bacterial frontal sinusitis. Treat as for meningitis	S. pneumoniae N. meningitides H. influenzae (rare) S. aureus (very rare)	**Ceftriaxone** 2 gm IV q12h + **Vanco** 30-60 mg/kg/d in 2-3 div doses, target AUC_{24} 400-600 µg/mL x h + **Dexamethasone**	**MER** 2 gm IV q8h + **Vanco** 30-60 mg/kg/d in 2-3 div doses, target AUC_{24} 400-600 µg/mL x h + **Dexamethasone**	• Diagnosis: MRI • Prognosis: bad; causes cortical vein thrombosis, hemorrhagic infarcts and brainstem herniation. • Anticoagulants not recommended
Jugular Vein, Lemierre's Syndrome: Complication of pharyngitis, tonsillitis, dental infection, EBV.	Fusobacterium necrophorum (anaerobe) Less often: Other Fusobacterium S. pyogenes Bacteroides sp.	**Ceftriaxone** 2 gm IV q24h + **Metro** 500 mg IV q8h	**Pip/tazo** 4.5 gm IV over 4 h q8h OR **IMP** 500 mg IV q6h (or other carbapenem)	• Add vanco for line-related infection • For F. necrophorum can use Clinda 600-900 mg IV q8h • Duration of therapy 3-6 weeks • Imaging: Hi-res CT scan • Role of anticoagulants unclear • Ref: *Cureus 2023;15:e43685*
Pelvic Vein: Includes ovarian vein and deep pelvic vein phlebitis	Aerobic gram-neg bacilli Streptococcus sp. Anaerobes	Antibiotics + anticoagulation (heparin, then coumadin) *Low prevalence of MDR GNB:* **Pip-tazo** 4.5 gm IV (over 4h) q8h or 4.5 gm IV q8h OR (**Ceftriaxone** 2 gm IV once daily + **Metro** 500 mg IV q8h)	*High prevalence of MDR GNB:* **MER** 1 gm IV q8h. If severe beta-lactam allergy: (**CIP** 400 mg IV q12h + **Metro** 500 mg IV q8h)	• Diagnosis: ovarian vein infection presents 1 week post-partum with fever & local pain; deep pelvic vein presents 3-5 days post-delivery with fever but no local pain. CT or MRI may help. • Treat until afebrile for 48 hrs & WBC normal • Coumadin for 6 weeks
Portal Vein (Pylephlebitis): Complication of diverticulitis, appendicitis and (rarely) other intra-abdominal infection	Aerobic gram-neg bacilli: E. coli, Klebsiella & Proteus most common Other: aerobic/anaerobic streptococci, B. fragilis, Clostridia	*Low prevalence of MDR GNB* (<20%): **Pip-tazo** 4.5 gm infused over 4h IV q8h OR (**CIP** 400 mg IV q12h + **Metro** 500 mg IV q8h)	*High prevalence of MDR GNB* (≥20%): *If ESBL producer:* **Meropenem** 1-2 gm IV q8h. *If KPC producer:* **Ceftaz-avi** or **MER-vabor** or **IMP-rele**. *If MBL producer:* **Ceftaz-avi** + **Aztreonam**.	• Diagnosis: Pain, fever, neutrophilia in pt with intra-abdominal infection. Abdominal CT scan • Pyogenic liver abscesses are a complication • No anticoagulants unless hypercoagulable disease (neoplasm) • Surgery on vein not indicated

Abbreviations on page 2. *NOTE: All dosage recommendations are for adults (unless otherwise indicated) and assume normal renal function. § Alternatives consider allergy, PK, compliance, local resistance, cost.

TABLE 2 – RECOMMENDED ANTIMICROBIAL AGENTS AGAINST SELECTED BACTERIA

See specific diseases or syndromes in *Table 1* or refer to pathogen-specific information found in *Sanford Guide digital content (Web or mobile app).*

TABLE 3 – SUGGESTED DURATION OF ANTIBIOTIC THERAPY FOR SELECTED CLINICAL SYNDROMES IN IMMUNOCOMPETENT PATIENTS

For a given clinical infection:

- Goal is selection of the right drug, in the right dose for the right period of time.
- Past traditional treatment durations were based on observational studies, expert opinion, and FDA approved " gold standard" regimens
- This Table summarizes the duration of therapy suggested for selected common clinical settings. See *Table 1* for other syndromes and for greater detail regarding the settings listed here.
    - Most are the traditional durations used in Guidelines or drug package inserts or expert opinion
    - If the traditional gold standard duration was found non-inferior to a shorter regimen in one or more Randomized Clinical Trials (RCT), the validating number of RCTs is shown.
    - Pertinent "Shorter is Better" references:
        - *https://doi.org/10.1016/j.cmi.2022.08.024*
        - *Ann Intern Med 2021 174:822*
- NOTE: Whatever duration is selected, cessation of therapy requires evidence of "source control" as manifest by resolution of clinical signs and symptoms plus trending, or resolved, biomarkers of inflammation.

CLINICAL SITUATION		DURATION OF THERAPY (Days)
SITE	**CLINICAL SETTING**	
Bacteremia	**GNB** bacteremia with source control	7 vs. 14 days (equal efficacy in 3 RCT)
Bone	Osteomyelitis, adult; acute child; acute; staph, strep and Enterobacterales child; acute; meningococci, haemophilus	**42-56** **21-28** until ESR normal **14-21**
Ear	Otitis media with effusion	<2 yrs: **10**; ≥2 yrs: **5–7**
GI *Also see Table 1*	Bacillary dysentery (shigellosis)/traveler's diarrhea	single dose, up to **3** days if no response
	Typhoid fever (S. typhi): Azithro Ceftriaxone FQ Chloramphenicol	**5–7** (children/adolescents) **7–14** (Short course ↑ effective) **7–10** **14**
	Helicobacter pylori	**14**
	Pseudomembranous enterocolitis (C. difficile)	**10**
Genital	Pelvic inflammatory disease	**14**
Heart	Pericarditis (purulent)	**28** or until resolution of S&S and biomarkers normalize
Joint, native	Septic arthritis (non-gonococcal): Adult Infant/child	**14–28** (equal efficacy in 3 RCT); **4 weeks** for S. aureus if bacteremia is present **10–14** (Response varies, stop when resolution of S&S and biomarkers normalize).
	Gonococcal arthritis/disseminated GC infection	**7** *(See Table 1, page 25)*
Kidney	Cystitis, acute	**3** (FQ or TMP-SMX) **5** (nitrofurantoin) **1** (fosfomycin)
	Pyelonephritis	**7** (CIP) **5** (Levo 750 mg) (8 RCT)
	Asymptomatic bacteriuria	no treatment unless pregnancy or urologic surgery
Intra-abdominal	Peritonitis, secondary	**4-7** (with source control) (1 RCT)
Lung	Pneumonia, pneumococcal, CAP	**3-5** vs **5-14** (equal efficacy in 14 RCT)
	Pneumonia, VAP, eg, Pseudomonas, GNB	**8-15** (equal efficacy in 2 RCT)
	Pneumonia, staphylococcal	**21-28** (variable, until biomarkers normalize)
	Pneumocystis pneumonia (PCP) in AIDS	**21**
	Other immunocompromised	**14**
	Chlamydia, mycoplasma	Azithro **1** dose vs. **3** days (no difference); **5** vs. **10** days (equal efficacy in 2 RCT)
	Legionella	**7-10** (longer if immunocompromised)
	Lung abscess	Usually **28–42**, but variable
Meninges	N. meningitidis H. influenzae S. pneumoniae Listeria meningoencephalitis, gp B strep, coliforms	**7** **7** **10–14** **21** (longer in immunocompromised)
	Child: relapses seldom occur until 3 or more days post-rx.	
Multiple systems	Brucellosis *(See Table 1, page 67)*	**42** (depends on site of infection)
	Tularemia *(See Table 1, pages 49, 67)*	**7-21** depending on severity
Muscle	Gas gangrene (clostridial)	**10** but depends on severity
Pharynx	Group A strep pharyngitis *Also see Pharyngitis, Table 1, page 53*	**10** (Pen VK), **5** (O Ceph 2/3, Azithro)
	Diphtheria (membranous) Carrier	**14** (Pen G, Erythro) **1 dose** (Pen G), **7-10** (Erythro)
Prostate	Chronic prostatitis	**30-90** (TMP-SMX), **28–42** (FQ)
Sinuses	Acute bacterial sinusitis (usually viral etiology)	**3-7** vs. **6-10** (equal efficacy 12 RCT)
Skin	Cellulitis, erysipelas, abscess	**5-7**
Systemic	Lyme disease	*See Table 1, page 65.*
	Rocky Mountain spotted fever *(See Table 1, page 66)*	**Until afebrile 2 days**

TABLE 4A – ANTIBACTERIAL ACTIVITY SPECTRA

The data shown in the table are intended to serve as a general overview of antibacterial usefulness based aggregation of information from approved package inserts, treatment guidelines and recommendations, in vitro activity, clinical trials data, predominant patterns of susceptibility or resistance and/or demonstrated clinical effectiveness. Variability in resistance patterns due to regional differences or as a consequent of clinical setting (e.g., community-onset vs. ICU-acquired infection) should be taken into account when using this table because local activity of certain agents can differ significantly from what is shown in the table.

Preferred (++): Agent is a first line therapy: reliably active in vitro, clinically effective, guideline recommended, recommended as a primary or acceptable alternative agent in the Sanford Guide. See pathogen page for specific recommendations.

Alternative (+): Agent is a potential alternative agent (active in vitro, possesses class activity comparable to known effective agents or a therapeutically interchangeable agents and hence likely to be clinically effective, but second line due to overly broad spectrum, toxicity, limited clinical experience, or paucity of direct evidence of effectiveness).

Limited Utility (±): Variable activity such that the agent, although clinically effective in some settings or types of infections is not reliably effective in others, or should be used in combination with another agent, and/or its efficacy is limited by resistance which has been associated with treatment failure.

Not Recommended (0): Agent is a poor alternative to other agents for one or more reasons: 1) lack of in vitro activity; 2) resistance to likely to be present or occur; 3) due to poor drug penetration to site of infection; 4) an unfavorable toxicity profile, particularly when there are other highly effective and safer alternatives; or 5) there are insufficient clinical data to support effectiveness.

	Penicillins											
	Penicillin G	Penicillin VK	Nafcillin	Oxacillin	Cloxacillin	Flucloxacillin	Dicloxacillin	Ampicillin	Amoxicillin	Amox-Clav	Amp-Sulb	Pip-Tazo
Aerobic gram-pos cocci												
E. faecalis (VS)	++	0	0	0	0	0	0	++	++	+	+	+
E. faecium (VS)	±	0	0	0	0	0	0	±	±	±	±	±
E. faecalis (VRE)	±	0	0	0	0	0	0	±	±	±	±	±
E. faecium (VRE)	±	0	0	0	0	0	0	±	±	±	±	±
S. aureus MSSA	±	±	++	++	++	++	++	±	±	+	+	+
S. aureus MRSA	0	0	0	0	0	0	0	0	0	0	0	0
Staph coag-neg (MS)	±	±	++	++	++	++	++	±	±	+	+	+
Staph coag-neg (MR)	0	0	0	0	0	0	0	0	0	0	0	0
S. epidermidis (MR)	0	0	0	0	0	0	0	0	0	0	0	0
S. epidermidis (MS)	±	±	++	++	++	++	++	±	±	+	+	+
S. lugdunensis	±	±	++	++	++	++	++	±	±	+	+	+
S. saprophyticus	±	±	+	+	+	+	+	±	±	++	+	+
S. anginosus gp	++	++	+	+	+	+	+	+	+	+	+	+
Strep. pyogenes gp (A)	++	++	+	+	+	+	+	+	+	+	+	+
Strep. agalactiae gp (B)	++	++	+	+	+	+	+	+	+	+	+	+
Strep. gp C, F, G	++	++	+	+	+	+	+	+	+	+	+	+
Strep. pneumoniae	++	++	+	+	+	+	+	+	+	+	+	+
Viridans Strep.	±	±	±	±	±	±	±	±	±	±	±	±

	Carbapenems						Mono	
	Doripenem	Ertapenem	Imp-cilastatin	Imp-cila-rele	Meropenem	Mero-Vabor	Aztreonam	Aztreo-Avibac
Aerobic gram-pos cocci								
E. faecalis (VS)	0	0	+	+	±	±	0	0
E. faecium (VS)	0	0	0	0	0	0	0	0
E. faecalis (VRE)	0	0	0	0	0	0	0	0
E. faecium (VRE)	0	0	0	0	0	0	0	0
S. aureus MSSA	+	+	+	+	+	+	0	0
S. aureus MRSA	0	0	0	0	0	0	0	0
Staph coag-neg (MS)	+	+	+	+	+	+	0	0
Staph coag-neg (MR)	0	0	0	0	0	0	0	0
S. epidermidis (MR)	0	0	0	0	0	0	0	0
S. epidermidis (MS)	+	+	+	+	+	+	0	0
S. lugdunensis	+	+	+	+	+	+	0	0
S. saprophyticus	+	+	+	+	+	+	0	0
S. anginosus gp	+	+	+	+	+	+	0	0
Strep. pyogenes gp (A)	+	+	+	+	+	+	0	0
Strep. agalactiae gp (B)	+	+	+	+	+	+	0	0
Strep. gp C, F, G	+	+	+	+	+	+	0	0
Strep. pneumoniae	+	+	+	+	+	+	0	0
Viridans Strep.	+	+	+	+	+	+	0	0

	Fluoroquinolone								
	Ciprofloxacin	Delafloxacin	Ofloxacin	Levofloxacin	Moxifloxacin	Norfloxacin	Prulifloxacin	Gemifloxacin	Gatifloxacin
Aerobic gram-pos cocci									
E. faecalis (VS)	±	+	±	+	+	+	±	+	+
E. faecium (VS)	0	0	0	0	±	0	0	±	±
E. faecalis (VRE)	0	0	0	0	0	0	0	0	0
E. faecium (VRE)	0	0	0	0	0	0	0	0	0
S. aureus MSSA	0	+	0	+	+	0	0	+	+
S. aureus MRSA	0	+	0	0	0	0	0	0	0
Staph coag-neg (MS)	0	+	0	+	+	0	0	+	+
Staph coag-neg (MR)	0	+	0	±	±	0	0	0	0
S. epidermidis (MR)	0	+	0	±	±	0	0	0	0
S. epidermidis (MS)	0	+	0	+	+	0	0	+	+
S. lugdunensis	0	+	+	+	+	0	0	+	+
S. saprophyticus	+	+	+	+	+	0	+	+	+
S. anginosus gp	±	+	±	+	+	0	±	+	+
Strep. pyogenes gp (A)	±	+	±	+	+	0	±	+	+
Strep. agalactiae gp (B)	±	+	±	+	+	0	±	+	+
Strep. gp C, F, G	±	+	±	+	+	0	±	+	+
Strep. pneumoniae	±	+	±	+	+	0	±	+	+
Viridans Strep.	0	+	0	+	+	0	0	+	+

	Parenteral Cephalosporins															
	Cefazolin	Cefotetan	Cefoxitin	Cefuroxime	Cefotaxime	Ceftizoxime	Cefoperazone	Ceftriaxone	Ceftazidime	Cefepime	Cefep-Enmeta	Ceftaz-Avibac	Ceftaroline	Ceftobiprole	Ceftol-Tazo	Cefiderocol
Aerobic gram-pos cocci																
E. faecalis (VS)	0	0	0	0	0	0	0	±	0	0	0	0	±	±	0	0
E. faecium (VS)	0	0	0	0	0	0	0	0	0	0	0	0	0	0	0	0
E. faecalis (VRE)	0	0	0	0	0	0	0	0	0	0	0	0	±	±	0	0
E. faecium (VRE)	0	0	0	0	0	0	0	0	0	0	0	0	0	0	0	0
S. aureus MSSA	++	+	+	+	+	+	+	+	0	+	+	0	+	+	0	0
S. aureus MRSA	0	0	0	0	0	0	0	0	0	0	0	0	+	+	0	0
Staph coag-neg (MS)	++	+	+	+	+	+	+	+	0	+	+	0	+	+	0	0
Staph coag-neg (MR)	0	0	0	0	0	0	0	0	0	0	0	0	+	+	0	0
S. epidermidis (MR)	0	0	0	0	0	0	0	0	0	0	0	0	+	+	0	0
S. epidermidis (MS)	++	+	+	+	+	+	+	+	0	+	+	0	+	+	0	0
S. lugdunensis	++	+	+	+	+	+	+	+	0	+	+	0	+	+	0	0
S. saprophyticus	++	+	+	+	+	+	+	+	0	+	+	0	+	+	0	0
S. anginosus gp	+	+	+	+	+	+	+	+	±	+	+	±	+	+	+	0
Strep. pyogenes gp (A)	+	+	+	+	+	+	+	+	+	+	+	+	+	+	+	0
Strep. agalactiae gp (B)	+	+	+	+	+	+	+	+	+	+	+	+	+	+	+	0
Strep. gp C, F, G	+	+	+	+	+	+	+	+	+	+	+	+	+	+	+	0
Strep. pneumoniae	+	+	+	+	+	+	+	+	+	+	+	+	+	+	+	0
Viridans Strep.	+	+	+	+	++	+	+	++	±	+	+	±	+	+	+	0

TABLE 4A (2)

	Penicillins											
	Penicillin G	Penicillin VK	Nafcillin	Oxacillin	Cloxacillin	Flucloxacillin	Dicloxacillin	Ampicillin	Amoxicillin	Amox-Clav	Amp-Sulb	Pip-Tazo
Aerobic gram-pos bacilli												
Arcanobacter. sp	+	+	0	0	0	0	0	+	+	+	+	+
C. diphtheriae	++	++	0	0	0	0	0	+	+	+	+	+
C. jeikeium	0	0	0	0	0	0	0	0	0	0	0	0
L. monocytogenes	+	0	0	0	0	0	0	++	+	+	+	+
Nocardia sp.	0	0	0	0	0	0	0	0	0	±	0	0
Aerobic GNB - Enterobacterales												
Aeromonas sp.	0	0	0	0	0	0	0	0	0	±	±	+
C. freundii	0	0	0	0	0	0	0	0	0	0	0	0
C. koseri	0	0	0	0	0	0	0	0	0	+	+	++
E. cloacae	0	0	0	0	0	0	0	0	0	0	0	0
E. coli (S)	0	0	0	0	0	0	0	±	±	+	+	++
E. coli, ESBL	0	0	0	0	0	0	0	0	0	0	0	0
E. coli, Klebs KPC	0	0	0	0	0	0	0	0	0	0	0	0
E. coli, Klebs MBL	0	0	0	0	0	0	0	0	0	0	0	0
K. aerogenes	0	0	0	0	0	0	0	0	0	0	0	0
K. oxytoca (S)	0	0	0	0	0	0	0	0	0	+	+	++
K. pneumoniae (S)	0	0	0	0	0	0	0	0	0	+	+	++
Klebsiella sp. (ESBL)	0	0	0	0	0	0	0	0	0	0	0	0
M. morganii	0	0	0	0	0	0	0	0	0	0	0	++
P. mirabilis	0	0	0	0	0	0	0	+	+	+	+	+
P. vulgaris	0	0	0	0	0	0	0	0	0	+	+	+
Providencia sp.	0	0	0	0	0	0	0	0	0	+	+	+
Salmonella sp.	0	0	0	0	0	0	0	±	±	0	0	0
S. marcescens	0	0	0	0	0	0	0	0	0	0	0	+
Shigella sp.	0	0	0	0	0	0	0	0	0	+	+	+
Y. enterocolitica	0	0	0	0	0	0	0	0	0	±	±	+

	Carbapenems						Mono	
	Doripenem	Ertapenem	Imp-cilastatin	Imp-cila-rele	Meropenem	Mero-Vabor	Aztreonam	Aztreo-Avibac
Aerobic gram-pos bacilli								
Arcanobacter. sp	+	+	+	+	+	+	0	0
C. diphtheriae	0	0	0	0	0	0	0	0
C. jeikeium	0	0	0	0	0	0	0	0
L. monocytogenes	0	0	0	0	±	±	0	0
Nocardia sp.	0	0	++	++	±	±	0	0
Aerobic GNB - Enterobacterales								
Aeromonas sp.	+	+	+	+	+	+	+	+
C. freundii	+	+	+	+	++	+	0	+
C. koseri	+	+	+	+	++	+	+	+
E. cloacae	+	+	+	+	+	+	0	+
E. coli (S)	+	+	+	+	+	+	+	+
E. coli, ESBL	+	++	++	+	++	+	0	+
E. coli, Klebs KPC	0	0	0	+	0	+	0	+
E. coli, Klebs MBL	0	0	0	0	0	0	0	+
K. aerogenes	+	+	+	+	+	+	+	+
K. oxytoca (S)	+	+	+	+	+	+	+	+
K. pneumoniae (S)	+	+	+	+	+	+	+	+
Klebsiella sp. (ESBL)	+	+	++	+	++	+	0	+
M. morganii	+	+	±	±	+	+	+	+
P. mirabilis	+	+	±	±	+	+	+	+
P. vulgaris	+	+	±	±	+	+	+	+
Providencia sp.	++	++	±	±	++	+	+	+
Salmonella sp.	0	+	+	+	+	+	0	+
S. marcescens	+	+	+	+	+	+	+	+
Shigella sp.	+	+	+	+	+	+	+	+
Y. enterocolitica	+	0	+	+	+	+	+	+

	Fluoroquinolone								
	Ciprofloxacin	Delafloxacin	Ofloxacin	Levofloxacin	Moxifloxacin	Norfloxacin	Prulifloxacin	Gemifloxacin	Gatifloxacin
Aerobic gram-pos bacilli									
Arcanobacter. sp	+	0	+	+	+	0	+	+	+
C. diphtheriae	0	0	0	0	0	0	0	0	0
C. jeikeium	0	0	0	0	±	0	0	±	0
L. monocytogenes	0	0	0	0	0	0	0	0	0
Nocardia sp.	0	0	0	0	0	0	0	0	0
Aerobic GNB - Enterobacterales									
Aeromonas sp.	+	+	+	+	+	0	+	+	+
C. freundii	+	+	+	+	+	+	+	+	+
C. koseri	+	+	+	+	+	+	+	+	+
E. cloacae	+	+	+	+	+	+	+	+	+
E. coli (S)	+	+	+	+	+	+	+	+	+
E. coli, ESBL	±	±	±	±	±	±	±	±	±
E. coli, Klebs KPC	0	0	0	0	0	0	0	0	0
E. coli, Klebs MBL	±	0	0	0	0	0	0	0	0
K. aerogenes	+	+	+	+	+	+	+	+	+
K. oxytoca (S)	+	+	+	+	+	+	+	+	+
K. pneumoniae (S)	+	+	+	+	+	+	+	+	+
Klebsiella sp. (ESBL)	±	±	±	±	±	±	±	±	±
M. morganii	+	+	+	+	+	+	+	+	+
P. mirabilis	+	+	+	+	+	+	+	+	+
P. vulgaris	+	+	+	+	+	+	+	+	+
Providencia sp.	+	+	+	+	+	+	+	±	±
Salmonella sp.	±	±	±	±	±	0	0	±	±
S. marcescens	+	+	+	+	+	0	+	+	+
Shigella sp.	++	±	±	++	±	0	±	±	±
Y. enterocolitica	++	+	+	++	+	0	++	0	+

	Parenteral Cephalosporins															
	Cefazolin	Cefotetan	Cefoxitin	Cefuroxime	Cefotaxime	Ceftizoxime	Cefoperazone	Ceftriaxone	Ceftazidime	Cefepime	Cefep-Enmeta	Ceftaz-Avibac	Ceftaroline	Ceftobiprole	Ceftol-Tazo	Cefiderocol
Aerobic gram-pos bacilli																
Arcanobacter. sp	+	+	+	+	+	+	0	+	+	+	+	+	0	0	0	0
C. diphtheriae	0	0	0	0	0	0	0	0	0	0	0	0	0	0	0	0
C. jeikeium	0	0	0	0	0	0	0	0	0	0	0	0	0	0	0	0
L. monocytogenes	0	0	0	0	0	0	0	0	0	0	0	0	0	0	0	0
Nocardia sp.	0	0	0	0	±	0	0	±	0	0	0	0	0	0	0	0
Aerobic GNB - Enterobacterales																
Aeromonas sp.	0	0	0	0	+	+	0	+	+	+	+	+	0	0	0	0
C. freundii	0	0	0	0	0	0	0	0	0	++	+	+	±	±	+	+
C. koseri	0	0	0	0	+	+	+	+	+	++	+	+	+	+	+	+
E. cloacae	0	0	0	0	0	0	0	0	0	+	+	+	+	+	+	+
E. coli (S)	+	+	+	+	+	+	+	++	+	+	+	+	+	+	+	+
E. coli, ESBL	0	+	+	0	0	0	0	0	0	0	+	+	0	0	+	+
E. coli, Klebs KPC	0	0	0	0	0	0	0	0	0	0	0	++	0	0	0	+
E. coli, Klebs MBL	0	0	0	0	0	0	0	0	0	0	0	0	0	0	0	+
K. aerogenes	0	0	0	0	0	0	0	0	0	+	+	+	±	±	+	+
K. oxytoca (S)	+	+	+	+	+	+	+	++	+	+	+	+	+	+	+	+
K. pneumoniae (S)	+	+	+	+	+	+	+	++	+	+	+	+	+	+	+	+
Klebsiella sp. (ESBL)	0	±	±	0	0	0	0	0	0	0	+	+	0	0	+	+
M. morganii	0	+	+	0	+	+	+	++	+	+	+	+	+	+	+	+
P. mirabilis	+	+	+	+	+	+	+	+	+	+	+	+	+	+	+	+
P. vulgaris	0	+	+	+	+	+	+	+	+	+	+	+	0	0	+	+
Providencia sp.	0	+	+	0	+	+	+	+	+	+	+	+	0	0	+	+
Salmonella sp.	0	0	0	0	+	+	+	+	+	+	+	+	0	0	0	0
S. marcescens	0	+	0	0	+	+	+	+	+	+	+	+	±	±	+	+
Shigella sp.	0	0	0	0	+	+	+	+	+	+	+	+	0	0	0	0
Y. enterocolitica	0	±	±	±	++	+	+	++	±	+	+	0	0	0	0	0

TABLE 4A (3)

Penicillins

Aerobic GNB - non-Enterobacterales	Penicillin G	Penicillin VK	Nafcillin	Oxacillin	Cloxacillin	Flucloxacillin	Dicloxacillin	Ampicillin	Amoxicillin	Amox-Clav	Amp-Sulb	Pip-Tazo
Bartonella sp.	0	0	0	0	0	0	0	0	0	0	0	0
B. pertussis	0	0	0	0	0	0	0	0	0	0	0	0
B. burgdorferi	+	0	0	0	0	0	0	++	++	+	+	0
Brucella sp.	0	0	0	0	0	0	0	0	0	0	0	0
C. jejuni	0	0	0	0	0	0	0	0	0	+	0	0
Capnocytophaga sp.	±	±	0	0	0	0	0	±	±	++	+	++
C. burnetii	0	0	0	0	0	0	0	0	0	0	0	0
Ehrlichia, Anaplas	0	0	0	0	0	0	0	0	0	0	0	0
Eikenella sp	±	±	0	0	0	0	0	±	±	+	+	+
F. tularensis	0	0	0	0	0	0	0	0	0	0	0	0
H. ducreyi	0	0	0	0	0	0	0	0	0	0	0	0
H. influenzae	0	0	0	0	0	0	0	±	±	++	++	+
Kingella sp.	+	+	0	0	0	0	0	+	+	+	+	+
K. granulomatis	0	0	0	0	0	0	0	0	0	0	0	0
Legionella sp.	0	0	0	0	0	0	0	0	0	0	0	0
Leptospira sp.	++	0	0	0	0	0	0	+	+	+	+	+
M. catarrhalis	0	0	0	0	0	0	0	0	0	++	+	+
N. meningitidis	+	0	0	0	0	0	0	++	++	0	0	+
P. multocida	++	++	0	0	0	0	0	++	++	++	++	+
R. rickettsii	0	0	0	0	0	0	0	0	0	0	0	0
V. cholera	0	0	0	0	0	0	0	0	0	0	0	0
V. parahaemolyticus	0	0	0	0	0	0	0	0	0	0	0	0
V. vulnificus	0	0	0	0	0	0	0	0	0	0	0	0
Y. pestis	0	0	0	0	0	0	0	0	0	0	0	0

Carbapenems / Mono

Aerobic GNB - non-Enterobacterales	Doripenem	Ertapenem	Imp-cilastatin	Imp-cila-rele	Meropenem	Mero-Vabor	Aztreonam	Aztreo-Avibac
Bartonella sp.	0	0	0	0	0	0	0	0
B. pertussis	0	0	0	0	0	0	0	0
B. burgdorferi	0	0	0	0	0	0	0	0
Brucella sp.	0	0	0	0	0	0	0	0
C. jejuni	+	+	+	+	+	+	0	0
Capnocytophaga sp.	+	+	+	+	+	+	0	0
C. burnetii	0	0	0	0	0	0	0	0
Ehrlichia, Anaplas	0	0	0	0	0	0	0	0
Eikenella sp	+	+	+	+	+	+	0	0
F. tularensis	0	0	0	0	0	0	0	0
H. ducreyi	0	0	0	0	0	0	0	0
H. influenzae	+	+	+	+	+	+	+	+
Kingella sp.	+	+	+	+	+	+	0	0
K. granulomatis	0	0	0	0	0	0	0	0
Legionella sp.	0	0	0	0	0	0	0	0
Leptospira sp.	+	+	+	+	+	+	+	+
M. catarrhalis	+	+	+	+	+	+	+	+
N. meningitidis	+	+	+	+	+	+	+	+
P. multocida	+	+	+	+	+	+	+	+
R. rickettsii	0	0	0	0	0	0	0	0
V. cholera	0	0	0	0	0	0	0	0
V. parahaemolyticus	0	0	0	0	0	0	0	0
V. vulnificus	0	0	0	0	0	0	0	0
Y. pestis	0	0	0	0	0	0	0	0

Fluoroquinolone

Aerobic GNB - non-Enterobacterales	Ciprofloxacin	Delafloxacin	Ofloxacin	Levofloxacin	Moxifloxacin	Norfloxacin	Prulifloxacin	Gemifloxacin	Gatifloxacin
Bartonella sp.	0	0	0	0	0	0	0	0	0
B. pertussis	0	0	0	0	0	0	0	0	0
B. burgdorferi	0	0	0	0	0	0	0	0	0
Brucella sp.	+	0	0	0	0	0	+	0	0
C. jejuni	+	+	+	+	+	0	+	+	+
Capnocytophaga sp.	±	0	±	±	0	0	±	0	0
C. burnetii	+	0	+	+	+	0	+	+	+
Ehrlichia, Anaplas	0	0	0	0	0	0	0	0	0
Eikenella sp	+	0	+	+	0	0	+	0	0
F. tularensis	++	0	0	0	0	0	++	0	0
H. ducreyi	++	0	0	+	0	0	++	0	0
H. influenzae	+	+	+	++	++	0	+	+	+
Kingella sp.	+	+	+	++	0	0	+	0	0
K. granulomatis	++	0	0	0	0	0	++	0	0
Legionella sp.	++	+	++	++	++	0	++	+	+
Leptospira sp.	+	+	+	+	+	0	+	+	+
M. catarrhalis	+	+	+	+	+	0	+	+	+
N. meningitidis	±	0	0	0	0	0	0	0	0
P. multocida	+	+	+	+	+	0	+	+	+
R. rickettsii	±	0	±	±	±	0	±	0	0
V. cholera	+	0	0	0	0	0	+	0	0
V. parahaemolyticus	+	0	+	+	0	0	+	0	0
V. vulnificus	+	0	+	+	0	0	+	0	0
Y. pestis	+	0	0	0	0	0	+	0	0

Parenteral Cephalosporins

Aerobic GNB - non-Enterobacterales	Cefazolin	Cefotetan	Cefoxitin	Cefuroxime	Cefotaxime	Ceftizoxime	Cefoperazone	Ceftriaxone	Ceftazidime	Cefepime	Cefep-Enmeta	Ceftaz-Avibac	Ceftaroline	Ceftobiprole	Ceftol-Tazo	Cefiderocol
Bartonella sp.	0	0	0	0	0	0	0	0	0	0	0	0	0	0	0	0
B. pertussis	0	0	0	0	0	0	0	0	0	0	0	0	0	0	0	0
B. burgdorferi	0	0	0	+	+	0	0	++	0	0	0	0	0	0	0	0
Brucella sp.	0	0	0	0	0	0	0	0	0	0	0	0	0	0	0	0
C. jejuni	0	0	0	0	0	0	0	0	0	0	0	0	0	0	0	0
Capnocytophaga sp.	0	0	0	0	+	0	0	+	+	+	+	+	0	0	0	0
C. burnetii	0	0	0	0	0	0	0	0	0	0	0	0	0	0	0	0
Ehrlichia, Anaplas	0	0	0	0	0	0	0	0	0	0	0	0	0	0	0	0
Eikenella sp	0	0	+	0	+	0	0	+	0	0	0	0	0	0	0	0
F. tularensis	0	0	0	0	0	0	0	0	0	0	0	0	0	0	0	0
H. ducreyi	0	0	0	0	0	0	0	++	0	0	0	0	0	0	0	0
H. influenzae	0	+	+	+	++	+	+	++	+	+	+	+	+	+	+	0
Kingella sp.	+	+	+	+	+	+	+	++	+	+	+	+	+	+	+	0
K. granulomatis	0	0	+	0	0	0	0	+	0	0	0	0	0	0	0	0
Legionella sp.	0	0	0	0	0	0	0	0	0	0	0	0	0	0	0	0
Leptospira sp.	0	0	0	0	++	0	0	++	0	0	0	+	0	0	0	0
M. catarrhalis	0	+	±	+	+	+	+	+	+	+	+	+	+	+	+	0
N. meningitidis	0	0	0	0	+	0	0	++	+	+	+	+	0	0	0	0
P. multocida	0	0	0	+	+	+	+	+	0	+	+	0	+	+	+	0
R. rickettsii	0	0	0	0	0	0	0	0	0	0	0	0	0	0	0	0
V. cholera	0	0	0	0	0	0	0	0	0	0	0	0	0	0	0	0
V. parahaemolyticus	0	0	0	0	+	+	0	+	+	+	+	+	0	0	0	0
V. vulnificus	0	0	0	0	+	+	0	+	+	+	+	+	0	0	0	0
Y. pestis	0	0	0	0	0	0	0	0	0	0	0	0	0	0	0	0

TABLE 4A (4)

	Penicillins												Carbapenems						Mono		Fluoroquinolone									Parenteral Cephalosporins															
	Penicillin G	Penicillin VK	Nafcillin	Oxacillin	Cloxacillin	Flucloxacillin	Dicloxacillin	Ampicillin	Amoxicillin	Amox-Clav	Amp-Sulb	Pip-Tazo	Doripenem	Ertapenem	Imp-cilastatin	Imp-cila-rele	Meropenem	Mero-Vabor	Aztreonam	Aztreo-Avibac	Ciprofloxacin	Delafloxacin	Ofloxacin	Levofloxacin	Moxifloxacin	Norfloxacin	Prulifloxacin	Gemifloxacin	Gatifloxacin	Cefazolin	Cefotetan	Cefoxitin	Cefuroxime	Cefotaxime	Ceftizoxime	Cefoperazone	Ceftriaxone	Ceftazidime	Cefepime	Cefep-Enmeta	Ceftaz-Avibac	Ceftaroline	Ceftobiprole	Ceftol-Tazo	Cefiderocol
Aerobic GNB non-fermenter																																													
A. baumannii	0	0	0	0	0	0	0	0	0	0	±	±	0	0	±	±	±	±	0	0	±	±	±	±	±	0	±	0	0	0	0	0	0	0	0	0	0	±	±	±	±	0	0	±	+
B. cepacia	0	0	0	0	0	0	0	0	0	0	0	0	±	0	±	±	±	±	0	0	±	+	0	±	±	0	0	0	0	0	0	0	0	0	0	0	0	±	±	±	+	0	0	±	+
P. aeruginosa	0	0	0	0	0	0	0	0	0	0	0	++	+	0	+	+	++	+	+	+	+	+	0	+	0	0	+	0	0	0	0	0	0	0	0	0	0	++	++	++	+	0	0	++	+
S. maltophilia	0	0	0	0	0	0	0	0	0	0	0	0	0	0	0	0	0	0	0	0	±	±	0	±	±	0	0	0	0	0	0	0	0	0	0	0	0	±	0	0	±	0	0	0	+
Aerobic - cell wall-deficient																																													
C. trachomatis	0	0	0	0	0	0	0	+	+	0	0	0	0	0	0	0	0	0	0	0	0	0	++	++	+	0	0	+	+	0	0	0	0	0	0	0	0	0	0	0	0	0	0	0	0
Chlamydophila sp.	0	0	0	0	0	0	0	0	0	0	0	0	0	0	0	0	0	0	0	0	+	0	+	+	+	0	+	+	+	0	0	0	0	0	0	0	0	0	0	0	0	0	0	0	0
M. pneumoniae	0	0	0	0	0	0	0	0	0	0	0	0	0	0	0	0	0	0	0	0	+	0	+	++	++	0	+	+	+	0	0	0	0	0	0	0	0	0	0	0	0	0	0	0	0
Anaerobic GNB																																													
B. fragilis	0	0	0	0	0	0	0	0	0	++	+	++	+	++	++	+	++	+	0	0	0	+	0	0	±	0	0	0	0	0	±	±	0	0	+	+	0	0	0	0	0	0	0	+	0
F. necrophorum	±	±	0	0	0	0	0	±	±	+	+	+	+	+	+	+	+	+	0	0	0	0	0	0	0	0	0	0	0	0	+	+	0	+	+	+	+	0	0	0	0	0	0	0	0
Prevotella sp.	±	±	0	0	0	0	0	±	±	+	+	+	+	+	+	+	+	+	0	0	0	0	0	±	+	0	0	0	0	0	+	+	0	0	+	+	0	0	0	0	0	0	0	+	0
Anaerobic gram-positive																																													
Actinomyces sp.	++	++	0	0	0	0	0	++	++	+	+	+	+	+	+	+	+	+	0	0	0	0	0	0	0	0	0	0	0	0	0	+	0	+	+	0	+	0	0	0	0	0	0	0	0
Clostridium sp.	++	+	0	0	0	0	0	+	+	+	+	+	+	+	+	+	+	+	0	0	0	+	0	0	0	0	0	0	0	0	+	+	0	+	+	0	+	0	0	0	0	0	0	0	0
C. acnes	++	+	0	0	0	0	0	+	+	+	+	+	+	+	+	+	+	+	0	0	±	0	±	±	±	0	±	0	0	+	+	+	+	+	+	0	+	+	+	+	+	+	+	+	0
Peptostreptococci	++	++	0	0	0	0	0	++	++	+	+	+	+	+	+	+	+	+	0	0	0	+	0	+	+	0	0	0	+	+	+	+	+	+	+	+	+	+	+	+	+	+	+	+	0

TABLE 4A (5)

	Oral Cephalosporins										Aminoglyco					Macrolides				Tetracyclines						Glyco/Lipo						Ox-lid		Poly			Other									
	Cefadroxil	Cephalexin	Cefaclor	Cefprozil	Cefurox-Axe	Cefixime	Ceftibuten	Cefpodoxime	Cefdinir	Cefditoren	Gentamicin	Tobramycin	Amikacin	Plazomicin	Clindamycin	Erythromycin	Azithromycin	Clarithromycin	Telithromycin	Doxycycline	Eravacycline	Minocycline	Omadacycline	Tetracycline	Tigecycline	Daptomycin	Vancomycin	Teicoplanin	Telavancin	Oritavancin	Dalbavancin	Linezolid	Tedizolid	Polymyxin B	Colistin	Lefamulin	Chloramphen	Fusidic Acid	Rif (comb)	TMP-SMX	Nitrofurantoin	Fosfomycin (IV)	Fosfomycin (po)	Pivmecillinam	Metronidazole	Pristinamycin
Aerobic gram-pos cocci																																														
E. faecalis (VS)	0	0	0	0	0	0	0	0	0	0	±	0	0	0	0	0	0	0	0	±	+	±	+	±	+	+	++	++	+	+	+	+	+	0	0	0	±	±	±	0	+	±	±	0	0	0
E. faecium (VS)	0	0	0	0	0	0	0	0	0	0	±	0	0	0	0	0	0	0	0	±	+	±	+	±	+	+	±	±	±	+	±	++	+	0	0	0	±	±	±	0	+	±	±	0	0	+
E. faecalis (VRE)	0	0	0	0	0	0	0	0	0	0	±	0	0	0	0	0	0	0	0	±	±	±	±	±	±	+	0	0	±	+	0	++	+	0	0	0	±	0	±	0	+	±	±	0	0	0
E. faecium (VRE)	0	0	0	0	0	0	0	0	0	0	±	0	0	0	0	0	0	0	0	±	±	±	±	±	±	+	0	0	±	+	0	++	+	0	0	0	±	0	±	0	+	±	±	0	0	+
S. aureus MSSA	+	+	+	+	+	0	0	+	+	+	±	0	0	0	+	±	±	±	+	+	+	+	+	+	+	+	+	+	+	+	+	+	+	0	0	+	+	+	±	+	±	±	0	0	0	+
S. aureus MRSA	0	0	0	0	0	0	0	0	0	0	±	0	0	0	±	0	0	0	0	+	+	+	+	±	+	++	++	+	+	+	+	++	+	0	0	+	0	+	±	+	±	±	0	0	0	+
Staph coag-neg (MS)	+	+	+	+	+	0	0	+	+	+	±	0	0	0	+	±	±	±	+	+	+	+	+	+	+	+	+	+	+	+	+	+	+	0	0	+	+	+	±	+	0	±	0	0	0	+
Staph coag-neg (MR)	0	0	0	0	0	0	0	0	0	0	±	0	0	0	±	0	0	0	±	±	+	±	+	±	+	++	++	++	+	+	+	++	+	0	0	0	+	+	±	+	0	±	0	0	0	+
S. epidermidis (MR)	0	0	0	0	0	0	0	0	0	0	±	0	0	0	±	0	0	0	±	±	+	±	+	±	+	++	++	++	+	+	+	++	+	0	0	0	+	+	±	+	0	±	0	0	0	+
S. epidermidis (MS)	+	+	+	+	+	0	0	+	+	+	±	0	0	0	+	±	±	±	+	+	+	+	+	+	+	+	+	+	+	+	+	+	+	0	0	+	+	+	±	+	0	±	0	0	0	+
S. lugdunensis	+	+	+	+	+	0	0	+	+	+	±	0	0	0	+	+	+	+	+	+	+	+	+	+	+	+	+	+	+	+	+	+	+	0	0	0	+	+	±	+	0	0	0	0	0	+
S. saprophyticus	++	++	++	+	+	0	0	+	+	+	0	0	0	0	+	±	±	±	0	+	+	+	+	+	+	+	+	+	+	0	0	0	0	0	0	0	+	0	0	+	+	±	±	+	0	0
S. anginosus gp	+	+	+	+	+	+	+	+	+	+	±	0	0	0	+	±	±	±	+	±	+	±	+	±	+	0	+	+	+	+	+	+	+	0	0	+	+	0	0	0	0	0	0	0	0	+
Strep. pyogenes gp (A)	+	+	+	+	+	+	+	+	+	+	0	0	0	0	±	±	±	±	+	0	+	0	+	0	+	+	+	+	+	+	+	+	+	0	0	+	+	0	0	±	0	0	0	0	0	+
Strep. agalactiae gp (B)	+	+	+	+	+	+	+	+	+	+	±	0	0	0	±	±	±	±	+	0	+	0	+	0	+	+	+	+	+	+	+	+	+	0	0	+	+	0	0	±	0	0	0	0	0	+
Strep. gp C, F, G	+	+	+	+	+	+	+	+	+	+	±	0	0	0	+	±	±	±	+	0	+	0	+	0	+	+	+	+	+	+	+	+	+	0	0	0	+	0	0	±	0	0	0	0	0	+
Strep. pneumoniae	+	+	+	+	+	+	+	+	+	+	0	0	0	0	+	±	±	±	+	±	+	±	+	±	+	±	+	+	+	0	0	+	+	0	0	+	+	0	0	±	0	0	0	0	0	+
Viridans Strep.	+	+	+	0	+	+	0	+	+	+	±	0	0	0	±	±	±	±	+	±	+	±	+	±	+	0	++	++	+	+	+	+	+	0	0	+	+	0	0	0	0	0	0	0	0	+
Aerobic gram-pos bacilli																																														
Arcanobacter. sp	+	+	+	+	+	+	+	+	+	0	0	0	0	0	++	++	++	++	+	++	+	+	+	+	+	+	++	+	+	0	0	+	0	0	0	0	0	0	0	0	0	0	0	0	0	+
C. diphtheriae	0	0	0	0	0	0	0	0	0	0	0	0	0	0	+	++	++	+	0	0	0	0	0	0	0	0	0	0	0	0	0	0	0	0	0	0	0	0	0	0	0	0	0	0	0	0
C. jeikeium	0	0	0	0	0	0	0	0	0	0	0	0	0	0	0	0	0	0	0	0	+	0	+	0	+	+	++	+	+	0	0	+	0	0	0	0	0	0	0	0	0	0	0	0	0	0
L. monocytogenes	0	0	0	0	0	0	0	0	0	0	±	0	0	0	0	0	0	0	0	0	0	0	0	0	0	0	0	0	0	0	0	+	0	0	0	0	0	0	0	+	0	0	0	0	0	0
Nocardia sp.	0	0	0	0	0	0	0	0	0	0	0	0	++	0	0	0	0	0	0	0	0	±	0	0	0	0	0	0	0	0	0	+	0	0	0	0	0	0	0	++	0	0	0	0	0	0

TABLE 4A (6)

	Oral Cephalosporins										Aminoglyco					Macrolides			
	Cefadroxil	Cephalexin	Cefaclor	Cefprozil	Cefurox-Axe	Cefixime	Ceftibuten	Cefpodoxime	Cefdinir	Cefditoren	Gentamicin	Tobramycin	Amikacin	Plazomicin	Clindamycin	Erythromycin	Azithromycin	Clarithromycin	Telithromycin
Aerobic GNB - enterobacterales																			
Aeromonas sp.	0	0	0	0	0	0	0	0	0	0	+	+	+	0	0	0	0	0	0
C. freundii	0	0	0	0	0	0	0	0	0	0	+	+	+	0	0	0	0	0	0
C. koseri	0	0	0	0	0	+	+	+	+	0	+	+	+	0	0	0	0	0	0
E. cloacae	0	0	0	0	0	0	0	0	0	0	+	+	+	0	0	0	0	0	0
E. coli (S)	±	±	±	+	+	+	+	+	+	0	+	+	+	0	0	0	±	0	0
E. coli, ESBL	0	0	0	0	0	0	0	0	0	0	±	±	±	+	0	0	0	0	0
E. coli, Klebs KPC	0	0	0	0	0	0	0	0	0	0	±	±	±	+	0	0	0	0	0
E. coli, Klebs MBL	0	0	0	0	0	0	0	0	0	0	±	±	±	+	0	0	0	0	0
K. aerogenes	0	0	0	0	0	0	0	0	0	0	+	+	+	0	0	0	0	0	0
K. oxytoca (S)	±	±	±	+	+	+	+	+	+	0	+	+	+	0	0	0	0	0	0
K. pneumoniae (S)	±	±	±	+	+	+	+	+	+	0	+	+	+	0	0	0	0	0	0
Klebsiella sp. (ESBL)	0	0	0	0	0	0	0	0	0	0	±	±	±	+	0	0	0	0	0
M. morganii	0	0	0	0	0	±	±	±	0	±	+	+	+	0	0	0	0	0	0
P. mirabilis	+	±	+	+	+	+	+	+	+	0	+	+	+	0	0	0	0	0	0
P. vulgaris	0	0	0	0	0	+	+	+	0	0	+	+	+	0	0	0	0	0	0
Providencia sp.	0	0	0	0	0	+	+	+	0	0	±	±	+	0	0	0	0	0	0
Salmonella sp.	0	0	0	0	0	+	0	0	0	0	0	0	0	0	0	0	+	0	0
S. marcescens	0	0	0	0	0	+	0	0	0	0	+	+	+	+	0	0	0	0	0
Shigella sp.	0	0	0	0	0	+	+	+	+	0	+	+	+	0	0	0	+	0	0
Y. enterocolitica	0	0	0	0	0	+	+	0	0	0	+	+	+	0	0	0	0	0	0
Aerobic GNB - non-enterobacterales																			
Bartonella sp.	0	0	0	0	0	0	0	0	0	0	++	0	0	0	0	+	++	++	0
B. pertussis	0	0	0	0	0	0	0	0	0	0	0	0	0	0	0	+	++	++	0
B. burgdorferi	0	0	0	0	++	0	0	0	0	0	0	0	0	0	0	+	+	+	0
Brucella sp.	0	0	0	0	0	0	0	0	0	0	+	0	0	0	0	0	0	0	0
C. jejuni	0	0	0	0	0	0	0	0	0	0	+	+	+	0	0	++	++	+	0

	Tetracyclines						Glyco/Lipo						Ox-lid		Poly			Other									
	Doxycycline	Eravacycline	Minocycline	Omadacycline	Tetracycline	Tigecycline	Daptomycin	Vancomycin	Teicoplanin	Telavancin	Oritavancin	Dalbavancin	Linezolid	Tedizolid	Polymyxin B	Colistin	Lefamulin	Chloramphen	Fusidic Acid	Rif (comb)	TMP-SMX	Nitrofurantoin	Fosfomycin (IV)	Fosfomycin (po)	Pivmecillinam	Metronidazole	Pristinamycin
Aerobic GNB - enterobacterales																											
Aeromonas sp.	+	+	+	+	0	+	0	0	0	0	0	0	0	0	0	0	0	+	0	0	+	0	0	0	0	0	0
C. freundii	0	+	0	+	0	+	0	0	0	0	0	0	0	0	0	0	0	0	0	0	±	±	+	+	±	0	0
C. koseri	0	+	0	+	0	+	0	0	0	0	0	0	0	0	0	0	0	0	0	0	±	±	+	+	+	0	0
E. cloacae	0	+	0	+	0	+	0	0	0	0	0	0	0	0	0	0	0	0	0	0	+	±	±	±	+	0	0
E. coli (S)	±	+	±	+	±	+	0	0	0	0	0	0	0	0	0	0	0	+	0	0	±	+	+	+	+	0	0
E. coli, ESBL	0	+	0	+	0	+	0	0	0	0	0	0	0	0	0	0	0	±	0	0	±	±	+	+	+	0	0
E. coli, Klebs KPC	0	+	0	+	0	+	0	0	0	0	0	0	0	0	±	±	0	0	0	0	±	±	±	±	0	0	0
E. coli, Klebs MBL	0	+	0	+	0	+	0	0	0	0	0	0	0	0	±	±	0	0	0	0	0	0	±	±	0	0	0
K. aerogenes	0	+	0	+	0	+	0	0	0	0	0	0	0	0	0	0	0	0	0	0	+	±	±	±	+	0	0
K. oxytoca (S)	±	+	±	+	±	+	0	0	0	0	0	0	0	0	0	0	0	+	0	0	±	+	+	+	±	0	0
K. pneumoniae (S)	±	+	±	+	±	+	0	0	0	0	0	0	0	0	0	0	0	+	0	0	±	+	+	+	+	0	0
Klebsiella sp. (ESBL)	0	+	0	+	0	+	0	0	0	0	0	0	0	0	0	0	0	±	0	0	±	±	+	+	+	0	0
M. morganii	0	0	0	0	0	0	0	0	0	0	0	0	0	0	0	0	0	0	0	0	±	0	0	0	?	0	0
P. mirabilis	0	0	0	0	0	0	0	0	0	0	0	0	0	0	0	0	0	0	0	0	±	0	+	+	?	0	0
P. vulgaris	0	0	0	0	0	0	0	0	0	0	0	0	0	0	0	0	0	±	0	0	±	0	±	±	?	0	0
Providencia sp.	0	0	0	0	0	0	0	0	0	0	0	0	0	0	0	0	0	0	0	0	±	0	+	+	?	0	0
Salmonella sp.	0	0	0	0	0	0	0	0	0	0	0	0	0	0	0	0	0	0	0	0	±	0	0	0	0	0	0
S. marcescens	0	+	0	+	0	+	0	0	0	0	0	0	0	0	0	0	0	0	0	0	+	0	±	±	0	0	0
Shigella sp.	±	+	±	+	0	+	0	0	0	0	0	0	0	0	0	0	0	+	0	0	±	0	0	0	0	0	0
Y. enterocolitica	+	0	0	0	0	0	0	0	0	0	0	0	0	0	0	0	0	0	0	0	+	0	0	0	0	0	0
Aerobic GNB - non-enterobacterales																											
Bartonella sp.	++	0	+	0	+	0	0	0	0	0	0	0	0	0	0	0	0	0	0	±	0	0	0	0	0	0	0
B. pertussis	0	0	0	0	0	0	0	0	0	0	0	0	0	0	0	0	0	0	0	0	+	0	0	0	0	0	0
B. burgdorferi	++	0	+	0	+	0	0	0	0	0	0	0	0	0	0	0	0	0	0	0	0	0	0	0	0	0	0
Brucella sp.	+	0	+	0	+	0	0	0	0	0	0	0	0	0	0	0	0	+	0	±	+	0	0	0	0	0	0
C. jejuni	±	0	±	0	±	0	0	0	0	0	0	0	0	0	0	0	0	0	0	0	0	0	0	0	0	0	0

TABLE 4A (7)

	Oral Cephalosporins										Aminoglyco				
	Cefadroxil	Cephalexin	Cefaclor	Cefprozil	Cefurox-Axe	Cefixime	Ceftibuten	Cefpodoxime	Cefdinir	Cefditoren	Gentamicin	Tobramycin	Amikacin	Plazomicin	Clindamycin
Aerobic GNB - Non-enterobacterales *(continued)*															
Capnocytophaga sp.	0	0	0	0	0	0	0	0	0	0	±	±	±	0	++
C. burnetii	0	0	0	0	0	0	0	0	0	0	0	0	0	0	0
Ehrlichia, Anaplas	0	0	0	0	0	0	0	0	0	0	0	0	0	0	0
Eikenella sp	0	0	0	0	0	0	0	0	0	0	±	0	0	0	0
F. tularensis	0	0	0	0	0	0	0	0	0	0	++	+	0	0	0
H. ducreyi	0	0	0	0	0	0	0	0	0	0	0	0	0	0	0
H. influenzae	0	0	±	+	+	+	+	+	+	+	0	0	0	0	0
Kingella sp.	0	±	0	+	+	+	+	+	+	+	+	0	0	0	0
K. granulomatis	0	0	0	0	0	0	0	0	0	0	+	0	0	0	0
Legionella sp.	0	0	0	0	0	0	0	0	0	0	0	0	0	0	0
Leptospira sp.	0	0	0	0	0	0	0	0	0	0	0	0	0	0	0
M. catarrhalis	0	0	±	+	+	+	+	+	+	+	0	0	0	0	0
N. meningitidis	0	0	0	0	0	0	0	0	0	0	0	0	0	0	0
P. multocida	0	0	0	0	+	+	0	+	+	0	±	±	±	0	0
R. rickettsii	0	0	0	0	0	0	0	0	0	0	0	0	0	0	0
V. cholera	0	0	0	0	0	0	0	0	0	0	0	0	0	0	0
V. parahaemolyticus	0	0	0	0	0	0	0	0	0	0	0	0	0	0	0
V. vulnificus	0	0	0	0	0	0	0	0	0	0	0	0	0	0	0
Y. pestis	0	0	0	0	0	0	0	0	0	0	++	0	0	0	0
Aerobic GNB non-fermenter															
A. baumannii	0	0	0	0	0	0	0	0	0	0	0	0	±	0	0
B. cepacia	0	0	0	0	0	0	0	0	0	0	0	0	0	0	0
P. aeruginosa	0	0	0	0	0	0	0	0	0	0	0	+	±	0	0
S. maltophilia	0	0	0	0	0	0	0	0	0	0	0	0	0	0	0

	Macrolides				Tetracyclines						Glyco/Lipo					
	Erythromycin	Azithromycin	Clarithromycin	Telithromycin	Doxycycline	Eravacycline	Minocycline	Omadacycline	Tetracycline	Tigecycline	Daptomycin	Vancomycin	Teicoplanin	Telavancin	Oritavancin	Dalbavancin
Aerobic GNB - Non-enterobacterales *(continued)*																
Capnocytophaga sp.	0	0	0	0	+	0	+	0	+	0	0	0	0	0	0	0
C. burnetii	+	+	+	0	++	0	+	0	+	0	0	0	0	0	0	0
Ehrlichia, Anaplas	0	0	0	0	++	0	+	0	+	0	0	0	0	0	0	0
Eikenella sp	0	0	0	0	+	0	+	0	+	0	0	0	0	0	0	0
F. tularensis	0	0	0	0	++	0	+	0	+	0	0	0	0	0	0	0
H. ducreyi	++	++	0	0	0	0	0	0	0	0	0	0	0	0	0	0
H. influenzae	0	+	+	+	+	+	+	+	+	+	0	0	0	0	0	0
Kingella sp.	0	0	0	0	+	+	+	+	+	+	0	0	0	0	0	0
K. granulomatis	++	++	+	0	++	0	+	0	+	0	0	0	0	0	0	0
Legionella sp.	++	++	++	+	+	+	+	+	+	+	0	0	0	0	0	0
Leptospira sp.	+	++	+	0	++	0	+	0	+	0	0	0	0	0	0	0
M. catarrhalis	+	+	+	+	+	0	+	0	+	0	0	0	0	0	0	0
N. meningitidis	0	0	0	0	0	0	0	0	0	0	0	0	0	0	0	0
P. multocida	0	+	0	0	+	+	+	+	+	+	0	0	0	0	0	0
R. rickettsii	0	0	±	0	++	0	+	0	+	0	0	0	0	0	0	0
V. cholera	+	+	0	0	+	0	+	0	+	0	0	0	0	0	0	0
V. parahaemolyticus	0	+	0	0	+	0	0	0	+	0	0	0	0	0	0	0
V. vulnificus	0	0	0	0	+	0	+	0	+	0	0	0	0	0	0	0
Y. pestis	0	0	0	0	+	0	+	0	+	0	0	0	0	0	0	0
Aerobic GNB non-fermenter																
A. baumannii	0	0	0	0	0	+	±	+	±	0	0	0	0	0	0	0
B. cepacia	0	0	0	0	0	0	±	0	±	0	0	0	0	0	0	0
P. aeruginosa	0	0	0	0	0	0	0	0	0	0	0	0	0	0	0	0
S. maltophilia	0	0	0	0	+	+	+	+	0	+	0	0	0	0	0	0

	Ox-lid		Poly			Other									
	Linezolid	Tedizolid	Polymyxin B	Colistin	Lefamulin	Chloramphen	Fusidic Acid	Rif (comb)	TMP-SMX	Nitrofurantoin	Fosfomycin (IV)	Fosfomycin (po)	Pivmecillinam	Metronidazole	Pristinamycin
Aerobic GNB - Non-enterobacterales *(continued)*															
Capnocytophaga sp.	0	0	0	0	0	+	0	0	±	0	0	0	0	0	0
C. burnetii	0	0	0	0	0	+	0	±	+	0	0	0	0	0	0
Ehrlichia, Anaplas	0	0	0	0	0	±	0	±	0	0	0	0	0	0	0
Eikenella sp	0	0	0	0	0	+	0	0	0	0	0	0	0	0	0
F. tularensis	0	0	0	0	0	+	0	0	0	0	0	0	0	0	0
H. ducreyi	0	0	0	0	0	0	0	0	0	0	0	0	0	0	0
H. influenzae	0	0	0	0	+	+	0	0	+	0	+	0	0	0	0
Kingella sp.	0	0	0	0	0	+	0	0	+	0	0	0	0	0	0
K. granulomatis	0	0	0	0	0	+	0	0	++	0	0	0	0	0	0
Legionella sp.	0	0	0	0	+	0	0	±	+	0	0	0	0	0	0
Leptospira sp.	0	0	0	0	0	+	0	0	0	0	0	0	0	0	0
M. catarrhalis	0	0	0	0	+	0	0	0	+	0	0	0	0	0	0
N. meningitidis	0	0	0	0	0	+	0	0	0	0	0	0	0	0	0
P. multocida	0	0	0	0	0	0	0	0	+	0	0	0	0	0	0
R. rickettsii	0	0	0	0	0	+	0	0	0	0	0	0	0	0	0
V. cholera	0	0	0	0	0	0	0	0	0	0	0	0	0	0	0
V. parahaemolyticus	0	0	0	0	0	+	0	0	0	0	0	0	0	0	0
V. vulnificus	0	0	0	0	0	+	0	0	0	0	0	0	0	0	0
Y. pestis	0	0	0	0	0	+	0	0	+	0	0	0	0	0	0
Aerobic GNB non-fermenter															
A. baumannii	0	0	±	±	0	0	0	0	±	0	0	0	0	0	0
B. cepacia	0	0	0	0	0	±	0	0	+	0	0	0	0	0	0
P. aeruginosa	0	0	±	±	0	0	0	0	0	0	±	±	0	0	0
S. maltophilia	0	0	±	±	0	+	0	0	++	0	0	0	0	0	0

TABLE 4A (8)

	Oral Cephalosporins										Aminoglyco					Macrolides			
	Cefadroxil	Cephalexin	Cefaclor	Cefprozil	Cefurox-Axe	Cefixime	Ceftibuten	Cefpodoxime	Cefdinir	Cefditoren	Gentamicin	Tobramycin	Amikacin	Plazomicin	Clindamycin	Erythromycin	Azithromycin	Clarithromycin	Telithromycin
Aerobic - cell wall-deficient																			
C. trachomatis	0	0	0	0	0	0	0	0	0	0	0	0	0	0	0	+	++	+	0
Chlamydophila sp.	0	0	0	0	0	0	0	0	0	0	0	0	0	0	0	+	+	+	+
M. pneumoniae	0	0	0	0	0	0	0	0	0	0	0	0	0	0	0	±	±	±	±
Anaerobic GNB																			
B. fragilis	0	0	0	0	0	0	0	0	0	0	0	0	0	0	0	0	0	0	0
F. necrophorum	0	0	0	0	0	0	0	0	0	0	0	0	0	0	+	0	0	0	0
Prevotella sp	0	0	0	0	0	0	0	0	0	0	0	0	0	0	+	±	±	±	0
Anaerobic gram-positive																			
Actinomyces sp.	0	0	0	0	0	0	0	0	0	0	0	0	0	0	++	++	+	+	0
Clostridium sp.	0	0	0	0	0	0	0	0	0	0	0	0	0	0	+	+	+	+	0
C. acnes	+	0	0	+	+	0	0	0	0	0	0	0	0	0	±	±	±	±	0
Peptostreptococci	+	+	+	+	+	+	+	+	0	0	0	0	0	0	+	±	±	±	0

	Tetracyclines						Glyco/Lipo						Ox-lid		Poly			Other									
	Doxycycline	Eravacycline	Minocycline	Omadacycline	Tetracycline	Tigecycline	Daptomycin	Vancomycin	Teicoplanin	Telavancin	Oritavancin	Dalbavancin	Linezolid	Tedizolid	Polymyxin B	Colistin	Lefamulin	Chloramphen	Fusidic Acid	Rif (comb)	TMP-SMX	Nitrofurantoin	Fosfomycin (IV)	Fosfomycin (po)	Pivmecillinam	Metronidazole	Pristinamycin
Aerobic - cell wall-deficient																											
C. trachomatis	++	0	+	0	+	0	0	0	0	0	0	0	0	0	0	0	0	0	0	0	0	0	0	0	0	0	0
Chlamydophila sp.	++	+	+	+	+	+	0	0	0	0	0	0	0	0	0	0	+	+	0	±	0	0	0	0	0	0	0
M. pneumoniae	++	+	++	+	++	+	0	0	0	0	0	0	0	0	0	0	+	0	0	0	0	0	0	0	0	0	0
Anaerobic GNB																											
B. fragilis	±	+	±	+	±	+	0	0	0	0	0	0	0	0	0	0	0	+	0	0	0	0	0	0	0	++	0
F. necrophorum	+	+	+	+	+	+	0	0	0	0	0	0	0	0	0	0	0	+	0	0	0	0	0	0	0	++	0
Prevotella sp	+	+	+	+	+	+	0	0	0	0	0	0	0	0	0	0	0	+	0	0	0	0	0	0	0	++	0
Anaerobic gram-positive																											
Actinomyces sp.	+	0	+	0	+	0	0	0	0	0	0	0	+	0	0	0	0	+	0	0	0	0	0	0	0	0	0
Clostridium sp.	+	+	+	+	+	+	±	+	+	+	+	+	+	0	0	0	0	+	0	0	0	0	0	0	0	+	0
C. acnes	+	+	+	+	+	+	+	+	+	+	+	+	+	0	0	0	0	0	0	0	±	0	0	0	0	0	0
Peptostreptococci	+	+	+	+	+	+	+	+	+	+	+	+	+	0	0	0	0	+	0	0	0	0	+	0	0	±	0

TABLE 4B – ANTIFUNGAL ACTIVITY SPECTRA

	Antifungal Drugs									
	Fluconazole	Itraconazole	Voriconazole	Posaconazole	Isavuconazonium sulfate	Anidulafungin	Caspofungin	Micafungin	Rezafungin	Amphotericin B
Fungi										
Aspergillus fumigatus	0	±	++	++	++	±	±	±	0	+
Aspergillus niger	0	±	++	++	++	±	±	±	0	+
Aspergillus terreus	0	±	++	++	++	±	±	±	0	0
Aspergillus flavus	0	±	++	++	++	±	±	±	0	+
Candida albicans	++	+	+	+	+	++	++	++	++	+
Candida auris	0	±	±	±	±	++	++	++	+	±
Candida dubliniensis	++	+	+	+	+	++	++	++	+	++
Candida glabrata	±	±	±	±	±	++	++	++	++	++
Candida guilliermondii	++	++	++	++	+	++	++	++	+	++
Candida krusei	0	0	+	+	+	++	++	++	+	++
Candida lusitaniae	++	+	+	+	+	++	++	++	+	0
Candida parapsilosis	++	+	+	+	+	+	+	+	++	++
Candida tropicalis	++	+	+	+	+	++	++	++	++	++
Cryptococcosis	++	+	+	+	+	0	0	0	0	++
Dematiaceous molds	0	++	++	+	+	±	±	±	0	+
Fusarium sp.	0	±	±	±	±	0	0	0	0	±
Mucormycosis	0	0	0	+	+	0	0	0	0	++
Scedo apiospermum	0	0	++	+	0	0	0	0	0	0
Lomentospora prolificans	0	0	+	0	0	0	0	0	0	0
Talaromyces marneffei	0	++	++	0	0	0	0	0	0	++
Trichosporon spp.	±	+	+	+	+	0	0	0	0	+
Dimorphic Fungi										
Blastomycosis	±	++	+	+	+	0	0	0	0	++
Coccidiomycosis	++	++	+	+	+	0	0	0	0	++
Histoplasmosis	±	++	+	+	+	0	0	0	0	++
Sporotrichosis	±	++	+	+	+	0	0	0	0	++

TABLE 5A – TREATMENT OPTIONS FOR SYSTEMIC INFECTION DUE TO MULTI-DRUG RESISTANT GRAM-POSITIVE BACTERIA

ORGANISM	RESISTANT TO	PRIMARY TREATMENT OPTIONS	ALTERNATIVE TREATMENT OPTIONS	COMMENTS
Enterococcus faecium; Enterococcus faecalis (Consultation suggested) For review of VRE treatment: *Infect Dis Clin North Am 30:415, 2016.*	Vancomycin (VRE), Ampicillin, Penicillin G, Gentamicin (high level resistance)	**E. faecium**, systemic infection, bacteremia: **Dapto** 10-12 mg/kg IV q24h + (**AMP** 2 gm IV q4h OR **Ceftaroline** 600 mg IV q8h) **Linezolid** 600 mg po/IV q12h OR **AMP** 2 gm IV q4h	**E. faecalis**: Resistance to AMP or Pen rare. If aminoglycoside resistance: **AMP** 2 gm IV q4h + **Ceftriaxone** 2 gm IV q12h. If Pen-resistant due to beta-lactamase (extremely rare): **Dapto** 8-12 mg/kg IV q12h + **Amp** 2 gm IV q 4h or **Ceftaroline** 600 mg IV q8h	Addition of a beta lactam to Dapto reverses Dapto resistance & impedes development of resistance. Linezolid preferred for treatment of VRE infections if Dapto MIC > 4 µg/ml. Oritavancin and tigecycline active against VRE in vitro but limited data on efficacy.
Staphylococcus aureus *(See Table 6 for more details)*	Vancomycin (VISA or VRSA) and all beta lactams (except Ceftaroline)	**Dapto** 10-12 mg/kg IV q24h or (**Dapto** 10-12 mg/kg IV q24h + **Ceftaroline** 600 mg IV q8h) *(AAC 56:5296, 2012)*	**Telavancin** 10 mg/kg IV q24h or **Linezolid** 600 mg IV/po q12h	**Confirm dapto susceptibility** as VISA strains may be non-susceptible. If prior vanco therapy (or persistent infection on vanco) there is significant chance of developing resistance to dapto *(JAC 66:1696, 2011).*
Streptococcus pneumoniae	Penicillin G (MIC ≥4 µg/mL)	If no meningitis: **Ceftriaxone** 2 gm IV once daily OR **Ceftaroline** 600 mg IV q12h OR **Linezolid** 600 mg IV/po q12h	Meningitis: **Vanco** 30-60 mg/kg/d in 2-3 div doses (target AUC24 400-600 µg/mL x h) + **Ceftriaxone** 2 gm q12h or **MER** 2 gm IV q8h	Ceftriaxone 2 gm IV q12h should also work for meningitis for strains with Ceftriaxone MIC ≤ 0.5 mcg/mL.

TABLE 5B – ANTIBACTERIAL TREATMENT: PRESUMED OR CONFIRMED ENTEROBACTERALES PRODUCING EXTENDED-SPECTRUM BETA-LACTAMASES (ESBL)

Recommendations assume in vitro susceptibility to drugs listed. ESBL production detected by phenotypic pattern of in vitro resistance: e.g., ceftriaxone MIC ≥2 µg/mL. Can confirm ESBL production with detection of ESBL genes: e.g., bla_{CTX-M}, bla_{SHV}. Ref: *IDSA 2023 Guidance on the Treatment of Antimicrobial Resistant Gram-Negative Infections, CID 18 Jul 2023, https://doi.org/10.1093/cid/ciad428*

ESBLs inactivate most penicillins, cephalosporins and aztreonam

Clinical Syndrome	Primary Therapy	Alternative Therapy	Comments
Cystitis (Cystitis over-diagnosed: confirm actual infection before treating.)	**Nitrofurantoin**; **TMP/SMX** if susceptible	Single dose **aminoglycoside**; **fosfomycin** if susceptible E. coli; **CIP** or **Levo**; **Erta**; **MER**; **IMP** **Pivmecillinam** 185 mg po tid x 3-7 days	Aminoglycoside single dose *(AAC 2019;63:e0216518)* Amox-clav, CIP, or Levo may work even for non-susceptible strains because of high urine concentrations. Try to reserve carbapenems for multidrug resistant bacteria.
Pyelonephritis or cUTI Any UTI in a male is complicated. Look for structural or functional disease of urinary tract.	**Erta**; **MER**; **IMP**	If suscept., switch from carbapenem to **CIP, Levo** or **TMP/SMX** if susceptible in vitro. Avoid Moxi (low urine concentrations). Ceftolozane-tazobactam also an option and carbapenem sparing	All have high concentrations in urine. Do not use nitrofurantoin or Fosfomycin (inadequate renal concentrations; doxycycline has low urine concentrations)
Non-urinary tract infections	**Erta**; **IMP**; **MER**	If susceptible in vitro plus source control, can switch to oral **CIP, Levo** or **TMP/SMX**	**Avoid both piperacillin/tazobactam and cefepime even if targeted organism is susceptible in vitro**

TABLE 5C – SUGGESTED SPECIFIC ANTIBACTERIAL THERAPY: CARBAPENEM-RESISTANT ENTEROBACTERALES

Expert panel does not recommend combination therapy for treatment of carbapenem-resistant Enterobacterales. Recommendations assume demonstrable in vitro susceptibility.
Ref: *IDSA 2023 Guidance on the Treatment of Antimicrobial Resistant Gram-Negative Infections, CID 18 Jul 2023, https://doi.org/10.1093/cid/ciad428*

Clinical Syndrome	Primary Therapy	Alternative Therapy	Comments
Cystitis (Cystitis over-diagnosed: confirm actual infection before treating.)	**Nitrofurantoin**; **CIP**, **Levo**, **TMP/SMX** if susceptible.	**Fosfomycin**, if susceptible *E. coli*; **Ceftaz-avi**; **Mero-vabor**; **IMP-rele** or **Cefiderocol** If susceptible: **CIP**, **Levo** or **TMP-SMX**	Colistin, only if no alternative; do not use polymyxin B (low urine concentrations) Erta resistant, Mero susceptible strains are not resistant due to production of carbapenemases
Pyelonephritis or cUTI	**Ceftaz-avi**; **MER-vabor**; **IMP-rele**, **cefiderocol** If Erta resistant, Mero susceptible and neg for carbapenemase, can use mero with extended (3 hr) infusion	Once daily **Gent** or another aminoglycoside (**Tobra**, **AMK**, **plazomicin**) If susceptible: **CIP**, **Levo** or **TMP-SMX**	Avoid meropenem alone if phenotypic or genotypic positive for production of carbapenemase
Non-UTI infection due to ertapenem-resistant but meropenem-susceptible organism	**MER** okay as resistance is not due to carbapenemase		Should have neg carbapenemase test result
Non-UTI infection due to resistance to both meropenem & ertapenem: possible serine carbapenemase KPC (Klebsiella-producing carbapenemase - *see Comment)*	**Ceftaz-avi**; **MER-vabor**; **IMP-rele**	**Cefiderocol**, caution, sparse data **Eravacycline** (if intra-abdominal infection)	Carbapenemase test not done or result not available. Treat as if carbapenemase-positive Majority of carbapenemase-producing Enterobacterales in U.S. are Klebsiella-producing carbapenemase (KPCs)
Metallo-beta-lactamase carbapenemase detected (see Comment)	**Ceftaz-avi** + **Aztreonam** ± **Cefiderocol** (only if susceptible in vitro: *CID 2022;75:1081 & 1085*)	**Eravacycline** (if intra-abdominal infection) (active in vitro, but sparse clinical data)	Example enzymes: NDM, VIM or IMP. Treatment listed also effective vs KPCs and OXA-48 enzymes
OXA-48-like carbapenemase producers detected	**Ceftaz-avi**	**Cefiderocol** **Eravacycline** (if intra-abdominal infection) (active in vitro, but sparse clinical data)	

TABLE 5D – TREATMENT OPTIONS FOR DIFFICULT TO TREAT PSEUDOMONAS AERUGINOSA

Assumes in vitro susceptibility to suggested drugs. **"Difficult to treat" means non-susceptibility to: piperacillin/tazobactam, ceftazidime, cefepime, aztreonam, meropenem, imipenem/cilastatin, ciprofloxacin, and levofloxacin.** Ref: *IDSA 2023 Guidance on the Treatment of Antimicrobial Resistant Gram-Negative Infections, CID 18 Jul 2023, https://doi.org/10.1093/cid/ciad428*

Clinical Syndrome	Primary Therapy	Alternative Therapy	Comments
Cystitis	**Ceftolo-tazo**; **Ceftaz-avi**; **IMP-rele; Cefiderocol**	**Tobramycin** or **Amikacin** x 1 dose	Note: avoid polymyxin B due to low concentrations in the urine
Pyelonephritis or cUTI	**Ceftolo-tazo**; **Ceftaz-avi**; **IMP-rele**; **Cefiderocol**	Once daily aminoglycoside: **Tobramycin, Amikacin, Plazomicin**	Avoid Fosfomycin due to resistance and low renal concentrations. Note absence of activity of MER-vabor
Infection other than the urinary tract	**Ceftolo-tazo**; **Ceftaz-avi**; **IMP-rele**	**Cefiderocol**	Combination therapy used for empiric therapy; not recommended for specific therapy. MER-vabor is NOT recommended

TABLE 5E – TREATMENT OPTIONS FOR AMP C BETA-LACTAMASE PRODUCING ENTEROBACTERALES, CARBAPENEM-RESISTANT ACINETOBACTER BAUMANNII, AND STENOTROPHOMONAS MALTOPHILIA

Treatment recommendations assume demonstrated in vitro susceptibility. Ref: *IDSA 2023 Guidance on the Treatment of Antimicrobial Resistant Gram-Negative Infections, CID 18 Jul 2023, https://doi.org/10.1093/cid/ciad428*

Pathogen(s) Detected	Microbiology: Resistance	Suggested Treatments		Comments	Other Rx options
		Primary	Alternative		
Amp C beta-lactamase producing Enterobacterales	Beta-lactamase production may be constitutive or inducible. Inducible AmpC production *E. cloacae, K. aerogenes, C. freundii*	**CFP** if MIC ≤ 2 **TMP/SMX**, **CIP**, or **Levo**	Avoid CFP if MIC >2. Use a carbapenem (**Erta**, **IMP** or **MER**)	Avoid ceftriaxone due to risk of inducing ß-lactamase production Avoid pip/tazo due to weak activity of tazobactam to block hydrolysis by Amp C	• Cystitis: TMP/SMX, nitrofurantoin, single-dose aminoglycoside • Systemic infection: fluoroquinolone
Carbapenem-resistant *Acinetobacter baumannii* (CRAB): moderate to severe infections	Often assoc. resistance to other beta-lactams, aminoglycosides, fluoroquinolones. No "standard of care" antibiotic regimen	(**Sulbactam** 1 gm IV + **Durlobactam** 1 gm IV + **IMP** 1 gm IV) q6h *(see Lancet ID 2023; 23:1072)*	**Cefiderocol** 2 gm IV over 3h q8h + **Minocycline** 200 mg IV/po q12h	Do not include rifampin or fosfomycin in combination therapies Combination therapy recommended for moderately severe or severe infection.	• Minocycline PK/PD results indicate FDA-approved max dose may be inadequate if MIC is > 1 µg/ml *(AAC 2021;65:e01809)*
Stenotrophomonas maltophilia: moderate to severe infection	Produces beta-lactamases that hydrolyze all beta-lactams. Resistant to aminoglycosides, tetracyclines, & FQs.	Combination therapy with any two of the following agents: **TMP-SMX** (8-12 mg/kg/d IV/po 2-3 divided doses), **Levo** (750 mg IV/po q24h), **Minocycline** (200 mg IV/po q12h), or **Cefiderocol** 2 g IV q8h infused over 3 hours) *(Clin Infect Dis 2024; Aug. 7, online ahead of print)*	**Ceftazidime-avibactam** 2.5 gm IV over 3h q8h + **Aztreonam** 2 gm IV over 2h q8h	No "standard of care" antibiotic regimen **For mild infections and polymicrobial infections** where the role of S. maltophilia is unclear: monotherapy with TMP-SMX, Levofloxacin, Minocycline, or Cefiderocol	Avoid ceftazidime alone regardless of in vitro susceptibility results

TABLE 6 – SUGGESTED MANAGEMENT OF SUSPECTED OR CULTURE-POSITIVE METHICILLIN-RESISTANT S. AUREUS INFECTIONS

IDSA Guidelines: *CID 52 (Feb 1):1, 2011.*

NOTE: Distinction between community and hospital strains of MRSA blurring.

CLINICAL ILLNESS	ABSCESS, NO IMMUNOSUPPRESSION, OUT-PATIENT CARE	PNEUMONIA	BACTEREMIA OR POSSIBLE ENDOCARDITIS OR BACTEREMIC SHOCK	TREATMENT FAILURE *(See footnote[2])*
Management *Drug doses in footnote[1].*	**TMP/SMX** 1 DS (2 DS if BMI >40) po bid OR **Clinda** 300 mg (450 mg for BMI >40) po tid *(NEJM 372:1093, 2015).* For larger abscesses, multiple lesions or systemic inflammatory response: **I&D** + (**Oritavancin** 1200 mg x 1 or **Dalbavancin** 1000 mg x 1 than 500 mg x 1 a wk later) an option for outpatient management of sicker patients with more extensive infection who might otherwise be admitted *(see NEJM 370:2180, 2014, NEJM 370:2169, 2014).*	**Vanco** IV or **Linezolid** IV	**Vanco** 30-60 mg/kg/d in 2-3 div doses, target AUC_{24} 400-600 µg/mL x h **Dapto** 8-12 mg/kg q24h.	**Dapto** 8-12 mg/kg IV q24h; confirm in vitro susceptibility as prior vanco therapy may select for daptomycin non-susceptibility (MIC >1 µg/mL) & some VISA strains are daptomycin non-susceptible. **Use combination therapy for bacteremia or endocarditis:** dapto + beta-lactam combination therapy [**Dapto** 8-12 mg/kg IV q24h + **Ceftaroline** 600 mg IV q8h] appears effective against MRSA strains as salvage therapy. **Linezolid** 600 mg IV/po q12h (Linezolid is bacteriostatic and should not be used as a single agent in suspected endovascular infection). **Telavancin** 10 mg/kg q24h IV.
Comments	**Fusidic acid** 500 mg tid (where available) + **RIF** also an option; do not use rifampin alone as resistance rapidly emerges. Patients not responding after 2-3 days should be evaluated for complicated infection and switched to **Vancomycin**.	Prospective study of **Linezolid** vs **Vanco** showed slightly higher cure rate with Linezolid, no difference in mortality *(CID 54:621, 2012).*	TMP-SMX **NOT** recommended in bacteremic pts; inferior to Vanco *(BMJ 350:2219, 2015).* Adjunctive rifampin did not improve outcomes in patients with *S. aureus* bacteremia *(Lancet 391:668, 2018).*	

[1] **Clindamycin:** 300 mg po tid. **Daptomycin:** 6 mg/kg IV q24h is the standard, FDA-approved dose for bacteremia and endocarditis but 8-12 mg/kg q24h is recommended by some and for treatment failures. **Doxycycline or Minocycline:** 100 mg po bid. **Linezolid:** 600 mg po/IV bid. **Rifampin:** Long serum half-life justifies dosing 600 mg po q24h; however, frequency of nausea less with 300 mg po bid. **TMP-SMX-DS:** Standard dose 8–10 mg per kg per day. For 70 kg person = 700 mg TMP component per day. **TMP-SMX** contains 160 mg TMP and 800 mg SMX. The dose for treatment of CA-MRSA skin and soft tissue infections (SSTI) is 1 DS tablet twice daily. **Vancomycin:** 30-60 mg/kg/d in 2-3 div doses, target AUC_{24} 400-600 µg/mL x h for serious infections.

[2] The median duration of bacteremia in endocarditis is 7-9 days in patients treated with vancomycin *(AnIM 115:674, 1991).* Longer duration of bacteremia, greater likelihood of endocarditis *(JID 190:1140, 2004).* Definition of failure unclear. Clinical response should be factored in. **Unsatisfactory clinical response especially if blood cultures remain positive >4 days.**

TABLE 7 – ANTIBIOTIC HYPERSENSITIVITY REACTIONS & DRUG DESENSITIZATION METHODS

Penicillin. Oral route (Pen VK) preferred. 1/3 pts develop transient reaction, usually mild. **Perform in ICU setting. Discontinue β-blockers. Have IV line, epinephrine, ECG, spirometer available.** Desensitization works as long as pt is receiving Pen; allergy returns after discontinuance. History of Steven-Johnson, exfoliative dermatitis, erythroderma are contraindications. Skin testing for evaluation of Pen allergy: Testing with major determinant (benzyl Pen polylysine) and minor determinants has negative predictive value (97-99%). Risk of systemic reaction to skin testing <1% *(Ann Allergy Asth Immunol 106:1, 2011)*. General refs: *CID 58:1140, 2014*.

- **Method:** Prepare dilutions using **Pen-VK** oral soln, 250 mg/5 mL. Administer each dose @ 15 min intervals in 30 mL water/flavored bev. After Step 14 observe pt for 30 min, then give full therapeutic dose by route of choice. Ref: *Allergy, Prin & Prac, Mosby, 1993, pg. 1726.*

Step	Dilution (mg/mL)	mL Administered	Dose/Step		Cumulative Dose Given	
			mg	units	mg	units
1	0.5	0.1	0.05	80	0.05	80
2	0.5	0.2	0.1	160	0.15	240
3	0.5	0.4	0.2	320	0.35	560
4	0.5	0.8	0.4	640	0.75	1,200
5	0.5	1.6	0.8	1,280	1.55	2,480
6	0.5	3.2	1.6	2,560	3.15	5,040
7	0.5	6.4	3.2	5,120	6.35	10,160
8	5	1.2	6	9,600	12.35	19,760
9	5	2.4	12	19,200	24.35	38,960
10	5	4.8	24	38,400	48.35	77,360
11	50	1	50	80,000	98.35	157,360
12	50	2	100	160,000	198.35	317,360
13	50	4	200	320,000	398.35	637,360
14	50	8	400	640,000	798.35	1,277,360

TMP-SMX. Perform in hospital/clinic. Refs: *CID 20:849, 1995; AIDS 5:311, 1991.*

- **Method:** Use **TMP-SMX** oral susp, (40 mg TMP/200 mg SMX)/5 mL. Take with 6 oz water after each dose. Corticosteroids, antihistaminics NOT used.

Hour	Dose (TMP/SMX) (mg)
	0.004/0.02
1	0.04/0.2
2	0.4/2
3	4/20
4	40/200
5	160/800

Penicillin. Parenteral (Pen G) route. Follow procedures/notes under Oral (Pen-VK) route. Ref: *Allergy, Prin & Prac, Mosby, 1993, pg. 1726.*

- **Method:** Administer **Pen G** IM, IV or sc as follows:

Step	Dilution (units/mL)	mL Administered	Dose/Step (units)	Cumulative Dose Given (units)
1	100	0.2	20	20
2		0.4	40	60
3		0.8	80	140
4	1,000	0.2	200	340
5		0.4	400	740
6		0.8	800	1,540
7	10,000	0.2	2,000	3,540
8		0.4	4,000	7,540
9		0.8	8,000	15,540
10	100,000	0.2	20,000	35,540
11		0.4	40,000	75,540
12		0.8	80,000	155,540
13	1,000,000	0.2	200,000	355,540
14		0.4	400,000	755,540
15		0.8	800,000	1,555,540

Ceftriaxone. Ref: *Allergol Immunopathol (Madr) 37:105, 2009.*

- **Method:** Infuse **Ceftriaxone** IV @ 20 min intervals as follows:

Day	Dose (mg)
1	0.001, then 0.01, then 0.1, then 1
2	1, then 5, then 10, then 50
3	100, then 250, then 500
4	1000

Desensitization Methods for Other Drugs (References)

- **Ceftazidime.** *Curr Opin All Clin Immunol 6(6): 476, 2006.*
- **Ceftazidime-avibactam.** *Fed Pract 2022:39:94*
- **Ceftaroline.** *Open Forum Infect Dis 2:1, 2015.*
- **Clindamycin.** *J Allergy Clin Immunol Pract 2018;6:2141.*
- **Colistin.** *Ann Allergy Asthma Immunol 2019;123:607.*
- **Daptomycin.** *Ann All Asthma Immun 100:87, 2008.*
- **Doxycycline.** *ID Cases 11:70, 2018; Ann Allergy Asthma Immunol 111:73, 2013.*
- **Entecavir.** *Ann Allergy Asthma Immunol 2019;123:312.*
- **Flucloxacillin.** *AAC 2018;62:e01371-18.*
- **Imipenem-Cilastatin.** *Ann Pharmacother 37:513, 2003.*
- **Liposomal Amphotericin B.** *J Allergy Clin Immunol Pract 5:181, 2017.*
- **Meropenem.** *Ann Pharmacother 37:1424, 2003.*
- **Metronidazole.** *Allergy Rhinol 5:1, 2014.*
- **Valganciclovir.** *Transplantation 98:e50, 2014.*
- **Vancomycin.** *Ann Pharmacother 2001;35:1458.*
- General review, including desensitization protocols for **Amp, Cefepime, CIP, Clarithro, Clinda, Dapto, Linezolid, Tobra** *(CID 58:1140, 2014)*.

TABLE 7 (2)

Ceftaroline. 12-step IV desensitization protocol. Ref: *Open Forum Infect Dis 2:1, 2015.*

- Method: Cumulative drug infused: 600 mg. Total time required for all 12 steps: 318 minutes.

Step	Conc (mg/mL)	Vol infused (mL)	Infusion duration (min)	Drug infused this step (mg)	Cumulative drug infused (mg)
1	0.0002	5	15	0.001	0.001
2	0.0002	15	15	0.003	0.004
3	0.002	5	15	0.01	0.014
4	0.002	15	15	0.03	0.04
5	0.02	5	15	0.1	0.14
6	0.02	15	15	0.3	0.4
7	0.2	5	15	1	1.4
8	0.2	15	15	3	4.4
9	2	5	15	10	14.4
10	2	15	15	30	44.4
11	2	25	15	50	94.4
12	2	255	153	510	604.4

Valganciclovir. 12-step oral desensitization protocol. Ref: *Transplantation 98:e50, 2014.*

- Method: Administer doses at 15-minute intervals; entire protocol takes 165 minutes. Cumulative dose administered: 453.6 mg

Step	Drug administered this step (mg)	Cumulative drug administered (mg)
1	0.1	0.1
2	0.2	0.3
3	0.4	0.7
4	0.8	1.5
5	1.6	3.1
6	3.5	6.6
7	7	13.6
8	14	27.6
9	28	55.6
10	58	113.6
11	115	228.6
12	225	453.6

TABLE 8A – PREGNANCY RISK AND SAFETY IN LACTATION

Note: Some drugs, e.g., Amikacin, Dapsone and Rifampin have activity in multiple categories. For space reasons, there is only one entry per drug in the table - the primary category for the drug. Example: Rifampin is found under Antimycobacterials.

Groups/Drugs	FDA Pregnancy Risk[1]	Use during Lactation
Antibacterials		
Amikacin	D	Probably safe, monitor infant for GI toxicity.
Amoxicillin	No evidence of toxicity in humans or animals	Milk concentrations low, adverse effects not expected. Monitor infant for GI toxicity.
Amoxicillin-clavulanate	No evidence of toxicity in humans or animals	Milk concentrations low, adverse effects not expected. Monitor infant for GI toxicity.
Ampicillin	No evidence of toxicity in humans or animals	Milk concentrations low, adverse effects not expected. Monitor infant for GI toxicity.
Ampicillin-sulbactam	No evidence of toxicity in humans or animals	Milk concentrations low, adverse effects not expected. Monitor infant for GI toxicity.
Azithromycin	Humans: no evidence of toxicity. Animals: some evidence of decreased viability and delayed development in rats.	Safe, monitor infant for GI toxicity.
Aztreonam	B	Milk concentrations low, adverse effects not expected. Monitor infant for GI toxicity.
Aztreonam-avibactam	No evidence of toxicity in humans or animals	Aztreonam: milk concentrations low. Avibactam: no data.
Cefaclor	No evidence of toxicity in humans or animals	Milk concentrations low, adverse effects not expected. Monitor infant for GI toxicity.
Cefadroxil	No evidence of toxicity in humans or animals	Milk concentrations low, adverse effects not expected. Monitor infant for GI toxicity.
Cefazolin	No evidence of toxicity in humans or animals	Milk concentrations low, adverse effects not expected. Monitor infant for GI toxicity.
Cefdinir	No evidence of toxicity in humans or animals	No data, but adverse effects not expected. Monitor infant for GI toxicity.
Cefditoren pivoxil	No evidence of toxicity in humans or animals	No data, but adverse effects not expected. Monitor infant for GI toxicity.
Cefepime	No evidence of toxicity in humans or animals	Milk concentrations low, adverse effects not expected. Monitor infant for GI toxicity.
Cefepime-enmetazobactam	Cefepime: No evidence of toxicity in humans or animals. Enmetazobactam: No data.	Milk concentrations low, adverse effects not expected. Monitor infant for GI toxicity.
Cefiderocol	No evidence of toxicity in humans or animals	No data, but adverse effects not expected. Monitor infant for GI toxicity.
Cefixime	No evidence of toxicity in humans or animals	Milk concentrations low, adverse effects not expected. Monitor infant for GI toxicity.
Cefmetazole	No evidence of toxicity in humans or animals	No data.
Cefoperazone	No evidence of toxicity in humans or animals	Milk concentrations low, adverse effects not expected. Monitor infant for GI toxicity.
Cefoperazone-sulbactam	No evidence of toxicity in humans or animals	Milk concentrations low, adverse effects not expected. Monitor infant for GI toxicity.
Cefotaxime	No evidence of toxicity in humans or animals	Milk concentrations low, adverse effects not expected. Monitor infant for GI toxicity.
Cefotetan	No evidence of toxicity in humans or animals	Milk concentrations low, adverse effects not expected. Monitor infant for GI toxicity.
Cefoxitin	No evidence of toxicity in humans or animals	Milk concentrations low, adverse effects not expected. Monitor infant for GI toxicity.
Cefpirome	No evidence of toxicity in humans or animals	No data.
Cefpodoxime proxetil	No evidence of toxicity in humans or animals	Milk concentrations low, adverse effects not expected. Monitor infant for GI toxicity.
Cefprozil	No evidence of toxicity in humans or animals	Milk concentrations low, adverse effects not expected. Monitor infant for GI toxicity.
Ceftaroline	No evidence of toxicity in humans or animals	No data, but adverse effects not expected. Monitor infant for GI toxicity.
Ceftazidime	No evidence of toxicity in humans or animals	Milk concentrations low, adverse effects not expected. Monitor infant for GI toxicity.
Ceftazidime-avibactam	No evidence of toxicity in humans or animals	Ceftazidime: milk concentrations low. Avibactam: no data.
Ceftibuten	No evidence of toxicity in humans or animals	Milk concentrations low, adverse effects not expected. Monitor infant for GI toxicity.
Ceftobiprole medocaril	No evidence of toxicity in humans or animals	No data, but adverse effects not expected. Monitor infant for GI toxicity.
Ceftizoxime	No evidence of toxicity in humans or animals	Milk concentrations low, adverse effects not expected. Monitor infant for GI toxicity.
Ceftolozane-tazobactam	No evidence of toxicity in humans or animals	Milk concentrations low, adverse effects not expected. Monitor infant for GI toxicity.
Ceftriaxone	No evidence of toxicity in humans or animals	Milk concentrations low, adverse effects not expected. Monitor infant for GI toxicity.
Cefuroxime	No evidence of toxicity in humans or animals	Milk concentrations low, adverse effects not expected. Monitor infant for GI toxicity.

Groups/Drugs	FDA Pregnancy Risk[1]	Use during Lactation
Antibacterials *(continued)*		
Cefuroxime axetil	No evidence of toxicity in humans or animals	Milk concentrations low, adverse effects not expected. Monitor infant for GI toxicity.
Cephalexin	No evidence of toxicity in humans or animals	Milk concentrations low, adverse effects not expected. Monitor infant for GI toxicity.
Chloramphenicol	C	Avoid use.
Ciprofloxacin	C	Avoid breastfeeding for 3-4 hrs after a dose, monitor infant for GI toxicity.
Clarithromycin	C	Safe, monitor for GI toxicity.
Clindamycin	Humans: no evidence of toxicity with 2nd or 3rd trimester use. Insufficient data with 1st trimester use. Animals: no evidence of toxicity.	Avoid use if possible, otherwise monitor infant for GI toxicity.
Cloxacillin	No evidence of toxicity in humans or animals	Milk concentrations low, adverse effects not expected. Monitor infant for GI toxicity.
Colistin (polymyxin E)	C	Probably safe with monitoring, but data limited.
Dalbavancin	No human data. Toxic in rats at 3.5x human exposure.	Probably safe with monitoring, but no data available.
Daptomycin	B	Probably safe with monitoring, but data limited.
Delafloxacin	No evidence of toxicity in humans or animals	No data, avoid use.
Dicloxacillin	No evidence of toxicity in humans or animals	Milk concentrations low, adverse effects not expected. Monitor infant for GI toxicity.
Doripenem	B	Probably safe with monitoring, but no data available.
Doxycycline	Avoid in 2nd and 3rd TM due to risk of permanent teeth discoloration or inhibition of bone growth. No evidence of substantial teratogenic risk if used in 1st TM, but data insufficient to conclude no risk.	Short-term use safe, monitor infant for GI toxicity.
Eravacycline	Avoid during 2nd and 3rd trimesters	Mfr suggests no breastfeeding during treatment and for 4 days after last dose. However, milk conc are likely low and absorption inhibited by calcium in breast milk. Short-term use is acceptable in nursing mothers; monitor infant for GI toxicity.
Ertapenem	Human data insufficient. Nontoxic in animals.	Safe, monitor infant for GI toxicity.
Erythromycin	B	Safe, monitor infant for GI toxicity.
Fidaxomicin	Human data insufficient. Nontoxic in animals.	Probably safe, but no data available.
Flucloxacillin	No evidence of toxicity in humans or animals	Safe, monitor infant for GI toxicity.
Fosfomycin PO	B	Probably safe with monitoring, but data limited.
Fosfomycin IV	No human data. No evidence of toxicity in animals.	Low quantities found in breast milk. Probably safe with monitoring of infant for GI toxicity, but data are limited.
Fusidic acid	-	Safety not established, avoid use.
Gatifloxacin	C	Short-term use safe, monitor infant for GI toxicity; avoid if possible.
Gemifloxacin	C	Short-term use safe, monitor infant for GI toxicity; avoid if possible.
Gentamicin	D	Probably safe, monitor infant for GI toxicity.
Imipenem-cilastatin	C	Safe, monitor infant for GI toxicity.
Imipenem-cilastatin-relebactam	Insufficient data in humans, evidence of embryofetal toxicity in animals	Safety not established, avoid use.
Isepamicin	D	Safety not established, avoid use.
Lefamulin	May cause fetal harm, based on toxicity in animal studies	Avoid use; pump and discard milk for tx duration and two days post.
Levofloxacin	C	Avoid breastfeeding for 4-6 hrs after a dose, monitor infant for GI toxicity.
Lincomycin	C	Safety not established, avoid use.
Linezolid	Humans: no evidence of toxicity Animals: embryo-fetal lethality in mice at 6.5x human exposure	Probably safe with monitoring for GI toxicity. Infant serum levels resulting from drug received through breast milk would be trivial.
Loracarbef	No evidence of toxicity in humans or animals	No data, but adverse effects not expected. Monitor infant for GI toxicity.
Meropenem	Humans: insufficient data to establish risk Animals: no evidence of toxicity	Probably safe with monitoring, but no data available.

Groups/Drugs	FDA Pregnancy Risk[1]	Use during Lactation
Antibacterials *(continued)*		
Meropenem-vaborbactam	No human data, toxic in animals	Probably safe with monitoring, but no data available.
Methenamine	Safety in early pregnancy not established, but appears safe in third trimester. No evidence of toxicity in animals.	Probably safe with monitoring, but data are limited.
Metronidazole	Human studies suggest (but cannot definitely establish) absence of risk. No evidence of toxicity in animals. *See footnote*[2]	Data and opinions conflict. Best to avoid IV/po therapy; topical/vaginal therapy likely safe.
Minocycline	D	Short-term use safe, monitor infant for GI toxicity.
Moxifloxacin	C	Short-term use safe, monitor infant for GI toxicity; avoid if possible.
Nafcillin	No evidence of toxicity in humans or animals	No data, but adverse effects not expected. Monitor infant for GI toxicity.
Netilmicin	D	Safety not established, avoid use.
Nitrofurantoin	Contraindicated at term (38-42 wks gestation), during labor and delivery, or when the onset of labor is imminent	Avoid if infant <8 days of age, or if G6PD-deficient (any age).
Ofloxacin	C	Avoid breastfeeding for 4-6 hrs after a dose, monitor infant for GI toxicity.
Omadacycline	Avoid during 2nd and 3rd trimesters	Mfr suggests no breastfeeding during treatment and for 4 days after last dose. However, milk conc are likely low and absorption inhibited by calcium in breast milk.
Oritavancin	No human data, no evidence of toxicity in animals	Probably safe with monitoring, but no data available; avoid if possible.
Oxacillin	No evidence of toxicity in humans or animals	Milk concentrations low, adverse effects not expected. Monitor infant for GI toxicity.
Penicillin G	No evidence of toxicity in humans or animals	Milk concentrations low, adverse effects not expected. Monitor infant for GI toxicity.
Piperacillin	Insufficient human data, evidence of fetotoxicity in animals	Milk concentrations low, adverse effects not expected. Monitor infant for GI toxicity.
Piperacillin-Tazobactam	Insufficient human data, evidence of fetotoxicity in animals	Milk concentrations low, adverse effects not expected. Monitor infant for GI toxicity.
Penicillin VK	No evidence of toxicity in humans or animals	Milk concentrations low, adverse effects not expected. Monitor infant for GI toxicity.
Pivmecillinam	No evidence of toxicity in humans or animals	Milk concentrations low, adverse effects not expected. Monitor infant for GI toxicity.
Plazomicin	Aminoglycosides are associated with fetal harm. No specific data for plazomicin.	Probably safe, monitor infant for GI toxicity.
Polymyxin B	C	Topical administration safe (no data with systemic use).
Quinupristin-dalfopristin	B	Probably safe with monitoring, but no data available; avoid if possible.
Retapamulin	B	Safety not established, avoid use.
Rifamycin SV	No human data, toxic in animals	No data, probably safe (since systemic absorption following oral administration is negligible).
Rifaximin	C	Probably safe with monitoring, but no data available; avoid if possible.
Sarecycline	Do not use (risk of fetal harm, tooth discoloration, inhibition of bone growth)	No data; avoid use.
Tedizolid	Insufficient data in humans. Fetal developmental toxicity in mice and rats.	Probably safe with monitoring, but no data available; avoid if possible.
Sulbactam + durlobactam	Sulbactam: No evidence of toxicity in humans or animals. Durlobactam: no human data, evidence of skeletal variations in mice.	No data regarding effects on the breastfed infant or milk production. Sulbactam is present in milk in low concentrations; no data for durlobactam.
Sulopenem etzadroxil-probenecid	Sulopenem: No data in humans, evidence of maternal toxicity in animals. Probenecid: No evidence of toxicity in humans.	Sulopenem: no data on presence in milk, effects on the breastfed infant, or effects on milk production. Probenecid: present in milk, no reports of adverse effects in breastfed infants.
Temocillin	No evidence of toxicity in humans or animals	No data.
Telavancin	Risk of fetal harm, based on animal studies. Avoid, unless benefit outweighs fetal risk.	Milk concentrations likely low, poorly absorbed. Safe, monitor infant for GI toxicity.
Telithromycin	C	Probably safe with monitoring, but no data available; avoid if possible.

Groups/Drugs	FDA Pregnancy Risk[1]	Use during Lactation
Antibacterials *(continued)*		
Tetracycline	D	Short-term use safe, monitor infant for GI toxicity.
Tigecycline	Humans: possible fetal toxicity Animals: fetal toxicity	Milk concentrations low, poor absorption of drug expected (calcium in milk). Short-term use safe, monitor infant for GI toxicity.
TMP-SMX	C	Risk of kernicterus in premature infants; avoid if infant G6PD-deficient.
Tobramycin	D	Probably safe, monitor infant for GI toxicity.
Vancomycin	C	Safe with monitoring.
Antibacterials (other)		
Bezlotoxumab	No human or animal data	No data, but milk concentrations are likely very low and adverse effects are not expected. Use in nursing mothers is acceptable.
Antibacterial combinations (H. pylori)		
Pylera	Contraindicated	Safety not established, avoid use.
Talicia	Not recommended	Safety not established, avoid use.
Voquezna	Triple Pak: not recommended. Dual Pak: No data.	Safety not established, avoid use.
Antifungals		
Amphotericin B (all products)	B	Probably safe, but no data available.
Anidulafungin	No human data; fetal toxicity in animals	Milk concentrations low, adverse effects not expected.
Caspofungin	Insufficient human data. Animal data suggest potential for fetal harm.	Milk concentrations low, adverse effects not expected.
Efinaconazole	No human data. Toxic in rats given sc only in supratherapeutic doses.	No data. Measurable breastmilk concentrations not likely.
Fluconazole	• Avoid if possible, especially high doses (6-12 mg/kg/day) for a prolonged period during first trimester. • The risk of miscarriage or congenital abnormalities with low doses (e.g., 150 mg x1) is unclear; CDC recommends topical azoles for VVC.	Safe with monitoring.
Flucytosine	C	Safety not established, avoid use.
Griseofulvin	X	Safety not established, avoid use.
Ibrexafungerp	Contraindicated (fetal harm in animals)	No data available.
Isavuconazonium sulfate	No human data; fetal harm in animals	Avoid use.
Itraconazole	No human data; fetal harm in animals	Little data available, avoid if possible.
Ketoconazole	C	Little data available, avoid if possible.
Micafungin	C	Safety not established, avoid use.
Oteseconazole	Contraindicated	Contraindicated.
Posaconazole	May cause fetal harm, based on animal data. Human data insufficient.	Safety not established, avoid use.
Rezafungin	No human data, no evidence of toxicity in animals	No human data, present in rat milk, avoid use if possible.
Terbinafine	No evidence of toxicity in animal or limited human studies	Milk concentrations low, adverse effects not expected. Monitor infant for liver toxicity.
Voriconazole	Can cause fetal harm. No data on voriconazole use in pregnancy are available. Advise use of effective contraception during treatment. Evidence of embryomortality, fetotoxicity, and teratogenicity in animals exist.	No data are available. If voriconazole is required by the mother, it is not a reason to discontinue breastfeeding. An alternate drug might be preferable.
Antimycobacterials		
Bedaquiline	Insufficient human data, no evidence of toxicity in animals	Safety not established, avoid use.
Capreomycin	C	Probably safe, monitor infant for GI toxicity.
Clofazimine	C	May color breastmilk pink; probably safe but avoid if possible.
Cycloserine	C	Probably safe, monitor infant for toxicity.
Dapsone	C	Safe, but avoid if infant G6PD-deficient.

Groups/Drugs	FDA Pregnancy Risk[1]	Use during Lactation
Antimycobacterials *(continued)*		
Delamanid	No human data, toxic in animals	Safety not established, avoid use.
Ethambutol	Safe	Probably safe, monitor infant for toxicity.
Ethionamide	C	Probably safe with monitoring, but data limited; avoid if possible.
Isoniazid (INH)	C	Safe, but mother and infant should receive pyridoxine.
Para-aminosalicylic acid (PAS)	C	Probably safe, monitor infant for toxicity.
Pretomanid	No human data, ↑ post-implantation loss in rats	No data available.
Pyrazinamide	C	Probably safe, monitor infant for toxicity.
Rifabutin	B	Probably safe, monitor infant for toxicity.
Rifampin	Humans: No well-controlled studies, does not appear to be teratogenic. Animals: Teratogenic in rodents, embryotoxic in rabbits.	Probably safe, monitor infant for toxicity. Breast milk may be stained a yellow, orange, red, or brown color.
Rifapentine	C	Probably safe, monitor infant for toxicity.
Streptomycin	D	Probably safe, monitor infant for GI toxicity.
Thalidomide	X	Safety not established, avoid use.
Antiparasitics		
Albendazole*	Category C. Limited data in pregnancy. Evidence suggests no difference in congenital abnormalities in the children of women accidentally treated with albendazole during MDA campaigns compared with those who were not. In MDA campaigns in countries where STH are common, WHO allows use in the 2nd and 3rd trimester. Balance the risk of treatment for the fetus with the risk of disease progression in the untreated woman.	Data limited. Minimally excreted in human milk. WHO: a single oral dose can be given safely to lactating women.
Artemether-lumefantrine	Can be used in all trimesters per WHO and CDC evidence review and policy[4]	No data on breastmilk excretion in humans but artemether and lumefantrine are transferred into rat milk indicating human milk presence.
Antimony, pentavalent	No data, but highly likely to be fetotoxic. Avoid use in pregnancy.	Milk concentrations low, adverse effects not expected (particularly if infant is >2 mon old). However, if nursing during therapy is withheld, breastfeeding can be reinstituted 24-48 hr after the last dose.
Artesunate (AS) (IV)	Can be used in all trimesters per WHO and CDC evidence review and policy[4]	Safety not established.
Atovaquone	Insufficient human data, no evidence of toxicity in animals	Data limited; probably safe, particularly if infant weighs at least 5 kg.
Atovaquone-Proguanil	Possibly safe, but no label change to date[5]	Data limited; probably safe, particularly if infant weighs at least 5 kg.
Benznidazole	Animal studies suggest risk of fetal harm. Pregnancy testing recommended for females of reproductive potential.	Milk concentrations low, adverse effects not expected. Use in nursing mothers is acceptable.
Chloroquine phosphate	C	Probably safe with monitoring, but data limited; avoid if possible.
Diethylcarbamazine	Do not use in pregnancy	No data, avoid use.
Dihydroartemisinin-piperaquine	Insufficient human data, avoid use	No data, avoid use.
Diloxanide furoate	No human data. No evidence of toxicity in animals.	Safety not established.
Eflornithine	Contraindicated, but use for HAT may be necessary as a rescue treatment[3]	Continue breastfeeding during treatment for HAT.[3]
Fexinidazole	Evidence of toxicity in rats and rabbits at supranormal doses. May be used after the first trimester for g-HAT.[3,6]	Continue breastfeeding during treatment for HAT.[3]
Fumagillin	No data	No data.

TABLE 8A (6)

Groups/Drugs	FDA Pregnancy Risk[1]	Use during Lactation
Antiparasitics *(continued)*		
Ivermectin	Category C. The available evidence (limited) suggests no difference in congenital abnormalities in the children of women who were accidentally treated during mass prevention campaigns with ivermectin compared with those who were not. The WHO excludes pregnant women from mass prevention campaigns that use ivermectin. Prescribe ivermectin only if the potential benefit to the woman justify the potential risk to the fetus.	Excreted in low concentrations in breast milk. Use only when the risk to the infant is outweighed by the risk of disease progression in the untreated mother.
Mebendazole	Category C. Limited data in pregnancy. Evidence suggests no difference in congenital abnormalities in the children of women accidentally treated with mebendazole during MDA campaigns compared with those who were not. In MDA campaigns in countries where STH are common, WHO allows use in the 2nd and 3rd trimester. Balance the risk of treatment for the fetus with the risk of disease progression in the untreated woman.	Minimally excreted in breast milk. WHO classifies mebendazole as safe during lactation.
Mefloquine	B	Probably safe, monitor infant for toxicity.
Melarsoprol	Contraindicated, but use for HAT may be necessary as a rescue treatment[3]	Continue breastfeeding during treatment for HAT.[3]
Miltefosine	D	Safety not established, avoid use.
Moxidectin	Humans: insufficient data Animals: no embryo/fetal toxicity	Safety not established; avoid use if possible.
Niclosamide	Category B. Limited data in pregnancy. Not systemically absorbed. Use if benefit outweighs risk.	Breast milk excretion unknown, but not systemically absorbed. Classified by WHO as compatible with breastfeeding.
Nifurtimox	Contraindicated, but use for HAT may be necessary as a rescue treatment[3]	Continue breastfeeding during treatment for HAT.[3]
Nitazoxanide	Category B. Usage data in pregnant women are limited, and embryo-fetal risk is unknown. Use if benefit outweighs risk.	Breast milk excretion unknown. Use with caution.
Paromomycin	Limited data. Non-absorbed, fetal risk low.	No data, but unlikely to be present in breast milk. Widely used for giardiasis in pregnancy.
Pentamidine	Limited data. Use only if the potential benefit justifies the potential risk to the fetus. WHO: May be administered to humans after the first trimester.[3]	Breast milk excretion unknown. WHO: Continue breastfeeding during treatment for HAT.[3]
Praziquantel	Category B. Available data suggest no difference in adverse birth outcomes in the children of women who were accidentally treated with PZQ during MDA campaigns compared with those who were not. In MDA campaigns for which the WHO has determined that the benefit of treatment outweighs the risk, WHO encourages the use of PZQ in any stage of pregnancy.	PZQ is excreted in low concentrations in breast milk. According to WHO guidelines for MDA campaigns, the use of PZQ during lactation is encouraged. In other clinical settings, balance the risk of treatment in lactating women with the risk of disease progression in the absence of treatment.
Primaquine	Avoid in pregnancy (risk of hemolysis if fetus G6PD-deficient)	Probably safe, monitor infant for toxicity.

Groups/Drugs	FDA Pregnancy Risk[1]	Use during Lactation
Antiparasitics *(continued)*		
Pyrantel pamoate	Category C. In mass treatment programs where benefit outweighs risk, WHO allows use in the 2nd and 3rd trimester. Balance the risk of treatment for the fetus with the risk of disease progression in the untreated woman.	Breast milk excretion unknown. WHO classifies pyrantel pamoate as compatible with breastfeeding, although data on use during lactation are limited.
Pyrimethamine	C	Safe with monitoring.
Pyronaridine-artesunate	Avoid in 1st trimester if possible (no data)	Safety not established.
Quinacrine	No human data; increased risk of fetal mortality in rats	No data, avoid use.
Quinine dihydrochloride	Use only if other effective antimalarials are unavailable	Probably safe, but avoid if infant G6PD-deficient.
Quinine sulfate	Use only if other effective antimalarials are unavailable	Probably safe, but avoid if infant G6PD-deficient.
Secnidazole	No human data, safe in animals	Safety not established, avoid breastfeeding for 96 hours after dose.
Spiramycin	No evidence of toxicity in humans	No data.
Sulfadoxine-pyrimethamine	Contraindicated in 1st trimester	Little data available, avoid use if possible.
Suramin	Insufficient human data, teratogenic in some animals. Avoid in pregnancy if possible.	No data, avoid use.
Tafenoquine	Not recommended (risk of hemolytic anemia if fetus G6PD-deficient)	Avoid breastfeeding x3 months after dose if infant G6PD-deficient or status unknown.
Tinidazole	Limited human data, but evidence of toxicity in animals. Contraindicated in 1st trimester, according to some experts.	Safety not established, avoid use.
Triclabendazole	No human data; no fetal toxicity in rats, rabbits	Safety not established, avoid use if possible.
Antivirals (coronavirus)		
Bamlanivimab + Etesevimab	No human data	No data. Follow clinical practice guidelines to avoid infant exposure to COVID-19.
Baricitinib (JAK inhibitor)	Insufficient data in humans, toxic in animals	No data. Follow clinical practice guidelines to avoid infant exposure to COVID-19.
Bebtelovimab	No human or animal data	No data. Follow clinical practice guidelines to avoid infant exposure to COVID-19.
Casirivimab + Imdevimab	No human data	No data. Follow clinical practice guidelines to avoid infant exposure to COVID-19.
Molnupiravir	Not recommended during pregnancy (embryo-fetal toxicity in animals, no human data)	No data. Follow clinical practice guidelines to avoid infant exposure to COVID-19.
Nirmatrelvir/RTV	Nirmatrelvir: no data in humans, evidence of embryo-fetal toxicity in animals. Ritonavir: No evidence of toxicity in humans or animals.	Milk concentrations of nirmatrelvir and ritonavir are low, adverse effects not expected. NIH endorses use during lactation.
Pemivibart	Insufficient data to assess risk	No data.
Remdesivir	No evidence of human toxicity in 2nd or 3rd trimester, insufficient data in 1st trimester. No evidence of toxicity in animals.	Parent drug and metabolite present in breast milk, no evidence of adverse effects on infant. Follow clinical practice guidelines to avoid infant exposure to COVID-19.
Sotrovimab	No human or animal data	No data. Follow clinical practice guidelines to avoid infant exposure to COVID-19.
Tixagevimab + Cilgavimab	No human data	No data. Follow clinical practice guidelines to avoid infant exposure to COVID-19.
Tocilizumab	Animal data: potential risk to fetus. Human data insufficient.	No data. Follow clinical practice guidelines to avoid infant exposure to COVID-19.
Tofacitinib (JAK inhibitor)	Insufficient data in humans, toxic in animals	No data. Follow clinical practice guidelines to avoid infant exposure to COVID-19.
Vilobelimab	No human data, no evidence of toxicity in animals	No data. Follow clinical practice guidelines to avoid infant exposure to COVID-19.

Groups/Drugs	FDA Pregnancy Risk[1]	Use during Lactation
Antivirals (Ebolavirus)		
Ansuvimab-zykl	Insufficient data to assess risk	Patients infected with Zaire ebolavirus should not breastfeed (potential for transmission).
Inmazeb	Humans, animals: no safety data	Patients infected with Zaire ebolavirus should not breastfeed (potential for transmission).
Antivirals (hepatitis B)		
Adefovir	Human data insufficient. Animals: No developmental toxicities observed at systemic exposures 23x higher in rats and 40x higher in rabbits (relative to exposure at human dosage).	Safety not established, avoid use if possible.
Entecavir	Human data insufficient. Animals: No developmental toxicities observed at systemic exposures 25x higher in rats and 200x higher in rabbits (relative to exposure at human dosage).	Safety not established, avoid use if possible.
Interferons	C	Probably safe, monitor infant for toxicity.
Telbivudine	B	Safety not established, avoid use if possible.
Tenofovir alafenamide fumarate (TAF)	No evidence of toxicity in humans or animals	Safety not established, avoid use if possible.
Antivirals (hepatitis C)		
Daclatasvir	No human data	Safety not established, avoid use if possible.
Ribavirin	Contraindicated (teratogenic and/or embryocidal)	No data, but probably safe with monitoring.
Simeprevir	C (X with RBV)	Safety not established, avoid use if possible.
Sofosbuvir	B (X with RBV)	Safety not established, avoid use if possible.
Antivirals (hep C combinations)		
Epclusa	No human data, safe in animals	Safety not established, avoid use if possible.
Harvoni	B	Safety not established, avoid use if possible.
Mavyret	No human data, safe in animals	Safety not established, avoid use if possible.
Technivie	B	Safety not established, avoid use if possible.
Viekira Pak	B	Safety not established, avoid use if possible.
Vosevi	No human data, safe in animals	Safety not established, avoid use if possible.
Zepatier	No human data, safe in animals	Safety not established, avoid use if possible.
Antivirals (herpesvirus)		
Acyclovir	B	Safe with monitoring.
Cidofovir	C	Avoid use.
Famciclovir	No evidence of toxicity in humans or animals	Safety not established, avoid use.
Foscarnet	C	Safety not established, avoid use.
Ganciclovir	C	Safety not established, avoid use.
Letermovir	Human data insufficient, toxic in rats at high exposures	Safety not established, avoid use.
Maribavir	Human data insufficient, decreased embryo-fetal survival in rats	No data, avoid use if possible.
Valacyclovir	Humans: no known drug-associated risk of major birth defects. Animals: no evidence of toxicity.	Safe with monitoring.
Valganciclovir	No human data. Embryo-fetal toxicity in animals.	Safety not established, avoid use.
Antivirals (influenza)		
Amantadine	C	Avoid use.
Baloxavir marboxil	No human data, safe in animals	Probably safe, but no data available.
Favipiravir	Teratogenic, do no administer	Avoid use.
Oseltamivir	Limited human data suggest no embryo-fetal toxicity. No evidence of toxicity in animals.	Probably safe (parent and carboxylate present in low levels, no evidence of toxicity from postmarketing data.
Peramivir	Human data insufficient, toxic in animals at high exposures	Safety not established, avoid use if possible.
Rimantadine	C	Avoid use.
Zanamivir	No evidence of toxicity in humans or animals	Probably safe, but no data.

Groups/Drugs	FDA Pregnancy Risk[1]	Use during Lactation
Antivirals (poxviruses)		
Brincidofovir	May cause fetal harm, based on animal data. No human data available.	Breastfeeding not recommended in patients with smallpox.
Tecovirimat	No human data, safe in animals	Safety not established, avoid use if possible.

[1] Capital letter = Old FDA risk category; Text = New FDA risk category.
[2] Metronidazole: ACOG allows use in pregnancy for severe disease due to G. duodenalis and E. histolytica
[3] WHO recommendation *(HAT guidelines, June 2024).*
[4] Recht J et al. Safety of artemisinin and non-artemisinin antimalarials in the first trimester of pregnancy: a review. *Geneva: WHO; 2023.*
[5] *J Travel Med 2019;26:tay138; Travel Med Infect Dis 2019;32:101519.*
[6] Given the rapid clinical evolution of r-HAT, treatment cannot usually be delayed. Clearly explain risk-benefit to patient and relatives.

TABLE 8B ANTIRETROVIRALS (ARV) – PREGNANCY AND LACTATION USE

Use of antiretrovirals during lactation: If on ART + suppressed VL throughout pregnancy, breastfeeding is a reasonable option after counseling about infant feeding options, risks and benefits.

Antiretrovirals	FDA Pregnancy Risk Category
Abacavir (ABC)	C
Atazanavir (ATV)	B
Cabotegravir (CAB)	Insufficient human data
Darunavir (DRV)	C
Didanosine (ddI)	B
Dolutegravir (DTG)	Preferred drug (all trimesters)
Doravirine (DOR)	No human data, safe in animals
Efavirenz (EFV)	FDA: avoid 1st trimester DHHS, WHO: safe all trimesters
Emtricitabine (FTC)	Humans, animals: no evidence of toxicity
Enfuvirtide (ENF/T20)	B
Etravirine (ETR)	B
Fosamprenavir (FPV)	C
Fostemsavir (FTR)	No human data, safe in animals
Ibalizumab-uiyk (IBA)	No human data. Animal data suggest immunosuppression in infants exposed in utero.
Indinavir (IDV)	C
Lamivudine (3TC)	C
Lenacapavir (LEN)	Insufficient human data. No evidence of toxicity in animals.
Maraviroc (MVC)	B
Nelfinavir (NFV)	B
Nevirapine (NVP)	B
Raltegravir (RAL)	Safe in humans (data for 400 mg bid only)
Rilpivirine (RPV)	No evidence of toxicity in humans or animals
Ritonavir (RTV)	B
Saquinavir (SQV)	B
Stavudine (d4T)	C
Tenofovir disoproxil fumarate (TDF)	Nontoxic in animals, humans
Tipranavir (TPV)	C
Zidovudine (ZDV/AZT)	C
Antiretroviral combinations	
Atripla (EFV/FTC/TDF)	D
Biktarvy (BIC/FTC/TAF)	No human data, safe in animals
Cabenuva (CAB/RPV)	Insufficient human data
Cimduo, Temixys (3TC/TDF)	Human: 3TC safe, TDF safe Animals: 3TC embryotoxic, TDF safe
Combivir (3TC/ZDV)	C
Complera/Eviplera (RPV/FTC/TDF)	B
Descovy (FTC/TAF)	No human data, nontoxic in animals
Dovato (DTG/3TC)	DTG: preferred drug 3TC: no human toxicity
Epzicom/Kivexa (ABC/3TC)	Nontoxic in humans, toxic in animals
Evotaz (ATV/cobi)	Not recommended (↓ATV/c exposure)
Genvoya (EVG/cobi/FTC/TAF)	Not recommended (↓EVG/c exposure)
Juluca (DTG/RPV)	DTG: preferred drug RPV: no human toxicity
Kaletra (LPV/RTV)	Nontoxic in humans, toxic in rats
Odefsey (RPV/FTC/TAF)	Humans: inadequate data Animals: nontoxic
Prezcobix (DRV/cobi)	Not recommended (↓DRV/c exposure)
Stribild (EVG/cobi/FTC/TDF)	Not recommended (↓EVG/c exposure)
Symfi, Symfi Lo (EFV/3TC/TDF)	Risk of fetal harm from EFV; avoid in first trimester
Symtuza (DRV/cobi/FTC/TAF)	Not recommended (↓DRV/c exposure)
Temixys (3TC/TDF)	Humans: 3TC safe, TDF safe Animals: 3TC embryotoxic, TDF safe
Triumeq (DTG/3TC/ABC)	Preferred combination
Trizivir (ABC/3TC/ZDV)	Nontoxic in humans, toxic in animals
Truvada (FTC/TDF)	B

TABLE 9A – SELECTED PHARMACOLOGIC FEATURES OF ANTIMICROBIAL AGENTS

For pharmacodynamics, see Table 9B; for Cytochrome P450 interactions, see Table 9C. Table terminology key at bottom of each page. Additional footnotes at end of Table 9A, page 135.

Groups/Drugs	PK/PD Index	Pharmaceutical Preparations	Food Rec (PO Drugs)[1]	Oral Abs (%)	Tmax (hr)	Peak Serum Conc (µg/mL)[2]	Peak Urine Conc (µg/mL)	Protein Binding (%)	Volume of Distribution (Vd)[3]	Avg Serum $T_{1/2}$ (hr)[4]	Elimination	Bile Pen (%)[5]	CSF/blood (%)[6]	Therapeutic Levels in CSF[7]	AUC (µg*hr/mL)[8]
Antibacterials															
Aminoglycosides/Aminocyclitols															
Amikacin	24-hr AUC/MIC	Injection, liposome inhalation susp	-	-	-	41-49 (15 mg/kg IV, SD)	No data	0-10	0.26 L/kg	2-3	Renal	10-60	0-30	No	110-145 (15 mg/kg, 0-inf)
Gentamicin	24-hr AUC/MIC	Injection, 0.1% cream, 0.1% ointment, 0.3% ointment, 0.3% eye drops	-	-	-	4-6 (1.7 mg/kg IV, SD)	No data	0-10	0.26 L/kg	2-3	Renal	10-60	0-30	No	70-100 (7 mg/kg, 0-inf)
Neomycin	No data	Tab (500 mg)	Tab ± food	<3	No data	No data	No data	No data	No data	No data	Negligible absorption	No data	No data	No data	No data
Netilmicin	24-hr AUC/MIC	Injection	-	-	-	4-8 (2 mg/kg IV, SD)	No data	0-10	0.26 L/kg	2-3	Renal	10-60	0-30	No	No data
Plazomicin	24-hr AUC/MIC	Injection	-	-	-	51-74 (15 mg/kg IV, SD)	No data	20	18-31 L	3.5	Renal	No data	No data	No data	226-257 (15 mg/kg, 0-inf)
Spectinomycin	No data	Injection	-	-	1	100 (2 gm IM, SD)	No data	Low	No data	1.5-2	Renal	No data	No data	No	No data
Tobramycin	24-hr AUC/MIC	Injection, 0.3% oph ointment, 0.3% eye drops, inhalation	-	-	-	4-6 (1.7 mg/kg IV, SD)	No data	0-10	0.26 L/kg	2-3	Renal	10-60	0-30	No	70-100 (7 mg/kg, 0-inf)
Antibodies (monoclonal, polyclonal)															
Anthrax immune globulin	No data	Injection	-	-	-	156.4 mU/mL (420 U IV, SD)	No data	No data	6.84 L	24-28 days	Catabolized	No data	No data	No data	2537 (420 U IV, 0-inf)
Bezlotoxumab	No data	Injection	-	-	-	185 (10 mg/kg IV, SD)	No data	No data	7.33 L	19 days	Catabolized	No data	No data	No data	53000 (10 mg/kg IV, 0-inf)
Obiltoxaximab	No data	Injection	-	-	-	400 (16 mg/kg IV, SD)	No data	No data	No data	≥16 days	Catabolized	No data	No data	No data	5170 (16 mg/kg IV, 0-inf)
Raxibacumab	No data	Injection	-	-	-	1020 (40 mg/kg IV, SD)	No data	No data	58-73 mL/kg (Vss)	16-19 days	Catabolized	No data	No data	No data	15846 µg*day/mL (40 mg/kg IV, 0-inf)

Food Effect (po dosing): + food = take with food, **no food** = take without food, **± food** = take with or without food; **Oral % AB** = % absorbed; **Peak Serum Level: SD** = after single dose, **SS** = steady state after multiple doses; **Volume of Distribution (Vd): V/F** = Vd/oral bioavailability, **Vss** = Vd at steady state, **Vss/F** = Vd at steady state/oral bioavailability; **CSF Penetration:** therapeutic efficacy comment based on dose, usual susceptibility or target organism & penetration into CSF; **AUC** = area under drug concentration curve; **24hr** = AUC 0-24; **Tmax** = time to max plasma concentration.

TABLE 9A (2) *(Footnotes at the end of table)*

Groups/Drugs	PK/PD Index	Pharmaceutical Preparations	Food Rec (PO Drugs)[1]	Oral Abs (%)	Tmax (hr)	Peak Serum Conc (µg/mL)[2]	Peak Urine Conc (µg/mL)	Protein Binding (%)	Volume of Distribution (Vd)[3]	Avg Serum T½ (hr)[4]	Elimination	Bile Pen (%)[5]	CSF/blood (%)[6]	Therapeutic Levels in CSF[7]	AUC (µg*hr/mL)[8]
Antibacterials *(continued)*															
Antifolates															
Sulfadiazine	No data	Tab (500 mg)	Tab ± food	No data	3-6	76.2 (1 gm po q6h, SS)	No data	80	39-41 L (V/F)	10	Renal	No data	32-65	Probable	280 (1 gm po q6h, 0-6h)
Trimethoprim	No data	Tab (100 mg) Oral soln 50 mg/5 ml (not in US)	Tab ± food	80	1-4	1 (100 mg po, SD)	No data	44	100-120 L (V/F)	8-15	Renal	100-200	50	No	No data
TMP-SMX	No data	SS tab (TMP 80 mg, SMX 400 mg) DS tab (TMP 160 mg, SMX 800 mg) Oral susp (TMP 40 mg + SMX 200 mg per 5 mL) Injection	Tab/susp ± food	TMP 70-90 SMX 70-90	po: TMP 1-4, SMX 1-4	TMP 1-2, SMX 40-60 (DS tab po q12h, SS) TMP 9, SMX 105 (160/800 mg IV q8h, SS)	No data	TMP 44, SMX 70	TMP 100-120 L, SMX 12-18 L	TMP 11, SMX 9	Renal	po 100-200, IV 40-70	TMP 50, SMX 40	Most meningococci: resistant Bacteriostatic vs. coliforms	No data
Beta-lactams															
Carbapenems															
Doripenem	T>MIC	Injection	-	-	-	23 (500 mg IV, SD)	601 (500 mg IV, SD)	8.1	16.8 L (Vss)	1	Renal	117 (0-611)	No data	No data	36.3 (500 mg, 0-inf)
Ertapenem	T>MIC	Injection	-	-	-	154 (1 gm IV, SD)	No data	95	0.12 L/kg (Vss)	4	Renal	10	No data	No data	572.1 (1 gm IV, 0-inf)
Imipenem-cilastatin	T>MIC	Injection	-	-	-	40 (500 mg IV, SD)	No data	15-25	0.23-0.31 L/kg	1	Renal	Minimal	8.5	Possibly[9]	42.2 (500 mg IV, 0-inf)
Imipenem-cilastatin-relebactam	Imi T>MIC, Rel 24-hr AUC/MIC	Injection	-	-	-	Imi 104.3 µM, Rel 64.0 µM (1.25 gm IV q6h, SS)	No data	Imi 20, Cil 40, Rel 22	Imi 24.3, Cil 13.8, Rel 19.0 L (Vss)	Imi 1, Cil 1, Rel 1.2	Renal	Imi minimal	Imi 8.5	Possibly (imi)[9]	Imi 573.9, Rel 427.3 µM-hr (SS, 0-24 hr)
Meropenem	T>MIC	Injection	-	-	-	49 (1 gm IV, SD)	No data	2	0.23-0.35 L/kg	1	Renal	3-300	21-39 (inflamed meninges)	Possibly[9]	72.5 (1 gm IV, 0-inf)
Meropenem-vaborbactam	T>MIC	Injection	-	-	-	Mer 43.4, Vab 55.6 (4 gm IV q8h, SS)	No data	Mer 2, Vab 33	Mer 20.2L, Vab 18.6 L (Vss)	Mer 1.22, Vab 1.68	Renal	No data	No data	No data	Mer 138, Vab 196 (SS, 0-8 hr)

Food Effect (po dosing): + food = take with food, **no food** = take without food, **± food** = take with or without food; **Oral % AB** = % absorbed; **Peak Serum Level: SD** = after single dose, **SS** = steady state after multiple doses; **Volume of Distribution (Vd): V/F** = Vd/oral bioavailability, **Vss** = Vd at steady state, **Vss/F** = Vd at steady state/oral bioavailability; **CSF Penetration:** therapeutic efficacy comment based on dose, usual susceptibility or target organism & penetration into CSF; **AUC** = area under drug concentration curve; **24hr** = AUC 0-24; **Tmax** = time to max plasma concentration.

TABLE 9A (3) *(Footnotes at the end of table)*

Groups/Drugs	PK/PD Index	Pharmaceutical Preparations	Food Rec (PO Drugs)[1]	Oral Abs (%)	Tmax (hr)	Peak Serum Conc (µg/mL)[2]	Peak Urine Conc (µg/mL)	Protein Binding (%)	Volume of Distribution (Vd)[3]	Avg Serum T½ (hr)[4]	Elimination	Bile Pen (%)[5]	CSF/blood (%)[6]	Therapeutic Levels in CSF[7]	AUC (µg*hr/mL)[8]
Antibacterials *(continued)*															
Cephalosporins (parenteral)															
1st gen IV															
Cefazolin	T>MIC	Injection	-	-	-	188 (1 gm IV, SD)	No data	73-87	0.19 L/kg	2	Renal	29-300	1-4	Possibly, with high doses	236 (1 gm IV, 0-inf)
2nd gen IV															
Cefmetazole	T>MIC	Injection	-	-	-	143 (2 gm IV, SD)	>2000 (2 gm IV, SD)	65-85	≈ 0.18 L/kg	1.1-1.5	Renal	No data	No data	No data	161 (2 gm IV, 0-inf)
Cefotetan	T>MIC	Injection	-	-	-	158 (1 gm IV, SD)	No data	88	10.3 L	3-4.6	Renal	2-21	No data	No data	504 (1 gm IV, 0-inf)
Cefoxitin	T>MIC	Injection	-	-	-	110 (1 gm IV, SD)	No data	65-79	16.1 L (Vss)	0.8	Renal	280	3	No	No data
Cefuroxime	T>MIC	Injection	-	-	-	100 (1.5 gm IV, SD)	No data	33-50	0.19 L/kg (Vss)	1.5	Renal	35-80	17-88	Marginal	150 (1.5 gm IV, 0-inf)
3rd gen IV, non-antipseudomonal															
Cefotaxime	T>MIC	Injection	-	-	-	100 (1 gm IV, SD)	No data	30-51	0.28 L/kg	1.5	Renal	15-75	10	Yes	70 (1 gm IV, 0-inf)
Ceftizoxime	T>MIC	Injection	-	-	-	60 (1 gm IV, SD)	No data	30	0.34 L/kg	1.7	Renal	34-82	No data	No data	85 (1 gm IV, 0-inf)
Ceftriaxone	T>MIC	Injection	-	-	-	150 (1 gm IV, SD)	995 (1 gm IV, SD)	85-95	5.8-13.5 L	8	Renal, biliary	200-500	8-16	Yes	1006 (1 gm IV, 0-inf)
IV, antipseudomonal															
Cefepime	T>MIC	Injection	-	-	-	164 (2 gm IV, SD)	No data	20	18 L (Vss)	2	Renal	10-20	10	Yes	284.8 (2 gm IV, 0-inf)
Cefepime-Enmetazobactam	T>MIC	Injection	-	-	-	Cefe: 99.8 Enme: 19.8 (2.5 gm [over 2 hr] q8h, SS)	No data	Cefe: 20 Enme: nil	Cefe: 20 L (Vss) Enme: 25.3 L (Vss)	Cefe: 2.7 Enme: 2.6	Cefe: renal Enme: renal	No data	No data	No data	Cefe: 379.5 Enme: 75.3 (2.5 gm [over 2 hr] q8h, 0-24h)
Cefiderocol	T>MIC	Injection	-	-	-	138 (2 gm IV q8h, SS)	No data	40-60	18 L	2-3	Renal	No data	44 (*JAC 2022; 77:1787*)	Possibly	394.7 (SS, 0-8 hr)

Food Effect (po dosing): + food = take with food, **no food** = take without food, **± food** = take with or without food; **Oral % AB** = % absorbed; **Peak Serum Level: SD** = after single dose, **SS** = steady state after multiple doses; **Volume of Distribution (Vd): V/F** = Vd/oral bioavailability, **Vss** = Vd at steady state, **Vss/F** = Vd at steady state/oral bioavailability; **CSF Penetration:** therapeutic efficacy comment based on dose, usual susceptibility or target organism & penetration into CSF; **AUC** = area under drug concentration curve; **24hr** = AUC 0-24; **Tmax** = time to max plasma concentration.

TABLE 9A (4) *(Footnotes at the end of table)*

Groups/Drugs	PK/PD Index	Pharmaceutical Preparations	Food Rec (PO Drugs)[1]	Oral Abs (%)	Tmax (hr)	Peak Serum Conc (µg/mL)[2]	Peak Urine Conc (µg/mL)	Protein Binding (%)	Volume of Distribution (Vd)[3]	Avg Serum T½ (hr)[4]	Elimination	Bile Pen (%)[5]	CSF/blood (%)[6]	Therapeutic Levels in CSF[7]	AUC (µg*hr/mL)[8]
Antibacterials/Cephalosporins (parenteral)/IV, antipseudomonal *(continued)*															
Cefoperazone	T>MIC	Injection	-	-	-	252 (2 gm over 15 min, SD)	>2200 (2 gm IV over 15 min, SD)	87-90	10.2-11.3 L	1.7-2.0	Biliary	Up to 100x serum conc	No data	No data	No data
Cefoperazone-sulbactam	T>MIC	Injection	-	-	-	Cef: 236.8 (1 gm IV over 5 min, SD) Sul: 130 (1 gm IV over 5 min, SD)	Cef: >2200 (2 gm IV over 15 min, SD)	Cef: 87-90	Cef: 10.2-11.3 L Sul: 18.0-27.6 L	Cef: 1.7-2.0 Sul: 1.0	Cef: Biliary (main) Sul: renal	Cef: Up to 100x serum conc	No data	No data	No data
Cefpirome	T>MIC	Injection	-	-	-	80 (1 gm IV, SD)	No data	10	21 L (Vss)	2	Renal	No data	5-15	No data	150 (1 gm IV, 0-inf)
Ceftazidime	T>MIC	Injection	-	-	-	69 (1 gm IV, SD)	No data	<10	0.24 L/kg (Vss)	1.9	Renal	13-54	20-40	Yes	127 (1 gm IV, 0-inf)
Ceftazidime-avibactam	T>MIC	Injection	-	-	-	Ceftaz: 90.4 Avi: 14.6 (2.5 gm IV q8h, SS)	No data	Ceftaz: <10 Avi: 5.7-8.2	Ceftaz: 17 L Avi: 22.2 L (Vss)	Ceftaz: 2.8 Avi: 2.7	Renal	Ceftaz: 13-54 Avi: no data	Ceftaz: 20-40 Avi: no data	Ceftaz: Yes Avi: no data	Ceftaz: 291 Avi: 38.2 (SS, 0-8 hr)
Ceftolozane-tazobactam	T>MIC	Injection	-	-	-	Ceftolo: 74.4 Tazo: 18 (1.5 gm IV q8h, SS)	No data	Ceftolo: 16-21 Tazo: 30	Ceftolo: 13.5 L Tazo: 18.2 L (Vss)	Ceftolo: 3.1 Tazo: 1.0	Renal	No data	Ceftolo: 20 Tazo: 20 *(AAC 2020; 65:e01698-20)*	Not likely	Ceftolo: 182 Tazo: 25 (SS, 0-8 hr)
IV, anti-MRSA															
Ceftaroline	T>MIC	Injection	-	-	-	21.3 (600 mg IV q12h, SS)	No data	20	20.3 L (Vss)	2.7	Renal	No data	<10	Maybe (at high doses) *(J Pediatr Pharmacol Ther 2020; 25:336)*	56.3 (SS, 0-12 hr)
Ceftobiprole medocaril	T>MIC	Injection	-	-	-	33.0 (667 mg IV q8h, SS)	No data	16	18 L (Vss)	3.3	Renal	No data	12% (conc 1.2 µg/mL) *(Heliyon 2024; 10:e27285)*	Possibly	102 (667 mg IV q8h, 0-8 h)

Food Effect (po dosing): + food = take with food, **no food** = take without food, **± food** = take with or without food; **Oral % AB** = % absorbed; **Peak Serum Level: SD** = after single dose, **SS** = steady state after multiple doses; **Volume of Distribution (Vd): V/F** = Vd/oral bioavailability, **Vss** = Vd at steady state, **Vss/F** = Vd at steady state/oral bioavailability; **CSF Penetration:** therapeutic efficacy comment based on dose, usual susceptibility or target organism & penetration into CSF; **AUC** = area under drug concentration curve; **24hr** = AUC 0-24; **Tmax** = time to max plasma concentration.

TABLE 9A (5) *(Footnotes at the end of table)*

Groups/Drugs	PK/PD Index	Pharmaceutical Preparations	Food Rec (PO Drugs)[1]	Oral Abs (%)	Tmax (hr)	Peak Serum Conc (µg/mL)[2]	Peak Urine Conc (µg/mL)	Protein Binding (%)	Volume of Distribution (Vd)[3]	Avg Serum T½ (hr)[4]	Elimination	Bile Pen (%)[5]	CSF/blood (%)[6]	Therapeutic Levels in CSF[7]	AUC (µg*hr/mL)[8]
Antibacterials *(continued)*															
Cephalosporins (oral)															
1st gen po															
Cefadroxil	T>MIC	Cap (500 mg) Tab (1 gm) Oral susp (250 mg/5 mL, 500 mg/5 mL)	All preps ± food	90	No data	16 (500 mg po, SD)	1800 (500 mg po, SD)	20	0.305 L/kg (V/F)	1.5	Renal	22	No data	No data	47.4 (500 mg po, 0-inf)
Cephalexin	T>MIC	Cap (250, 500, 750 mg) Tab (250, 500 mg) Oral susp (125 mg/5 mL, 250 mg/5 mL)	Cap/tab/susp ± food	90	1	18 (500 mg po, SD)	2200 (500 mg po, SD)	5-15	0.38 L/kg (V/F)	1	Renal	216	No data	No data	29 (500 mg po, 0-inf)
2nd gen po															
Cefaclor	T>MIC	Cap (250, 500 mg) Extended-release (ER) tab (500 mg) Chewtab (125, 187, 250, 375 mg) Oral susp (125 mg/5 mL, 187 mg/5 mL, 250 mg/5 mL, 375 mg/5 mL)	Cap/chewtab/susp ± food ER tab + food	93 (ER no data)	Cap/chewtab/susp 0.5-1.0 ER tab 2.5	13 (500 mg po, SD) 8.4 (500 mg ER po, SD)	900 (500 mg po, SD)	22-25	0.33 L/kg (V/F)	0.8	Renal	>60	No data	No data	20.5 (500 mg po, 0-inf)
Cefprozil	T>MIC	Tab (250, 500 mg), oral susp (125 mg/5 mL, 250 mg/5 mL)	All preps ± food	95	1.5	10.5 (500 mg po, SD)	No data	36	0.23 L/kg (Vss/F)	1.5	Renal	No data	No data	No data	25.7 (500 mg po, 0-inf)
Cefuroxime axetil	T>MIC	Tab (250, 500 mg) Oral susp (125 mg/5 mL, 250 mg/5 mL) (oral susp not available in US)	Susp + food Tab ± food	52	2.5	4.1 (250 mg po, SD)	No data	50	0.66 L/kg (V/F)	1.5	Renal	35-80	No data	No data	12.9 (250 mg po, 0-inf)

Food Effect (po dosing): + food = take with food, **no food** = take without food, **± food** = take with or without food; **Oral % AB** = % absorbed; **Peak Serum Level: SD** = after single dose, **SS** = steady state after multiple doses; **Volume of Distribution (Vd): V/F** = Vd/oral bioavailability, **Vss** = Vd at steady state, **Vss/F** = Vd at steady state/oral bioavailability; **CSF Penetration:** therapeutic efficacy comment based on dose, usual susceptibility or target organism & penetration into CSF; **AUC** = area under drug concentration curve; **24hr** = AUC 0-24; **Tmax** = time to max plasma concentration.

TABLE 9A (6) *(Footnotes at the end of table)*

Groups/Drugs	PK/PD Index	Pharmaceutical Preparations	Food Rec (PO Drugs)[1]	Oral Abs (%)	Tmax (hr)	Peak Serum Conc (µg/mL)[2]	Peak Urine Conc (µg/mL)	Protein Binding (%)	Volume of Distribution (Vd)[3]	Avg Serum T½ (hr)[4]	Elimination	Bile Pen (%)[5]	CSF/blood (%)[6]	Therapeutic Levels in CSF[7]	AUC (µg*hr/mL)[8]
Antibacterials/Cephalosporins (oral)/2nd gen po *(continued)*															
Loracarbef	T>MIC	Cap (200, 400 mg) Oral susp (100 mg/5 mL, 200 mg/5 mL)	All preps no food	90	No data	8 (200 mg po, SD)	No data	25	0.33 L/kg (V/F)	1.2	Renal	No data	No data	No data	10.6 (200 mg po, 0-inf)
3rd gen po															
Cefdinir	T>MIC	Cap (300 mg) Oral susp (125 mg/5 mL, 250 mg/5 mL)	All preps ± food	Caps 16-21 Susp 25	2-4	1.6 (300 mg po, SD)	No data	60-70	0.35 L/kg (V/F)	1.7	Renal	No data	No data	No data	7.1 (300 mg po, 0-inf)
Cefditoren pivoxil	T>MIC	Tab (200, 400 mg)	Tab + food	16	1.5-3.0	4 (400 mg po, SD)	No data	88	9.3 L (Vss/F)	1.6	Renal	No data	No data	No data	20 (400 mg po, 0-inf)
Cefixime	T>MIC	Cap (400 mg) Chewtab (100, 200 mg) Oral susp (100 mg/5 mL, 200 mg/5 mL, 500 mg/5 mL)	All preps ± food	50	4	3-5 (400 mg po, SD)	No data	65	0.93 L/kg (V/F)	3	Renal, biliary	800	No data	No data	25.8 (400 mg po, 0-inf)
Cefpodoxime proxetil	T>MIC	Tab (100, 200 mg), oral susp (50 mg/5 mL, 100 mg/5 mL)	Tab + food, Susp ± food	46	2-3	2.3 (200 mg po, SD)	49-196 (50-800 mg po, SD; *IJAA 1994; 4:37*)	40	0.7 L/kg (V/F)	2.5	Renal	115	No data	No data	14.5 (200 mg po, 0-inf)
Ceftibuten	T>MIC	Cap (400 mg), oral susp (90 mg/5 mL, 180 mg/5 mL)	All preps no food	80	2.6	15 (400 mg po, SD)	No data	65	0.21 L/kg (V/F)	2.5	Renal	No data	No data	No data	73.7 (400 mg po, 0-inf)
Monobactams															
Aztreonam	T>MIC	Injection	-	-	-	90 (1 gm IV, SD)	Avg: 3500-6600 (1-2 gm IV, SD)	56	12.6 L (Vss)	2	Renal	115-405	3-52	No data	271 (1 gm IV, 0-inf)
Aztreonam-avibactam	T>MIC	Injection	-	-	-	Az: 54.2 Avi: 11.0 (1.5 gm/0.5 gm IV q6h, SS)[13]	No data	Az: 38 Avi: 8	Az: 20 L (Vss) Avi: 24 L (Vss)	Az: 2-3 Avi: 2-3	Az: renal Avi: renal	Az: 115-405 Avi: no data	Az: 3-52 Avi: no data	Az: no data Avi: no data	Az: 833 Avi: 161 (1.5 gm/0.5 gm IV q6h, 0-24h)[13]

Food Effect (po dosing): + food = take with food, **no food** = take without food, **± food** = take with or without food; **Oral % AB** = % absorbed; **Peak Serum Level: SD** = after single dose, **SS** = steady state after multiple doses; **Volume of Distribution (Vd): V/F** = Vd/oral bioavailability, **Vss** = Vd at steady state, **Vss/F** = Vd at steady state/oral bioavailability; **CSF Penetration:** therapeutic efficacy comment based on dose, usual susceptibility or target organism & penetration into CSF; **AUC** = area under drug concentration curve; **24hr** = AUC 0-24; **Tmax** = time to max plasma concentration.

TABLE 9A (7) *(Footnotes at the end of table)*

Groups/Drugs	PK/PD Index	Pharmaceutical Preparations	Food Rec (PO Drugs)[1]	Oral Abs (%)	Tmax (hr)	Peak Serum Conc (μg/mL)[2]	Peak Urine Conc (μg/mL)	Protein Binding (%)	Volume of Distribution (Vd)[3]	Avg Serum T½ (hr)[4]	Elimination	Bile Pen (%)[5]	CSF/blood (%)[6]	Therapeutic Levels in CSF[7]	AUC (μg*hr/mL)[8]
Antibacterials *(continued)*															
Penicillins (natural)															
Penicillin G	T>MIC	Injection	-	-	-	20 (2 mill units IV, SD)	No data	65	0.35 L/kg	0.5	Renal	500	5-10	Yes	No data
Penicillin VK	T>MIC	Tab (250, 500 mg), oral soln (125 mg/5 mL, 250 mg/5 mL)	All preps no food	60-73	No data	5-6 (500 mg po, SD)	No data	65	No data	0.5	Renal	No data	No data	No data	No data
Penicillins (amino)															
Amoxicillin	T>MIC	Cap (250, 500 mg), tab (500, 875 mg), chewtab (125, 250 mg), extended-release (ER) tab (775 mg), oral susp (125 mg/5 mL, 200 mg/5 mL, 250 mg/5 mL, 400 mg/5 mL)	Standard preps ± food ER tab + food	80	Cap/tab/ chewtab/ susp: 1-2 ER tab: 3.1	5.5-7.5 (500 mg po, SD) 6.6 (775 mg ER po, SD)	No data	17-20	0.36 L/kg	1.2-1.5	Renal	100-3000	13-14	Yes (IV only)	22 (500 mg po, 0-inf) 29.8 (775 mg ER po, 0-inf)

Food Effect (po dosing): + food = take with food, **no food** = take without food, **± food** = take with or without food; **Oral % AB** = % absorbed; **Peak Serum Level: SD** = after single dose, **SS** = steady state after multiple doses; **Volume of Distribution (Vd): V/F** = Vd/oral bioavailability, **Vss** = Vd at steady state, **Vss/F** = Vd at steady state/oral bioavailability; **CSF Penetration:** therapeutic efficacy comment based on dose, usual susceptibility or target organism & penetration into CSF; **AUC** = area under drug concentration curve; **24hr** = AUC 0-24; **Tmax** = time to max plasma concentration.

TABLE 9A (8) *(Footnotes at the end of table)*

Groups/Drugs	PK/PD Index	Pharmaceutical Preparations	Food Rec (PO Drugs)[1]	Oral Abs (%)	Tmax (hr)	Peak Serum Conc (µg/mL)[2]	Peak Urine Conc (µg/mL)	Protein Binding (%)	Volume of Distribution (Vd)[3]	Avg Serum T½ (hr)[4]	Elimination	Bile Pen (%)[5]	CSF/blood (%)[6]	Therapeutic Levels in CSF[7]	AUC (µg*hr/mL)[8]
Antibacterials/Penicillins (amino) *(continued)*															
Amoxicillin-clavulanate*	T>MIC	Tab (250 mg/125 mg, 500 mg/125 mg, 875 mg/125 mg) Chewtab (200 mg/28.5 mg, 400 mg/57 mg) Extended-release (ER) tab (1000 mg/ 62.5 mg) Oral susp per 5 mL (125 mg/31.25 mg, 250 mg/62.5 mg, 200 mg/28.5 mg, 400 mg/57 mg, 600 mg/42.9 mg) Injection (500 mg/100 mg, 1000 mg/200 mg, 2000 mg/200 mg)	Standard preps ± food ER + food	Amox: 80 Clav: 30-98	ER: amox 1.5, clav 1.03	Standard: amox 11.6, clav 2.2 (875 mg/ 125 mg, SD) ER: amox 17, clav 2.1 (2000 mg/ 125 mg, SD) IV: amox 105.4, clav 28.5 (1000 mg/ 200 mg, SD)	No data	Amox: 18 Clav: 25	Amox: 0.36 L/kg Clav: 0.21 L/kg	Amox: 1-1.4 Clav: 1	Amox: renal Clav: hepatic metabolism	Amox: 100-3000	No data	No data	Standard: amox 26.8, clav 5.1 (875 mg/ 125 mg) ER: amox 71.6, clav 5.3 (2000 mg/ 125 mg) IV: amox 76.3, clav 27.9 (1000 mg/ 200 mg) (All are 0-inf)
Ampicillin	T>MIC	Cap (250, 500 mg) Oral susp (125 mg/5 mL, 250 mg/5 mL) Injection	-	-	-	100 (2 gm IV, SD)	No data	18-22	0.29 L/kg	1.2	Renal	100-3000	13-14	Yes	120 (2 gm IV, 0-inf)
Ampicillin-sulbactam	T>MIC	Injection	-	-	-	Amp: 109-150 sulb: 48-88 (3 gm IV, SD)	No data	Amp: 28 sulb: 38	Amp: 0.29 L/kg sulb: 0.3 L/kg	Amp: 1.4 sulb: 1.7	Renal	Amp: 100-3000	No data	No data	Amp: 120 sulb: 71 (3 gm IV, 0-inf)
Penicillins (penicillinase-resistant)															
Cloxacillin	T>MIC	Cap (250, 500 mg) Injection	Cap no food	50	1-1.5	7.5-14 (500 mg po, SD)	No data	95	0.1 L/kg	0.5	Renal, other	No data	1.8 *(CMI 2020; 26:1415.e1)*	Possibly	No data
Dicloxacillin	T>MIC	Cap (250, 500 mg)	Cap no food	37	1-1.5	10-17 (500 mg po, SD)	No data	98	0.1 L/kg	0.7	Renal, biliary	5-8	No data	No data	No data

Food Effect (po dosing): + food = take with food, **no food** = take without food, **± food** = take with or without food; **Oral % AB** = % absorbed; **Peak Serum Level: SD** = after single dose, **SS** = steady state after multiple doses; **Volume of Distribution (Vd): V/F** = Vd/oral bioavailability, **Vss** = Vd at steady state, **Vss/F** = Vd at steady state/oral bioavailability; **CSF Penetration:** therapeutic efficacy comment based on dose, usual susceptibility or target organism & penetration into CSF; **AUC** = area under drug concentration curve; **24hr** = AUC 0-24; **Tmax** = time to max plasma concentration.

TABLE 9A (9) *(Footnotes at the end of table)*

Groups/Drugs	PK/PD Index	Pharmaceutical Preparations	Food Rec (PO Drugs)[1]	Oral Abs (%)	Tmax (hr)	Peak Serum Conc (μg/mL)[2]	Peak Urine Conc (μg/mL)	Protein Binding (%)	Volume of Distribution (Vd)[3]	Avg Serum T½ (hr)[4]	Elimination	Bile Pen (%)[5]	CSF/blood (%)[6]	Therapeutic Levels in CSF[7]	AUC (μg*hr/mL)[8]
Antibacterials/Penicillins (penicillinase-resistant) *(continued)*															
Flucloxacillin	T>MIC	Cap (250, 500 mg), oral syrup (125 mg/5 mL, 250 mg/5 mL, injection)	Cap no food	50	po: 1	10 (250 mg, SD)	No data	95	No data	0.75	Renal	No data	No data	No data	No data
Nafcillin	T>MIC	Injection	-	-	-	30 (500 mg IV, SD)	No data	90-94	27.1 L (Vss)	0.5-1.0	Biliary	>100	9-20	Yes w/high doses	18.1 (500 mg IV, 0-inf)
Oxacillin	T>MIC	Injection	-	-	-	43 (500 mg IV, SD)	No data	90-94	0.4 L/kg	0.5-0.7	Renal	25	10-15	Yes w/high doses	No data
Temocillin	T>MIC	Injection	-	-	-	150-200 (2 gm IV, SD)	No data	70-85	0.2 L/kg	4	Renal	800-1000	8-15	No data	785 (2 gm IV, 0-inf)
Penicillins (antipseudomonal)															
Piperacillin	T>MIC	Injection	-	-	-	242 (3 gm IV, SD)	No data	16	0.24 L/kg	1	Renal	>100	30	No data	242 (3 gm IV q6h, 0-6h)
Piperacillin-Tazobactam	T>MIC	Injection	-	-	-	Pip: 242 Tazo: 24.2 (3.375 gm IV, SD)	No data	Pip: 16 Tazo: 48	Pip: 0.24 L/kg Tazo: 0.4 L/kg	Pip: 1 Tazo: 1	Renal	>100	No data	No data	Pip: 242 Tazo: 25 (3.375 gm IV, 0-inf)
Penicillins (other)															
Pivmecillinam	T>MIC	US: Tab (185 mg)	Tab ± food	25-35	1.5	1.7 (185 mg po, SD)	>200 (400 mg HCl salt, SD)	<25	51 L	1	Renal	No data	No data	No data	214 μg*min/mL (185 mg po, 0-8 hr)

Food Effect (po dosing): **+ food** = take with food, **no food** = take without food, **± food** = take with or without food; **Oral % AB** = % absorbed; **Peak Serum Level: SD** = after single dose, **SS** = steady state after multiple doses; **Volume of Distribution (Vd): V/F** = Vd/oral bioavailability, **Vss** = Vd at steady state, **Vss/F** = Vd at steady state/oral bioavailability; **CSF Penetration:** therapeutic efficacy comment based on dose, usual susceptibility or target organism & penetration into CSF; **AUC** = area under drug concentration curve; **24hr** = AUC 0-24; **Tmax** = time to max plasma concentration.

TABLE 9A (10) *(Footnotes at the end of table)*

Groups/Drugs	PK/PD Index	Pharmaceutical Preparations	Food Rec (PO Drugs)[1]	Oral Abs (%)	Tmax (hr)	Peak Serum Conc (µg/mL)[2]	Peak Urine Conc (µg/mL)	Protein Binding (%)	Volume of Distribution (Vd)[3]	Avg Serum T½ (hr)[4]	Elimination	Bile Pen (%)[5]	CSF/blood (%)[6]	Therapeutic Levels in CSF[7]	AUC (µg*hr/mL)[8]
Antibacterials *(continued)*															
Fluoroquinolones[*]															
Ciprofloxacin	24-hr AUC/MIC	Tab (100, 250, 500, 750 mg) Ext-rel tab (500, 1000 mg) Oral susp (50 mg/mL, 100 mg/mL) 0.3% oph soln 0.3% oph ointment 0.2% otic soln 6% otic susp (intratympanic) Cipro 0.3%/dex 0.1% otic susp Cipro 0.3%/ fluocin 0.025% otic soln Cipro 0.2%/hc 1% otic susp	All preps ± food (no dairy products)	70	Tab, susp: 1-2 ER tab: 1-4	3.6 (750 mg po q12h, SS) 1.6-3.1 (500-1000 mg ER po q24h, SS) 4.6 (400 mg IV q12h, SS)	394 (500 mg po, SD)	20-40	2.4 L/kg	4 (ER tab 6.6)	Renal, some biliary	2800-4500	26	Inadequate for strepto-cocci *(CID 2000; 31:1131)*	31.6 (750 mg po q12h, 0-24 hr) 8 (500 mg ER po q24h, 0-24 hr) 25.4 (400 mg IV q12h, 0-24 hr)
Delafloxacin	24-hr AUC/MIC	Tab (450 mg) Injection	Tab ± food	59	1	9.3 (300 mg IV q12h, SS) 7.45 (450 mg po q12h, SS)	No data	84	30-48 L (Vss)	4.2-8.5	Renal, some fecal	No data	No data	No data	23.4 (300 mg IV q12h, 0-12 hr) 30.8 (450 mg po q12h, 0-12 hr)
Gatifloxacin	24-hr AUC/MIC	Tab (200, 400 mg) 0.5% oph soln Injection	Tab ± food	96	No data	4.2-4.6 (400 mg po/ IV q24h, SS)	No data	20	1.8 L/kg (Vss)	7-8	Renal	No data	36	No data	35 (400 mg po/IV q24h, 0-24 hr)
Gemifloxacin	24-hr AUC/MIC	Tab (320 mg)	Tab ± food	71	0.5-2.0	1.6 (320 mg po q24h, SS)	No data	55-73	1.7-12.1 L/kg (Vss/F)	7	Fecal, some renal	No data	No data	No data	9.9 (320 mg po q24h, 0-24 hr)

Food Effect (po dosing): + food = take with food, **no food** = take without food, **± food** = take with or without food; **Oral % AB** = % absorbed; **Peak Serum Level: SD** = after single dose, **SS** = steady state after multiple doses; **Volume of Distribution (Vd): V/F** = Vd/oral bioavailability, **Vss** = Vd at steady state, **Vss/F** = Vd at steady state/oral bioavailability; **CSF Penetration:** therapeutic efficacy comment based on dose, usual susceptibility or target organism & penetration into CSF; **AUC** = area under drug concentration curve; **24hr** = AUC 0-24; **Tmax** = time to max plasma concentration.

TABLE 9A (11) *(Footnotes at the end of table)*

Groups/Drugs	PK/PD Index	Pharmaceutical Preparations	Food Rec (PO Drugs)[1]	Oral Abs (%)	Tmax (hr)	Peak Serum Conc (µg/mL)[2]	Peak Urine Conc (µg/mL)	Protein Binding (%)	Volume of Distribution (Vd)[3]	Avg Serum T½ (hr)[4]	Elimination	Bile Pen (%)[5]	CSF/blood (%)[6]	Therapeutic Levels in CSF[7]	AUC (µg*hr/mL)[8]
Antibacterials/Fluoroquinolones *(continued)*															
Levofloxacin	24-hr AUC/MIC	Tab (250, 500, 750 mg) Oral soln (25 mg/mL) 0.5% oph soln Injection	Tab ± food, soln no food	99	po: 1.6	8.6 (750 mg po q24h, SS) 12.1 (750 mg IV q24h, SS)	521-771 (500 mg po/IV q24h, SS)	24-38	244 L (Vss)	7	Renal	No data	30-50	No data	90.7 (750 mg po q24h, 0-24 hr) 108 (750 mg IV q24h, 0-24 hr)
Moxifloxacin	24-hr AUC/MIC	Tab (400 mg) 0.5% oph soln Injection	Tab ± food	89	po: 1-3	4.2-4.6 (400 mg po/IV q24h, SS)	No data	30-50	2.2 L/kg	10-14	Metabolized, biliary, renal	No data	>50	Yes *(CID 2009; 49:1080)*	48 (400 mg po q24h, 0-24 hr) 38 (400 mg IV q24h, 0-24 hr)
Norfloxacin	24-hr AUC/MIC	Tab (400 mg)	Tab no food	30-40	1	1.5 (400 mg po, SD)	No data	10-15	1.7 L/kg	3-4	Metabolized, biliary, renal	700	No data	No	6.4 (400 mg po, 0-inf)
Ofloxacin	24-hr AUC/MIC	Tab (200, 300, 400 mg) 0.3% oph soln 0.3% otic soln	Tab ± food	98	1-2	4.6-6.2 (400 mg po q12h, SS)	No data	32	1-2.5 L/kg	7	Renal	No data	No data	No data	82.4 (400 mg po q12h, 0-24 hr)
Prulifloxacin	24-hr AUC/MIC	Tab (600 mg)	Tab ± food	No data	1	Ulifloxacin 1.6 (600 mg po, SD)	No data	45	1231 L	10.6-12.1	Fecal	No data	Negligible	No	7.3 (600 mg po, 0-inf)
Glyco-, Lipoglyco-, Lipopeptides															
Dalbavancin	24-hr AUC/MIC	Injection	-	-	-	280-300 (1 gm IV, SD)	No data	93-98	0.11 L/kg *(Drugs 2010; 70:859)*	147-258 (terminal)	Renal, fecal	No data	No data	No data	23443 (1 gm IV, 0-inf)
Daptomycin	24-hr AUC/MIC	Injection	-	-	-	57.8-183.7 (4-12 mg/kg IV q24h, SS)	No data	92	0.1 L/kg (Vss)	8-9	Renal	No data	0-8	No data	494-1277 (4-12 mg/kg IV q24h, 0-24 hr)
Oritavancin	24-hr AUC/MIC	Injection	-	-	-	148 (1200 mg IV over 1 hr, SD)	No data	85	87.6 L	245 (terminal)	Renal, fecal	No data	No data	No	1460 (1200 mg IV over 1 hr, 0-72 hr)
Teicoplanin	24-hr AUC/MIC	Injection	-	-	-	70 (6 mgkg IV q24h, SS)	No data	90-95	0.9-1.6 L/kg (Vss)	70-100	Renal	No data	negligible	No	500-600 (6 mg/kg IV, 0-inf)

Food Effect (po dosing): + food = take with food, **no food** = take without food, **± food** = take with or without food; **Oral % AB** = % absorbed; **Peak Serum Level: SD** = after single dose, **SS** = steady state after multiple doses; **Volume of Distribution (Vd): V/F** = Vd/oral bioavailability, **Vss** = Vd at steady state, **Vss/F** = Vd at steady state/oral bioavailability; **CSF Penetration:** therapeutic efficacy comment based on dose, usual susceptibility or target organism & penetration into CSF; **AUC** = area under drug concentration curve; **24hr** = AUC 0-24; **Tmax** = time to max plasma concentration.

TABLE 9A (12) *(Footnotes at the end of table)*

Groups/Drugs	PK/PD Index	Pharmaceutical Preparations	Food Rec (PO Drugs)[1]	Oral Abs (%)	Tmax (hr)	Peak Serum Conc (μg/mL)[2]	Peak Urine Conc (μg/mL)	Protein Binding (%)	Volume of Distribution (Vd)[3]	Avg Serum T½ (hr)[4]	Elimination	Bile Pen (%)[5]	CSF/blood (%)[6]	Therapeutic Levels in CSF[7]	AUC (μg*hr/mL)[8]
Antibacterials/Glyco-, Lipoglyco-, Lipopeptides *(continued)*															
Telavancin	24-hr AUC/MIC	Injection	-	-	-	108 (10 mg/kg IV q24h, SS)	No data	90	0.13 L/kg (Vss)	8.1	Renal	Low	No data	No data	780 (10 mg/kg IV q24h, 0-24 hr)
Vancomycin	24-hr AUC/MIC	Injection, cap (125, 250 mg), oral soln (25 mg/mL, 50 mg/mL)	-	-	-	10-20 (SS)	No data	55	0.7 L/kg	4-6	Renal	No data	7-14	High doses required	400-600 (0-24 hr)
H. pylori combination products															
Pylera	Bis: no data Metro: 24-hr AUC/MIC Tetra: 24-hr AUC/MIC	Cap (Bismuth subcitrate K 140 mg, metronidazole 125 mg, tetracycline 125 mg)	Cap after meals, qhs	Bis: no data Metro: good Tetra: 60-90	Bis: no data Metro: 1-2 Tetra: no data	Bis: 0.017 (420 mg, SD) Metro: 8.7 (375 mg, SD) Tetra: 0.77 (375 mg, SD)	No data	Bis: >90 Metro: <20 Tetra: 20-65	Bis: no data Metro: 0.6-0.85 L/kg Tetra: 1.3 L/kg	Bis: 120 Metro: 6-14 Tetra: 6-12	Bis: biliary, renal Metro: metabolism, some renal Tetra: biliary, renal	Bis: no data Metro: 100 Tetra: 200-3200	Bis: no data Metro: 45-89 Tetra: poor	Bis: no data Metro: no data Tetra: no	Bis: 0.057 (420 mg, 0-inf) Metro: 84.4 (375 mg, 0-inf) Tetra: 10 (375 mg, 0-inf)
Talicia	Omep: no data Amox: T>MIC Rifabutin: 24-hr AUC/MIC	Cap (omeprazole 10 mg, amoxicillin 250 mg, rifabutin 12.5 mg)	Cap + food	Omep: no data Amox: no data Rifabutin: no data	Omep: 1.25 Amox: 2 Rifabutin: 3	Omep: 1.28 (40 mg q8h, SS) Amox: 15.9 (1 gm q8h, SS) Rifabutin: 0.088 (50 mg q8h, SS)	No data	Omep: 95 Amox: 20 Rifabutin: 85	Omep: no data Amox: 0.36 L/kg Rifabutin: 9.3 L/kg (Vss)	Omep: 1 Amox: 1.4 Rifabutin: 34	Omep: metabolized Amox: renal Rifabutin: metabolism, renal	Omep: no data Amox: 100-3000 Rifabutin: 300-500	Omep: no data Amox: 13-14 Rifabutin: 30-70	Omep: no data Amox: yes Rifabutin: no data	Omep: 7.16 (40 mg q8h, 0-24h) Amox: 145.8 (1 gm q8h, 0-24h) Rifabutin: 1.32 (50 mg q8h, 0-24h)
Voquezna (Triple Pak, Dual Pak)	Vono: no data Amox: T>MIC Clari: 24-hr AUC/MIC	Vonoprazan 20 mg tab Amoxicillin 500 mg cap Clarithromycin 500 mg tab	Vono ± food Amox ± food Clari ± food	Vono: no data Amox: 80 Clari: 50	Vono: 3.0 Amox: 1-2 Clari: 2-2.5	Vono: 0.038 (20 mg q12h, SS) Amox: 5.5-7.5 (500 mg, SD) Clari: 3-4 (500 mg q8-12h, SS)	No data	Vono: 85-88 Amox: 20 Clari: 65-70	Vono: 782.7 L (V/F) Amox: 0.36 L/kg Clari: 4 L/kg	Vono: 6.8 Amox: 1 Clari: 5-7	Vono: metabolized Amox: renal Clari: metabolism, renal	Vono: no data Amox: 100-3000 Clari: 7000	Vono: no data Amox: 13-14 Clari: no data	Vono: no data Amox: yes Clari: no data	Vono: 0.272 (20 mg q12h, 0-12h) Amox: 22 (500 mg, 0-inf) Clari: 20 (500 mg q12h, 0-24h)

Food Effect (po dosing): + food = take with food, **no food** = take without food, **± food** = take with or without food; **Oral % AB** = % absorbed; **Peak Serum Level: SD** = after single dose, **SS** = steady state after multiple doses; **Volume of Distribution (Vd): V/F** = Vd/oral bioavailability, **Vss** = Vd at steady state, **Vss/F** = Vd at steady state/oral bioavailability; **CSF Penetration:** therapeutic efficacy comment based on dose, usual susceptibility or target organism & penetration into CSF; **AUC** = area under drug concentration curve; **24hr** = AUC 0-24; **Tmax** = time to max plasma concentration.

TABLE 9A (13) *(Footnotes at the end of table)*

Groups/Drugs	PK/PD Index	Pharmaceutical Preparations	Food Rec (PO Drugs)[1]	Oral Abs (%)	Tmax (hr)	Peak Serum Conc (μg/mL)[2]	Peak Urine Conc (μg/mL)	Protein Binding (%)	Volume of Distribution (Vd)[3]	Avg Serum T½ (hr)[4]	Elimination	Bile Pen (%)[5]	CSF/blood (%)[6]	Therapeutic Levels in CSF[7]	AUC (μg*hr/mL)[8]
Antibacterials *(continued)*															
Macrolides, Azalides, Lincosamides, Ketolide															
Azithromycin	24-hr AUC/MIC	Tab (250, 500, 600 mg) Oral susp (1 gm pkt) Oral susp (100 mg/5 mL, 200 mg/5 mL) 1% oph soln Injection	All preps ± food	37	po 2.5	0.4 (500 mg po, SD) 3.6 (500 mg IV, SD)	No data	7-51	31.1-33.3 L/kg	68	Biliary	High	No data	No data	4.3 (500 mg po, 0-inf) 9.6 (500 mg IV, 0-24 hr, pre-SS)
Clarithromycin	24-hr AUC/MIC	Tab (250, 500 mg) Extended-release tab (500 mg) Oral susp (125 mg/5 mL, 250 mg/5 mL)	Tab/susp ± food ER tab + food	50	Tab 2.0-2.5 ER tab 5-8	3-4 (500 mg po q12h, SS) 2-3 (1 gm ER po q24h, SS)	No data	65-70	4 L/kg	5-7	Metabolized (active metab), renal	7000	No data	No data	20 (500 mg po q12h, 0-24 hr)
Clindamycin	24-hr AUC/MIC	Cap (75, 150, 300 mg), oral soln (75 mg/5 mL), topical (gel, cream, lotion), vaginal supp, vaginal gel, injection	Cap/soln ± food	90	0.75	2.5 (150 mg po, SD) 14.1 (900 mg IV q8h, SS)	No data	85-94	1.1 L/kg	2.4	Metabolized	250-300	No data	No	No data

<u>Food Effect</u> (po dosing): + food = take with food, **no food** = take without food, **± food** = take with or without food; **Oral % AB** = % absorbed; **<u>Peak Serum Level</u>: SD** = after single dose, **SS** = steady state after multiple doses; **<u>Volume of Distribution (Vd)</u>: V/F** = Vd/oral bioavailability, **Vss** = Vd at steady state, **Vss/F** = Vd at steady state/oral bioavailability; **<u>CSF Penetration</u>:** therapeutic efficacy comment based on dose, usual susceptibility or target organism & penetration into CSF; **AUC** = area under drug concentration curve; **24hr** = AUC 0-24; **Tmax** = time to max plasma concentration.

TABLE 9A (14) *(Footnotes at the end of table)*

Groups/Drugs	PK/PD Index	Pharmaceutical Preparations	Food Rec (PO Drugs)[1]	Oral Abs (%)	Tmax (hr)	Peak Serum Conc (μg/mL)[2]	Peak Urine Conc (μg/mL)	Protein Binding (%)	Volume of Distribution (Vd)[3]	Avg Serum T½ (hr)[4]	Elimination	Bile Pen (%)[5]	CSF/blood (%)[6]	Therapeutic Levels in CSF[7]	AUC (μg*hr/mL)[8]
Antibacterials/Macrolides, Azalides, Lincosamides, Ketolide *(continued)*															
Erythromycin (base, ethylsuccinate, lactobionate)	24-hr AUC/MIC	Base tab (250, 500 mg), delayed-release (DR) tab (250, 333, 500 mg), DR cap (250 mg), ethylsuccinate tab (400 mg), ethylsuccinate oral susp (200 mg/5 mL, 400 mg/5 mL), 2% topical gel/pad/soln, 0.5% oph ointment, lactobionate injection	Base no food DR/ ethylsucc ± food	18-45	DR preps 3	0.1-2.0 (500 mg base po, SD) 3-4 (500 mg IV, SD)	No data	70-74	0.6 L/kg	2-4	Biliary	No data	2-13	No	No data
Fidaxomicin	No data	Tab (200 mg), oral susp (40 mg/mL)	Tab/susp ± food	Minimal	No data	0.005 (200 mg po, SD)	No data	No data	No data	2	Fecal	No data	No data	No	0.063 (200 mg po, 0-inf)
Lincomycin	24-hr AUC/MIC	Injection	-	-	-	15.9 (600 mg IV over 2hr, SD) 11.6 (600 mg IM, SD)	No data	70-75	No data	5.4	Metabolized	No data	Poor	No data	No data
Telithromycin	24-hr AUC/MIC	Tab (300, 400 mg)	Tab ± food	57	1	2.3 (800 mg po q24h, SS)	No data	60-70	2.9 L/kg	10	Metabolized, biliary, renal	7	-	-	12.5 (24 hr)
Miscellaneous Antibacterials															
Chloramphenicol	No data	Injection (no po in US)	Cap ± food	High	No data	18 (1 gm po q6h, SS)	No data	25-50	0.8 L/kg	4.1	Metabolized	No data	45-89	Yes	No data
Fosfomycin IV	T>MIC	Injection (disodium salt)	-	-	-	552 (8 gm q8h, SS) (healthy volunteers)	No data	Negligible	0.3 L/kg	2.0	Renal	No data	20-50	Yes	3679 (8 gm q8h, 0-24h) (healthy volunteers)
Fosfomycin PO	T>MIC	3 gm sachet	Sachet ± food	trometh 40	2	26.1 (3 gm po, SD)	4400 (0-4 hr after 3 gm)	Negligible	136.1 L (Vss/F)	5.7	Renal	No data	20-50	No	145-193 (3 gm po, 0-inf)

Food Effect (po dosing): + food = take with food, **no food** = take without food, **± food** = take with or without food; **Oral % AB** = % absorbed; **Peak Serum Level: SD** = after single dose, **SS** = steady state after multiple doses; **Volume of Distribution (Vd): V/F** = Vd/oral bioavailability, **Vss** = Vd at steady state, **Vss/F** = Vd at steady state/oral bioavailability; **CSF Penetration:** therapeutic efficacy comment based on dose, usual susceptibility or target organism & penetration into CSF; **AUC** = area under drug concentration curve; **24hr** = AUC 0-24; **Tmax** = time to max plasma concentration.

TABLE 9A (15) *(Footnotes at the end of table)*

Groups/Drugs	PK/PD Index	Pharmaceutical Preparations	Food Rec (PO Drugs)[1]	Oral Abs (%)	Tmax (hr)	Peak Serum Conc (µg/mL)[2]	Peak Urine Conc (µg/mL)	Protein Binding (%)	Volume of Distribution (Vd)[3]	Avg Serum T½ (hr)[4]	Elimination	Bile Pen (%)[5]	CSF/blood (%)[6]	Therapeutic Levels in CSF[7]	AUC (µg*hr/mL)[8]
Antibacterials/Miscellaneous *(continued)*															
Fusidic acid	No data	Tab (250 mg), oral susp (50 mg/5 mL), 2% cream/ ointment, 1% oph soln, injection	Tab + food	91	2-4	30 (500 mg po, SD)	No data	95-99	0.3 L/kg	15	Biliary	100-200	No data	No data	442 (500 mg po, 0-inf)
Methenamine	No data	Hippurate tab (1 gm) Mandelate tab (500 mg, 1 gm)	Tab ± food	No data	1-2	No data	No data	No data	No data	4	Renal	No data	No data	No data	No data
Nitrofurantoin	No data	Macrocrystalline cap (25, 50, 100 mg) Oral susp (25 mg/5 mL) Slow-release cap (100 mg)	All preps + food	80-90	No data	<1 (100 mg, SD)	50-200 (100 mg, SD)	No data	No data	0.5-2.0	Renal, metabolism	No data	No data	No	1-3 (100 mg, 0-inf)
Sulopenem etzadroxil-probenecid	T>MIC	Tablet (500 mg sulo/500 mg prob)	Tab + food	Sulo: 64 Prob: no data	Sulo: 2 Prob: 2	Sulo: 2.7 Prob: 30.4 (500 mg/500 mg, SD)	No data	Sulo: 11 Prob: no data	Sulo: 92.1 L Prob: 11.9 L	Sulo: 1.3 Prob: 3.8	Sulo: metabolized, renal	No data	No data	No data	Sulo: 7.4 Prob: 237 (500 mg/500 mg, 0-inf)
Nitroimidazoles															
Metronidazole	24-hr AUC/MIC	Tab (250, 500 mg) Cap (375 mg) Oral susp (500 mg/5 mL) Injection Cream (0.75%) Gel (0.75%, 1%) Lotion (0.75%) Vaginal gel (0.75%)	All preps ± food	100	0.75-2.33	20-25 (500 mg IV q6h, SS) Oral susp: 10-13 (500 mg, SD)	No data	20	0.6-0.85 L/kg	6-14	Metabolized; renal excretion of parent + metabolites	100	45-89	No data	560 (500 mg IV q6h, 0-24 hr) 144-146 (500 mg po susp, 0-inf)
Secnidazole	No data	Oral granules (2 gm packets)	Granules ± food	No data	4	45.4 (2 gm po, SD)	No data	<5	42 L	17	Metabolized	No data	No data	No data	1331.6 (2 gm po, 0-inf)

Food Effect (po dosing): + food = take with food, **no food** = take without food, **± food** = take with or without food; **Oral % AB** = % absorbed; **Peak Serum Level: SD** = after single dose, **SS** = steady state after multiple doses; **Volume of Distribution (Vd): V/F** = Vd/oral bioavailability, **Vss** = Vd at steady state, **Vss/F** = Vd at steady state/oral bioavailability; **CSF Penetration:** therapeutic efficacy comment based on dose, usual susceptibility or target organism & penetration into CSF; **AUC** = area under drug concentration curve; **24hr** = AUC 0-24; **Tmax** = time to max plasma concentration.

TABLE 9A (16) *(Footnotes at the end of table)*

Groups/Drugs	PK/PD Index	Pharmaceutical Preparations	Food Rec (PO Drugs)[1]	Oral Abs (%)	Tmax (hr)	Peak Serum Conc (μg/mL)[2]	Peak Urine Conc (μg/mL)	Protein Binding (%)	Volume of Distribution (Vd)[3]	Avg Serum T½ (hr)[4]	Elimination	Bile Pen (%)[5]	CSF/blood (%)[6]	Therapeutic Levels in CSF[7]	AUC (μg*hr/mL)[8]
Antibacterials *(continued)*															
Oxazolidinones															
Linezolid	24-hr AUC/MIC	Tab (600 mg) Oral susp (100 mg/5 mL) Injection	Tab/susp ± food	100	1-2	15-20 (600 mg IV/ po q12h, SS)	No data	31	40-50 L (Vss)	5	Metabolized, renal	No data	60-70	Yes *(AAC 2006; 50:3971)*	179 (600 mg IV q12h, 0-24 hr) 276 (600 mg po q12h, 0-24 hr)
Tedizolid phosphate (phosphate)	24-hr AUC/MIC	Tab (200 mg), injection	Tab ± food	91	3	3.0 (200 mg IV q24h, SS) 2.2 (200 mg po q24h, SS)	No data	70-90	67-80 L (Vss)	12	Fecal	No data	No data	No data	29.2 (200 mg IV q24h, 0-24 hr) 25.6 (200 mg po q24h, 0-24 hr)
Pleuromutilins															
Lefamulin	24-hr AUC/MIC	Tab (600 mg) Injection	Tab no food	25	po: 0.88-2.0	3.6 (150 mg IV q12h, SS) 2.24 (600 mg po q12h, SS)	No data	94.8-97.1	86.1 L (Vss)	8	Metabolized	No data	No data	No data	28.6 (150 mg IV q12h, 0-24 hr) 32.7 (600 mg po q12h, 0-24 hr)
Retapamulin	No data	1% ointment	-	-	-	Low, not always measurable	No data	94	No data	No data	Metabolized	No data	No data	No data	No data
Polymyxins															
Colistin (polymyxin E)	Free AUC/MIC	Injection	-	-	-	0.83 (30 mg CBA IV, SD) *(CPT 2011; 89:875)*	No data	≈ 50	0.17 L/kg *(CPT 2011; 89:875)*	6.3-12	Renal	No data	Poor	No	11.5-225 (CBA 75-410 mg/ day IV, 0-24 hr)
Polymyxin B	Free AUC/MIC	Injection, topical (in combination)	-	-	-	2.8 (1.5 mg/ kg IV q12h, avg conc at SS)	No data	60	No data	4.5-6 (old data)	Nonrenal	No data	No data	No data	66.9 (1.5 mg/kg IV q12h, 0-24 hr)

Food Effect (po dosing): + food = take with food, **no food** = take without food, **± food** = take with or without food; **Oral % AB** = % absorbed; **Peak Serum Level: SD** = after single dose, **SS** = steady state after multiple doses; **Volume of Distribution (Vd): V/F** = Vd/oral bioavailability, **Vss** = Vd at steady state, **Vss/F** = Vd at steady state/oral bioavailability; **CSF Penetration:** therapeutic efficacy comment based on dose, usual susceptibility or target organism & penetration into CSF; **AUC** = area under drug concentration curve; **24hr** = AUC 0-24; **Tmax** = time to max plasma concentration.

TABLE 9A (17) *(Footnotes at the end of table)*

Groups/Drugs	PK/PD Index	Pharmaceutical Preparations	Food Rec (PO Drugs)[1]	Oral Abs (%)	Tmax (hr)	Peak Serum Conc (µg/mL)[2]	Peak Urine Conc (µg/mL)	Protein Binding (%)	Volume of Distribution (Vd)[3]	Avg Serum T½ (hr)[4]	Elimination	Bile Pen (%)[5]	CSF/blood (%)[6]	Therapeutic Levels in CSF[7]	AUC (µg*hr/mL)[8]
Antibacterials *(continued)*															
Rifamycins															
Rifamycin SV	24-hr AUC/MIC	Tab (194 mg)	Tab ± food (no alcohol)	Negligible	-	Negligible	No data	80	No data	No data	Fecal	No data	No data	No data	No data
Rifaximin	No data	Tab (200, 550 mg)	Tab ± food	<0.4	1	0.0007-0.002 (200 mg po q8h, SS)	No data	67.5	No data	2-5	Negligible absorption	No data	No data	No data	0.008 (200 mg po, 0-inf)
Streptogramins															
Pristinamycin	24-hr AUC/MIC	Tab (250, 500 mg)	Tab + food	No data	PIA 3.25, PIIA 3.08	PIA 0.76 (2 gm po, SD) PIIA 0.58 (2 gm po, SD)	No data	No data	No data	PIA 4.03, PIIA 2.83	Biliary	No data	No data	No data	PIA 2.2 (2 gm po, 0-inf) PIIA 1.21 (2 gm po, 0-inf)
Quinupristin-dalfopristin	24-hr AUC/MIC	Injection	-	-	-	Quin: 3.2 Dalf: 8 (7.5 mg/kg IV q8h, SS)	No data	Quin> Dalf (not quantified)	Quin: 0.45 Dalf: 0.24 (L/kg, Vss)	Quin: 0.85 Dalf: 0.7	Biliary	No data	No data	No data	Quin: 7.2 Dalf: 10.6 (7.5 mg/kg IV q8h, 0-24 hr)
Tetracyclines, Glycylcyclines															
Doxycycline	24-hr AUC/MIC	Monohydrate: Cap (50, 75, 100, 150 mg) Tab (100, 150 mg) Delayed-release cap (40 mg) Oral susp (25 mg/5 mL) Hyclate: Cap (100 mg) Tab (20, 50, 75, 100, 150 mg) DR tab (50, 60, 75, 80, 100, 120, 150, 200 mg) Injection	Tab/cap/ susp + food	90	2 (not DR)	1.5-2.1 (100 mg po, SD)	No data	>90	0.7 L/kg	18-24	Biliary, renal	200-3200	26	No	31.7 (100 mg po, 0-inf)
Eravacycline	24-hr AUC/MIC	Injection	-	-	-	1.825 (1 mg/kg IV q12h, SS)	No data	79-90	321 L (Vss)	20	Metabolized	No data	No data	No data	6.31 (1 mg/kg IV q12h, 0-12 hr)

Food Effect (po dosing): + food = take with food, **no food** = take without food, **± food** = take with or without food; **Oral % AB** = % absorbed; **Peak Serum Level: SD** = after single dose, **SS** = steady state after multiple doses; **Volume of Distribution (Vd): V/F** = Vd/oral bioavailability, **Vss** = Vd at steady state, **Vss/F** = Vd at steady state/oral bioavailability; **CSF Penetration:** therapeutic efficacy comment based on dose, usual susceptibility or target organism & penetration into CSF; **AUC** = area under drug concentration curve; **24hr** = AUC 0-24; **Tmax** = time to max plasma concentration.

TABLE 9A (18) *(Footnotes at the end of table)*

Groups/Drugs	PK/PD Index	Pharmaceutical Preparations	Food Rec (PO Drugs)[1]	Oral Abs (%)	Tmax (hr)	Peak Serum Conc (µg/mL)[2]	Peak Urine Conc (µg/mL)	Protein Binding (%)	Volume of Distribution (Vd)[3]	Avg Serum $T_{1/2}$ (hr)[4]	Elimination	Bile Pen (%)[5]	CSF/blood (%)[6]	Therapeutic Levels in CSF[7]	AUC (µg*hr/mL)[8]
Antibacterials/Tetracyclines, Glycylcyclines *(continued)*															
Minocycline	24-hr AUC/MIC	Tab/cap (50, 75, 100 mg), extended-release tab (45, 55, 65, 80, 90, 105, 115, 135 mg), 1 gm pwd for subgingival use, 4% topical foam, injection	Cap/tab/ ER tab ± food	No data	2.1	2.0-3.5 (200 mg po, SD) 4.2 (200 mg IV, SD)	No data	76	80-114 L (Vss)	16	Biliary	200-3200	No data	No data	48.3 (200 mg po, 0-inf)
Omadacycline	24-hr AUC/MIC	Tab (150 mg), injection	Tab no food	34.5	po: 2.5	2.12 (100 mg IV q24h, SS) 0.95 (300 mg po q24h, SS)	No data	20	190 L (Vss)	15.5-16.8	Fecal	No data	No data	No data	12.14 (100 mg IV q24h, 0-24 hr) 11.16 (300 mg po q24h, 0-24 hr)
Sarecycline	24-hr AUC/MIC	Tab (60, 100, 150 mg)	Tab ± food	No data	1.5-2.0	No data	No data	62.5-74.7	91.4-97.0 (Vss)	21-22	Fecal, renal	No data	No data	No data	No data
Tetracycline	24-hr AUC/MIC	Cap (250, 500 mg)	Cap no food	No data	2-4	1.5-2.2 (250 mg po, SD)	No data	20-65	1.3 L/kg	6-12	Biliary, renal	200-3200	Poor	No	30 (250 mg po, 0-inf)
Tigecycline	24-hr AUC/MIC	Injection	-	-	-	0.63 (50 mg IV q12h, SS)	No data	71-89	7-9 L/kg (Vss)	42	Biliary, renal	138	5.9-10.6	No	4.7 (50 mg IV q12h, 0-24 hr)
Antifungals															
Allylamines															
Terbinafine	No data	Tab (250 mg), 1% cream	Tab ± food	>70	2	1 (250 mg po, SD)	No data	>99	950 L (Vss)	36	Metabolized	No data	No data	No data	4.56 (250 mg po, 0-inf)
Benzofuran															
Griseofulvin	No data	Microsize tab (500 mg) Microsize oral susp (125 mg/5 mL) Ultramicrosize tab (125, 250 mg)	Tab/susp + food (high fat)	27-72 (best with ultramicrosize)	4	0.6-0.67 (250 mg ultra po, SD) 0.5-2.0 (500 mg micro po, SD)	No data	No data	No data	9-24	Metabolized	No data	No data	No data	8.6-9.0 (250 mg ultra po, 0-inf)

Food Effect (po dosing): + food = take with food, **no food** = take without food, **± food** = take with or without food; **Oral % AB** = % absorbed; **Peak Serum Level: SD** = after single dose, **SS** = steady state after multiple doses; **Volume of Distribution (Vd): V/F** = Vd/oral bioavailability, **Vss** = Vd at steady state, **Vss/F** = Vd at steady state/oral bioavailability; **CSF Penetration:** therapeutic efficacy comment based on dose, usual susceptibility or target organism & penetration into CSF; **AUC** = area under drug concentration curve; **24hr** = AUC 0-24; **Tmax** = time to max plasma concentration.

TABLE 9A (19) *(Footnotes at the end of table)*

Groups/Drugs	PK/PD Index	Pharmaceutical Preparations	Food Rec (PO Drugs)[1]	Oral Abs (%)	Tmax (hr)	Peak Serum Conc (µg/mL)[2]	Peak Urine Conc (µg/mL)	Protein Binding (%)	Volume of Distribution (Vd)[3]	Avg Serum $T_{1/2}$ (hr)[4]	Elimination	Bile Pen (%)[5]	CSF/blood (%)[6]	Therapeutic Levels in CSF[7]	AUC (µg*hr/mL)[8]
Antifungals *(continued)*															
Polyenes															
Amphotericin B	Cmax/MIC	Injection (deoxycholate, ABLC, liposomal)	-	-	-	Deoxy: 0.5-3.5 (0.4-0.7 mg/kg q24h, SS) ABLC: 1.0-2.5 (5 mg/kg q24h, SS) Lipo: 83 (5 mg/kg q24h, SS)	No data	Deoxy: 91-95 ABLC, lipo: no data	Deoxy: 4 L/kg ABLC: 131 L/kg Lipo: 0.1-0.4 L/kg (Vss)	Deoxy: 24 ABLC: 173 Lipo: 6.8	Renal (slow); metabolized?	No data	Poor	No	Deoxy: 17 (0.4-0.7 mg/kg q24h, 0-24 hr) ABLC: 14 (5 mg/kg q24h, 0-24 hr) Lipo: 555 (5 mg/kg q24h, 0-24 hr)
Antimetabolite															
Flucytosine	T>MIC	Cap (250, 500 mg)	Cap ± food	78-90	2	30-40 (2.5 gm po, SD)	No data	≈4	0.6 L/kg	3-5	Renal	No data	60-100	Yes	No data
Azoles															
Efinaconazole	No data	10% topical soln (4 mL, 8 mL)	-	-	-	0.67 ng/mL (after 28 days)	No data	No data	No data	29.9	No data	No data	No data	No data	12.15 ng*hr/mL (after 28 days)
Fluconazole	24-hr AUC/MIC	Tab (50, 100, 150, 200 mg) Oral susp (10 mg/mL, 40 mg/mL) Injection	Tab/susp ± food	>90	po: 1-2	6.7-14 (400-800 mg, SD)	At least 10x plasma conc	11-12	50 L (V/F)	30	Renal	No data	80	Yes	140 (3 mg/kg, 0-inf)
Isavuconazonium sulfate	24-hr AUC/MIC	Cap (74.5, 186 mg) Injection	Cap ± food	98	po: 2-3	3.3 (372 mg po, SD)	No data	>99	450 L (Vss)	130	Metabolized	No data	No data	No data	112.2 (372 mg po, 0-inf)
Itraconazole	24-hr AUC/MIC	Cap (65, 100 mg), tab (200 mg), oral soln (10 mg/mL), injection (not in US)	Cap/tab + food, po soln no food	55	Itra 2.0, OH-itra 5.3	Itra 2.0, OH-itra 2.0 (200 mg po soln q24h, SS)	No data	99.8	796 L	35-40	Metabolized	No data	0	No data	Itra 29.3, OH-itra 45.2 (200 mg po soln q24h, 0-24 hr)
Ketoconazole	24-hr AUC/MIC	Tab (200 mg)	Tab + food	Variable	1-2	3.5 (200 mg po, SD)	No data	99	1.2 L/kg	8	Metabolized, biliary	No data	<10	No data	12 (200 mg po q24h, 0-24 hr)

Food Effect (po dosing): + food = take with food, **no food** = take without food, **± food** = take with or without food; **Oral % AB** = % absorbed; **Peak Serum Level: SD** = after single dose, **SS** = steady state after multiple doses; **Volume of Distribution (Vd): V/F** = Vd/oral bioavailability, **Vss** = Vd at steady state, **Vss/F** = Vd at steady state/oral bioavailability; **CSF Penetration:** therapeutic efficacy comment based on dose, usual susceptibility or target organism & penetration into CSF; **AUC** = area under drug concentration curve; **24hr** = AUC 0-24; **Tmax** = time to max plasma concentration.

TABLE 9A (20) *(Footnotes at the end of table)*

Groups/Drugs	PK/PD Index	Pharmaceutical Preparations	Food Rec (PO Drugs)[1]	Oral Abs (%)	Tmax (hr)	Peak Serum Conc (μg/mL)[2]	Peak Urine Conc (μg/mL)	Protein Binding (%)	Volume of Distribution (Vd)[3]	Avg Serum T½ (hr)[4]	Elimination	Bile Pen (%)[5]	CSF/blood (%)[6]	Therapeutic Levels in CSF[7]	AUC (μg*hr/mL)[8]
Antifungals/Azoles *(continued)*															
Oteseconazole	No data	Cap (150 mg)	Cap + food	No data	5-10	2.8 (post-treatment)	No data	99.5-99.7	423 L	138 days (terminal)	Biliary, renal	No data	No data	No data	64.2 (end of tx, 0-24 hr)
Posaconazole	24-hr AUC/MIC	Delayed-release (DR) tab (100 mg), DR oral susp (30 mg/mL), oral susp (40 mg/mL), injection	All preps + food	Oral susp ≈50 DR tab ≈50 DR susp 70-80	Oral susp 3-5 DR tab 4-5 Injection 1.5	0.2-1.0 (oral susp 200 mg, SD) 2.1-2.9 (DR tab 300 mg q24h, SS) 3.3 (300 mg IV q24h, SS)	No data	98-99	226-295 L	20-66	Metabolized	No data	Variable, 0.4-237 *(Drugs 2020; 80:671)*	Possibly *(JAC 2005; 56:745)*	9.1 (400 mg oral susp q12h, 0-12 hr) 37.9 (300 mg DR tab q24h, 0-24 hr) 36.1 (300 mg IV q24h, 0-24 hr)
Voriconazole	24-hr AUC/MIC	Tab (50, 200 mg) Oral susp (40 mg/mL) Injection	Tab/susp no food	96	1-2	4.77 (4 mg/kg IV q12h)	No data	58	4.6 L/kg (Vss)	Variable (non-linear PK)	Metabolized	No data	22-100	Yes *(CID 2003; 37:728)*	33.9 (4 mg/kg IV q12h, 0-12h)
Echinocandins															
Anidulafungin	24-hr AUC/MIC	Injection	-	-	-	7.2 (100 mg IV q24h, SS)	No data	>99	30-50 L	26.5	Slow hydrolysis	No data	No data	No data	112 (100 mg IV q24h, 0-24 hr)
Caspofungin	24-hr AUC/MIC	Injection	-	-	-	8.7 (50 mg IV q24h, SS)	No data	97	9.7 L (Vss)	β-phase: 9-11 γ-phase: 40-50	Slow hydrolysis, N-acetylation	No data	No data	No data	87.3 (50 mg IV q24h, 0-24 hr)
Micafungin	24-hr AUC/MIC	Injection	-	-	-	10.1 (100 mg IV q24h, SS)	No data	>99	0.39 L/kg	15-17	Metabolism, fecal	No data	No data	No data	97 (100 mg IV q24h, 0-24 hr)
Rezafungin	No data	Injection	-	-	-	11.8 (400 mg then 200 mg wkly, on day 15)	No data	87.5 to >98.6	67 L	152 (terminal)	Fecal	No data	No data	No data	667 (400 mg then 200 mg wkly, 0-168 hr)
Triterpenoids															
Ibrexafungerp	No data	Tab (150 mg)	Tab ± food	No data	4-6	0.44-0.63 (after 2nd 300 mg dose)	No data	>99	600 L (Vss)	20	Metabolism, biliary	No data	No data	No data	6.8-9.9 (300 mg q12h, 0-24h)

Food Effect (po dosing): + food = take with food, **no food** = take without food, **± food** = take with or without food; **Oral % AB** = % absorbed; **Peak Serum Level: SD** = after single dose, **SS** = steady state after multiple doses; **Volume of Distribution (Vd): V/F** = Vd/oral bioavailability, **Vss** = Vd at steady state, **Vss/F** = Vd at steady state/oral bioavailability; **CSF Penetration:** therapeutic efficacy comment based on dose, usual susceptibility or target organism & penetration into CSF; **AUC** = area under drug concentration curve; **24hr** = AUC 0-24; **Tmax** = time to max plasma concentration.

TABLE 9A (21) *(Footnotes at the end of table)*

Groups/Drugs	PK/PD Index	Pharmaceutical Preparations	Food Rec (PO Drugs)[1]	Oral Abs (%)	Tmax (hr)	Peak Serum Conc (μg/mL)[2]	Peak Urine Conc (μg/mL)	Protein Binding (%)	Volume of Distribution (Vd)[3]	Avg Serum T½ (hr)[4]	Elimination	Bile Pen (%)[5]	CSF/blood (%)[6]	Therapeutic Levels in CSF[7]	AUC (μg*hr/mL)[8]
Antimycobacterials															
First line, tuberculosis															
Ethambutol	No data	Tab (100, 400 mg)	Tab + food	80	2-4	2-6 (25 mg/kg, SD)	No data	10-30	6 L/kg (Vss/F)	4	Renal	No data	10-50	No	29.6 (25 mg/kg po, 0-inf)
Isoniazid (INH)	No data	Tab (100, 300 mg), oral soln (10 mg/mL), injection	Tab/oral soln no food	100	1-2	3-5 (300 mg po, SD)	No data	<10	0.6-1.2 L/kg (V/F)	0.7-4.0	Acetylation, dehydrazination	No data	up to 90	Yes	20.1 (300 mg po, 0-inf)
Pyrazinamide	No data	Tab (500 mg)	Tab ± food	95	2	30-50 (20-25 mg/kg po, SD)	No data	5-10	No data	10-16	Renal	No data	100	Yes	500 (20-25 mg/kg po, 0-inf)
Rifabutin	No data	Cap (150 mg)	Cap + food	20	2.5-4.0	0.2-0.6 (300 mg po, SD)	No data	85	9.3 L/kg (Vss)	32-67	Metabolism, renal	300-500	30-70	No data	4.0 (300 mg po q24h, 0-24 hr)
Rifampin	24-hr AUC/MIC	Cap (150, 300 mg) Injection	Cap no food	70-90	1.5-2.0	7 (600 mg po, SD)	No data	80	0.65 L/kg	1.5-5.0	Metabolism, biliary, fecal	10,000	7-56	Yes	40-60 (600 mg po q24h, 0-24 hr)
Rifapentine	No data	Tab (150 mg)	Tab + food	No data	4.8	15 (600 mg po q72h, SS)	No data	98	70 L	13.2-14.1	Feces (parent, metabolite)	No data	No data	No data	320 (600 mg po q72hr, 0-72 hr)
Streptomycin	24-hr AUC/MIC	Injection	-	-	-	25-50 (15 mg/kg IM, SD)	No data	0-10	0.26 L/kg	2-3	Renal	10-60	0-30	No	No data
Second line, tuberculosis															
Bedaquiline	No data	Tab (100 mg)	Tab + food	No data	5	3.3 (during wk 2)	No data	>99	≈60 x total body water (Vss)	24-30 (terminal half-life 4-5 mo)	Metabolism, fecal	No data	Undetectable *(JAC 2016; 62:523)*	No	22 (0-24 hr, after 8 wk)
Capreomycin	No data	Injection	-	-	1-2	30 (1 gm IM, SD)	No data	No data	0.4 L/kg	2-5	Renal	No data	Negligible	No	No data
Clofazimine	No data	Cap (50, 100 mg)	Cap + food	70	No data	2 (200 mg po, SD)	No data	No data	1300 L	up to 70 days	Biliary, fecal	No data	Negligible	No	2.5-5.0 (200 mg po, 0-inf)
Cycloserine	No data	Cap (250 mg)	Cap no food	70-90	1-2	20-35 (250-500 mg po q12h, SS)	No data	No data	No data	10	Renal	No data	≈100	Yes	No data

Food Effect (po dosing): + food = take with food, **no food** = take without food, **± food** = take with or without food; **Oral % AB** = % absorbed; **Peak Serum Level: SD** = after single dose, **SS** = steady state after multiple doses; **Volume of Distribution (Vd): V/F** = Vd/oral bioavailability, **Vss** = Vd at steady state, **Vss/F** = Vd at steady state/oral bioavailability; **CSF Penetration:** therapeutic efficacy comment based on dose, usual susceptibility or target organism & penetration into CSF; **AUC** = area under drug concentration curve; **24hr** = AUC 0-24; **Tmax** = time to max plasma concentration.

TABLE 9A (22) *(Footnotes at the end of table)*

Groups/Drugs	PK/PD Index	Pharmaceutical Preparations	Food Rec (PO Drugs)[1]	Oral Abs (%)	Tmax (hr)	Peak Serum Conc (μg/mL)[2]	Peak Urine Conc (μg/mL)	Protein Binding (%)	Volume of Distribution (Vd)[3]	Avg Serum $T_{1/2}$ (hr)[4]	Elimination	Bile Pen (%)[5]	CSF/blood (%)[6]	Therapeutic Levels in CSF[7]	AUC (μg*hr/mL)[8]
Antimycobacterials/Second line, tuberculosis *(continued)*															
Delamanid	No data	Film-coated tab (50 mg), dispersible tab (25 mg)	Tab + food	25-47	4-5	No data	No data	≥99.5	2100 L (V/F)	30-38	Fecal	No data	No data	No data	No data
Ethionamide	No data	Tab (250 mg)	Tab ± food	≈100	1	2.2 (250 mg po, SD)	No data	30	93.5 L	2	Hepatic metabolism	No data	≈100	Yes	7.7 (250 mg po, 0-inf)
Kanamycin	24-hr AUC/MIC	Injection	-	-	-	25-50 (15 mg/kg IM, SD)	No data	0-10	0.26 L/kg	2-3	Renal	10-60	0-30	No	No data
Para-aminosalicylic acid (PAS)	No data	Granules (4 gm packets)	Granules + food	No data	8	9-35 (4 gm po, SD)	No data	50-60	0.9-1.4 L/kg (V/F)	0.75-1.0	Renal	No data	10-50	Marginal	108 (4 gm po, 0-inf)
Pretomanid	No data	Tab (200 mg)	Tab + food	No data	5	2.0 (200 mg po, SD)	No data	86.4	97 L (V/F)	17.4	Metabolized	No data	No data	No data	53.0 (200 mg po, 0-inf)
Thalidomide	No data	Cap (50, 100, 150, 200 mg)	Cap no food	No data	2-5	2.8-3.4 (400 mg po, SD)	No data	55-66	120 L (V/F)	5.5-7.3	Metabolized	No data	No data	No data	36.4-46.4 (400 mg po, 0-inf)
Antiparasitics															
Antimalarials															
Artemether-lumefantrine	No data	Tab (artemether 20 mg, lumefantrine 120 mg)	Tab + food	No data	Art 1.5-2 Lum 6-8	Art 0.06-0.08 (4 tabs po, SD) DHA 0.09-0.1 (4 tabs po, SD) Lum 7.4-9.8 (4 tabs po, SD)	No data	Art 95.4 DHA 47-76 Lum 99.7	ND	Art 1.6-2.2 DHA 1.6-2.2 Lum 101-119	ART, DHA, Lum: nonrenal	No data	No data	No data	Art 0.15-0.26 (4 tabs po, 0-inf) DHA 0.29 (4 tabs po, 0-inf) Lum 158-243 (4 tabs po, 0-inf)
Artesunate (AS)	No data	Injection	-	-	-	AS 3.3 (after multiple doses) DHA 3.1 (after multiple doses)	No data	AS 93 DHA 93	AS 68.5L DHA 59.7 L	AS 0.3 DHA 1.3	AS: esterases DHA: glucuronidation	No data	AS <10 DHA <10	No data	AS 0.7 (2.4 mg/kg IV, 0-inf) DHA 3.5 (2.4 mg/kg IV, 0-inf)
Atovaquone-Proguanil	No data	Tab (Atova 250/Pro 100 mg, Atova 62.5/Pro 25 mg)	Tab + food	Atova: 23 Pro: no data	Atova: no data Pro: no data	Atova: no data Pro: no data	No data	Atova: >99 Pro: 75	Atova: 8.8 L/kg (V/F) Pro: 1617-2502 L (V/F)	Atova: 48-72 Pro: 12-21	Atova: fecal Pro: metabolism, renal	No data	No data	No data	Atova: no data Pro: no data

Food Effect (po dosing): + food = take with food, **no food** = take without food, **± food** = take with or without food; **Oral % AB** = % absorbed; **Peak Serum Level: SD** = after single dose, **SS** = steady state after multiple doses; **Volume of Distribution (Vd): V/F** = Vd/oral bioavailability, **Vss** = Vd at steady state, **Vss/F** = Vd at steady state/oral bioavailability; **CSF Penetration:** therapeutic efficacy comment based on dose, usual susceptibility or target organism & penetration into CSF; **AUC** = area under drug concentration curve; **24hr** = AUC 0-24; **Tmax** = time to max plasma concentration.

TABLE 9A (23) *(Footnotes at the end of table)*

Groups/Drugs	PK/PD Index	Pharmaceutical Preparations	Food Rec (PO Drugs)[1]	Oral Abs (%)	Tmax (hr)	Peak Serum Conc (µg/mL)[2]	Peak Urine Conc (µg/mL)	Protein Binding (%)	Volume of Distribution (Vd)[3]	Avg Serum T½ (hr)[4]	Elimination	Bile Pen (%)[5]	CSF/blood (%)[6]	Therapeutic Levels in CSF[7]	AUC (µg*hr/mL)[8]
Antiparasitics/Antimalarials *(continued)*															
Chloroquine phosphate	No data	Tab (500 mg) =300 mg base	Tab + food	90	1-6	0.06-0.09 (300 mg po base, SD)	No data	55	100-1000 L/kg	45-55 days (terminal)	Metabolism, renal	No data	No data	No data	No data
Dihydroartemisinin-piperaquine	No data	Tab (DHA 20 mg/PPQ 160 mg) Tab (DHA 40 mg/PPQ 320 mg)	Tab no food	No data	DHA: 1-2 PPQ: 5	DHA: 0.75 (dose not known) PPQ: 0.18 (dose not known)	No data	DHA: 44-93 PPQ: >99	DHA: 0.8 L/kg PPQ: 730 L/kg	DHA: 1 hr PPQ: 22 days	DHA: glucuronidation PPQ: biliary	No data	No data	No data	DHA: 2 (dose not known, 0-inf) PPQ: 1.7 (dose not known, 0-24h)
Hydroxychloroquine sulfate	No data	Tab (200 mg) =155 mg base	Tab + food	>90	3-4	50.3 ng/mL (200 mg po, SD)	No data	No data	No data	40-50 days (terminal)	Metabolism, renal	No data	No data	No data	No data
Mefloquine	No data	Tab (250 mg)	Tab + food	No data	17	0.5-1.2 (1250 mg po, SD)	No data	98	20 L/kg	13-24 days	Biliary, fecal	No data	No data	No data	No data
Primaquine (phosphate)	No data	Tab (26.3 mg [15 mg base])	Tab + food	No data	2-3	0.18-0.2 (30 mg base q24h, SS)	No data	No data	3 L/kg	3.7-9.6	Hepatic metabolism	No data	No data	No data	1.2-1.6 (30 mg base, 0-inf)
Pyronaridine-artesunate	No data	Tab: pyr 180 mg, AS 60 mg Granules: pyr 60 mg, AS 20 mg	Tab ± food	No data	Pyr: 2-8 AS: 0.5-1 DHA: 1-2	Pyr: 0.23 (720 mg q24h x3 days) Highly variable	No data	Pyr: 92-25 AS: 62-93 DHA: 62-93	Pyr: ≈26,000L (Vss/F) Highly variable	Pyr: 14-18 days AS: 0.5 hr DHA: 0.8 hr	Pyr: metabolism, fecal AS: esterases DHA: glucuronidation	No data	No data	No data	1134 ng*day/mL (720 mg q24h x3 days, 0-inf) Highly variable
Quinacrine	No data	Tab (100 mg) (must be compounded in US)	Take with liquids after a meal	100	Rapid	No data	No data	80-90	No data	5-14 days	Renal	No data	No data	No data	No data
Quinine dihydrochloride	No data	Injection	-	-	IV: 1-1.1	3-3.5 (10 mg/kg IV, SD)	No data	80-90	0.45-4.24 L/kg	8-10	Hepatic metabolism	No data	Poor	No	No data
Quinine sulfate	No data	Cap (324 mg)	Cap + food	76-88	2.8	3.2 (648 mg po, SD)	No data	69-92	2.5-7.1 L/kg (V/F)	9.7-12.5	Hepatic metabolism	No data	2-7	No	28 (648 mg po, 0-inf)

Food Effect (po dosing): **+ food** = take with food, **no food** = take without food, **± food** = take with or without food; **Oral % AB** = % absorbed; **Peak Serum Level: SD** = after single dose, **SS** = steady state after multiple doses; **Volume of Distribution (Vd): V/F** = Vd/oral bioavailability, **Vss** = Vd at steady state, **Vss/F** = Vd at steady state/oral bioavailability; **CSF Penetration:** therapeutic efficacy comment based on dose, usual susceptibility or target organism & penetration into CSF; **AUC** = area under drug concentration curve; **24hr** = AUC 0-24; **Tmax** = time to max plasma concentration.

TABLE 9A (24) *(Footnotes at the end of table)*

Groups/Drugs	PK/PD Index	Pharmaceutical Preparations	Food Rec (PO Drugs)[1]	Oral Abs (%)	Tmax (hr)	Peak Serum Conc (µg/mL)[2]	Peak Urine Conc (µg/mL)	Protein Binding (%)	Volume of Distribution (Vd)[3]	Avg Serum T½ (hr)[4]	Elimination	Bile Pen (%)[5]	CSF/blood (%)[6]	Therapeutic Levels in CSF[7]	AUC (µg*hr/mL)[8]
Antiparasitics/Antimalarials *(continued)*															
Sulfadoxine-pyrimethamine	No data	Tab (sulfadoxine 500 mg, pyrimethamine 25 mg)	Tab post meal	No data	Sul: 4 Pyr: 4	Sul: 60 (500 mg po, SD) Pyr: 0.2 (25 mg po, SD)	No data	Sul: 90 Pyr: 90	Sul: 0.14 L/kg Pyr: 2.3 L/kg	Sul: 200 Pyr: 100	Sul: renal Pyr: metabolized	No data	No data	No	No data
Tafenoquine	No data	Tab (100, 150 mg)	Tab + food	No data	12-15	0.15 (200 mg po, SD)	No data	>99.5	1600-2500 L	15 days (terminal)	Slow metabolism	No data	No data	No data	70 (200 mg po, 0-inf)
Antiparasitics, Other															
Albendazole	No data	Tab (200 mg)	Tab + food	Poor	Sulfoxide: 2-5	Sulfoxide: 0.5-1.6 (400 mg po, SD)	No data	70	No data	8-12	Metabolized	Sulfoxide: 100	No data	No data	No data
Antimony, pentavalent	No data	Injection	-	-	IM: 0.5-2	38 (20 mg/kg IV q24h, SS)	No data	No data	≈260 L (Vss)	elim 2 hr, terminal 1-3 days	Renal	No data	No data	No data	65.4 (10 mg/kg SD, 0-inf)
Atovaquone	No data	Oral susp (750 mg/5 mL)	Susp + food	47	No data	24 (750 mg q12h, SS) (HIV-infected patients)	No data	99.9	0.6 L/kg (Vss)	67-78	Fecal	No data	No data	No data	801 (750 mg po, 0-inf) (healthy subjects)
Benznidazole	No data	Tab (12.5 mg, 100 mg)	Tab + food	92	2.9	2.2 (100 mg po, SD)	No data	44	39.2 L (V/F)	13.3	Renal, fecal	No data	No data	No data	51.3 (100 mg po, 0-inf)
Dapsone	No data	Tab (25, 100 mg), 5% gel	Tab ± food	70-100	2-6	1.1 (100 mg po q24h, SS)	No data	70	1.5 L/kg	10-50	Metabolized	No data	No data	No data	52.6 (100 mg po q24h, 0-24 hr)
Diethylcarbamazine	No data	Tab (100 mg)	Tab + food	80-85	1-2	1.93 (6 mg/kg po, SD)	No data	No data	3-5 L/kg	9	Metabolism (N-oxide) Renal	No data	No data	No data	23.8 (6 mg/kg po, 0-inf)
Diloxanide furoate	No data	Tab (500 mg)	Tab + food	No data	2	No data	No data	No data	No data	3-6?	Renal, fecal	No data	No data	No data	No data
Eflornithine	No data	Injection	-	-	-	50-90 nmol/L (100 mg/kg IV q6h, SS)	No data	Negligible	No data	3.3	Renal	No data	60-90	Yes	No data

<u>Food Effect</u> (po dosing): + food = take with food, **no food** = take without food, **± food** = take with or without food; **Oral % AB** = % absorbed; **<u>Peak Serum Level</u>: SD** = after single dose, **SS** = steady state after multiple doses; **Volume of Distribution (Vd): V/F** = Vd/oral bioavailability, **Vss** = Vd at steady state, **Vss/F** = Vd at steady state/oral bioavailability; **CSF Penetration:** therapeutic efficacy comment based on

TABLE 9A (25) *(Footnotes at the end of table)*

Groups/Drugs	PK/PD Index	Pharmaceutical Preparations	Food Rec (PO Drugs)[1]	Oral Abs (%)	Tmax (hr)	Peak Serum Conc (μg/mL)[2]	Peak Urine Conc (μg/mL)	Protein Binding (%)	Volume of Distribution (Vd)[3]	Avg Serum T½ (hr)[4]	Elimination	Bile Pen (%)[5]	CSF/blood (%)[6]	Therapeutic Levels in CSF[7]	AUC (μg*hr/mL)[8]
Antiparasitics/Other *(continued)*															
Fexinidazole	No data	Tab (600 mg)	Tab + food	No data	Fex/M1 4 M2 6	Fex 0.5 (≥35 kg regimen, SS) M1 5.9 (≥35 kg regimen, SS) M2 12.5 (≥35 kg regimen, SS)	No data	Fex 98 M1 41 M2 57	Fex 3222 L (apparent Vd, day 4)	Fex 15 M1 16 M2 23	Metabolism, fecal	No data	M1 53 M2 36	Yes	Fex 7.0 (≥35 kg regimen, 0-24 hr) M1 84.2 (≥35 kg regimen, 0-24 hr) M2 252.4 (≥35 kg regimen, 0-24 hr)
Fumagillin	No data	Cap (20 mg) Ophthalmic soln	Cap no food	No data	No data	No data	No data	No data	No data	No data	No data	No data	No data	No data	No data
Iodoquinol	No data	Tab (650 mg)	Tab + food	Poor	No data	No data	No data	No data	No data	No data	Metabolism, fecal	No data	No data	No data	No data
Ivermectin	No data	Tab (3 mg)	Tab no food	60	4	0.05-0.08 (12 mg po, SD)	No data	93	3-3.5 L/kg	20	Metabolism, fecal	No data	No data	No data	No data
Mebendazole	No data	Tab (100 mg, 500 mg) (may be chewed)	Tab ± food	Minimal	2-4	0.014 fasting, 0.056 fed (500 mg po, SD)	No data	90-95	1-2 L/kg	3-6	Metabolized	No data	No data	No data	175 fasting, 456 fed (ng*hr/mL, 500 mg po, 0-inf)
Melarsoprol	No data	Injection	-	-	-	2-4 (2.2 mg/kg IV, SD)	No data	80	No data	<0.5 (parent)	Metabolized	No data	5	No data	No data
Miltefosine	No data	Cap (50 mg)	Cap + food	No data	2-8, up to 24	76 (50 mg po q8h, after 23 days)	No data	95	No data	7-31 days *(AAC 2008; 52:2855)*	Metabolism (phospholipase D?)	No data	2-4 *(Parasitol Res 2015; 114:4431)*	Unlikely	486 (50 mg po q8h, 0-8 hr)
Moxidectin*	No data	Tab (2 mg)	Tab ± food	↑ AUC with food (44%)[12]	4	0.059-0.063 (8 mg po, SD)	No data	No data	2421 L	23.3 days (terminal)	Nonrenal Minimal hepatic metabolism	No data	No data	No data	2.7-3.4 (8 mg po, 0-inf)
Niclosamide*	No data	500 mg chewable tabs	Tab ± food	Negligible	No data	No data	No data	No data	No data	No data	No data	No data	No data	No data	No data
Nifurtimox	No data	Tab (30 mg, 120 mg)	Tab + food	No data	4	425-568 ng/mL (120 mg po, SD)	No data	42	No data	2.4-3.6	Metabolism (nitroreductases)	No data	No data	No data	1676-2670 ng*hr/mL (120 mg po, 0-inf)

Food Effect (po dosing): + food = take with food, **no food** = take without food, **± food** = take with or without food; **Oral % AB** = % absorbed; **Peak Serum Level: SD** = after single dose, **SS** = steady state after multiple doses; **Volume of Distribution (Vd): V/F** = Vd/oral bioavailability, **Vss** = Vd at steady state, **Vss/F** = Vd at steady state/oral bioavailability; **CSF Penetration:** therapeutic efficacy comment based on dose, usual susceptibility or target organism & penetration into CSF; **AUC** = area under drug concentration curve; **24hr** = AUC 0-24; **Tmax** = time to max plasma concentration.

TABLE 9A (26) *(Footnotes at the end of table)*

Groups/Drugs	PK/PD Index	Pharmaceutical Preparations	Food Rec (PO Drugs)[1]	Oral Abs (%)	Tmax (hr)	Peak Serum Conc (µg/mL)[2]	Peak Urine Conc (µg/mL)	Protein Binding (%)	Volume of Distribution (Vd)[3]	Avg Serum T½ (hr)[4]	Elimination	Bile Pen (%)[5]	CSF/blood (%)[6]	Therapeutic Levels in CSF[7]	AUC (µg*hr/mL)[8]
Antiparasitics/Other *(continued)*															
Nitazoxanide	No data	Tab (500 mg), oral susp (100 mg/5 mL)	Tab/susp + food	Susp 70% of tab	Tizox: 1-4 Tizox gluc: 1-4	Tizox: 9-11 (500 mg po, SD) Tizox gluc: 7.3-10.5 (500 mg po, SD)	No data	Tizox: 99	No data	Tizox: 1.3-1.8	Conjugation, fecal, renal	No data	No data	No data	Tizox: 39.5-41.9 (500 mg po, 0-inf) Tizox gluc: 46.5-63 500 mg po, 0-inf)
Paromomycin	No data	Cap (250 mg)	Cap + food	Negligible	No data	No data	No data	No data	No data	2-3	Fecal	No data	No data	No data	No data
Pentamidine	No data	Injection, inhalation	-	-	IM: 1	0.6 (4 mg/kg IV, SD)	No data	69	200-400 L/kg (Vss)	terminal 11-12 days	Metabolism	No data	Poor	No	0.75 (3 mg/kg IV, 0-inf)
Praziquantel	No data	Tab (600 mg)	Tab + food	80-100	1-3	0.83 (40 mg/kg po, SD)	No data	≈80	8000 L (V/F)	0.8-1.5	Metabolism	No data	10-20	No data	3.02 (40 mg/kg po, 0-inf)
Pyrantel pamoate	No data	Oral susp (50 mg/mL base)	Susp ± food	Poor	1-3	0.05-0.13 (11 mg/kg po, SD)	No data	No data	No data	No data	Fecal	No data	No data	No data	No data
Pyrimethamine	No data	Tab (25 mg)	Tab ± food	High	2-6	0.1-0.3 (25 mg po, SD)	No data	87	3 L/kg	96	Metabolized	No data	Good *(AIDS 1992; 6:1040)*	No data	No data
Spiramycin	No data	Cap (250, 500 mg)	Cap ± food	30-39	No data	0.4-1.4 (1 gm po, SD)	No data	10-25	>300 L	4.5-6.2	Fecal-biliary	No data	Poor	No	No data
Suramin	No data	Injection	-	-	No data	>100 (persists for several weeks)	No data	≈99.7	No data	44-54 days	Renal	No data	Negligible	No	No data
Tinidazole	No data	Tab (250, 500 mg)	Tab + food	48	1.6	48 (2 gm po, SD)	No data	12	50 L	13	Metabolism, renal	No data	No data	No data	902 (2 gm po, 0-inf)

Food Effect (po dosing): + food = take with food, **no food** = take without food, **± food** = take with or without food; **Oral % AB** = % absorbed; **Peak Serum Level: SD** = after single dose, **SS** = steady state after

TABLE 9A (27) *(Footnotes at the end of table)*

Groups/Drugs	PK/PD Index	Pharmaceutical Preparations	Food Rec (PO Drugs)[1]	Oral Abs (%)	Tmax (hr)	Peak Serum Conc (µg/mL)[2]	Peak Urine Conc (µg/mL)	Protein Binding (%)	Volume of Distribution (Vd)[3]	Avg Serum T½ (hr)[4]	Elimination	Bile Pen (%)[5]	CSF/blood (%)[6]	Therapeutic Levels in CSF[7]	AUC (µg*hr/mL)[8]
Antiparasitics/Other *(continued)*															
Triclabendazole	No data	Tab (250 mg)	Tab + food	No data	Tricla: 3-4 Sulfoxide: 3-4	Tricla: 1.16 µmol/mL (10 mg/kg po, SD) Sulfoxide: 38.6 µmol/mL (10 mg/kg po, SD) Sulfone: 2.29 µmol/mL (10 mg/kg po, SD)	No data	Tricla: 96.7 Sulfoxide: 98.4 Sulfone: 98.8	Sulfoxide 1 L/kg	Tricla: 8 Sulfoxide: 14 Sulfone: 11	No human data	No data	No data	No data	Tricla: 5.72 µmol*hr/L (10 mg/kg, 0-inf) Sulfoxide: 386 µmol*hr/L (10 mg/kg, 0-inf) Sulfone: 30.5 µmol*hr/L (10 mg/kg, 0-inf)
Antivirals (non-HIV)															
Coronavirus															
Bamlanivimab + Etesevimab	No data	Injection	-	-	-	Bam: 196 (700 mg IV, SD) Ete: 504 (1400 mg IV, SD)	No data	No data	Bam: 5.58 L (Vss) Ete: 4.36 L (Vss)	Bam: 17.6 days Ete: 25.1 days	Catabolized (similar to IgG)	No data	No data	No data	No data
Baricitinib (JAK inhibitor)	No data	Tab (1, 2 mg)	Tab ± food	80	1	No data	No data	50	76 L	12	Primarily renal	No data	No data	No data	No data
Bebtelovimab	No data	Injection	-	-	-	59.8 (175 mg IV, SD)	No data	No data	4.61 L (Vss)	11.5 days	Catabolized (similar to IgG)	No data	No data	No data	522 µg*day/mL (175 mg IV, 0-inf)
Casirivimab + Imdevimab	No data	Injection	-	-	-	Cas: IV 192, SC 55.6 (600 mg, SD) Imd: IV 198, SC 52.7 (600 mg, SD)	No data	No data	No data	Cas: 31.8 days Imd: 26.9 days	Catabolized (similar to IgG)	No data	No data	No data	Cas: 2580 mg*day/L (600 mg IV, 0-inf) Imd: 1990 mg*day/L (600 mg IV, 0-inf)
Molnupiravir	No data	Cap (200 mg)	Cap ± food	No data	1.5	2.33 (800 mg po q12h, SS)	No data	≈0	142 L	3.3 (N-hydroxycytidine)	Metabolism	No data	No data	No data	8.26 (800 mg po q12h, 0-12 hr)

__Food Effect__ **(po dosing): + food** = take with food, **no food** = take without food, **± food** = take with or without food; **Oral % AB** = % absorbed; **__Peak Serum Level__: SD** = after single dose, **SS** = steady state after multiple doses; **__Volume of Distribution (Vd)__: V/F** = Vd/oral bioavailability, **Vss** = Vd at steady state, **Vss/F** = Vd at steady state/oral bioavailability; **__CSF Penetration__:** therapeutic efficacy comment based on dose, usual susceptibility or target organism & penetration into CSF; **AUC** = area under drug concentration curve; **24hr** = AUC 0-24; **Tmax** = time to max plasma concentration.

TABLE 9A (28) *(Footnotes at the end of table)*

Groups/Drugs	PK/PD Index	Pharmaceutical Preparations	Food Rec (PO Drugs)[1]	Oral Abs (%)	Tmax (hr)	Peak Serum Conc (µg/mL)[2]	Peak Urine Conc (µg/mL)	Protein Binding (%)	Volume of Distribution (Vd)[3]	Avg Serum T½ (hr)[4]	Elimination	Bile Pen (%)[5]	CSF/blood (%)[6]	Therapeutic Levels in CSF[7]	AUC (µg*hr/mL)[8]
Antivirals (non-HIV)/Coronavirus *(continued)*															
Nirmatrelvir + Ritonavir	No data	Tab (Nir 150 mg, RTV 100 mg)	Tabs ± food	No data	Nir: 3 RTV: 3.98	Nir: 2.21 (150 mg po, SD)	No data	Nir: 69 RTV: 98-99	Nir: 104.7 L (Vz/F) RTV: 112.4 L (Vz/F)	Nir: 6.05 RTV: 6.15	Nir: renal RTV: metabolized (CYP3A4)	No data	No data	No data	Nir: 23.01 (150 mg po, 0-inf)
Pemivibart	No data	Injection	-	-	-	1750 (4500 mg IV, SD)	No data	No data	5.54 L (Vss)	44.8 days	Catabolized (similar to IgG)	No data	No data	No data	36,600 (4500 mg IV, 0-3 mon)
Remdesivir	No data	Injection	-	-	No data	Rem: 2.23 (100 mg IV q24h, SS) GS-441524: 0.14 (100 mg IV q24h, SS)	No data	Rem: 88-93.6 GS-441524: 2	No data	Rem: 1 GS-441524: 27	GS-441524: Renal	No data	No data	No data	Rem: 1.56 (100 mg IV q24h, 0-24 hr) GS-441524: 2.23 (100 mg IV q24h, 0-24 hr)
Sotrovimab	No data	Injection	-	-	-	137 (500 mg IV, SD)	No data	No data	No data	No data	Catabolized (similar to IgG)	No data	No data	No data	No data
Tixagevimab + Cilgavimab	No data	Injection	-	-	Tix: 14.9 days Cil: 15 days	Tix: 21.9 (300 mg IM, SD) Cil: 20.3 (300 mg IM, SD)	No data	No data	Tix: 7.7 L Cil: 8.7 L	Tix: 87.9 days Cil: 82.9 days	Catabolized (similar to IgG)	No data	No data	No data	Tix: 1408 µg*day/mL (300 mg IM, 0-84 d) Cil: 1307 µg*day/mL (300 mg IM, 0-84 d)
Tocilizumab	No data	Injection	-	-	-	151 (8 mg/kg IV, SD)	No data	No data	8.75 L	21.5 days (terminal)	Catabolized (similar to IgG)	No data	No data	No data	No data
Tofacitinib (JAK inhibitor)	No data	Tab (5, 10 mg), XR tab (11, 22 mg), oral soln (1 mg/mL)	All preps ± food	74	0.8	84.7 ng/mL (10 mg po q12h, SS)	No data	40	87 L	3	Hepatic metabolism, renal	No data	No data	No data	539.6 ng*hr/mL (10 mg po q12h, 0-24 hr)

Food Effect (po dosing): **+ food** = take with food, **no food** = take without food, **± food** = take with or without food; **Oral % AB** = % absorbed; **Peak Serum Level**: **SD** = after single dose, **SS** = steady state after

TABLE 9A (29) *(Footnotes at the end of table)*

Groups/Drugs	PK/PD Index	Pharmaceutical Preparations	Food Rec (PO Drugs)[1]	Oral Abs (%)	Tmax (hr)	Peak Serum Conc (µg/mL)[2]	Peak Urine Conc (µg/mL)	Protein Binding (%)	Volume of Distribution (Vd)[3]	Avg Serum T½ (hr)[4]	Elimination	Bile Pen (%)[5]	CSF/blood (%)[6]	Therapeutic Levels in CSF[7]	AUC (µg*hr/mL)[8]
Antivirals (non-HIV) *(continued)*															
Ebola virus															
Ansuvimab-zykl	No data	Injection	-	-	-	No data	No data	No data	No data	≈24 days	Catabolized (similar to IgG)	No data	No data	No data	No data
Inmazeb (atoltivimab + maftivimab + odesivimab)	No data	Injection	-	-	-	Ato: 1220 (50 mg/kg IV, SD) Maf: 1280 (50 mg/kg IV, SD) Ode: 1260 (50 mg/kg IV, SD)	No data	No data	Ato: 58.2 mL/kg (Vss) Maf: 57.6 mL/kg (Vss) Ode: 56 mL/kg (Vss)	Ato: 21.2 days Maf: 22.3 days Ode: 25.3 days	Catabolized (similar to IgG)	No data	No data	No data	Ato: 17100 µg*day/mL (50 mg/kg IV, 0-inf) Maf: 18700 µg*day/mL (50 mg/kg IV, 0-inf) Ode: 25600 µg*day/mL (50 mg/kg IV, 0-inf)
Hepatitis B															
Adefovir	No data	Tab (10 mg)	Tab ± food	59	1.75	0.02 (10 mg po, SD)	No data	≤4	0.35-0.39 L/kg (Vss)	7.5	Renal	No data	No data	No data	0.22 (10 mg po, 0-inf)
Entecavir	No data	Tab (0.5, 1 mg), oral soln (0.05 mg/mL)	Tab/soln no food	100	0.5-1.5	4.2 ng/mL (0.5 mg po q24h, SS)	No data	13	>0.6 L/kg (V/F)	128-149 (terminal)	Renal	No data	No data	No data	0.014 (0.5 mg po q24h, 0-24 hr)
Interferons	No data	Injection	-	-	-	18-116 IU/mL (alfa-2b 5 million IU/m², SD)	No data	No data	12-40 L (smaller if pegylated)	2-3 (longer if pegylated)	Catabolized	No data	No data	No data	No data
Telbivudine	No data	Tab (600 mg), oral soln (100 mg/5 mL)	Tab/soln ± food	No data	2	3.7 (600 mg po q24h, SS)	No data	3.3	>0.6 L/kg (V/F)	40-49	Renal	No data	No data	No data	26.1 (600 mg po q24h, 0-24 hr)
Tenofovir alafenamide fumarate (TAF)	No data	Tab (25 mg)	Tab + food	No data	0.48	0.27 (25 mg po q24h, SS)	No data	80	No data	0.51	Metabolized	No data	No data	No data	0.27 (25 mg po q24h, 0-24 hr)

Food Effect (po dosing): + food = take with food, **no food** = take without food, **± food** = take with or without food; **Oral % AB** = % absorbed; **Peak Serum Level: SD** = after single dose, **SS** = steady state after multiple doses; **Volume of Distribution (Vd): V/F** = Vd/oral bioavailability, **Vss** = Vd at steady state, **Vss/F** = Vd at steady state/oral bioavailability; **CSF Penetration:** therapeutic efficacy comment based on dose, usual susceptibility or target organism & penetration into CSF; **AUC** = area under drug concentration curve; **24hr** = AUC 0-24; **Tmax** = time to max plasma concentration.

TABLE 9A (30) *(Footnotes at the end of table)*

Groups/Drugs	PK/PD Index	Pharmaceutical Preparations	Food Rec (PO Drugs)[1]	Oral Abs (%)	Tmax (hr)	Peak Serum Conc (µg/mL)[2]	Peak Urine Conc (µg/mL)	Protein Binding (%)	Volume of Distribution (Vd)[3]	Avg Serum T½ (hr)[4]	Elimination	Bile Pen (%)[5]	CSF/blood (%)[6]	Therapeutic Levels in CSF[7]	AUC (µg*hr/mL)[8]
Antivirals (non-HIV) *(continued)*															
Hepatitis C															
Daclatasvir	No data	Tab (30, 60, 90 mg)	Tab ± food	67	2	0.18 (Cmin, 60 mg po q24h, SS)	No data	99	47 (Vss)	12-15	Metabolism	No data	No data	No data	11 (60 mg po q24h, 0-24 hr)
Ribavirin	No data	Cap (200 mg) Tab (200mg) Oral soln (40 mg/mL) Inhalation soln (6 gm vials)	All preps + food	64	2	3.7 (600 mg po q12h, SS)	No data	Minimal	2825 L (V/F)	44 (terminal 298)	Metabolism, renal	No data	No data	No data	228 (600 mg po q12h, 0-12 hr)
Simeprevir	No data	Cap (150 mg) where available outside US	Cap + food	No data	4-6	No data	No data	>99.9	No data	41	Biliary	No data	No data	No data	57.5 (150 mg po q24h, 0-24 hr)
Sofosbuvir	No data	Tab (200, 400 mg), oral pellets (150, 200 mg)	Tab ± food	No data	Sofos: 0.5-2 GS-331007: 3.5-4	Sofos: 0.6 (400 mg po q24h, SS) GS-331007: 1.4 (400 mg po q24h, SS)	No data	Sofos: 61-65 GS-331007: minimal	No data	Sofos: 0.5-0.75 GS-331007: 27	Sofos: metabolism GS-331007: renal	No data	No data	No data	Sofos: 0.9-1.3 (400 mg po q24h, 0-24h) GS-331007: 12 (400 mg po q24h, 0-24h)
Hepatitis C combinations															
Elbasvir + Grazoprevir (Zepatier)	No data	Tab (Elb 50 mg, Grazo 100 mg)	Tab ± food	No data	Elb: 3 Grazo: 2	Elb: 0.121 (50 mg po q24h, SS) Grazo: 0.165 (100 mg po q24h, SS)	No data	Elb: >99.9 Grazo: >98.8	Elb: 680 L Grazo: 1250 L	Elb: 24 Grazo: 31	Elb: metabolism, fecal Grazo: metabolism, fecal	No data	No data	No data	Elb: 1.92 (50 mg po q24h, 0-24 hr) Grazo: 1.42 (100 mg po q24h, 0-24 hr)
Glecaprevir + Pibrentasvir (Mavyret)	No data	Tab (Gleca 100 mg, Pibrent 40 mg)	Tab + food	No data	Gleca: 5 Pibrent: 5	Gleca: 0.6 (300 mg po q24h, SS) Pibrent: 0.11 (120 mg po q24h, SS)	No data	Gleca: 97.5 Pibrent: >99.9	No data	Gleca: 6 Pibrent: 13	Gleca: biliary-fecal Pibrent: biliary-fecal	No data	No data	No data	Gleca: 4.8 (300 mg po q24h, 0-24 hr) Pibrent: 1.43 (120 mg po q24h, 0-24 hr)

Food Effect (po dosing): + food = take with food, **no food** = take without food, **± food** = take with or without food; **Oral % AB** = % absorbed; **Peak Serum Level: SD** = after single dose, **SS** = steady state after multiple doses; **Volume of Distribution (Vd): V/F** = Vd/oral bioavailability, **Vss** = Vd at steady state, **Vss/F** = Vd at steady state/oral bioavailability; **CSF Penetration:** therapeutic efficacy comment based on dose, usual susceptibility or target organism & penetration into CSF; **AUC** = area under drug concentration curve; **24hr** = AUC 0-24; **Tmax** = time to max plasma concentration.

TABLE 9A (31) *(Footnotes at the end of table)*

Groups/Drugs	PK/PD Index	Pharmaceutical Preparations	Food Rec (PO Drugs)[1]	Oral Abs (%)	Tmax (hr)	Peak Serum Conc (μg/mL)[2]	Peak Urine Conc (μg/mL)	Protein Binding (%)	Volume of Distribution (Vd)[3]	Avg Serum T½ (hr)[4]	Elimination	Bile Pen (%)[5]	CSF/blood (%)[6]	Therapeutic Levels in CSF[7]	AUC (μg*hr/mL)[8]
Antivirals (non-HIV)/Hepatitis C combinations *(continued)*															
Ledipasvir + Sofosbuvir (Harvoni)	No data	Tab (Ledip 90 mg, Sofos 400 mg)	Tab ± food	No data	Ledip: 4-4.5 Sofos: 0.8-1 GS-331007: 3.5-4	Ledip: 0.3 (90 mg po q24h, SS) Sofos: 0.62 (400 mg po q24h, SS) GS-331007: 0.71 (400 mg po q24h, SS)	No data	Ledip: >99.8 Sofos: 61-65 GS-331007: minimal	No data	Ledip: 47 Sofos: 0.5 GS-331007: 27	Ledip: biliary-fecal Sofos: metabolism GS-331007: renal	No data	No data	No data	Ledip: 7.3 (90 mg po q24h, 0-24 hr) Sofos: 1.3 (400 mg po q24h, 0-24 hr) GS-331007: 12 (400 mg po q24h, 0-24 hr)
Ombitasvir + Paritaprevir + RTV (Technivie)	No data	Tab (Ombit 12.5 mg, Parita 75 mg, RTV 50 mg)	Tab + food	Ombit: 48 Parita: 53	Ombit: 5 Parita: 4-5 RTV: 4-5	Ombit: 0.082 (25 mg po q24h, SS) Parita: 0.19 (150 mg po q24h, SS) RTV: 0.54 (100 po q24h, SS)	No data	Ombit: 99.9 Parita: 97-98.6 RTV: >99	Ombit: 173 L (Vss) Parita: 103 L (Vss) RTV: 21.5 L (V/F)	Ombit: 21-25 Parita: 5.5 RTV: 4	Ombit: biliary Parita: metabolism RTV: metabolism	No data	No data	No data	Ombit: 1.24 (25 mg po q24h, 0-24 hr) Parita: 2.28 (150 mg po q24h, 0-24 hr) RTV: 6.1 (100 mg po q24h, 0-24 hr)
Ombitasvir + Paritaprevir + RTV + Dasabuvir (Viekira Pak)	No data	Tab (Ombit 12.5 mg, Parita 75 mg, RTV 50 mg), Tab (Dasa 250 mg) XR (Ombit 8.33 mg, Parita 50 mg, RTV 33.33 mg, Dasa 200 mg)	All tabs + food	Ombit: 48 Parita: 53 Dasa: 70	Ombit: 5 (XR 5) Parita: 4-5 (XR 5) RTV: 4-5 (XR 4) Dasa: 4 (XR 8)	Ombit: 0.068 (25 mg po q24h, SS) Parita: 0.26 (150 mg po q24h, SS) RTV: 0.68 (100 mg po q24h, SS) Dasa: 0.67 (250 mg po q12h SS)	No data	Ombit: 99.9 Parita: 97-98.6 RTV: >99 Dasa: >99.5	Ombit: 173 L (Vss) Parita: 103 L (Vss) RTV: 21.5 L (V/F) Dasa: 149 L (Vss)	Ombit: 21-25 Parita: 5.5 RTV: 4 Dasa: 5.5-6	Ombit: biliary Parita: metabolism RTV: metabolism Data: metabolism	No data	No data	No data	Ombit: 1 (25 mg po q24h, 0-24h) Parita: 2.22 (150 mg po q24h, 0-24h) RTV: 6.2 (100 mg po q24h, 0-24h) Dasa: 3.24 (250 mg po q12h, 0-12h)

Food Effect (po dosing): + food = take with food, **no food** = take without food, **± food** = take with or without food; **Oral % AB** = % absorbed; **Peak Serum Level: SD** = after single dose, **SS** = steady state after multiple doses; **Volume of Distribution (Vd): V/F** = Vd/oral bioavailability, **Vss** = Vd at steady state, **Vss/F** = Vd at steady state/oral bioavailability; **CSF Penetration:** therapeutic efficacy comment based on dose, usual susceptibility or target organism & penetration into CSF; **AUC** = area under drug concentration curve; **24hr** = AUC 0-24; **Tmax** = time to max plasma concentration.

TABLE 9A (32) *(Footnotes at the end of table)*

Groups/Drugs	PK/PD Index	Pharmaceutical Preparations	Food Rec (PO Drugs)[1]	Oral Abs (%)	Tmax (hr)	Peak Serum Conc (µg/mL)[2]	Peak Urine Conc (µg/mL)	Protein Binding (%)	Volume of Distribution (Vd)[3]	Avg Serum T½ (hr)[4]	Elimination	Bile Pen (%)[5]	CSF/blood (%)[6]	Therapeutic Levels in CSF[7]	AUC (µg*hr/mL)[8]
Antivirals (non-HIV)/Hepatitis C combinations *(continued)*															
Velpatasvir + Sofosbuvir (Epclusa)	No data	Tab (Velpat 100 mg, Sofos 400 mg)	Tab ± food	No data	Velpat: 3 Sofos: 0.5-1	Velpat: 0.26 (100 mg po q24h, SS) Sofos: 0.57 (400 mg po q24h, SS) GS-331007: 0.9 (400 mg po q24h, SS)	No data	Velpat: >99.5 Sofos: 61-65	No data	Velpat: 15 Sofos: 0.5 GS-331007: 25	Velpat: biliary Sofos: metabolism GS-331007: renal	No data	No data	No data	Velpat: 2.98 (100 mg q24h, 0-24h) Sofos: 1.3 (400 mg q24h, 0-24h) GS-331007: 14.4 (400 mg q24h, 0-24h)
Velpatasvir + Sofosbuvir + Voxilaprevir (Vosevi)	No data	Tab (Velpat 100 mg, Sofos 400 mg, Voxila 100 mg)	Tab + food	No data	Velpat: 4 Sofos: 2 Voxila: 4	Velpat: 0.31 (100 mg po q24h, SS) Sofos: 0.68 (400 mg po q24h, SS) GS-331007: 0.74 (400 mg po q24h, SS) Voxila: 0.19 (100 mg po q24h, SS)	No data	Velpat: >99 Sofos: 61-65 Voxila: >99	No data	Velpat: 17 Sofos: 0.5 GS-331007: 29 Voxila: 33	Velpat: biliary Sofos: metabolism GS-331007: renal Voxila: biliary	No data	No data	No data	Velpat: 4.04 (100 mg q24h, 0-24h) Sofos: 1.67 (400 mg q24h, 0-24h) GS-331007: 12.8 (400 mg q24h, 0-24h) Voxila: 2.58 (100 mg q24h, 0-24h)
Herpesvirus															
Acyclovir	No data	Tab (200, 400, 800 mg) Oral susp (200 mg/5 mL) Buccal tab (50 mg) 5% ointment 5% cream 3% ophthalmic ointment Injection	Tab/susp ± food	10-20	1.5-2	1.21 (400 mg po q12h, SS) 22.9 (10 mg/kg IV q8h, SS)	No data	9-33	0.7 L/kg	2.5-3.5	Renal	No data	No data	No data	7.4 (400 mg po q12h, 0-24h)

Food Effect (po dosing): + food = take with food, **no food** = take without food, **± food** = take with or without food; **Oral % AB** = % absorbed; **Peak Serum Level: SD** = after single dose, **SS** = steady state after multiple doses; **Volume of Distribution (Vd): V/F** = Vd/oral bioavailability, **Vss** = Vd at steady state, **Vss/F** = Vd at steady state/oral bioavailability; **CSF Penetration:** therapeutic efficacy comment based on [illegible] **AUC** = area under drug concentration curve; **24hr** = AUC 0-24; **Tmax** = time to max plasma concentration

TABLE 9A (33) *(Footnotes at the end of table)*

Groups/Drugs	PK/PD Index	Pharmaceutical Preparations	Food Rec (PO Drugs)[1]	Oral Abs (%)	Tmax (hr)	Peak Serum Conc (µg/mL)[2]	Peak Urine Conc (µg/mL)	Protein Binding (%)	Volume of Distribution (Vd)[3]	Avg Serum T½ (hr)[4]	Elimination	Bile Pen (%)[5]	CSF/blood (%)[6]	Therapeutic Levels in CSF[7]	AUC (µg*hr/mL)[8]
Antivirals (non-HIV)/Herpesvirus *(continued)*															
Cidofovir	No data	Injection	(Probenecid ± food)	-	1.1	19.6 (5 mg/kg IV, SD)	No data	<6	0.41 L/kg (Vss)	2.6	Renal	No data	Undetectable	No	40.8 (5 mg/kg IV, 0-inf)
Famciclovir	No data	Tab (125, 250, 500 mg)	Tab ± food	77	Penciclovir 0.9	3-4 (500 mg po, SD)	No data	<20	Penciclovir 1.1 L/kg	Penciclovir 2-3	Penciclovir: renal	No data	No data	No data	Penciclovir 8.9 (500 mg, 0-inf)
Foscarnet	No data	Injection	-	-	-	155 (60 mg/kg IV, SD)	No data	4	0.41-0.52 L/kg	3 (terminal 18-88)	Renal	No data	No data	No data	2195 µM*hr (60 mg/kg, 0-inf)
Ganciclovir	No data	Cap (250, 500 mg), 4.5 mg intravitreal implant, 0.15% oph gel, injection	Cap + food	Cap 5%	No data	8.3 (5 mg/kg IV, SD)	No data	1-2	0.7 L/kg (Vss)	3.5	Renal	No data	24-70	No data	24.5 (5 mg/kg IV, 0-inf)
Letermovir	No data	Tab (240, 480 mg) Injection	Tab ± food	94 (healthy subjects)	po 1.5-3.0	13 (480 mg po q24h, SS) (healthy subjects)	No data	99	45.5 L (Vss)	12	Fecal	No data	No data	No data	71.5 (480 mg po q24h, 0-24h) (healthy subjects)
Maribavir	No data	Tab (200 mg)	Tab ± food	No data	1-3	17.2 (400 mg po q12h, SS)	No data	98	27.3 L (Vss)	4.3	Hepatic metabolism	No data	No data	No data	128 (400 mg q12h, 0-12h)
Valacyclovir	No data	Tab (500 mg, 1 gm)	Tab ± food	55	No data	5.6 (1 gm po, SD) (acyclovir)	No data	9-33 (acyclovir)	0.7 L/kg (acyclovir)	2.5-3.2 (acyclovir)	Renal: filtration, secretion (acyclovir)	No data	No data	No data	19.5 (1 gm po, 0-inf) (acyclovir)
Valganciclovir	No data	Tab (450 mg), oral soln (50 mg/mL)	Tab/soln + food	59	Gan 1-3	Gan 5.6 (900 mg po q24h, SS)	No data	Gan 1-2	Gan 0.7 L/kg (Vss)	Gan 4	Ganciclovir: renal	No data	No data	No	Gan 29.1 (900 mg po q24h, 0-24h)
Influenza															
Amantadine	No data	Tab (100 mg), cap (100 mg), oral soln (50 mg/5 mL)	All preps ± food	No data	2-4	0.22 (100 mg po, SD)	No data	67	3-8 L/kg	16	Renal	No data	No data	No data	No data

Food Effect (po dosing): **+ food** = take with food, **no food** = take without food, **± food** = take with or without food; **Oral % AB** = % absorbed; **Peak Serum Level**: **SD** = after single dose, **SS** = steady state after multiple doses; **Volume of Distribution (Vd)**: **V/F** = Vd/oral bioavailability, **Vss** = Vd at steady state, **Vss/F** = Vd at steady state/oral bioavailability; **CSF Penetration**: therapeutic efficacy comment based on dose, usual susceptibility or target organism & penetration into CSF; **AUC** = area under drug concentration curve; **24hr** = AUC 0-24; **Tmax** = time to max plasma concentration.

TABLE 9A (34) *(Footnotes at the end of table)*

Groups/Drugs	PK/PD Index	Pharmaceutical Preparations	Food Rec (PO Drugs)[1]	Oral Abs (%)	Tmax (hr)	Peak Serum Conc (μg/mL)[2]	Peak Urine Conc (μg/mL)	Protein Binding (%)	Volume of Distribution (Vd)[3]	Avg Serum T½ (hr)[4]	Elimination	Bile Pen (%)[5]	CSF/blood (%)[6]	Therapeutic Levels in CSF[7]	AUC (μg*hr/mL)[8]
Antivirals (non-HIV)/Influenza *(continued)*															
Baloxavir marboxil	No data	Tab (40, 80 mg) Oral susp (2 mg/mL)	Tab/susp ± food	No data	Bal 4	Bal 0.069 (40 mg po, SD)	No data	Bal 92.9-93.9	Bal 1180 L (V/F)	Bal 79.1	Fecal	No data	No data	No data	Bal 5.52 (40 mg po, 0-inf)
Favipiravir	No data	Tab (200 mg) where available outside US	Tab + food (?)	No data	1.5	64.7 (600 mg po q12h, SS)	No data	54	No data	5.6	Metabolized	No data	No data	No	554 (600 mg po q12h, 0-12h)
Laninamivir octanoate	No data	Inhalation (where available outside US)	-	-	4	Lan 0.024 (40 mg inh, SD)	No data	Lan <0.01	No data	Lan 64.7	-	No data	No data	No data	Lan 0.745 (40 mg inh, 0-inf)
Oseltamivir	No data	Cap (30, 45, 75 mg) Oral susp (6 mg/mL)	Cap/susp ± food	75	No data	Carboxylate 0.35 (75 mg po q12h, SS)	No data	3	Carboxylate 23-26 L (Vss)	Carboxylate 6-10	Carboxylate: renal	No data	Carboxylate 3.5	No data	Carboxylate 5.4 (75 mg po q12h, 0-24h)
Peramivir	No data	Injection	-	-	-	46.8 (600 mg IV, SD)	No data	<30	12.56 L	20	Renal	No data	No data	No data	102.7 (600 mg IV, 0-inf)
Rimantadine	No data	Tab (100 mg)	Tab ± food	No data	6	0.05-0.14 (100 mg po, SD)	No data	40	No data	25.4	Metabolism	No data	No data	No data	No data
Poxviruses															
Brincidofovir	No data	Tab (100 mg), oral susp (10 mg/mL)	Tab/susp no food	Tab 13.4 Susp 16.8	3	Brin 0.48 (200 mg po, SD)	No data	>99.9	1230 L	19.3	Metabolism, renal, fecal	No data	No data	No data	Brin 3.4 (200 mg po, 0-inf)
Tecovirimat	No data	Cap (200 mg), injection	Cap + food	No data	po 4-6	2.16 (600 mg po q12h, SS) 2.63 (200 mg IV q12h, SS)	No data	77-82	po 1030 L (Vz/F) IV 383 L (Vz/F)	po 19 IV 21	Metabolism	No data	No data	No data	29.8 (600 mg po q12h, 0-24h) 39.4 (200 mg IV q12h, 0-24h)
RSV															
Nirsevimab-alip	No data	Injection	-	IM bioavailability: 84%	6 days	No data	No data	No data	447 mL (5 kg infant)	71 days (terminal)	Catabolized into small peptides	No data	No data	No data	No data

Food Effect (po dosing): **+ food** = take with food, **no food** = take without food, **± food** = take with or without food; **Oral % AB** = % absorbed; **Peak Serum Level: SD** = after single dose, **SS** = steady state after multiple doses; **Volume of Distribution (Vd): V/F** = Vd/oral bioavailability, **Vss** = Vd at steady state, **Vss/F** = Vd at steady state/oral bioavailability; **CSF Penetration:** therapeutic efficacy comment based on dose, usual susceptibility or target organism & penetration into CSF; **AUC** = area under drug concentration curve; **24hr** = AUC 0-24; **Tmax** = time to max plasma concentration.

TABLE 9A (35) *(Footnotes at the end of table)*

Groups/Drugs	PK/PD Index	Pharmaceutical Preparations	Food Rec (PO Drugs)[1]	Oral Abs (%)	Tmax (hr)	Peak Serum Conc (μg/mL)[2]	Peak Urine Conc (μg/mL)	Protein Binding (%)	Volume of Distribution (Vd)[3]	Avg Serum T½ (hr)[4]	Elimination	Bile Pen (%)[5]	CSF/blood (%)[6]	Therapeutic Levels in CSF[7]	AUC (μg*hr/mL)[8]
Antivirals (non-HIV)/RSV *(continued)*															
Palivizumab	No data	Injection	-	-	-	72 (30 days post dose 4)	No data	-	-	24.5 days	Catabolized (similar to IgG)	No data	No data	No data	No data

1 Refers to adult oral preparations unless otherwise noted; + food = take with food, no food = take without food, ± food = take with or without food.
2 SD = after a single dose, SS = at steady state.
3 V/F = Vd/oral bioavailability; Vss = Vd at steady state; Vss/F = Vd at steady state/oral bioavailability.
4 Assumes CrCl >80 mL/min.
5 (Peak concentration in bile/peak concentration in serum) x 100. If blank, no data.
6 CSF concentrations with inflammation.
7 Judgment based on drug dose and organism susceptibility. CSF concentration ideally ≥10x MIC.
8 AUC = area under serum concentration vs. time curve. KEY: 0-inf = AUC 0 to infinity; 0-xh = AUC 0 to x hours.
9 Concern over seizure potential.
10 Take all oral FQs 2-4 hours before sucralfate or any multivalent cation (calcium, iron, zinc).
11 CPE (CNS Penetration Effectiveness) value: 1=low penetration, 2-3=intermediate penetration, 4=highest penetration *(Letendre et al, CROI 2010, abs #430).*
12 *Am J Trop Med Hyg 2021;86:122.*
13 Doses infused over 3 hours.

Food Effect (po dosing): + food = take with food, **no food** = take without food, **± food** = take with or without food; **Oral % AB** = % absorbed; **Peak Serum Level: SD** = after single dose, **SS** = steady state after multiple doses; **Volume of Distribution (Vd): V/F** = Vd/oral bioavailability, **Vss** = Vd at steady state, **Vss/F** = Vd at steady state/oral bioavailability; **CSF Penetration:** therapeutic efficacy comment based on dose, usual susceptibility or target organism & penetration into CSF; **AUC** = area under drug concentration curve; **24hr** = AUC 0-24; **Tmax** = time to max plasma concentration.

TABLE 9A (36) *(Footnotes at the end of table)*

Groups/Drugs	Class	Pharmaceutical Preparations	Food Rec[1]	Oral Abs (%)	Tmax (hr)	Peak Serum Conc (μg/mL)[2]	Protein Binding (%)	Volume of Distribution (Vd)[3]	Avg Serum T½ (hr)[4]	Elimination	Intracell T½ (hr)	CSF/blood (%)[6]	CPE[11]	AUC (μg*hr/mL)[8]
Antiretrovirals														
NRTIs														
Abacavir (ABC)	NRTI	Tab (300 mg) Oral soln (20 mg/mL)	Tab/soln ± food	83	1.3	4.3 (600 mg q24h, SS)	50	0.86 L/kg	1.5	Metabolized (non-CYP)	20.6	36	3	12 (600 mg q24h, 0-24h)
Didanosine (ddI)	NRTI	EC cap (125, 200, 250, 400 mg) Pwd for oral soln (10 mg/mL)	All preps no food	30-40	2	No data	<5	308-363 L	1.6	Metabolism, renal	25-40	No data	2	2.6 (400 mg EC q24h, 0-24h)
Emtricitabine (FTC)	NRTI	Cap (200 mg) Oral soln (10 mg/mL)	Cap/soln ± food	cap 93 soln 75	1-2	1.8 (200 mg [cap] q24h, SS)	<4	No data	≈10	Renal	39	No data	3	10 (200 mg q24h, 0-24 h)
Lamivudine (3TC)	NRTI	Tab (150, 300 mg) Oral soln (10 mg/mL)	Tab/soln ± food	86	No data	2.6 (300 mg q24h, SS)	<36	1.3 L/kg	5-7	Renal, metabolism	18	No data	2	11 (300 mg, 0-inf)
Stavudine (d4T)	NRTI	Cap (15, 20, 30, 40 mg) Oral soln (1 mg/mL)	Cap/soln ± food	86	1	0.54 (40 mg q12h, SS)	<5	46 L	1.2-1.6	Metabolism, renal	3.5	20	2	2.6 (40 mg q12h, 0-24h)
Tenofovir disoproxil fumarate (TDF)	NRTI	Tab (150, 200, 250, 300 mg) Oral pwd (40 mg/scoop)	Tab ± food Pwd + food	39 w/food 25 fasting	1	0.3 (300 mg, SD)	<7	1.2-1.3 L/kg (Vss)	17	Renal	>60	No data	1	2.3 (300 mg, 0-inf)
Zidovudine (ZDV/AZT)	NRTI	Tab (300 mg) Cap (100 mg) Oral syrup (10 mg/mL) Injection	Tab/cap/ syrup ± food	60	0.5-1.5	1-2 (300 mg po, SD)	<38	1.6 L/kg	0.5-3	Metabolized	11	2	4	2.1 (300 mg po, 0-inf)
NNRTIs														
Doravirine (DOR)	NNRTI	Tab (100 mg)	Tab ± food	64	2	0.962 (100 mg q24h, SS)	76	60.5 L (Vss)	15	Metabolized	No data	No data	No data	16.1 (100 mg q24h, 0-24h)
Efavirenz (EFV)	NNRTI	Cap (50, 200 mg) Tab (600 mg)	Cap/tab no food	42	3-5	4.1 (600 mg q24h, SS)	99	252 L (V/F)	40-55	Metabolized	No data	No data	3	184 μM*hr (600 mg q24h, 0-24h)
Etravirine (ETR)	NNRTI	Tab (25, 100, 200 mg)	Tab + food	No data	2.5-4.0	0.3 (200 mg q12h, SS)	99.9	No data	41	Metabolized	No data	No data	2	9 (200 mg q12h, 0-24h)

TABLE 9A (37) *(Footnotes at the end of table)*

Groups/Drugs	Class	Pharmaceutical Preparations	Food Rec[1]	Oral Abs (%)	Tmax (hr)	Peak Serum Conc (μg/mL)[2]	Protein Binding (%)	Volume of Distribution (Vd)[3]	Avg Serum T½ (hr)[4]	Elimination	Intracell T½ (hr)	CSF/blood (%)[6]	CPE[11]	AUC (μg*hr/mL)[8]
Antiretrovirals/NNRTIs *(continued)*														
Nevirapine (NVP)	NNRTI	Tab (200 mg) XR tab (100, 400 mg) Oral susp (10 mg/mL)	Tab/susp ± food	>90	4	2 (200 mg, SD)	60	1.21 L/kg (Vss)	25-30	Metabolized	No data	63	4	110 (200 mg q12h, 0-24h)
Rilpivirine (RPV)	NNRTI	Tab (25 mg) Dispersible peds tab (2.5 mg)	All preps + food	No data	4-5	0.1-0.2 (25 mg, SD)	99.7	152 L	45-50	Metabolized	No data	No data	No data	2.4 (25 mg q24h, 0-24h)
PIs, Boosting Agents														
Atazanavir (ATV)	Protease inhibitor	Cap (150, 200, 300 mg) Oral powder (50 mg)	Cap/pwd + food	Good if pH low	2.5	2.3 (400 mg q24h, SS)	86	88.3 L (V/F)	≈7	Metabolized	No data	No data	2	22.3 (400 mg q24h, 0-24h)
Cobicistat (COBI or c)	CYP3A inhibitor	Tab (150 mg)	Tab + food	No data	3.5	0.99 (150 mg q24h, SS)	97-98	No data	3-4	Metabolized	No data	No data	No data	7.6 (150 mg q24h, 0-24h)
Darunavir (DRV)	Protease inhibitor	Tab (75, 150, 600, 800 mg) Oral susp (100 mg/mL)	Tab/susp + food	82	2.5-4	3.5 (600 mg q12h, SS) (w/RTV 100 mg q12h)	95	2 L/kg	15	Metabolized	No data	No data	3	116.8 (600 mg q12h, 0-24h) (w/ RTV 100 mg q12h)
Fosamprenavir (FPV)	Protease inhibitor	Tab (700 mg) Oral susp (50 mg/mL)	Tab ± food Susp (adults) no food Susp (peds) + food	No data	2.5	6 (700 mg q12h, SS) (w/RTV 100 mg q12h)	90	No data	7.7	Metabolized	No data	No data	3	79.2 (700 mg q12h, 0-24h) (w/ RTV 100 mg q12h)
Indinavir (IDV)	Protease inhibitor	Cap (100, 200, 400 mg)	Cap + food	65	0.8 fasting	20.2 μM (800 mg q12h, SS) (w/RTV 100 mg q12h)	60	No data	1.2-2	Metabolism, fecal	No data	11	4	249 μM*h (800 mg q12h, 0-24h) (w/RTV 100 mg q12h)
Nelfinavir (NFV)	Protease inhibitor	Tab (250, 625 mg)	Tab/pwd + food	20-80	No data	3-4 (1250 mg q12h, SS)	98	2-7 L/kg (V/F)	3.5-5	Metabolism, fecal	No data	0	1	53 (1250 mg q12h, 0-24h)
Ritonavir (RTV)	Protease inhibitor	Tab (100 mg) Oral pwd (100 mg pkts)	All preps + food	65	No data	No data	98-99	0.41 L/kg (V/F)	3-5	Metabolized	No data	No data	1	No data
Saquinavir (SQV)	Protease inhibitor	Cap (200 mg) Tab (500 mg)	Cap/tab + food	4	No data	0.37 (1000 mg q12h, SS) (w/RTV 100 mg q12h)	97	700 L (Vss)	1-2	Metabolized	No data	No data	1	29.2 (1000 mg q12h, 0-24h) (w/ RTV 100 mg q12h)

TABLE 9A (38) *(Footnotes at the end of table)*

Groups/Drugs	Class	Pharmaceutical Preparations	Food Rec[1]	Oral Abs (%)	Tmax (hr)	Peak Serum Conc (µg/mL)[2]	Protein Binding (%)	Volume of Distribution (Vd)[3]	Avg Serum T½ (hr)[4]	Elimination	Intracell T½ (hr)	CSF/blood (%)[6]	CPE[11]	AUC (µg*hr/mL)[8]
Antiretrovirals/PIs, Boosting Agents *(continued)*														
Tipranavir (TPV)	Protease inhibitor	Cap (250 mg) Oral soln (100 mg/mL)	Cap/soln + food	Low	3	47-57 (500 mg q12h, SS) (w/RTV 200 mg q12h)	99.9	7.7-10 L	5.5-6	Fecal	No data	No data	1	1600 µM*h (500 mg q12h, 0-24h) (w/RTV 200 mg q12h)
INSTIs														
Cabotegravir (CAB)	INSTI	Tab (30 mg) Injection	Tab + food	No data	po 3 IM 7 days	8 (30 mg po q24h, SS) 4 (600 mg IM q2 mon, SS)	>99.8	No data	po 41 IM 5.6-11.5 wk	Metabolized	No data	0.3	No data	145 (30 mg po q24h, 0-24h) 3764 (600 mg IM q2 mon, 0-2 mon)
Dolutegravir (DTG)	INSTI	Tab (10, 25, 50 mg) Oral susp tab (5 mg)	All preps ± food	No data	2-3	3.67 (50 mg q24h, SS)	>99	17.4 L (V/F)	14	Metabolized	No data	No data	4	53.6 (50 mg q24h, 0-24h)
Raltegravir (RAL)	INSTI	Tab (400, 600 mg) Chewtab (25, 100 mg) Oral susp granules (10 mg/mL)	All preps ± food	No data	1.5-3	4.5 µM (400 mg q12h, SS) 15.7 µM (1200 mg q24h, SS)	83	287 L (Vss/F)	9	Glucuronidation	No data	1-53.5 (median 5.8)	3	14.3 µM*h (400 mg q12h, 0-12h) 55.3 µM*h (1200 mg q24h, 0-24h)
Fusion, Entry Inhibitors														
Enfuvirtide (ENF/T20)	Fusion inhibitor	Injection	-	84 (sc % ab)	4-8	5 (90 mg sc q12h, SS)	92	5.5 L (Vss)	3.8	Catabolism	No data	No data	1	97.4 (90 mg sc q12h, 0-24h)
Maraviroc (MVC)	CCR5 receptor antagonist	Tab (25, 75, 150, 300 mg) Oral soln (20 mg/mL)	All preps ± food	33	0.5-4	0.3-0.9 (300 mg q12h, SS)	76	194 L	14-18	Metabolized	No data	No data	3	3 (300 mg q12h, 0-24h)
Attachment Inhibitor														
Fostemsavir (FTR)	Attachment inhibitor	Ext-rel tab (600 mg)	Tab ± food	26.9	2	1.77 (600 mg q12h, SS)	88.4	29.5 L (Vss)	11	Metabolized	No data	No data	No data	12.9 (600 mg q12h, 0-12h)
Ibalizumab-uiyk (IBA)	Monoclonal antibody	Injection	-	-	-	No data	No data	4.8 L	Dose-dependent	Catabolized (similar to IgG)	No data	No data	No data	No data
Capsid Inhibitor														
Lenacapavir (LEN)	HIV-1 capsid inhibitor	Tab (300 mg) Injection	Tab ± food	6-10	po 4 hr sc 77-84 days	0.087-0.097 (end of month 6)	>98.5	po 19240 L (V/F) sc 9500-11700 L	po 10-12 days sc 8-12 wks	Fecal, metabolism	No data	No data	No data	234.3 (2-day initiation, 0-6 mon)

TABLE 9A (39) *(Footnotes at the end of table)*

Groups/Drugs	Class	Pharmaceutical Preparations	Food Rec[1]	Oral Abs (%)	Tmax (hr)	Peak Serum Conc (μg/mL)[2]	Protein Binding (%)	Volume of Distribution (Vd)[3]	Avg Serum T½ (hr)[4]	Elimination	Intracell T½ (hr)	CSF/blood (%)[6]	CPE[11]	AUC (μg*hr/mL)[8]
Antiretroviral Combination Products														
Atripla (EFV/FTC/TDF)	NNRTI + 2 NRTI	Tab: EFV 600 mg + FTC 200 mg + TDF 300 mg	Tab no food	EFV: 42 FTC: 93 TDF: 25	EFV: 3-5 FTC: 1-2 TDF: 1	EFV: 12.9 μM (600 mg q24h, SS) FTC: 1.8 (200 mg q24h, SS) TDF: 0.3 (300 mg, SD)	EFV: >99.5 FTC: <4 TDF: <0.7	EFV: 252 L (V/F) FTC: no data TDF: 1.2-1.3 L/kg (Vss)	EFV: 40-55 FTC: 10 TDF: 17	EFV: Metabolized FTC: Renal TDF: Renal	EFV: no data FTC: 39 TDF: >60	EFV: no data FTC: no data TDF: no data	EFV: 3 FTC: 3 TDF: 1	EFV: 184 μM*hr (600 mg q24h, 0-24h) FTC: 10 (200 mg q24h, 0-24h) TDF: 2.3 (300 mg q24h, 0-24h)
Biktarvy (BIC/FTC/TAF)	INSTI + 2 NRTI	Tab: BIC 50 mg + FTC 200 mg + TAF 25 mg	Tab ± food	BIC: no data FTC: no data TAF: no data	BIC: 2-4 FTC: 1.5-2 TAF: 0.5-2	BIC: 6.15 (50 mg q24h, SS) FTC: 2.13 (200 mg q24h, SS) TAF: 0.121 (25 mg q24h, SS)	BIC: >99 FTC: <4 TAF: ≈80	BIC: no data FTC: no data TAF: no data	BIC: 17.3 FTC: 10.4 TAF: 0.51	BIC: Metabolized FTC: Renal TAF: Metabolized	BIC: no data FTC: 39 TAF: no data	BIC: no data FTC: no data TAF: no data	BIC: no data FTC: 3 TAF: no data	BIC: 102 (50 mg q24h, 0-24h) FTC: 12.3 (200 mg q24h, 0-24h) TAF: 0.142 (25 mg q24h, 0-24h)
Cabenuva (CAB/RPV)	INSTI + NNRTI (co-packaged)	CAB 400 mg/ RPV 600 mg inj kit CAB 600 mg/ RPV 900 mg inj kit	-	-	CAB: 7 days RPV: 3-4 days	CAB: 4.2 (400 mg IM, SD) RPV: 0.12 (600 mg IM, SD)	CAB: >99.8 RPV: 99.7	CAB: no data RPV: no data	CAB: 5.6-11.5 wk RPV: 13-28 wk	CAB: Metabolized RPV: Metabolized	CAB: no data RPV: no data	CAB: 0.3 RPV: 1	CAB: no data RPV: no data	CAB: 2415 (400 mg IM qmon, 0-1 mon) RPV: 65.6 (600 mg IM qmon, 0-1 mon)
Cimduo, Temixys (3TC/TDF)	2 NRTI	Tab: 3TC 300 mg + TDF 300 mg	Tab ± food	3TC: 86 TDF: 39 (w/food) TDF: 25 (fasting)	3TC: no data TDF: 1	3TC: 2.6 (300 mg, SD) TDF: 0.3 (300 mg, SD)	3TC: <36 TDF: <0.7	3TC: 1.3 L/kg TDF: 1.2-1.3 L/kg (Vss)	3TC: 5-7 TDF: 17	3TC: Renal, metabolism TDF: Renal	3TC: 18 TDF: >60	3TC: no data TDF: no data	3TC: 2 TDF: 1	3TC: 11 (300 mg, 0-inf) TDF: 2.3 (300 mg, 0-inf)
Combivir (3TC/ZDV)	2 NRTI	Tab: 3TC 150 mg + ZDV 300 mg	Tab ± food	3TC: 86 ZDV: 64	3TC: rapid ZDV: 0.5-1.5	3TC: 2.04 (300 mg q24h, SS) ZDV: 1-2 (300 mg, SD)	3TC: <36 ZDV: <38	3TC: 1.3 L/kg ZDV: 1.6 L/kg	3TC: 5-7 ZDV: 0.5-3	3TC: Renal, metabolism ZDV: Metabolized	3TC: 18 ZDV: 11	3TC: no data ZDV: 2	3TC: 2 ZDV: 4	3TC: 11 (300 mg, 0-inf) ZDV: 2.1 (300 mg, 0-inf)
Complera/Eviplera (RPV/FTC/TDF)	NNRTI + 2 NRTI	Tab: RPV 25 mg + FTC 200 mg + TDF 300 mg	Tab + food	RPV: no data FTC: 93 TDF: 39	RPV: 4-5 FTC: 1-2 TDF: 1	RPV: 0.1-0.2 (25 mg, SD) FTC: 1.8 (200 mg q24h, SS) TDF: 0.3 (300 mg, SD)	RPV: 99.7 FTC: <4 TDF: <0.7	RPV: 152 L FTC: no data TDF: no data	RPV: 50 FTC: 10 TDF: 17	RPV: Metabolized FTC: Renal TDF: Renal	RPV: no data FTC: 39 TDF: >60	RPV: no data FTC: no data TDF: no data	RPV: no data FTC: 3 TDF: 1	RPV: 2.2 (25 mg q24h, 0-24h) FTC: 10 (200 mg q24h, 0-24h) TDF: 2.3 (300 mg, 0-inf)

TABLE 9A (40) *(Footnotes at the end of table)*

Groups/Drugs	Class	Pharmaceutical Preparations	Food Rec[1]	Oral Abs (%)	Tmax (hr)	Peak Serum Conc (µg/mL)[2]	Protein Binding (%)	Volume of Distribution (Vd)[3]	Avg Serum T½ (hr)[4]	Elimination	Intracell T½ (hr)	CSF/blood (%)[6]	CPE[11]	AUC (µg*hr/mL)[8]
Antiretroviral Combination Products *(continued)*														
Delstrigo (DOR/3TC/TDF)	NNRTI + 2 NRTI	Tab: DOR 100 mg + 3TC 300 mg + TDF 300 mg	Tab ± food	DOR: 64 3TC: 86 TDF: 25	DOR: 2 3TC: no data TDF: 1	DOR: 0.962 (100 mg q24h, SS) 3TC: 2.04 (300 mg q24h, SS) TDF: 0.3 (300 mg q24h, SS)	DOR: 76 3TC: <36 TDF: <0.7	DOR: 60.5 L (Vss) 3TC: 1.3 L/kg (Vss) TDF: 1.3 L/kg (Vss)	DOR: 15 3TC: 5-7 TDF: 17	DOR: Metabolized 3TC: Renal, metabolism TDF: Renal	DOR: no data 3TC: 18 TDF: >60	DOR: no data 3TC: no data TDF: no data	DOR: no data 3TC: 2 TDF: 1	DOR: 16.1 (100 mg q24h, 0-24h) 3TC: 8.87 (300 mg q24h, 0-24h) TDF: 2.29 (300 mg q24h, 0-24h)
Descovy (FTC/TAF)	2 NRTI	Tab: FTC 200 mg + TAF 25 mg	Tab ± food	FTC: no data TAF: no data	FTC: 3 TAF: 1	FTC: 2.1 (200 mg q24h, SS) TAF: 0.16 (10 mg q24h, SS) Tenofovir: 0.02 (10 mg q24h, SS)	FTC: <4 TAF: ≈80	FTC: no data TAF: no data	FTC: 10 TAF: 0.51	FTC: Renal TAF: Metabolized	FTC: 39 TAF: no data	FTC: no data TAF: no data	FTC: 3 TAF: no data	FTC: 11.7 (200 mg q24h, 0-24h) TAF: 0.21 (10 mg q24h, 0-24h) Tenofovir: 0.29 (10 mg q24h, 0-24h)
Dovato (DTG/3TC)	INSTI + NRTI	Tab: DTG 50 mg + 3TC 300 mg	Tab ± food	DTG: no data 3TC: 86	DTG: 2.5 3TC: 1	DTG: 3.67 (50 mg q24h, SS) 3TC: 2.04 (300 mg q24h, SS)	DTG: >99 3TC: 36	DTG: 17.4 L (V/F) 3TC: 1.3 L/kg	DTG: 14 3TC: 5-7	DTG: Metabolized 3TC: Renal, metabolism	DTG: no data 3TC: 18	DTG: no data 3TC: no data	DTG: no data 3TC: 2	DTG: 53.6 (50 mg q24h, 0-24h) 3TC: 8.87 (300 mg q24h, 0-24h)
Epzicom/Kivexa (ABC/3TC)	2 NRTI	Tab: ABC 600 mg + 3TC 300 mg	Tab ± food	ABC: 86 3TC: 86	ABC: 1.3 3TC: no data	ABC: 4.26 (600 mg, SD) 3TC: 2.04 (300 mg q24h, SS)	ABC: 50 3TC: <36	ABC: 0.86 L/kg 3TC: 1.3 L/kg	ABC: 1.45 3TC: 5-7	ABC: Metabolized (non-CYP) 3TC: Renal, metabolism	ABC: 20.6 3TC: 18	ABC: no data 3TC: no data	ABC: 3 3TC: 2	ABC: 11.95 (600 mg, 0-inf) 3TC: 8.87 (300 mg q24h, 0-24h)
Evotaz (ATV/cobi)	PI + booster	Tab: ATV 300 mg + Cobi 150 mg	Tab + food	ATV: no data Cobi: no data	ATV: 3.5 Cobi: 3	ATV: 3.91 (300 mg q24h, SS) Cobi: 1.5 (150 mg q24h, SS)	ATV: 86 Cobi: 97-98	ATV: 88.3 L (V/F) Cobi: no data	ATV: 7.5 Cobi: 3-4	ATV: Metabolized Cobi: Metabolized	ATV: no data Cobi: no data	ATV: no data Cobi: no data	ATV: 2 Cobi: no data	ATV: 46.1 (300 mg q24h, 0-24h) Cobi: 11.1 (150 mg q24h, 0-24h)

TABLE 9A (41) *(Footnotes at the end of table)*

Groups/Drugs	Class	Pharmaceutical Preparations	Food Rec[1]	Oral Abs (%)	Tmax (hr)	Peak Serum Conc (µg/mL)[2]	Protein Binding (%)	Volume of Distribution (Vd)[3]	Avg Serum T½ (hr)[4]	Elimination	Intracell T½ (hr)	CSF/blood (%)[6]	CPE[11]	AUC (µg*hr/mL)[8]
Antiretroviral Combination Products *(continued)*														
Genvoya (EVG/cobi/FTC/TAF)	INSTI + booster + 2 NRTI	Tab: EVG 150 mg + Cobi 150 mg + FTC 200 mg + TAF 10 mg	Tab + food	EVG: no data Cobi: no data FTC: no data TAF: no data	EVG: 4 Cobi: 3 FTC: 3 TAF: 1	EVG: 2.1 (150 mg q24h, SS) Cobi: 1.5 (150 mg q24h, SS) FTC: 2.1 (200 mg q24h, SS) TAF: 0.16 (10 mg q24h, SS) Tenofovir: 0.02 (10 mg q24h, SS)	EVG: ≈99 Cobi: ≈98 FTC: <4 TAF: ≈80	EVG: no data Cobi: no data FTC: no data TAF: no data	EVG: 12.9 Cobi: 3.5 FTC: 10 TAF: 0.51	EVG: Metabolized Cobi: Metabolized FTC: Renal TAF: Metabolized	EVG: no data Cobi: no data FTC: 39 TAF: no data	EVG: no data Cobi: no data FTC: no data TAF: no data	EVG: no data Cobi: no data FTC: 3 TAF: no data	EVG: 22.8 (150 mg q24h, 0-24h) Cobi: 9.5 (150 mg q24h, 0-24h) FTC: 11.7 (200 mg q24h, 0-24h) TAF: 0.21 (10 mg q24h, 0-24h) Tenofovir: 0.29 (10 mg q24h, 0-24h)
Juluca (DTG/RPV)	INSTI + NNRTI	Tab: DTG 50 mg + RPV 25 mg	Tab + food	DTG: no data RPV: no data	DTG: 3 RPV: 4	DTG: 3.67 (50 mg q24h, SS) RPV: 0.13 (25 mg q24h, SS)	DTG: ≈99 RPV: ≈99	DTG: 17.4 L (V/F) RPV: 152 L	DTG: 14 RPV: 50	DTG: Metabolized RPV: Metabolized	DTG: no data RPV: no data	DTG: no data RPV: no data	DTG: no data RPV: no data	DTG: 53.6 (50 mg q24h, 0-24h) RPV: 2.2 (25 mg q24h, 0-24h)
Kaletra (LPV/RTV)	PI + booster	Tab (LPV 100 mg/RTV 25 mg) Tab (LPV 200 mg/RTV 50 mg) Oral soln (LPV 80 mg/RTV 20 mg per mL)	Tab ± food Soln + food	no data	LPV 4.4	LPV 9.8 (400 mg/100 mg q12h, SS)	LPV >98 RTV 98-99	LPV 16.9 L (V/F) RTV 0.41 L/kg (V/F)	LPV 6.9 RTV 3-5	LPV: Metabolized RTV: Metabolized	no data	no data	LPV 3 RTV 1	LPV 185.2 (400 mg/100 mg q12h, 0-24h)
Odefsey (RPV/FTC/TAF)	NNRTI + 2 NRTI	Tab: RPV 25 mg + FTC 200 mg + TAF 25 mg	Tab + food	RPV: no data FTC: no data TAF: no data	RPV: 4 FTC: 3 TAF: 1	RPV: 0.1-0.2 (25 mg, SD) FTC: 2.1 (200 mg q24h, SS) TAF: 0.16 (10 mg q24h, SS) Tenofovir: 0.02 (10 mg q24h, SS)	RPV: ≈99 FTC: <4 TAF: ≈80	RPV: 152 L FTC: no data TAF: no data	RPV: 50 FTC: 10 TAF: 0.51	RPV: Metabolized FTC: Renal TAF: Metabolized	RPV: no data FTC: 39 TAF: no data	RPV: no data FTC: no data TAF: no data	RPV: no data FTC: no data TAF: no data	RPV: 2.2 (25 mg q24h, 0-24h) FTC: 11.7 (200 mg q24h, 0-24h) TAF: 0.21 (10 mg q24h, 0-24h) Tenofovir: 0.29 (10 mg q24h, 0-24h)

TABLE 9A (42) *(Footnotes at the end of table)*

Groups/Drugs	Class	Pharmaceutical Preparations	Food Rec[1]	Oral Abs (%)	Tmax (hr)	Peak Serum Conc (μg/mL)[2]	Protein Binding (%)	Volume of Distribution (Vd)[3]	Avg Serum T½ (hr)[4]	Elimination	Intracell T½ (hr)	CSF/blood (%)[6]	CPE[11]	AUC (μg*hr/mL)[8]
Antiretroviral Combination Products *(continued)*														
Prezcobix (DRV/cobi)	PI + booster	Tab: DRV 800 mg + Cobi 150 mg	Tab + food	DRV: no data Cobi: no data	DRV: 4-4.5 Cobi: 4-5	DRV: 7.74 (800 mg q24h, SS) Cobi: 0.99 (150 mg q24h, SS)	DRV: 95 Cobi: 97-98	DRV: no data Cobi: no data	DRV: 7 Cobi: 3.5-4	DRV: Metabolized Cobi: Metabolized	DRV: no data Cobi: no data	DRV: no data Cobi: no data	DRV: 3 Cobi: no data	DRV: 100.1 (800 mg q24h, 0-24h) Cobi: no data
Stribild (EVG/cobi/FTC/TDF)	INSTI + booster + 2 NRTI	Tab: EVG 150 mg + Cobi 150 mg + FTC 200 mg + TDF 300 mg	Tab + food	EVG: no data Cobi: no data FTC: no data TDF: no data	EVG: 4 Cobi: 3 FTC: 3 TDF: 2	EVG: 1.7 (150 mg q24h, SS) Cobi: 1.1 (150 mg q24h, SS) FTC: 1.9 (200 mg q24h, SS) TDF: 0.45 (300 mg q24h, SS)	EVG: ≈99 Cobi: ≈98 FTC: <4 TDF: <0.7	EVG: no data Cobi: no data FTC: no data TDF: no data	EVG: 12.9 Cobi: 3.5 FTC: 10 TDF: 12-18	EVG: Metabolized Cobi: Metabolized FTC: Renal TDF: Renal	EVG: no data Cobi: no data FTC: 39 TDF: no data	EVG: no data Cobi: no data FTC: no data TDF: no data	EVG: no data Cobi: no data FTC: 3 TDF: no data	EVG: 23.0 (150 mg q24h, 0-24h) Cobi: 8.3 (150 mg q24h, 0-24h) FTC: 12.7 (200 mg q24h, 0-24h) TDF: 4.4 (300 mg q24h, 0-24h)
Symfi, Symfi Lo (EFV/3TC/TDF)	NNRTI + 2 NRTI	Symfi: EFV 600 mg + 3TC 300 mg + TDF 300 mg Symfi Lo: EFV 400 mg + 3TC 300 mg + TDF 300 mg	Tab no food	EFV: 42 3TC: >80 TDF: 25	EFV: 3-5 3TC: no data TDF: 1	EFV: 12.9 μM (600 mg q24h, SS) 3TC: 2.6 (300 mg, SD) TDF: 0.3 (300 mg, SD)	EFV: >99.5 3TC: <36 TDF: <0.7	EFV: 252 L (V/F) 3TC: 1.3 L/kg TDF: 1.2-1.3 L/kg (Vss)	EFV: 40-55 3TC: 5-7 TDF: 17	EFV: Metabolized 3TC: Renal, metabolism TDF: Renal	EFV: no data 3TC: 18 TDF: >60	EFV: no data 3TC: no data TDF: no data	EFV: 3 3TC: 2 TDF: 1	EFV: 184 μM*hr (600 mg q24h, 0-24h) 3TC: 11.0 (300 mg, 0-inf) TDF: 2.3 (300 mg, 0-inf)
Symtuza (DRV/cobi/FTC/TAF)	PI + booster + 2 NRTI	Tab: DRV 800 mg + Cobi 150 mg + FTC 200 mg + TAF 10 mg	Tab + food	DRV: no data Cobi: no data FTC: no data TAF: no data	DRV: 3 Cobi: 3 FTC: 1.5 TAF: 0.5	DRV: 8.83 (800 mg q24h, SS) Cobi: 1.13 (150 mg q24h, SS) FTC: 2.06 (200 mg q24h, SS) TAF: 0.16 (10 mg q24h, SS) Tenofovir: 0.019 (10 mg q24h, SS)	DRV: 95 Cobi: 97-98 FTC: <4 TAF: ≈80	DRV: no data Cobi: no data FTC: no data TAF: no data	DRV: 9.4 Cobi: 3.2 FTC: 7.5 TAF: 0.5	DRV: Metabolized Cobi: Metabolized FTC: Renal TAF: Metabolized	DRV: no data Cobi: no data FTC: 39 TAF: no data	DRV: no data Cobi: no data FTC: no data TAF: no data	DRV: 3 Cobi: no data FTC: 3 TAF: no data	DRV: 87.9 (800 mg q24h, 0-24h) Cobi: 8.75 (150 mg q24h, 0-24h) FTC: 11.9 (200 mg q24h, 0-24h) TAF: 0.13 (10 mg q24h, 0-24h) Tenofovir: 0.34 (10 mg q24h, 0-24h)

TABLE 9A (43) *(Footnotes at the end of table)*

Groups/Drugs	Class	Pharmaceutical Preparations	Food Rec[1]	Oral Abs (%)	Tmax (hr)	Peak Serum Conc (µg/mL)[2]	Protein Binding (%)	Volume of Distribution (Vd)[3]	Avg Serum T½ (hr)[4]	Elimination	Intracell T½ (hr)	CSF/blood (%)[6]	CPE[11]	AUC (µg*hr/mL)[8]
Antiretroviral Combination Products *(continued)*														
Triumeq (DTG/3TC/ABC)	INSTI + 2 NRTI	Tab: ABC 600 mg + DTG 50 mg + 3TC 300 mg	Tab ± food	ABC: 83 DTG: no data 3TC: 86	ABC: 1.3 DTG: 2-3 3TC: rapid	ABC: 4.26 (600 mg, SD) DTG: 3.67 (50 mg q24h, SS) 3TC: 2.04 (300 mg q24h, SS)	ABC: 50 DTG: ≈99 3TC: <36	ABC: 0.86 L/kg DTG: 17.4 L (V/F) 3TC: 1.3 L/kg	ABC: 1.54 DTG: 14 3TC: 5-7	ABC: Metabolized (non-CYP) DTG: Metabolized 3TC: Renal, metabolism	ABC: 20.6 DTG: no data 3TC: 18	ABC: 36 DTG: no data 3TC: no data	ABC: 3 DTG: 4 3TC: 2	ABC: 11.95 (600 mg q24h, 0-24h) DTG: 53.6 (50 mg q24h, 0-24h) 3TC: 8.87 (300 mg q24h, 0-24h)
Trizivir (ABC/3TC/ZDV)	3 NRTI	Tab: ABC 300 mg + 3TC 150 mg + ZDV 300 mg	Tab ± food	ABC: 86 3TC: 86 ZDV: 64	ABC: 1.3 3TC: no data ZDV: 0.5-1.5	ABC: 4.26 (600 mg, SD) 3TC: 2.04 (300 mg q24h, SS) ZDV: 1-2 (300 mg, SD)	ABC: 50 3TC: <36 ZDV: <38	ABC: 0.86 L/kg 3TC: 1.3 L/kg ZDV: 1.6 L/kg	ABC: 1.45 3TC: 5-7 ZDV: 0.5-3	ABC: Metabolized (non-CYP) 3TC: Renal, metabolism ZDV: Metabolized	ABC: 20.6 3TC: 18 ZDV: 11	ABC: 36 3TC: no data ZDV: 2	ABC: 3 3TC: 2 ZDV: 4	ABC: 11.95 (600 mg q24h, 0-24h) 3TC: 11 (300 mg, 0-inf) ZDV: 2.1 (300 mg, 0-inf)
Truvada (FTC/TDF)	2 NRTI	Tab: FTC 200 mg + TDF 300 mg Tab: FTC 167 mg + TDF 250 mg Tab: FTC 133 mg + TDF 200 mg Tab: FTC 100 mg + TDF 150 mg	Tab ± food	FTC: 92 TDF: 25 (fasting)	FTC: 1-2 TDF: 1	FTC: 1.8 (200 mg q24h, SS) TDF: 0.3 (300 mg, SD)	FTC: <4 TDF: <0.7	FTC: no data TDF: 1.2-1.3 L/kg (Vss)	FTC: 10 TDF: 17	FTC: Renal TDF: Renal	FTC: 39 TDF: >60	FTC: no data TDF: no data	FTC: 3 TDF: 1	FTC: 10.0 (200 mg, 0-inf) TDF: 2.3 (300 mg, 0-inf)

[1] Refers to adult oral preparations unless otherwise noted; + food = take with food, no food = take without food, ± food = take with or without food.
[2] SD = after a single dose, SS = at steady state.
[3] V/F = Vd/oral bioavailability; Vss = Vd at steady state; Vss/F = Vd at steady state/oral bioavailability.
[4] Assumes CrCl >80 mL/min.
[5] (Peak concentration in bile/peak concentration in serum) x 100. If blank, no data.
[6] CSF concentrations with inflammation.
[7] Judgment based on drug dose and organism susceptibility. CSF concentration ideally ≥10x MIC.
[8] AUC = area under serum concentration vs. time curve. KEY: 0-inf = AUC 0 to infinity; 0-xh = AUC 0 to x hours.
[9] Concern over seizure potential *(see Table 10B)*.
[10] Take all oral FQs 2-4 hours before sucralfate or any multivalent cation (calcium, iron, zinc).
[11] CPE (CNS Penetration Effectiveness) value: 1=low penetration, 2-3=intermediate penetration, 4=highest penetration *(Letendre et al, CROI 2010, abs #430)*.

TABLE 9B – PHARMACODYNAMICS OF ANTIBACTERIALS*

Antibacterial activity	Post-antibiotic effect (PAE)	Drugs	Goal of therapy	PK/PD parameter
Bactericidal, time-dependent	Short for gram-positive cocci, none to short for gram-negative bacilli (except carbapenems, which have a PAE against many gram-negative bacilli)	Beta-lactams, vancomycin	Enhance duration of exposure	Time above MIC
Bactericidal, concentration-dependent	Prolonged (also concentration-dependent)	Aminoglycosides, fluoroquinolones, daptomycin, colistin, metronidazole, azithromycin (?), ketolides	Enhance antibiotic concentrations	Cmax/MIC, AUC_{24}/MIC
Bacteriostatic	Moderate to prolonged	Macrolides, clindamycin, streptogramins, tetracyclines, tigecycline, linezolid	Enhance amount of antibiotic	AUC_{24}/MIC

TABLE 9C – ENZYME -AND TRANSPORTER- MEDIATED INTERACTIONS OF ANTIMICROBIALS

>50% of all drugs are metabolized by one or more members of the CYP450 enzyme system. The Metabolism of a drug that is a substrate of a particular CYP enzyme may be induced (accelerated) by another drug, resulting in under dosing and therapeutic failure. Conversely the Metabolism of a drug may be inhibited (slowed) by another drug, resulting in overdosing and toxicity. A drug may act as a substrate for more than one enzyme, or it may inhibit or induce multiple enzymes. Inhibition tends to be a relatively quick process related to the dose of the inhibitor, whereas induction occurs more slowly. Risk is amplified when two or more drugs that are enzyme inhibitors or inducers are administered. CYP450 enzymes commonly involved in drug interactions include CYP3A4, CYP2C9/19, CYP1A2, and CYP2D6.

Drug transporter systems may also be involved in drug interactions. Transporters are found in many tissues, such as the kidney and GI tract, and they work to pump drugs into cells (influx) or out of cells (efflux). Examples of important drug transporters systems include P-glycoprotein (PGP), organic anion transporter (OAT), and organic cation transporter (OCT).

Knowledge of these enzymes is useful in understanding clinically relevant drug interactions and can also assist in predicting previously unrecognized interactions. With respect to specific antimicrobials, always check for drug-drug interactions when ordering these inhibitors that may cause elevated serum concentrations: macrolides, ciprofloxacin, metronidazole, TMP-SMX, isoniazid, azole antifungals, antiretrovirals, and anti-HCV drugs. Nafcillin, rifamycins, and certain antiretrovirals are known to induce Metabolism and lead to treatment failure. If a drug interaction is recognized and no suitable alternative regimen exists, check serum concentration of the affected drug (if available), adjust dose, and monitor for toxicity.

BCRP: Breast Cancer Resistance Protein. **CYP450 Nomenclature:** e.g. 3A4: 3 = family; A = subfamily; 4 gene. **OAT:** Organic Anion Transporter. **OATP:** Organic Anion Transporter Polypeptide. **OCT:** Organic Cation Transporter. **PGP:** P-glycoprotein. **UGT:** Uridine Diphosphate Glucuronosyltransferase

Groups/Drugs	Drug is a substrate of CYP450	Drug is a substrate of Transporter	CYP450 Inhibited by drug	Transporter Inhibited by drug	CYP450 Induced by drug	Transporter Induced by drug	Impact on Serum Drug Concentrations1
Antibacterials							
Amoxicillin		OAT					
Ampicillin		OAT					
Azithromycin		PGP		PGP (weak)			mild ↑
Aztreonam		OAT1, OAT3					
Aztreonam-avibactam		Az: OAT1, OAT3 Avi: OAT1, OAT3					
Ceftobiprole medocaril				OATP1B1, OATP1B3			↑
Cephalexin		MATE1					
Chloramphenicol			2C19, 3A4				↑
Ciprofloxacin			1A2; 3A4 (minor)				↑
Clarithromycin	3A4		3A4	PGP, OAT			↑
Clindamycin	3A4						
Dicloxacillin					2C9, 2C19, 3A4	PGP (intestinal)	↓
Eravacycline	3A4						

TABLE 9C (2)

Groups/Drugs	Drug is a substrate of CYP450	Drug is a substrate of Transporter	CYP450 Inhibited by drug	Transporter Inhibited by drug	CYP450 Induced by drug	Transporter Induced by drug	Impact on Serum Drug Concentrations1
Antibacterials *(continued)*							
Erythromycin	3A4	PGP	3A4	PGP, OAT			↑
Flucloxacillin					3A4?	PGP?	↓
Fusidic acid	3A4		3A4	BCRP, OATP1B1			↑
Imipenem-cilastatin[2]		Imi: OAT1, OAT3					
Imipenem-cilastatin-relebactam[2]		Imi: OAT1, OAT3 Rele: OAT3, OAT4, MATE1, MATE2K					
Lefamulin	3A4		3A4				↑
Levofloxacin				MATE, OCT2			↑
Meropenem[2]		OAT1, OAT3					
Meropenem-vaborbactam[2]		OAT1, OAT3					
Metronidazole			2C9				↑
Nafcillin					2C9 (?), 3A4		↓
Norfloxacin			1A2 (weak)				mild ↑
Omadacycline		PGP					
Oritavancin			2C9 (weak), 2C19 (weak)		2D6 (weak), 3A4 (weak)		mild ↑ or ↓
Penicillin G		OAT					
Penicillin VK		OAT					
Pivmecillinam		OAT3, MATE1, MATE2-K					
Plazomicin				MATE1, MATE2-K			↑
Pristinamycin			3A4				↑
Quinupristin-dalfopristin			3A4				↑
Retapamulin	3A4						
Rifampin	-	PGP, OATP1B1	-	OAT, OATP1B1	1A2, 2B6, 2C8, 2C9, 2C19, 2D6 (weak), 3A4	PGP, UGT enzymes	↓
Rifaximin	3A4	PGP, OATP1A2, OATP1B1/3		PGP (in vitro only)	3A4		Minimal clinically relevant effects expected
Sarecycline				PGP			↑
Sulbactam		OAT1					
Sulopenem etzadroxil-probenecid		Sulopenem: OAT3 Probenecid: BCRP		Probenecid: OAT1/3			↑
Tedizolid phosphate				BCRP (gut)			↑
Telithromycin			3A4	PGP (?)			↑
Tigecycline		PGP					
TMP-SMX	SMX: 2C9 (major), 3A4		TMP: 2C8; SMX: 2C9				↑
Trimethoprim			2C8				↑

TABLE 9C (3)

Groups/Drugs	Drug is a substrate of CYP450	Drug is a substrate of Transporter	CYP450 Inhibited by drug	Transporter Inhibited by drug	CYP450 Induced by drug	Transporter Induced by drug	Impact on Serum Drug Concentrations1
Antifungals							
Fluconazole			2C9, 2C19, 3A4				↑
Ibrexafungerp	3A4		2C8, 3A4	PGP, OATP1B3			Short treatment duration for VVC limits clinical impact on other drugs
Isavuconazonium sulfate	3A4		3A4	PGP, OCT2			↑
Itraconazole	3A4		3A4	PGP			↑
Ketoconazole	3A4		3A4	PGP			↑
Oteseconazole				BCRP			↑
Posaconazole		PGP	3A4	PGP			↑
Terbinafine	Multiple		2D6				↑
Voriconazole	2C9, 2C19, 3A4		2C9, 2C19, 3A4				↑
Antimycobacterials (Rifampin listed above)							
Bedaquiline	3A4						
Delamanid	3A4						
Isoniazid (INH)			2C19, 3A4		2E1		↑ or ↓
Pretomanid	3A4			OAT3			↑
Rifabutin	3A4				3A4		↓
Rifapentine					2C9, 3A4		↓
Thalidomide	2C19						
Antiparasitics							
Artemether-lumefantrine	Art: 3A4 Lum: 3A4		Lum: 2D6		Art: 2B6, 2C19, 3A4 (all weakly)		↑ or ↓
Artesunate (AS)		AS: BCRP, PGP DHA: UGT1A9, UGT2B7	DHA: 1A2 (weak)	AS: OATP1B1 (weak), OAT3 (weak)			↑
Chloroquine phosphate	2C8, 2D6		2D6				↑
Dapsone	3A4						
Dihydroartemisinin-piperaquine	PPQ: 3A4, weak 2C19		DHA: 1A2, 2C19 PPQ: 3A4, 2C19		PPQ: 2E1?		↑ or ↓
Fexinidazole			1A2, 2B6, 2C19, 2D6, 3A4/5	OATP1B1/3, OCT2, OAT1, OAT3, MATE1, MATE2-K	1A2, 2B6		↑ or ↓
Halofantrine	3A4		2D6				↑
Ivermectin	3A4						
Mefloquine	3A4	PGP		PGP			↑
Praziquantel	3A4						
Primaquine	2D6, others?						
Proguanil	2C19						

TABLE 9C (4)

Groups/Drugs	Drug is a substrate of CYP450	Drug is a substrate of Transporter	CYP450 Inhibited by drug	Transporter Inhibited by drug	CYP450 Induced by drug	Transporter Induced by drug	Impact on Serum Drug Concentrations1
Antiparasitics *(continued)*							
Pyronaridine-artesunate		AS: BCRP, PGP DHA: UGT1A9, UGT2B7	DHA: 1A2 (weak) Pyr: 2D6	AS: OATP1B1 (weak), OAT3 (weak) Pyr: PGP			↑
Quinacrine	3A4/5	PGP	2E1				↑
Quinine sulfate	main 3A4, also 1A2, 2C9, 2D6		2D6				↑
Tafenoquine				OCT, MATE1, MATE2K			↑
Tinidazole	3A4						
Triclabendazole			2C19				↑
Antivirals							
Antivirals (coronavirus)							
Baricitinib		PGP, OAT3, BCRP, MATE2-K					
Nirmatrelvir	3A4	PGP	3A4	PGP			↑
Remdesivir	2C8, 2D6, 3A4	PGP, OATP1B1	3A4	OATP1B1/3, BSEP, MRP4, NTCP			Minimal clinically relevant effects expected
Tofacitinib	3A4						
Antivirals (hepatitis B)							
Entecavir		OCT2					↑
Antivirals (hepatitis C)							
Daclatasvir	3A4	PGP		PGP, OATP1B1/3, BCRP			↑
Dasabuvir	3A4	PGP, OATP1B1	2C8	UGT1A1, OATP1B1, OATP1B3			↑
Elbasvir	3A4	PGP		BCRP			↑
Glecaprevir		PGP, BCRP, OATP1B1/3	1A2 (weak), 3A4 (weak)	PGP, BCRP, OATP1B1/3, UGT1A1 (weak)			↑
Grazoprevir	3A4	PGP, OATP1B1/3	3A4 (weak)	BCRP			↑
Ledipasvir		PGP, BCRP		PGP, BCRP			↑
Ombitasvir	3A4	PGP		2C8, UGT1A1			↑
Paritaprevir	2C8, 2D6, 3A4	PGP		UGT1A1, OATP1B1			↑
Pibrentasvir		PGP, BCRP	1A2 (weak), 3A4 (weak)	PGP, BCRP, OATP1B1/3, UGT1A1 (weak)			↑
Simeprevir	3A4	PGP, OATP1B1/3	1A2 (weak), 3A4 (gut only)	PGP, OATP1B1/3			↑
Sofosbuvir		PGP, BCRP					
Velpatasvir	2B6, 2C8, 3A4	PGP, BCRP, OATP1B1/3		PGP, BCRP, OATP1B1/3, OATP2B1			↑

TABLE 9C (5)

Groups/Drugs	Drug is a substrate of CYP450	Drug is a substrate of Transporter	CYP450 Inhibited by drug	Transporter Inhibited by drug	CYP450 Induced by drug	Transporter Induced by drug	Impact on Serum Drug Concentrations1
Antivirals *(continued)*							
Antivirals (herpesvirus)							
Acyclovir		OAT1, OAT3					
Cidofovir		OAT1, OAT3					
Letermovir	2D6 (minor), 3A (minor)	OATP1B1/3, PGP, UGT1A1/3	2C8, 3A	OATP1B1/3	2B6, 2C9, 2C19		↑ or ↓
Maribavir	3A4 (major), 1A2 (minor)		3A4 (weak)	PGP, BCRP			↑
Valacyclovir		OAT1, OAT3					
Antivirals (influenza)							
Baloxavir marboxil		PGP					
Favipiravir			2C8				↑
Antivirals (poxviruses)							
Brincidofovir		OATP1B1/3	1A2, 2B6, 2C8/9, 2C19, 2D6, 4F2	BCRP, MRP2, BSEP, OATP1B1, OAT1, OAT3			↑
Tecovirimat		UGT1A1, 1A4	2C8 (weak), 2C19 (weak)	BCRP (weak)	3A4 (weak)		↑ or ↓
Antiretrovirals							
Atazanavir (ATV)	3A4	PGP	1A2, 2C8, 3A4	UGT1A1			↑
Bictegravir (BIC)	3A4	UGT1A1		OCT2, MATE1			↑
Cabotegravir (CAB)		PGP, BCRP		OAT1, OAT3			↑
Cobicistat (COBI or c)	2D6, 3A4		2D6, 3A4	PGP, BCRP, OATP1B1, OATP1B3			↑
Darunavir (DRV)	3A4		3A4				↑
Dolutegravir (DTG)	3A4	UGT1A1, UGT1A3, UGT1A9, BCRP, PGP		OCT2, MATE1			↑
Efavirenz (EFV)	2B6, 3A4		2B6, 2C9, 2C19		2C19, 3A4		↑ or ↓
Elvitegravir (EVG)	CYP3A4	UGT1A1/3		PGP (weak)	2C9 (weak)		mild ↑ or ↓
Etravirine (ETR)	2C9, 2C19, 3A4		2C9; 2C19 (weak)		3A4		↑ or ↓
Fosamprenavir (FPV)	3A4		3A4				↑
Fostemsavir (FTR)	3A4	PGP, BCRP		OATP1B1/3, BCRP			↑
Lamivudine (3TC)		PGP, BCRP, MATE1, MATE2-K, OCT2					
Lenacapavir (LEN)	3A	PGP, UGT1A1	3A	PGP, BCRP			↑
Lopinavir (LPV)	3A4						
Maraviroc (MVC)	3A4	PGP	2D6				↑
Nevirapine (NVP)	2B6, 3A4				2B6, 3A4		↓
Raltegravir (RAL)		UGT					

TABLE 9C (6)

Groups/Drugs	Drug is a substrate of CYP450	Drug is a substrate of Transporter	CYP450 Inhibited by drug	Transporter Inhibited by drug	CYP450 Induced by drug	Transporter Induced by drug	Impact on Serum Drug Concentrations1
Antiretrovirals *(continued)*							
Rilpivirine (RPV)	3A4						
Ritonavir (RTV)	3A4	PGP	2D6, 3A4	PGP	1A2, 2B6, 2C9, 2C19, 3A4 (long term)	PGP (long term), UGT	↑ or ↓
Tenofovir alafenamide fumarate (TAF)		PGP, BCRP					
Tenofovir disoproxil fumarate (TDF)		PGP, BCRP					
Non-Antimicrobial Drugs (found in H. pylori combination products)							
Omeprazole	2C19, 3A4		2C19				↑
Vonoprazan	3A4/5, 2B6, 2C9, 2C19, 2D6		2B6, 2C19, 3A4/5				↑

[1] Refers to serum concentrations of companion drugs that may be affected by the listed antimicrobial. ↑=increase, ↓=decrease.
[2] Carbapenems decrease valproic acid concentrations by inhibiting acylpeptide hydrolase (interrupting enterohepatic recycling).

TABLE 10A – ANTIBIOTIC DOSAGE* AND SIDE-EFFECTS

CLASS, AGENT, GENERIC NAME (TRADE NAME)	USUAL ADULT DOSAGE*	ADVERSE REACTIONS, COMMENTS
NATURAL PENICILLINS		
Benzathine penicillin G (Bicillin L-A)	**600,000–1.2 million units IM q2–4 wks**	**Allergic reactions a major issue.** 10% of all hospital admissions give history of pen allergy; but only 10% have allergic reaction if given penicillin. Why? Possible reasons: inaccurate history, waning immunity with age, aberrant response during viral illness. If given, **Bicillin C-R IM (procaine Pen + benzathine Pen)** could be reaction to procaine. **Most serious reaction is immediate IgE-mediated anaphylaxis;** incidence only 0.05% but 5-10% fatal. Other IgE-mediated reactions: urticaria, angioedema, laryngeal edema, bronchospasm, abdominal pain with emesis, or hypotension. All appear within 4 hrs. Can form IgE antibody against either the beta-lactam ring or the R-group side chain. **Morbilliform rash after 72 hrs is not IgE-mediated and not serious.** **Serious late allergic reactions:** Coombs-positive hemolytic anemia, neutropenia, thrombocytopenia, serum sickness, interstitial nephritis, hepatitis, eosinophilia, drug fever. **Cross-allergy to cephalosporins and carbapenems** varies from 0-11%. One factor is similarity, or lack of similarity, of side chains. **For pen desensitization,** *see Table 7.* For skin testing, suggest referral to allergist. High **CSF** concentrations cause seizures. Reduce dosage with renal impairment, *see Table 17A.* Allergy refs: *CID 59:1113, 2014; JAC 69:20-43, 2014; CID 58:1140, 2014.*
Penicillin G	**Low: 600,000–1.2 million units IM per day** **High: ≥20 million units IV q24h(=12 gm) div q4h**	
Penicillin V (250 & 500 mg caps)	**0.25–0.5 gm po bid, tid, qid before meals & at bedtime.** Pen V preferred over Pen G for oral therapy due to greater acid stability.	
PENICILLINASE-RESISTANT PENICILLINS		
Dicloxacillin (Dynapen) **(250 & 500 mg caps)**	**0.125–0.5 gm po q6h before meals**	Blood levels ~2 times greater than cloxacillin so preferred for po therapy. Hemorrhagic cystitis reported. Acute abdominal pain with GI bleeding without antibiotic-associated colitis also reported. Can impede warfarin.
Flucloxacillin[NUS] (Floxapen, Lutropin, Staphcil)	**0.25–0.5 gm po q6h** **1–2 gm IV q4h**	Cholestatic hepatitis occurs in 1:15,000 exposures: more frequently in age >55 yrs, females and therapy >2 wks duration. Can appear wks after end of therapy and take wks to resolve *(JAC 66:1431, 2011).* **Recommendation: use only in severe infection.**
Nafcillin (Unipen, Nafcil)	**1–2 gm IV/IM q4h.** Due to >90% protein binding, need 12 gm/day for bacteremia.	Extravasation can result in tissue necrosis. With 200–300 mg per kg per day hypokalemia may occur. **Reversible neutropenia (over 10% with ≥21-day rx, occasionally WBC <1000 per mm³).** Can impede warfarin effect.
Oxacillin (Prostaphlin)	**1–2 gm IV/IM q4h.** Due to >90% protein binding, need 12 gm/day for bacteremia.	**Hepatic dysfunction with ≥12 gm per day.** LFTs usually ↑ 2–24 days after start of rx, reversible. In children, more rash and liver toxicity with oxacillin as compared to nafcillin *(CID 34:50, 2002).*
AMINOPENICILLINS		
Amoxicillin (Amoxil, Polymox)	**250 mg–1 gm po tid**	IV available in UK & Europe. IV amoxicillin rapidly converted to ampicillin. Rash with infectious mono– *see Ampicillin.* Increased risk of cross-allergenicity with oral cephalosporins with identical side-chains: cefadroxil, cefprozil.
Amoxicillin extended release (Moxatag)	**One 775 mg tab po once daily**	Allergic reactions, C. difficile associated diarrhea, false positive test for urine glucose with clinitest.
Amoxicillin-clavulanate (Augmentin) **Amox-clav extra-strength peds suspension (ES-600)** **AM-CL-ER—extended release adult tabs**	*See Comment for adult products* **Peds Extra-Strength susp.: 600/42.9 per 5 mL. Dose: 90/6.4 mg/kg div bid.** For adult formulations, *see Comments* IV amox-clav available in Europe	With bid regimen, less clavulanate & less diarrhea. In pts with immediate allergic reaction to Amox-clav, ⅓ due to Clav component *(J Allergy Clin Immunol 125:502, 2010).* **Hepatotoxicity linked to clavulanic acid; Amox-clav causes 13-23% of drug-induced liver injury. Onset delayed. Usually mild; rare liver failure** *(Gastroenterol 148:1340, 2015; NEJM 381:264, 2019).* **Comparison adult Augmentin dosage regimens:** Augmentin 500/125 1 tab po tid Augmentin 875/125 1 tab po bid Augmentin-XR 1000/62.5 2 tabs po bid
Ampicillin (Principen) (250 & 500 mg caps)	**0.25–0.5 gm po q6h** **50–200 mg/kg IV/day div q6h**	A maculopapular rash occurs (not urticarial), **not true penicillin allergy,** in 65–100% pts with infectious mono, 90% with chronic lymphocytic leukemia, and 15–20% in pts taking allopurinol. EBV-associated rash does not indicate permanent allergy; post-EBV no rash when challenged. Increased risk of true cross-allergenicity with oral cephalosporins with identical side chains: cefaclor, cephalexin, loracarbef.

TABLE 10A (2)

CLASS, AGENT, GENERIC NAME (TRADE NAME)	USUAL ADULT DOSAGE*	ADVERSE REACTIONS, COMMENTS
AMINOPENICILLINS *(continued)*		
Ampicillin-sulbactam (Unasyn)	**1.5-3 gm IV q6h. For resistant Acinetobacter, 8 gm Amp/4 gm sulb IV over 4 hr q8h in combination with Meropenem and Polymyxin B.**	Supplied in vials: amp 2 gm, sulbactam 1 gm. Adjust dose for renal insufficiency, *see Table 17A*. For combination regimen dosing (Amp-sulb + MER + Polymyxin B), *see Table 1, page 44*).
ANTIPSEUDOMONAL PENICILLINS		
Piperacillin-tazobactam (Zosyn) Prolonged infusion dosing, *See also Table 10D*. Obesity dosing, *see Table 17C*.	**Prolonged infusion (preferred method):** 4.5 gm (over 4 hours) IV q8h. Old dose (except *P. aeruginosa*): 3.375 gm IV q6h or 4.5 gm q8h. Old *P. aeruginosa* dose: 3.375 gm q4h or 4.5 gm q6h. Infuse all over 30 min.	• Cystic fibrosis + *P. aeruginosa* infection: 300-400 mg/kg/day (div q6h) For obesity dosing adjustment *see Table 17C, page 321*. Documented drug-induced thrombocytopenia *(J Thrombo Haemostasis 11:169, 2012)*. Does Pip-tazo + vanco increase risk of renal injury (increased Cr)? Cr increase may reflect competition of Pip-tazo for tubular secretion of Cr *(CID 71:426, 2020)*
Temocillin[NUS]	**2 gm IV q12h.**	Semi-synthetic penicillin stable in presence of classical & ESBLs plus AmpC beta-lactamases. Source: *www.eumedica.be*
CARBAPENEMS/THIOPENEMS. Review: *AAC 55:4943, 2011.* **NOTE: Cross allergenicity: In studies of pts with history of Pen-allergy but no confirmatory skin testing, 0-11% had allergic reactions with cephalosporin therapy** *(JAC 54:1155, 2004)*. **In better studies, pts with positive skin tests for Pen allergy were given Carbapenem: no reaction in 99%** *(J Allergy Clin Immunol 124:167, 2009)*. Of 12 pts with IgE-mediated reaction to ceph, 2 suffered rash & 1 an IgE reaction when given a carbapenem *(CID 59:1113, 2014)*. Incidence of carbapenem-resistant GNB highest in Georgia, Maryland & New York *(JAMA 314:1455 & 1479, 2015)*.		
Doripenem (Doribax) Ref: *CID 49:291, 2009. For prolonged infusion dosing, see Table 10D*	Intra-abdominal & complicated UTI: **500 mg IV q8h (1-hr infusion).** For prolonged infusion, *see Table 10D, page 167*. Do not use for pneumonia	Most common adverse reactions (≥5%): Headache, nausea, diarrhea, rash & phlebitis. Seizure reported in post-marketing surveillance. Can lower serum valproic acid levels. Adjust dose if renal impairment. Somewhat more stable in solution than **IMP** or **MER** *(JAC 65:1023, 2010; CID 49:291, 2009)*. FDA safety announcement (01/05/12): Trial of DORI for the treatment of VAP stopped early due to safety concerns. Compared to IMP, patients treated with DORI were observed to have excess mortality and poorer cure rate. **NOTE: DORI is not approved to treat any type of pneumonia; DORI is not approved for doses greater than 500 mg q8h.**
Ertapenem (Invanz)	**1 gm IV/IM q24h.**	**Lidocaine** diluent for IM use; ask about lidocaine allergy. Standard dosage may be inadequate in obesity (BMI ≥40). Reports of DRESS (drug rash eosinophilia systemic symptoms) Syndrome. Visual hallucinations reported *(NZ Med J 122:76, 2009)*. No predictable activity vs. *P. aeruginosa*.
Imipenem - cilastatin (Primaxin, Tienam) Ref: *JAC 58:916, 2006*	**0.5 gm IV q6h**; for P. aeruginosa: 1 gm q6–8h *(see Comment)*.	For P. aeruginosa, increase dosage to 3 or 4 gm per day div. q8h or q6h. Continuous infusion of carbapenems more efficacious & safer *(AAC 49:1881, 2005)*. **Seizures:** risk of seizure low but greatest with carbapenems. No diff between IMP and MER *(JAC 69:2043, 2014)*. Cilastatin blocks enzymatic degradation of Imipenem in lumen of renal proximal tubule & also prevents tubular toxicity. Compared to MER, more in vitro resistance to IMP vs. Proteus sp., Providencia sp., Morganella sp. *(Can ID Med Micro 2014,25:285)*
Imipenem-cilastatin-relebactam (Recarbrio)	**1.25 gm IV over 30 min q6h** Adjust dose if CrCl < 90 mL/min	**Seizure risk:** avoid concomitant valproic acid or divalproex sodium. C. diff toxin-mediated diarrhea reported. Active vs. KPC-producing GNB.
Meropenem (Merrem)	**0.5–1 gm IV q8h. Up to 2 gm IV q8h for meningitis. Prolonged infusion** in critically ill: If CrCl ≥50: 2 gm (over 3 hr) q8h If CrCl 30-49: 1 gm (over 3 hr) q8h If CrCl 10-29: 1 gm (over 3 hr) q12h *(Inten Care Med 37:632, 2011)*.	**Seizures:** In meta-analysis, risk of seizure low but greatest with carbapenems among beta-lactams. No diff between IMP and MER *(JAC 69:2043, 2014)*. Comments: Does not require a dehydropeptidase inhibitor (cilastatin). Activity vs aerobic gm-neg. slightly ↑ over IMP, activity vs staph & strep slightly ↓; anaerobes: B. ovatus, B. distasonis more resistant to meropenem.

(See page 2 for abbreviations)

*NOTE: all dosage recommendations are for adults (unless otherwise indicated) & assume normal renal function.

TABLE 10A (3)

CLASS, AGENT, GENERIC NAME (TRADE NAME)	USUAL ADULT DOSAGE*	ADVERSE REACTIONS, COMMENTS
CARBAPENEMS *(continued)*		
Meropenem-vaborbactam (Vabomere)	4 gm (2 gm meropenem + 2 gm vaborbactam) IV q8h infused over 3 hrs (with estimated eGFR >50 mL/min).	Combination of Meropenem with vaborbactam. Vaborbactam inhibits common serine beta-lactamases, ESBLs, KPCs, and AmpC but not metallo-beta-lactamases or oxacillinases with carbapenemase activity. Approved for the treatment of complicated urinary tract infections in patients age ≥18 years caused by *E. coli, K. pneumoniae, E. cloacae*, and other susceptible aerobic gram-negative bacilli. **Contraindicated:** if known hypersensitivity to meropenem or beta lactams. **AEs:** hypersensitivity reactions, seizure potential, C. diff-associated diarrhea, thrombocytopenia, neuromotor impairment, phlebitis (infusion site), diarrhea, headache. **Major interactions:** valproic acid (concomitant use not recommended), probenecid.
Sulopenem Etzadroxil-Probenecid	1 tablet po q12h x5 days. (1 tablet = 500 mg sulopenem etzadroxil + 500 mg probenecid)	**Most common AE:** GI (nausea, vomiting, diarrhea). **Other AE:** Hypersensitivity (rash, angioedema, anaphylaxis), headache, *C. difficile*-associated diarrhea. **May cause gout exacerbation.** When used in pts with gout history, institute measures to reduce uric acid stone development, such as increased fluids and urinary tract alkalinization. Contraindicated in pts with known uric acid stones. **May interfere with copper sulfate urine glucose tests,** resulting in a false-positive for glycosuria.
MONOBACTAMS		
Aztreonam (Azactam)	**1 gm q8h–2 gm IV q6h.**	Can be used in pts with allergy to penicillins/cephalosporins with exception of Ceftazidime as **side-chains of Aztreonam and Ceftazidime are identical.** PK/PD *(JAC 2016,71:2704)*.
Aztreonam for Inhalation (Cayston)	**75 mg inhaled tid x 28 days.** Use bronchodilator before each inhalation.	Improves respiratory symptoms in CF pts colonized with P. aeruginosa. Alternative to inhaled Tobra. AEs: bronchospasm, cough, wheezing. So far, no emergence of other resistant pathogens. Ref: *Chest 135:1223, 2009.*
CEPHALOSPORINS (1st parenteral, then oral drugs). NOTE: Prospective data demonstrate correlation between use of cephalosporins (esp. 3rd generation) and ↑ risk of C. difficile toxin-induced diarrhea. May also ↑ risk of colonization with vancomycin-resistant enterococci. *See Oral Cephalosporins, page 154,* **for important note on cross-allergenicity.**		
1st Generation, Parenteral		
Cefazolin (Ancef, Kefzol)	**1-1.5 gm IV/IM q8h, occasionally 2 gm IV q8h for serious infections, e.g., MSSA bacteremia (max. 12 gm/day)**	**Do not give into lateral ventricles—seizures!** No activity vs. MRSA. Very low risk of cross-allergenicity with other cephalosporins or beta-lactams.
2nd Generation, Parenteral (Cephamycins): May be active in vitro vs. ESBL-producing aerobic gram-negative bacilli. Do not use as there are no clinical data for efficacy.		
Cefotetan (Cefotan)	**1–3 gm IV/IM q12h. (max. dose not >6 gm q24h).**	Increasing resistance of B. fragilis, Prevotella bivia, Prevotella disiens (most common in pelvic infections); do not use for intra-abdominal infections. Methylthiotetrazole (MTT) side chain can inhibit vitamin K activation. Avoid alcohol-disulfiram reaction.
Cefoxitin (Mefoxin)	**1 gm q8h–2 gm IV/IM q6-8h.**	Increasing resistance of B. fragilis isolates.
Cefuroxime (Kefurox, Ceftin, Zinacef)	**0.75–1.5 gm IV/IM q8h.**	Improved activity against H. influenzae compared with 1st generation cephalosporins. *See Cefuroxime axetil for oral preparation.*
3rd Generation, Parenteral – Use correlates with incidence of C. difficile toxin diarrhea; most are inactivated by ESBLs and amp C cephalosporinase from aerobic gram-negative bacilli.		
Cefoperazone-Sulbactam[NUS] (Sulperazon)	**Usual dose (Cefoperazone comp) 1–2 gm IV q12h;** if larger doses, do not exceed 4 gm/day of sulbactam.	In SE Asia & elsewhere, used to treat intra-abdominal, biliary, & gyn. infections. Other uses due to broad spectrum of activity. Possible clotting problem due to side-chain.
Cefotaxime (Claforan)	**1 gm q8–12h to 2 gm IV q4h.**	Maximum daily dose: 12 gm; give as 4 gm IV q8h. Similar to ceftriaxone but, unlike ceftriaxone, but requires multiple daily doses.
Ceftizoxime (Cefizox)	From **1-2 gm IV q8-12h** up to **2 gm IV q4h.**	Maximum daily dose: 12 gm; can give as 4 gm IV q8h
Ceftobiprole[NUS] Similar activity to ceftaroline, incl MRSA	**0.5 gm IV over 2 hrs q8h**	Associated with caramel-like taste disturbance. Ref.: *Clin Microbiol Infections 13(Suppl 2):17 & 25, 2007.* Hydrolyzed by ESBL & AmpC cephalosporinase.

(See page 2 for abbreviations)

*NOTE: all dosage recommendations are for adults (unless otherwise indicated) & assume normal renal function.

TABLE 10A (4)

CLASS, AGENT, GENERIC NAME (TRADE NAME)	USUAL ADULT DOSAGE*	ADVERSE REACTIONS, COMMENTS
CEPHALOSPORINS/3rd Generation, Parenteral *(continued)*		
Ceftriaxone (Rocephin)	Commonly used IV dosage in adults: **1-2 gm once daily** Purulent meningitis: **2 gm q12h.** Can give **IM** in 1% lidocaine. 500 mg IV single dose for *N. gonorrhea (MMWR 69:1911, 2020)*	**"Pseudocholelithiasis"** 2° to sludge in gallbladder by ultrasound (50%), symptomatic (9%) *(NEJM 322:1821, 1990)*. More likely with ≥2 gm per day with pt on total parenteral nutrition and not eating *(AnIM 115:712, 1991)*. Has led to cholecystectomy *(JID 17:356, 1995)* and gallstone pancreatitis *(Ln 17:662, 1998)*. Can cause drug-induced thrombocytopenia *(J Thrombo & Haemo 2012,11:169)*. Combination of Ceftriaxone & Lansoprazole led to 1.4 x increased risk of increased QTc to >500 msec *(J Am Coll Cardio 2016,68:1756)*. For Ceftriaxone Desensitization, *see Table 7, page 89*.
Antipseudomonal		
Cefepime (Maxipime) For obesity dosing, *see Table 17C*	**Usual dose: 1–2 gm IV q8-12h.** **Prolonged infusion dosing:** Initial dose: 15 mg/kg over 30 min, then immediately begin: If CrCl >60: 6 gm (over 24 hr) daily If CrCl 30-60: 4 gm (over 24 hr) daily If CrCl 11-29: 2 gm (over 24 hr) daily	Active vs P. aeruginosa and many strains of Enterobacter, Serratia, C. freundii resistant to Ceftazidime, Cefotaxime, Aztreonam. More active vs MSSA than 3rd generation cephalosporins. Not "porin-dependent". Neutropenia after 14 days rx *(Scand J Infect Dis 42:156, 2010)*. Failures vs. E. cloacae bacteremia with MIC of 4-8 mcg/mL *(AAC 2015,59:7558)*. **FDA warning:** non-convulsive status epilepticus, especially in pts with renal insufficiency when doses not adjusted. Seizure activity resolved after drug discontinuation and/or hemodialysis. Postulated mechanism: binding to GABA receptors *(JAC 75:718, 2020)*.
CefpiromeNUS (HR 810)	**1–2 gm IV q12h**	Active against Enterobacterales and aerobic Gram-positive cocci (not enterococci or MRSA). Has activity against some P. aeruginosa. No useful activity against anaerobic bacilli.
Ceftazidime (Fortaz, Tazicef)	**Usual dose: 1–2 gm IV/IM q8–12h.** **Prolonged infusion dosing:** Initial dose: 15 mg/kg over 30 min, then immediately begin: If CrCl >50: 6 gm (over 24 hr) daily If CrCl 31-50: 4 gm (over 24 hr) daily If CrCl 10-30: 2 gm (over 24 hr) daily *(AAC 49:3550, 2005; Infect 37:418, 2009)*.	Often used in healthcare-associated infections, where P. aeruginosa is a consideration. Use may result in ↑ incidence of C. difficile-assoc. diarrhea and/or selection of vancomycin-resistant E. faecium. Risk of cross-allergenicity with aztreonam (same side chain).
Ceftolozane-tazobactam (Zerbaxa)	*See below*	
Anti-staphylococcal (MRSA)		
Ceftaroline fosamil (Teflaro)	**600 mg IV q12h (5-60 min infusion)** Pneumonia/bacteremia 600 mg IV q8hNAI. *See Comment*	**Avid binding to PBP 2a; active vs. MRSA.** Inactivated by Amp C & ESBL enzymes. Approved for MRSA skin and skin structure infections and used for MRSA pneumonia and bacteremia, but not approved indications *(J Infect Chemother 19:42, 2013)*. Active in vitro vs. VISA, VRSA. Refs: *CID 52:1156, 2011.* Used successfully for bacteremia and bone/joint infections, but NAI *(AAC 58:2541, 2014)*. Risk of neutropenia *(JAC 71:2010, 2016; AAC 60: 264, 2016)*.
Anti-ESBL resistant GNB		
Ceftolozane-tazobactam (Zerbaxa) Ref: *CID 2016,63:234*	1.5 gm (1/0.5 gm) IV q8h for gm-neg complicated UTI & complicated intra-abdominal (add Metro 500 mg IV q8h) infection	Infuse over 1 hr. Active vs. P. aeruginosa *(AAC 2017,61:e0046517)* and many gm-neg bacteria producing ESBLs. Cross-reaction in Beta-lactam allergic pts. Decreased efficacy w/ CrCl 30-50 mL/min. **Also approved for hospital-acquired & ventilator-associated pneumonia at higher dose: 3 gm IV over 1 hr q8h.**
Anti-ESBL and Serine-carbapenemase resistant GNB		
Ceftazidime-avibactam (Avycaz)	2.5 gm (2 gm Ceftazidime/0.5 gm avibactam) IV over 2 hrs q8h for gram-negative complicated UTI & add metronidazole 500 mg IV q8h for complicated intra-abdominal infection. Also approved for suscept GNB causing nosocomial pneumonia.	Active against ESBL- & KPC-producing aerobic gm-neg bacilli. No activity vs. GNB-producing metallo-carbapenemases. Decreased efficacy in pts with w/ CrCl 30-50 mL/min (in clinical trials).

(See page 2 for abbreviations)

*NOTE: all dosage recommendations are for adults (unless otherwise indicated) & assume normal renal function.

TABLE 10A (5)

CLASS, AGENT, GENERIC NAME (TRADE NAME)	USUAL ADULT DOSAGE*	ADVERSE REACTIONS, COMMENTS
CEPHALOSPORINS *(continued)*		
Anti-ESBL, Amp C, Serine & Metallo Carbapenemase GNB		
Cefiderocol (Fetroja) See FDA-approved package insert Phase 3 studies of MBL-producing pathogens *(CID 2022;75:1081 & 1085)*	Adult: 2 gm IV over 3 hrs q8h x 7-14 days Adjust dose for renal impairment (see Table 17A) Peds: no data	Siderophore cephalosporin FDA-approved for treatment of adults with complicated UTI, VABP, VHABP. Stable in vitro in presence of virtually all cephalosporinases and carbapenemases. Reserve for use in pts. with limited or no treatment options. Not active vs. gram positive and anaerobic bacteria. **Note:** In randomized trial of cefiderocol vs. best available therapy for pneumonia, bacteremia, complicated UTI due to carbapenem-resistant GNB, higher all-cause mortality in the pneumonia subgroup with Cefiderocol, but not statistically significant *(Lancet Infect Dis 2021; 21:226)*. In a double-blind RCT *(Lancet Infect Dis 2021;21:213)* Cefiderocol was non-inferior to Meropenem for Gram-negative HAP/VAP/HCAP; in 16 patients with Acinetobacter spp. with Meropenem MICs > 64 µg/mL, day 14 all-cause mortality was 0% (0/5) in the Cefiderocol group and 46% (5/11) in the Meropenem group.
Oral Cephalosporins		**Cross-Allergenicity: Patients with a history of IgE-mediated allergic reactions to penicillin (e.g., bronchospasm anaphylaxis, angioneurotic edema, immediate urticaria) should not receive a cephalosporin.** If the history is a "measles-like" rash to penicillin, available data suggest a 5–10% risk of rash in such patients; there is no enhanced risk of anaphylaxis. • In pts with history of Pen "reaction" and no skin testing, 0.2-8.4% react to a cephalosporin *(Aller Asthma Proc 26:135, 2006)*. If positive Pen G skin test, only 2% given a cephalosporin will react. Can predict with cephalosporin skin testing, but not easily available *(An IM 141:16, 2004; AJM 125:572, 2008)*. • IgE antibodies against either ring structure or side chains; 80% pts lose IgE over 10 yrs post-reaction *(J Aller Clin Immunol 103:918, 1999)*. Amox, Cefadroxil, Cefprozil have similar side chains; Amp, Cefaclor, Cephalexin, Cefadrine have similar side chains. • If Pen/Ceph skin testing not available or clinically no time, proceed with cephalosporin if history does not suggest IgE-mediated reaction, prior reaction more than 10 yrs ago or cephalosporin side chain differs from implicated Pen. Any of the cephalosporins can result in **C. difficile toxin**-mediated diarrhea/enterocolitis. There are **few drug-specific adverse effects, e.g.:** **Cefaclor:** Serum sickness-like reaction 0.1–0.5%--arthralgia, rash, erythema multiforme but no adenopathy, proteinuria or demonstrable immune complexes. **Cefdinir:** Drug-iron complex causes red stools in roughly 1% of pts. **Cefditoren pivoxil:** Hydrolysis yields pivalate. Pivalate absorbed (70%) & becomes pivaloylcarnitine which is renally excreted; 39–63% **↓ in serum carnitine concentrations.** Carnitine involved in fatty acid (FA) metabolism & FA transport into mitochondria. Effect transient & reversible. Contraindicated in patients with carnitine deficiency or those in whom inborn errors of metabolism might result in clinically significant carnitine deficiency. Also contains caseinate (milk protein); **avoid if milk allergy** (not same as lactose intolerance). Need gastric acid for optimal absorption. **Cefpodoxime:** There are rare reports of acute liver injury, bloody diarrhea, pulmonary infiltrates with eosinophilia. **Cephalexin:** Can cause false-neg. urine dipstick test for leukocytes.
1st Generation, Oral		
Cefadroxil (Duricef) (500 mg caps, 1 gm tabs)	**0.5–1 gm po q12h.**	
Cephalexin (Keflex) (250 & 500 mg tabs)	**0.25–1 gm po q6h (max 4 gm/day).**	
2nd Generation, Oral		
Cefaclor (Ceclor, Raniclor) (250 & 500 mg caps)	**0.25–0.5 gm po q8h.**	
Cefprozil (Cefzil) (250 & 500 mg tabs)	**0.25–0.5 gm po q12h.**	
Cefuroxime axetil po (Ceftin)	**0.125–0.5 gm po q12h.**	
3rd Generation, Oral		
Cefdinir (Omnicef) (300 mg cap)	**300 mg po q12h or 600 mg q24h.**	
Cefditoren pivoxil (Spectracef)	**400 mg po bid.**	
Cefixime (Suprax) (400 mg tab)	**0.4 gm po q12–24h.**	
Cefpodoxime proxetil (Vantin)	**0.1–0.2 gm po q12h.**	
Ceftibuten (Cedax) (400 mg tab)	**0.4 gm po q24h.**	

(See page 2 for abbreviations)

*NOTE: all dosage recommendations are for adults (unless otherwise indicated) & assume normal renal function.

TABLE 10A (6)

CLASS, AGENT, GENERIC NAME (TRADE NAME)	USUAL ADULT DOSAGE*	ADVERSE REACTIONS, COMMENTS
AMINOGLYCOSIDES AND RELATED ANTIBIOTICS – *See Table 10C, page 166, and Table 17A, page 288*		
GLYCOPEPTIDES, LIPOGLYCOPEPTIDES, LIPOPEPTIDES		
Dalbavancin (Dalvance, Xydalba)	**1000 mg IV over 30 min; one week later, 500 mg IV over 30 min or 1500 mg IV over 30 min x 1 dose.** Avoid use with saline, drug may precipitate out of solution.	**If CrCl<30**: 750 mg IV initial dose, then one week later 375 mg IV. **Hemodialysis:** Dose as for normal renal function Red man syndrome can occur with rapid infusion. Potential cross-reaction in those with hypersensitivity to other glycopeptides. No activity vs. VRE. Concomitant statins increase risk of myopathy/rhabdo *(CID 67:1356, 2018)*.
Daptomycin (Cubicin) Resistance: *JAC 2018,73:1.* Case series success in treating right- & left-sided endocarditis with higher dose of 8-10 mg/kg/day *(JAC 68:936 & 2921, 2013)*. In retrospective study, better survival in VRE bacteremia if dosed at ≥ 10 mg/kg/day *(CID 2017,64:605)*.	**Skin/soft tissue: 4 mg per kg IV over 2 or 30 minutes q24h** **Bacteremia/right-sided endocarditis: 6 mg per kg IV over 2 or 30 minutes q24h; up to 12 mg/kg IV q24h under study** **Morbid obesity:** base dose on total body weight *(AAC 51:2741, 2007)*, for other dosing recommendations, *see Table 17C, page 321.* Dapto + ceftaroline may work as salvage therapy in pts with refractory MRSA bacteremia *(AAC 57:66, 2013; AAC 56:5296, 2012)*.	**Pneumonia:** Dapto should not be used to treat pneumonia unless hematogenous in origin and is FDA approved for right-sided endocarditis with or without septic embolization/hematogenous pneumonia due to S. aureus. **Dapto Resistance:** Can occur de novo, after or during Vanco therapy, or after or during Dapto therapy *(CID 50(Suppl 1):S10, 2010)*. As Dapto MIC increases, MRSA more susceptible to TMP-SMX, nafcillin, oxacillin *(AAC 54:5187, 2010; CID 53:158, 2011)*. **Potential muscle toxicity:** Suggest weekly CPK; DC dapto if CPK exceeds 10x normal level or if symptoms of myopathy and CPK >1,000. Package insert: stop statins during dapto rx *(CID 2022;75:1416)*. Dapto interferes with protime reagents & artificially prolongs the PT. *(Blood Coag & Fibrinolysis 19:32, 2008)*. **NOTE:** Dapto well-tolerated at doses up to 12 mg/kg q24h x 14d *(AAC 50:3245, 2006)*. **Immune thrombocytopenia** reported *(AAC 56:6430, 2012)*. Reversible neutropenia with long-term use reported *(CID 56:1353, 2013)*. **Eosinophilic pneumonia**/chronic steroid-dep pneumonia reported *(CID 50:737, 2010; CID 50:e63, 2010)*.
Oritavancin (Orbactiv, Kimyrsa) Review: *CID 61:627, 2015*	Two formulations. **Orbactiv**: 1200 mg IV (over 3 hr) x1 dose, dilute in D5W only (not NS). **Kimyrsa**: 1200 mg IV (over 1 hr) x1 dose, dilute in D5W or NS.	Artificially increases PT & INR x 24 hr&aPTT x 48 hr. **Drug-drug interactions with warfarin:** ↑ warfarin serum levels. Acute urticarial has occurred. No dose adjustment for renal or hepatic insuff. Not removed by hemodialysis. In vitro activity vs. VRE *(AAC 56:1639, 2012)*.
Teicoplanin (Targocid) (where available)	**For septic arthritis—maintenance dose 12 mg/kg per day; S. aureus endocarditis— trough serum levels >20 mcg/mL required (12 mg/kg q12h times 3 loading dose, then 12 mg/kg q24h)**	Hypersensitivity: fever (at 3 mg/kg 2.2%, at 24 mg per kg 8.2%), skin reactions 2.4%. Marked ↓ platelets (high dose ≥15 mg per kg per day). Red neck syndrome less common than with vancomycin.
Telavancin (Vibativ) Lipoglycopeptide Ref: *CID 60:787, 2015; CID 61(Suppl 2), 2015*	10 mg/kg IV q24h if CrCl >50 mL/min. Infuse each dose over 1 hr.	**Avoid during pregnancy: teratogenic in animals.** Do pregnancy test before therapy. Adverse events: **dysgeusia (taste) 33%;** nausea 27%; vomiting 14%; headache 14%; ↑ creatinine (3.1%); foamy urine (13%); flushing if infused rapidly. In clin trials, **evidence of renal injury** in 3% telavancin vs. 1% vanco. In practice, renal injury reported in 1/3 of 21 complicated pts *(JAC 67:723, 2012)*. Interferes with PT, aPTT & INR for 18 hrs post-infusion.

(See page 2 for abbreviations)

*NOTE: all dosage recommendations are for adults (unless otherwise indicated) & assume normal renal function.

TABLE 10A (7)

CLASS, AGENT, GENERIC NAME (TRADE NAME)	USUAL ADULT DOSAGE*	ADVERSE REACTIONS, COMMENTS
GLYCOPEPTIDES, LIPOGLYCOPEPTIDES, LIPOPEPTIDES *(continued)*		
Vancomycin (Vancocin, Firvanq) **IV:** *S. aureus* bacteremia, endocarditis, invasive infection **PO:** *C. difficile* colitis **Intrathecal:** Meningitis **Refs: Updated dosing guidelines:** *Am J Health Sys Pharm 2020;77:835; Clin Infect Dis 2020; 70:1536 & 1546; Crit Care Med 2020; 48:912* Discussion of trough Vanco levels vs. calculation of AUC_{24} *(CID 2021;72:1497 & 1502)* **For AUC calculator**, *see Sanford Guide mobile app or web.sanfordguide.com* (based on trapezoidal model using 2 levels: peak and trough)	***S. aureus* bacteremia** & other susceptible gram-positive cocci: **Target level is AUC_{24} 400-600 µg/mL x h** **Loading Dose Recommended:** Use actual body weight: 20-30 mg/kg IV at 10-15 mg/min (max 3 gm), then either intermittent infusion (II) or continuous infusion (CI) **Intermittent Infusion Regimen:** Start first maintenance dose 12 hrs from start of loading dose: 15-20 mg/kg IV over 60 min, then repeat q12h. After 24-48 hrs, draw peak & trough serum levels to calculate AUC_{24} (use Sanford Guide AUC calculator). Adjust dose to attain AUC_{24} 400-600 mcg·hr/mL **Continuous Infusion (CI) Regimen:** Immediately after end of loading dose, start 30-40 mg/kg/day by CI. Within a few hrs, draw random serum level: AUC = serum level x 24. Adjust dose to attain AUC_{24} 400-600 mcg·hr/mL. **Morbid Obesity Regimen:** BMI > 30 kg/m². Give loading dose, then start first maintenance dose 8 hrs from start of loading dose. Intermittent infusion: 15-20 mg/kg IV over 2-3 hrs, then revert to q8h. After 24-48 hrs, draw peak & trough serum levels to calculate AUC_{24} (use Sanford Guide AUC calculator). No data on continuous infusion dosing in morbid obesity. **C. difficile colitis:** 125 mg po q6h x 10 days. Note: no absorption of oral vancomycin **Intrathecal Dose for Meningitis:** Infant: 5-10 mg/day Child & Adult: 10-20 mg/day. Target CSF concentration of 10-20 mcg/mL	**Optimizing Vancomycin PK:** now prefer dose that optimizes AUC_{24} with **target of 400-600 µg/mL x h** *(See updated guidelines – Refs)*. No need to divide AUC_{24} by MIC. Four methods for calculating AUC_{24}: 1. Use trough level: previously used method, but least reliable and no longer preferred 2. Draw steady state (24-48 hrs) peak and trough levels: use **Sanford Guide Vancomycin AUC calculator***, based on trapezoidal model, to determine AUC_{24}. Requires 2 levels. 3. Draw peak and trough serum levels after first dose and use Bayesian model calculator, if available. Accurate based on a single level but software can be expensive. Incremental benefit over 2 levels (above) debatable. 4. If continuous infusion, draw random serum level and multiply by duration of infusion (hrs), e.g., 23 or 24 **Oral Formulation:** FDA-approved oral solution: (Firvanq) 25/50 mg/mL (expensive). Compounded solution: 5 gm of powder used for IV form + 47.5 mL sterile water + 0.2 gm saccharin + 0.05 gm stevia powder + 40 mL glycerin & enough cherry syrup to yield 100 mL for 50 mg/mL. For 125 mg po, use 2.5 mL q6h. **AEs: Skin: red flushing reaction**, secondary to non-specific histamine release with too rapid an infusion. Not true allergy. OK to re-infuse at slower rate. **IgA bullous dermatitis**, immune mediated. Drug reaction: with eosinophilia + system signs & symptoms: genetic predisposition *(J Allergy Clin Immunol 2019;144:183)*; like Steven-Johnson without mucous membrane involvement. **Drug fever, immune neutropenia, thrombocytopenia. Dose dependent nephrotoxicity:** AUC_{24} > 600 mcg-hr/mL increases risk; Vanco + Pip-tazo may increase serum creatinine, likely due to benign competition between piperacillin & creatinine for tubular secretion *(CID 71:426, 2020)*. * *https://web.sanfordguide.com* or Sanford Guide mobile app

*NOTE: all dosage recommendations are for adults (unless otherwise indicated) & assume normal renal function.

CLASS, AGENT, GENERIC NAME (TRADE NAME)	USUAL ADULT DOSAGE*	ADVERSE REACTIONS, COMMENTS
CHLORAMPHENICOL, CLINDAMYCIN(S), ERYTHROMYCIN GROUP, KETOLIDES, OXAZOLIDINONES		
Chloramphenicol (Chloromycetin)	**50-100 mg/kg/day po/IV div q6h (max 4 gm/day)**	No oral drug distrib in U.S. Hematologic (↓ RBC ~1/3 pts, aplastic anemia 1:21,600 courses). Gray baby syndrome in premature infants, anaphylactoid reactions, optic atrophy or neuropathy (very rare), digital paresthesias, minor disulfiram-like reactions. Recent review suggests Chloro is probably less effective than current alternatives for serious infection: respiratory tract, enteric, meningitis *(JAC 70:979, 2015)*.
Clindamycin (Cleocin)	**0.15–0.45 gm po q6h. 600–900 mg IV/IM q8h.** In obese child, calc dose based on total body wt *(AAC 2017,61:e0201416)*	Based on number of exposed pts, these drugs are the most frequent cause of **C. difficile toxin-mediated diarrhea**. In most severe form can cause pseudomembranous colitis/toxic megacolon. Available as caps, IV sol'n, topical (for acne) & intravaginal suppositories & cream. **Used to inhibit synthesis of toxic shock syndrome toxins.**
Lincomycin (Lincocin)	**0.6 to 1 gm IV q8-12h**	Rarely used. Risk of C difficile. Requires appropriate dilution and infusion time based on dose (see Package Insert).
Erythromycin Group (Review drug interactions before use)		**Gastroparesis:** Erythro is alt drug for rx of gastroparesis. Initiates peristalsis by binding to motilin receptors & improves gastric emptying for approx 2 wks; then effect lost due to tachyphylaxis. Erythro dose: 1.5-3 mg/kg IV over 45 min q6h or 250 mg po liquid susp bid. Ref: *Gastro Clin NA 2015,44:97.* **Frequent drug-drug interactions:** Major concern is prolonged QT_c interval on EKG. **Prolonged QTc:** Erythro, clarithro & azithro all increase risk of ventricular tachycardia via increase in QTc interval. Can be congenital or acquired *(NEJM 358:169, 2008)*. Caution if positive family history of sudden cardiac death, electrolyte abnormalities or concomitant drugs that prolong QTc. **↑ risk QTc >500 msec! Risk amplified by other drugs** [macrolides, antiarrhythmics, & drug-drug interactions *(see FQs page 159 for list)*]. *www.qtdrugs.org & www.torsades.org*. Ref: *Am J Med 128:1362, 2015.* Cholestatic hepatitis in approx. 1:1000 adults (not children) given E estolate. **Drug-drug interactions of note:** Erythro or clarithro with statins: high statin levels, rhabdomyolysis *(Ann Int Med 158:869, 2013)*; concomitant clarithro & colchicine (gout) can cause fatal colchicine toxicity (pancytopenia, renal failure) *(CID 41:291, 2005)*. Concomitant clarithro & Ca++ channel blockers increase risk of hypotension, kidney injury *(JAMA 310:2544, 2013)*. Hypoglycemia with concomitant sulfonylureas *(JAMA Int Med 174:1605, 2014)*. **Transient reversible tinnitus or deafness** with ≥4 gm per day of erythro IV in pts with renal or hepatic impairment. Reversible sensorineural hearing loss with Azithro *(J Otolaryngol 36:257, 2007)*. Dosages of oral erythro preparations expressed as base equivalents. Variable amounts of erythro esters required to achieve same free erythro serum level. **Azithromycin** reported to exacerbate symptoms of myasthenia gravis. **FDA alerts**: clarithromycin use associated with increased cardio- and cerebro-vascular events; azithromycin use to prevent bronchiolitis obliterans after donor stem cell transplant associated with increased cancer relapse and death.
Azithromycin (Zithromax) **Azithromycin ER** (Zmax)	**po preps:** Tabs 250 & 600 mg. Peds suspension: 100 & 200 mg per 5 mL. Adult ER suspension: 2 gm. Dose varies with indication, *see Table 1*, Acute otitis media *(page 12)*, acute exac. chronic bronchitis *(page 42)*, Comm.-acq. pneumonia *(pages 43–44)*, & sinusitis *(page 55)*. **IV:** 0.5 gm per day.	
Erythromycin Base and esters (Erythrocin) IV name: E. lactobionate	**0.25 gm q6h–0.5 gm po/IV q6h:** **15–20 mg/kg up to 4 gm q24h. Infuse over 30+ min.**	
Clarithromycin (Biaxin) or clarithro extended release (Biaxin XL)	**0.5 gm po q12h.** **Extended release: Two 0.5 gm tabs po per day.**	
Fidaxomicin (Dificid) (200 mg tab)	**One 200 mg tab po bid x 10 days with or without food**	Approved for C. difficile toxin-mediated diarrhea, including hypervirulent NAP1/B1/027 strains. Minimal GI absorption; high fecal concentrations. Limited activity vs. normal bowel flora. In trial vs. po Vanco, lower relapse rate vs. non-NAP1 strains than Vanco *(NEJM 364:422, 2011)*. Despite absence of GI absorption, 12 pts developed allergic reactions; known macrolide allergy in 3 of 12 *(CID 58:537, 2014)*.
Ketolides: **Telithromycin** (Ketek) *(Med Lett 46:66, 2004; Drug Safety 31:561, 2008)*	**Two 400 mg tabs po q24h.** 300 mg tabs available.	Drug warnings: acute liver failure & serious liver injury post treatment. *(AnIM 144:415, 447, 2006)*. **Uncommon: blurred vision** 2° slow accommodation; may cause exacerbation of **myasthenia gravis (Black Box Warning: Contraindicated in this disorder)**. Liver, eye and myasthenia complications may be due to inhibition of nicotinic acetylcholine receptor at neuromuscular junction *(AAC 54:5399, 2010)*. Potential QT_c prolongation. Several **drug-drug interactions** *(NEJM 355:2260, 2006)*. No longer marketed in US.
Tedizolid phosphate (Sivextro) Ref: *CID 61:1315, 2015.*	**200 mg IV/po once daily. Infuse IV over 1 hr.**	**IV dose reconstituted in 250 mL of normal saline;** incompatible with lactated ringers as non-soluble in presence of divalent cations. SST clinical trial result *(JAMA 309:559 & 609, 2013)*. Excreted by liver. No adjustment for renal insufficiency. Weak inhibitor of monoamine oxidase, hence risk of serotonin syndrome, but low risk *(AAC 57:3060, 2013)*. Low risk of thrombocytopenia at therapeutic doses *(AAC 2016,71:2553)*.

(See page 2 for abbreviations)

*NOTE: all dosage recommendations are for adults (unless otherwise indicated) & assume normal renal function.

TABLE 10A (9)

CLASS, AGENT, GENERIC NAME (TRADE NAME)	USUAL ADULT DOSAGE*	ADVERSE REACTIONS, COMMENTS
CHLORAMPHENICOL, CLINDAMYCIN(S), ERYTHROMYCIN GROUP, KETOLIDES, OXAZOLIDINONES *(continued)*		
Linezolid (Zyvox) (600 mg tab) Review: *JAC 66(Suppl 4):3, 2011*	**po or IV dose: 600 mg q12h.** Available as 600 mg tabs, oral suspension (100 mg per 5 mL), & IV solution. Special populations Refs: Renal insufficiency *(J Infect Chemother 17:70, 2011; AAC 63:e00605, 2019)*; Liver transplant *(CID 42:434, 2006)*; Cystic fibrosis *(AAC 48:281, 2004)*; Burns *(J Burn Care Res 31:207, 2010)*. Obesity: clinical failure with standard dose in 265 kg patient *(Ann Pharmacother 47:e25, 2013)*.	**Reversible myelosuppression:** thrombocytopenia, anemia, & neutropenia reported. Most often after >2 wks of therapy. Increased risk on hemodialysis or peritoneal dialysis *(Int J Antimicrob Ag 36:179, 2010; JAC doi:10.1093/jac/dkv184)* **Lactic acidosis; peripheral neuropathy, optic neuropathy:** After 4 or more wks of therapy. Data consistent with time and dose-dependent inhibition of intramitochondrial protein synthesis *(Pharmacotherapy 27:771, 2007)*. Neuropathy, not reversible. Mitochondrial toxicity *(AAC 2017;61:e00542-17)*. **Inhibitor of monoamine oxidase;** risk of severe hypertension if taken with foods rich in tyramine. Avoid concomitant pseudoephedrine, phenylpropanolamine, and caution with SSRIs[1]. **Serotonin syndrome** (fever, agitation, mental status changes, tremors). Risk with concomitant SSRIs: *(CID 42:1578 and 43:180, 2006)*. Incidence low *(AAC 57:5901, 2013)*. Other: black hairy tongue, acute interstitial nephritis *(IDCP 17:61, 2009)*, teeth staining *(CID 2016,62:617)*. **Rhabdomyolysis:** case probably related to linezolid in a patient receiving linezolid as a component of multi-drug therapy for XDR tuberculosis *(CID 54:1624, 2012)*. **Resistance:** Linezolid resistant S. epidermidis and MRSA due to mutation of the 23S rRNA binding site *(JAC 68:4, 2013)*.
TETRACYCLINES		
Doxycycline (Vibramycin, Doryx, Monodox, Adoxa, Periostat) (20, 50, 75, 100 mg tab)	**Adult: 100 mg po/IV q12h; Child (regardless of age): 4.4 mg/kg/day po/IV divided bid x max of 21 days** (considered safe, *AAP Redbook 2018; J Ped 2015;166:1246)*.	Similar to other tetracyclines. ↑ nausea on empty stomach. Erosive esophagitis, esp. if taken at bedtime; **take with lots of water.** Phototoxicity & photo-onycholysis occur but less than with tetracycline. Deposition in teeth less than with tetracycline *(JAC 2017;72:2887)*. Can be used in patients with renal failure. Pseudotumor cerebri (intracranial hypertension) can occur. *Comments:* Effective in treatment and prophylaxis for malaria, leptospirosis, typhus fevers.
Eravacycline (Xerava) Activity similar to omadacycline & tigecycline, see *Table 4A*)	1 mg/kg IV infused over 60 min q12h x 4-14 days (increase to 1.5 mg/kg if co-administered with strong CYP3A4 inducer, e.g., RIF). Severe liver disease: 1 mg/kg IV q12h x 1 day, then 1 mg/kg IV q24h.	Approved for complicated intra-abdominal infections in adults. **Warnings**: life-threatening hypersensitivity reactions if known tetracycline allergy; Pregnancy (2nd/3rd trimester) risk of tooth discoloration and bone growth inhibition. **Common AEs**: infusion site reactions, nausea, vomiting.
Minocycline (Minocin, Dynacin) (50, 75, 100 mg cap; 45, 90, 135 mg ext rel tab; IV prep) Contains Mg++. Monitor serum Mg++ levels if renal impairment.	**200 mg po/IV loading dose, then 100 mg po/IV q12h** IV minocycline available.	**Vestibular symptoms** (30–90% in some groups, none in others): vertigo 33%, ataxia 43%, nausea 50%, vomiting 3%, women more frequently than men. Hypersensitivity pneumonitis, reversible, ~34 cases reported *(BMJ 310:1520, 1995)*. Can cause slate-grey **pigmentation** of the skin and other tissues with long-term use. **Intracranial hypertension** can occur. *Comments:* More effective than other tetracyclines vs staph and in prophylaxis of meningococcal disease. P. acnes: many resistant to other tetracyclines, not to mino. Induced autoimmunity reported in children treated for acne *(J Ped 153:314, 2008)*. Active vs Nocardia asteroides, Mycobacterium marinum and many acinetobacter isolates.
Omadacycline (Nuzyra) Activity similar to eravacycline & tigecycline, see *Table 4A*)	**CABP:** Loading: 200 mg IV (over 60 min) on day 1, or 100 mg IV (over 30 min) q12h x2 doses on day 1, or 300 mg po q12h x2 doses on day 1. Maintenance: 100 mg IV (over 30 min) q24h, or 300 mg po q24h. **ABSSSI:** Loading: 200 mg IV (over 60 min) on day 1, or 100 mg IV (over 30 min) q12h x2 doses on day 1, or 450 mg po q24h on days 1 and 2. Maintenance: 100 mg IV (over 30 min) q24h, or 300 mg po q24h.	Duration: 7-14 days. Breastfeeding not recommended during treatment and for 4 days after last dose. Fast for 4 hrs before dosing. No food for 2 hrs after dosing; no dairy products, antacids, multivitamins for 4 hrs after dosing. **Contraindication:** known tetracycline hypersensitivity. **Warnings:** Higher mortality risk in CAP vs. Moxi. Tooth discoloration/enamel dysplasia in 2nd half of pregnancy. Inhibition of bone growth in 2nd/3rd trimesters. AEs: diarrhea, nausea, vomiting, constipation; infusion site reactions; increased AST, ALT, GGT; hypertension; headache; insomnia. Ref: *CID 69:180, 2019*.

[1] **SSRI** = selective serotonin reuptake inhibitors, e.g., fluoxetine (Prozac).

*NOTE: all dosage recommendations are for adults (unless otherwise indicated) & assume normal renal function.

TABLE 10A (10)

CLASS, AGENT, GENERIC NAME (TRADE NAME)	USUAL ADULT DOSAGE*	ADVERSE REACTIONS, COMMENTS
TETRACYCLINES *(continued)*		
Tetracycline, Oxytetracycline (Sumycin) (250, 500 mg cap) *(CID 36:462, 2003)*	**0.25–0.5 gm po q6h, 0.5–1 gm IV q12h**	GI (oxy 19%, tetra 4), anaphylactoid reaction (rare), deposition in teeth, negative N balance, hepatotoxicity, enamel agenesis, pseudotumor cerebri/encephalopathy. Outdated drug: Fanconi syndrome. **Contraindicated in pregnancy, hepatotoxicity in mother, transplacental to fetus.** *Comments:* **Pregnancy:** IV dosage over 2 gm per day may be associated with fatal hepatotoxicity. (Ref: *JAC 66:1431, 2011*).
Tigecycline (Tygacil) Meta-analysis & editorial: *Ln ID 11:804 & 834, 2011.* Also *CID 54:1699 & 1710, 2012.*	**100 mg IV initially, then 50 mg IV q12h with po food, if possible to decrease risk of nausea.** **If severe liver dis. (Child Pugh C):** 100 mg IV initially, then 25 mg IV q12h	Derivative of tetracycline. High incidence of nausea (25%) & vomiting (20%) but only 1% of pts discontinued therapy. Pregnancy Category D. Do not use in children under age 18. Like other tetracyclines, may cause photosensitivity, pseudotumor cerebri, pancreatitis, a catabolic state (elevated BUN) and maybe hyperpigmentation *(CID 45:136, 2007)*. Decreases serum fibrinogen *(AAC 59:1650, 2015)*. **Tetracycline, minocycline & tigecycline** associated with acute pancreatitis *(Int J Antimicrob Agents, 34:486, 2009)*. **Black Box Warning:** In meta-analysis of clinical trials, all cause mortality higher in pts treated with tigecycline (2.5%) vs. 1.8% in comparators. Cause of mortality risk difference of 0.6% (95% CI 0.1, 1.2) not established. Tigecycline should be reserved for use in situations when alternative treatments are not suitable *(FDA MedWatch Sep 27, 2013)*. Poor result due to low serum levels *(AAC 56:1065 & 1466, 2012)*; high doses superior to low doses for *HAP (AAC 57:1756, 2013)*.
FLUOROQUINOLONES (FQs): All can cause false-positive urine drug screen for opiates *(Pharmacother 26:435, 2006)*. Toxicity review: *Drugs Aging 27:193, 2010.*		
Ciprofloxacin (Cipro) and **Ciprofloxacin-extended release** (Cipro XR, Proquin XR) (100, 250, 500, 750 mg tab; 500 mg ext rel tab)	Usual Parenteral Dose: **400 mg IV q12h** For P. aeruginosa: **400-600 mg IV q8h** *(JAC 74:1662, 2019)* Uncomplicated Urethritis/cystitis (Oral) Dose: **250 mg po bid or CIP XR 500 mg po once daily** Other Indications (Oral): **500-750 mg po bid**	FQs are a common precipitant of **C. difficile toxin-mediated diarrhea.** **Children:** No FQ approved for use under age 16 based on joint cartilage injury in immature animals. Articular SEs in children est. at 2–3% *(LnID 3:537, 2003)*. The exception is anthrax. Pathogenesis believed to involve FQ chelation of Mg++ and damaging chondrites *(AAC 51:1022, 2007; Int J Antimicrob Agents 33:194, 2009)*. No evidence of cartilage damage with Levo in children *(Pediatrics 134:e146, 2014)*. **CNS toxicity:** Poorly understood. Varies: lightheadedness, confusion, seizures. Trouble with attention/memory. Peripheral neuropathy occurs: rapid onset, potentially permanent injury. **Gemi skin rash:** Macular rash after 8–10 days of rx. Incidence of rash with ≤5 days of therapy only 1.5%. Frequency highest females, < age 40, treated 14 days (22.6%). In men, < age 40, treated 14 days, frequency 7.7%. Mechanism unclear. Indication to DC therapy. Ref: *Diag Micro Infect Dis 68:140, 2010.* **Hypoglycemia/hyperglycemia (Dysglycemia):** Increased risk, esp. of hypoglycemia in diabetic pts from any of the marketed FQs *(CID 57:971, 2013)*. **Thrombocytopenia** in critically ill *(J Thrombo Haemostasis 11:169, 2012)*. **Opiate screen false-positives:** FQs can cause false-positive urine assay for opiates *(Ann Pharmacotherapy 38:1525, 2004)*. **Photosensitivity:** *See Table 10B, page 165.* **QT_c (corrected QT) interval prolongation:** ↑ QT_c (>500 msec or >60 msec from baseline) is considered possible with any FQ (except Delaflox). ↑ QT_c can lead to torsades de pointes and ventricular fibrillation. Overall risk is 4.7/10,000 person yrs *(CID 55:1457, 2012)*. Risk low with current marketed drugs. Risk ↑ in women, ↓ K^+, ↓ mg^{++}, bradycardia. (Refs.: *CID 43:1603, 2006*). Major problem is ↑ risk with concomitant drugs.
Delafloxacin (Baxdela) 450 mg tablets IV for injection *(CID 2019;68:1058)*	**300 mg IV q12h infused over 1 hr** **450 mg po q12h** Treat 5-14 days (skin, skin structure), 5-10 days (CAP) Can switch from IV to po during course of rx	
Gatifloxacin (Tequin) (where available) *See comments*	**200–400 mg IV/po q24h**. *(See comment)* Ophthalmic solution (Zymar)	
Gemifloxacin (Factive) (320 mg tab)	**320 mg po q24h**.	
Levofloxacin (Levaquin) (250, 500, 750 mg tab)	**250–750 mg po/IV q24h.** For most indications, 750 mg is preferred dose. po therapy: avoid concomitant dairy products, multivitamins, iron, antacids due to chelation by multivalent cations & interference with absorption. No dose adjustment for morbid obesity.	**Avoid concomitant drugs with potential to prolong QTc** *(See Table 10G)*.

(See page 2 for abbreviations)

*NOTE: all dosage recommendations are for adults (unless otherwise indicated) & assume normal renal function.

TABLE 10A (11)

CLASS, AGENT, GENERIC NAME (TRADE NAME)	USUAL ADULT DOSAGE*	ADVERSE REACTIONS, COMMENTS
FLUOROQUINOLONES (FQs) *(continued)*		
Moxifloxacin (Avelox)	**400 mg po/IV q24h.** Note: no need to increase dose for morbid obesity *(JAC 66:2330, 2011)*. Ophthalmic solution (Vigamox)	**Tendinopathy:** Over age 60, approx. 2–6% of all Achilles tendon ruptures attributable to use of FQ *(ArIM 163:1801, 2003)*. ↑ risk with concomitant steroid, renal disease or post-transplant (heart, lung, kidney) *(CID 36:1404, 2003)*. **Chelation:** Risk of chelation of oral FQs by multivalent cations **(Ca++, Mg++, Fe++, Zn++)**. Avoid dairy products, multivitamins *Clin Pharmacokinet 40 (Suppl 1) 33:2001)*. **Allergic Reactions:** Rare (1:50,000). IgE-mediated: urticaria, anaphylaxis. 3 pts with Moxi had immediate reactions but tolerated CIP *(Ann Pharmacother 44:740, 2010)*. **Myasthenia gravis:** Any of the FQs may exacerbate muscle weakness in pts. with myasthenia gravis. **Retinal detachment:** Inconsistent data. **Carpal tunnel syndrome:** Pharmacoepidemiological study found increased risk of CTS with FQ use *(CID 65: 684, 2017)*. **Pseudotumor cerebri:** Significant risk ratio (4-6) reported *(Neurology 2017;89:892)*. **Aortic aneurysm tear:** Hazard ratio 1.2-2.9 *(BMJ 360:K678, 2018)*.
Ofloxacin (Floxin)	**200–400 mg po bid.** Ophthalmic solution (Ocuflox)	
Prulifloxacin (where available) Ref: *Drugs 64:2221, 2004.*	Tablets: 250 and 600 mg. Usual dose: **600 mg po once daily**	**Contraindications:** persons with celiac disease, pregnancy, nursing mothers, persons with seizure disorder **AEs:** similar to other FQs
PLEUROMUTILINS		
Lefamulin (Xenleta)	Adult: **600 mg po q8h or 150 mg IV q12h** Extend dosing interval if severe hepatic impairment	**AEs:** nausea, vomiting, diarrhea (including C. diff toxin colitis); more frequent with oral dosing. **Pregnancy:** may cause fetal harm; check for pregnancy before use. Breastfeeding safety unknown. **DDI:** Many due to CYP450 transporter interactions. Can increase QTc esp if interaction increases Lefamulin or other drug serum levels.
Retapamulin	Topical agent, *see page 164*	
POLYMYXINS (POLYPEPTIDES) Note: Proteus sp., Providencia sp, Serratia sp., B. cepacia are intrinsically resistant to polymyxins. Guideline: *Pharmacotherapy 39:10, 2019*		
Polymyxin B (Poly-Rx) 1 mg = 10,000 international units **Where available, Polymyxin B preferred over Colistin.**	Doses based on actual body weight. ***LOADING DOSE:*** 2.5 mg/kg IV over 2 hrs. ***MAINTENANCE DOSE:*** 12 hrs later 1.5 mg/kg over 1 hr, then repeat q12h. No dose reduction for renal insufficiency. **Intrathecal therapy for meningitis:** 5 mg/day into CSF x 3-4 days, then 5 mg every other day x 2 or more weeks.	**Adverse effects: Neurologic:** rare, but serious, is neuromuscular blockade; other, circumoral paresthesias, extremity numbness, blurred vision, drowsy, irritable, ataxia; can manifest as respiratory arrest *(Chest 141:515, 2012)*. **Renal:** reversible acute tubular necrosis. Renal injury in 42% (Polymyxin B) vs. 60% (Colistin) *(CID 57:1300, 2013)*. **Skin:** Hyperpigmentation in 8% of 249 pts *(J Clin Pharm Ther 2017;42:573)*. PK study showed no need to reduce dose for renal insufficiency *(CID 57:524, 2013)*. **Polymyxin B preferred over Colistin (except for UTI)** *(see Comment under Colistin for discussion)*. Combination therapy (polymyxin + carbapenem) failed in controlled clinical trial *(LnID 2018,18:391)*.

*NOTE: all dosage recommendations are for adults (unless otherwise indicated) & assume normal renal function.

TABLE 10A (12)

CLASS, AGENT, GENERIC NAME (TRADE NAME)	USUAL ADULT DOSAGE*	ADVERSE REACTIONS, COMMENTS

POLYMYXINS (POLYPEPTIDES) *(continued)*

Colistin, Polymyxin E
(Colymycin)

Polymyxin E (Colistin) and Polymyxin B are polymyxin class parenteral antibiotics active against multi-drug resistant (MDR) gram negative bacilli, e.g., *A. baumannii*, *P. aeruginosa*, *E. coli*, *K. pneumoniae*.

Resistance issues:
Serratia sp, Proteus sp., Providencia sp., Morganella sp., and B. cepacia are intrinsically resistant to polymyxins. Pan-resistant strains of Enterobacterales, including resistance to colistin mediated by plasmid-encoded gene mcr-1 *(AAC 60: 2443, 2016)* have been identified worldwide.

Colistin is the preferred polymyxin for:
Urinary tract infections (UTIs) & Adjunctive inhalation therapy for pneumonia caused by MDR gram-negative bacilli.

For all other indications, Polymyxin B: equivalent efficacy, faster attainment of target serum conc, less inter-patient variability in PK, no dose adjustment for renal impairment and lower risk of renal toxicity *(AAC 60: 2443, 2016; and AAC 2017:61: e02319-16)*)

Formulation and conversion: Colistin is formulated as a prodrug, colistimethate (CMS). Product vials may be labeled as international units (IU) or mg of prodrug or mg of **colistin base activity (CBA)** of active drug. **Always dose based on the CBA**. *To avoid dosing errors read product labels carefully!* **Conversions** *(CID 2014, 58:139)*: 1 mg CBA = 30,000 IU CMS; 33 mg CBA = 1,000,000 IU CMS; 1 mg CBA = 2.4 mg CMS.

Dosing recommendations continue to evolve. At present, there are 3 sets of dosing guidance: **PK Study Group:** creatinine clearance (CrCl)-based dosing *(CID 2017;64:565)*; **European Medicines Agency (EMA):** CrCl-based dosing *(CID 2016, 62:552)*; **U.S. FDA:** weight- and CrCl-based dosing, as found in the package insert (June 2016). Complicated calculation-based dosing has been replaced by simpler PK-based dosing using CrCl levels as benchmarks. The PK Study Group recommendations use finer divisions between CrCl levels; the EMA recommendations use broader divisions. *See Comments.*

For **severe systemic infection** and patients not on dialysis of any kind (Note: for dosing in patients on intermittent hemodialysis or CRRT, see Table 17A):

1. **Loading Dose:** Administer a Colistin loading dose IV, then begin daily maintenance dosing 12 hours later. Loading dose formula: 4 x body weight in kg. Use lower of ideal or actual weight. May result in loading dose > 300 mg CBA. Start daily maintenance dose 12 hrs. later.
2. **Maintenance Dose: Then, Total Daily maintenance dose: Divide daily dose to bid or tid** (from Total Daily maintenance dose table (Comments): Editors prefer PK Study Group). Once daily dosing not recommended due to potential for toxicity and lack of efficacy data.

Other adult dosing:
Inhaled therapy: 50-75 mg CBA in 3-4 mL saline via vibrating mesh nebulizer 2-3 times/day: concentration in lung epithelial lining is 100-1000x greater with inhaled dosing vs. IV dosing alone

Meningitis (intraventricular or intrathecal dose): 10 mg/day x several weeks; intrathecal dose often combined with IV dosing

Pediatric dosing:
Systemic Infection: 2.5-5 mg/kg/day in 2-4 divided doses (based on ideal body weight).
Cystic Fibrosis: 3-8 mg/kg/day in 3 divided doses (based on ideal body weight).

Note: Resistance and allergy issues. The plasmid-encoded colistin resistance gene, mcr-1, has been found in E. coli and Klebsiella sp. Resistance is due to modification of the lipid A target of the polymyxins. Strains may also produce metallo-carbapenemases, resulting in pan-resistance *(Infect Dis Clin NA 2020.doi.org/10.1016/jidc.2020.08.003)*. For carbapenem-allergic patients, no clear alternatives for a companion drug with colistin. Combination therapy with Rifampin did not improve clinical response or 30-day mortality in patients with Acinetobacter infections *(CID 2013, 57:349; Epidemiol Infect 2013, 141:1214)*. In vitro and in vivo exposure to polymyxins results in rapid selection of resistant sub-populations. In vitro, minocycline prevented emergence of resistance and augmented Colistin activity but no clinical trial data. Tigecycline may function similarly, but no data.

Nephrotoxicity *(Pharmacotherapy 35:28, 2015)*: Reversible acute tubular necrosis due to localization of drug in proximal tubular cells: *AAC 2017; 61:e02319-16*. Depending on criteria, incidence of toxicity varies, average around 25%. Risk factors: length of therapy, daily dose, and cumulative dose; exposure to concomitant nephrotoxins; obesity, diabetes mellitus, age and hypertension. In animal models, high dose ascorbic acid and melatonin prevented toxicity. In critically ill, the benefit of patient salvage may exceed the risk of nephrotoxicity.
Neurotoxicity: Frequent vertigo, facial paresthesias, abnormal vision, confusion, ataxia. Rarely, neuromuscular blockade results in respiratory failure; may unmask or exacerbate myasthenia gravis. In cystic fibrosis patients, 29% experienced paresthesias, ataxia or both.
Other: Maybe hyper-pigmentation *(CID 45:136, 2007)*.
Discussion and critiques of current dosing recommendations. The PK Study Group favors the EMA recommendations over the current (June 2016) U.S. FDA approved dosing *(CID 2016, 62:552)*. The weight- and CrCl-based approach in the FDA approved dosing is more complicated than either the PK Study Group or EMA recommendations. The PK Study Group recommendations are based on PK study of 214 critically ill patients *(CID 2017; 64:565)*. In patients with CrCl >80 mL/min, EMA recommended doses failed to achieve target serum concentration in 66% of patients versus less than 10% in patients with CrCl < 80 mL/min *(CID 2016, 62:552)* due to rapid renal clearance of colistimethate prodrug with less time for conversion of prodrug to active colistin.

Total Daily maintenance dose:

CrCl (mL/min)	PK Study Group (doses div bid or tid)*	EMA (doses div bid or tid)*	U.S. FDA (Wt - IBW)*
≥90	360 mg/day	300 mg/day	2.5-5 mg/kg/day div 2-4 doses
80 to <90	340 mg/day		
70 to <80	300 mg/day		2.5-3.8 mg/kg/day div 2 doses
60 to <70	275 mg/day		
50 to <60	245 mg/day		
40 to <50	220 mg/day	183-250 mg/day	2.5 mg/kg once daily or div bid
30 to <40	195 mg/day		
20 to <30	175 mg/day	150-183 mg/day	1.5 mg/kg q36h
10 to <20	160 mg/day		
5 to <10	145 mg/day	117 mg/day	N/R
<5	130 mg/day		

* All doses are stated as colistin base activity (CBA) in mg.
IBW = ideal body weight

(See page 2 for abbreviations)

*NOTE: all dosage recommendations are for adults (unless otherwise indicated) & assume normal renal function.

TABLE 10A (13)

CLASS, AGENT, GENERIC NAME (TRADE NAME)	USUAL ADULT DOSAGE*	ADVERSE REACTIONS, COMMENTS
MISCELLANEOUS AGENTS		
Fosfomycin po (Monurol) Fosfomycin tromethamine	Adult: **3 gm po x 1** (uncomplicated UTI) **or 3 gm po q3d x 3** (complicated UTI) **or x 7 days** (prostatitis). Child: **2 gm po x 1** (UTI)	**AEs:** diarrhea (more common than with TMP-SMX or nitrofurantoin), headache. Large sodium load. Active vs. susceptible gram-negative bacilli.
Fosfomycin IV (Ivozfo) Fosfomycin disodium (Available in Canada, Europe, Australia) US: emergency single patient IND from FDA (1-888-300-4374)	Adult: **12-24 gm IV daily div q8-12h** (osteo, complicated UTI, nosocomial pneumonia); **16-24 gm IV daily div q6-8h** (meningitis). Child: *see Table 16*	
Fusidic acid (Fucidin, Taksta) (where available)	**500 mg po/IV tid (Denmark & Canada)** **US: loading dose of 1500 mg po bid x 1 day, then 600 mg po bid**	Activity vs. MRSA of importance. Approved outside the U.S.; currently in U.S. clinical trials. Ref for proposed US regimen: *CID 52 (Suppl 7):S520, 2011.*
Methenamine hippurate (Hiprex, Urex)	**1 gm po bid**	Nausea and vomiting, skin rash or dysuria. Overall ~3%. Methenamine requires (pH ≤ 5.5) urine to liberate formaldehyde. Useful in suppressive therapy after infecting organisms cleared; do not use for pyelonephritis. *Comment:* Do not force fluids; may dilute formaldehyde. Of no value in pts with chronic Foley. If urine pH >5.5, co-administer ascorbic acid (1–2 gm q4h) to acidify the urine; cranberry juice (1200–4000 mL per day) has been used, results ±. Do not use concomitantly with sulfonamides (precipitate), or in presence of renal or severe hepatic dysfunction.
Methenamine mandelate (Mandelamine)	**1 gm po qid**	
Metronidazole (Flagyl) (250, 375, 500 mg tab/cap) Prevotella sp: some resistance *(JAC 2018,73:265).*	Anaerobic infections: **usually IV, 7.5 mg per kg (~500 mg) q6h (not to exceed 4 gm q24h).** With long T½, **can use IV at 15 mg per kg q12h.** If life-threatening, use loading dose of **IV 15 mg per kg. Oral dose: 500 mg qid; extended release tabs** available 750 mg Giardia, amebiasis: *See Table 13*	**Common AEs:** nausea (12%), metallic taste, "furry" tongue. **Avoid alcohol during 48 hrs after last dose to avoid disulfiram reaction (N/V, flushing, tachycardia, dyspnea).** Neurologic AEs with high dose/long Rx: peripheral, autonomic and optic neuropathy. **Aseptic meningitis, encephalopathy, seizures & reversible cerebellar lesion** reported *(NEJM 374:1465, 2016); CID 2017,64:525.* Possible association of po metronidazole with acute pancreatitis *(Clin Epidemiol 10:1573, 2018).* Risk of hypoglycemia with concomitant sulfonylureas. Can use IV sol'n as enema for *C. diff colitis.* **Resistant anaerobic organisms:** Actinomycetes, Peptostreptococci. **Once-daily IV dosing** of 1,500 mg: based on long serum T1/2; standard in Europe *(JAC 19:410, 2007).* **Safe to use in pregnancy** *(Curr Drug Safety 2015,10:170).*
Nitazoxanide	*See Table 13B, page 218*	
Nitrofurantoin Systematic rev: *JAC 70:2456, 2015*	Active UTI: **Furadantin/Macrodantin 50-100 mg po qid x 5-7 days OR Macrobid 100 mg po bid x 5-7 days** Dose for long-term UTI suppression: **50–100 mg at bedtime**	Absorption ↑ with meals. Increased activity in acid urine, much reduced at pH 8 or over. Nausea and vomiting, **peripheral neuropathy,** pancreatitis. **Pulmonary reactions** (with chronic rx): acute ARDS type, **chronic desquamative interstitial pneumonia with fibrosis**. Intrahepatic cholestasis & **hepatitis** similar to chronic active hepatitis. Hemolytic anemia in G6PD deficiency. Drug rash, eosinophilia, systemic symptoms (DRESS) hypersensitivity syndrome reported *(Neth J Med 67:147, 2009).* Should not be used in infants <1 month of age. Birth defects: increased risk reported *(Arch Ped Adolesc Med 163:978, 2009).*
Rifampin (Rimactane, Rifadin) (150, 300 mg cap) **Use in combination only**	**300 mg po/IV bid or 600 mg po/IV qd.** Rapid selection of resistant bacteria if used as monotherapy	Causes orange-brown discoloration of sweat, urine, tears, contact lens. **Many important drug-drug interactions**. Immune complex flu-like syndrome: fever, headache, myalgias, arthralgia--especially with intermittent rx. Drug induced immune thrombocytopenia *(J Thrombosis & Haemostasis 2012,11:169).* Can cause interstitial nephritis. Risk-benefit of adding RIF to standard therapies for S. aureus endocarditis *(AAC 52:2463, 2008).* *See also, Antimycobacterial Agents, Table 12B, page 198.*
Rifamycin (Aemcolo)	Tablets: 194 mg. Adult: **2 tabs bid x 3 days**	Approved for *E. coli* induced traveler's diarrhea; do not use if fever and/or bloody stools.
Rifaximin (Xifaxan) (200, 550 mg tab)	Traveler's diarrhea: **200 mg tab po tid** times 3 days. Hepatic encephalopathy: **550 mg tab po bid.** C. diff diarrhea as "chaser": **400 mg po tid**	For traveler's diarrhea and hepatic encephalopathy *(AAC 54:3618, 2010; NEJM 362:1071, 2010).* In general, adverse events equal to or less than placebo. Monitor INR in those taking warfarin. Systemic exposure may increase with severe hepatic disease or P-glycoprotein inhibitors.

(See page 2 for abbreviations)

*NOTE: all dosage recommendations are for adults (unless otherwise indicated) & assume normal renal function.

TABLE 10A (14)

CLASS, AGENT, GENERIC NAME (TRADE NAME)	USUAL ADULT DOSAGE*	ADVERSE REACTIONS, COMMENTS
MISCELLANEOUS AGENTS *(continued)*		
Secnidazole (Solosec)	2 gm packet (granules): sprinkle on applesauce, yogurt or pudding and consume mixture within 30 min without chewing granules. Follow with glass of water to aid swallowing	Nitroimidazole for treatment of bacterial vaginosis in adults. Vulvo-vaginal candidiasis may develop requiring antifungal therapy. Potential carcinogenicity seen in rodent studies. Avoid chronic use. **AEs:** Vulvo-vaginal candidiasis (≥2%), headache, nausea, dysgeusia, vomiting, diarrhea, abdominal pain, vulvo-vaginal pruritus.
Sulfonamides [e.g., sulfisoxazole (Gantrisin), sulfamethoxazole (Gantanol), (Truxazole), sulfadiazine]	Dose varies with indications. *See Nocardia & Toxoplasmosis*	**CNS:** fever, headache, dizziness; **Derm:** mild rash to life threatening Stevens-Johnson syndrome, toxic epidermal necrolysis *(Brit J Derm 2016,174:1194)*, photosensitivity; **Hem:** agranulocytosis, aplastic anemia; **Cross-allergenicity:** other sulfa drugs, sulfonylureas, diuretics, crystalluria (esp. sulfadiazine-need ≥1500 mL po fluid/day); **Other:** serum sickness, hemolysis if G6PD def, polyarteritis, SLE reported.
Tinidazole (Tindamax)	**Tabs 250, 500 mg. 2 gm po once or once daily depending on indication** (amebiasis, giardiasis, trichomoniasis, bacterial vaginosis)	**Adverse reactions:** metallic taste 3.7%, nausea 3.2%, anorexia/vomiting 1.5%. All higher with multi-day dosing. Avoid alcohol during & for 3 days after last dose; cause disulfiram reaction, flushing, N/V, tachycardia.
Trimethoprim (Trimpex, Proloprim, and others) (100, 200 mg tab)	**100 mg po q12h or 200 mg po q24h.**	**CNS:** drug fever, aseptic meningitis; **Derm:** rash (3-7% at 200 mg/day), phototoxicity, Stevens-Johnson syndrome (rare), toxic epidermal necrolysis (rare); **Renal:** ↑ K+, ↓ Na+, ↑ Cr; Hem: neutropenia, thrombocytopenia, methemoglobinemia. ACE inhibitors & aldactone increase serum K+. Higher incidence & severity when combined. Increased risk of death. *BMJ 2014, 349:g6196*. Mechanism: *JAMA 2015,314:2406*.
Trimethoprim (TMP)-Sulfamethoxazole (SMX) (Bactrim, Septra, Sulfatrim, Cotrimoxazole) Single-strength (SS) is 80 TMP/400 SMX, double-strength (DS) 160 TMP/800 SMX	**Standard po rx: 1 DS tab bid.** **P. jirovecii: IV rx (base on TMP component): standard 8–10 mg per kg IV per day divided q6h, q8h, or q12h.**	Adverse reactions in 10%: GI: nausea, vomiting, anorexia. Skin: Rash, urticaria, photosensitivity. More serious (1–10%): TMP, ACE inhibitors & aldactone increase serum K+. Higher incidence of severity when combined. Increased risk of death *(BMJ 349:g6196, 2014)*. **Stevens-Johnson syndrome & toxic epidermal necrolysis.** Skin reactions may represent toxic metabolites of SMX rather than allergy *(Ann Pharmacotherapy 32:381, 1998)*. Daily ascorbic acid 0.5–1.0 gm may promote detoxification *(JAIDS 36:1041, 2004)*. Risk of **hypoglycemia** with concomitant sulfonylureas. **Sweet's Syndrome** can occur. Hyperkalemia: Both TMP & ACE inhibitors can block renal tubular secretions of K+ & lead to dangerous hyperkalemia *(BMJ 349:g6196, 2014)*. TMP one etiology of **aseptic meningitis.** Report of psychosis during treatment of PCP *(JAC 66:1117, 2011)*. TMP-SMX contains sulfites and may trigger asthma in sulfite-sensitive pts. Frequent drug cause of thrombocytopenia. No cross allergenicity with other sulfonamide non-antibiotic drugs *(NEJM 349:1628, 2003)*. **For TMP-SMX desensitization,** *see Table 7, page 89.*
Topical Antimicrobial Agents Active vs. S. aureus & Strep. pyogenes *(CID 49:1541, 2009)*. **Review of topical antiseptics, antibiotics** *(CID 49:1541, 2009)*.		
Bacitracin (Baciguent)	20% bacitracin zinc ointment, apply 1-5 x/day.	Active vs. staph, strep & clostridium. Contact dermatitis occurs. Available without prescription.
Fusidic acid ointment	**2% ointment, apply tid**	Available in Canada and Europe *(Leo Laboratories)*. Active vs. S. aureus & S. pyogenes.
Mupirocin (Bactroban)	**Skin cream or ointment 2%: Apply tid times 10 days. Nasal ointment 2%: apply bid times 5 days.**	Skin cream: itch, burning, stinging 1–1.5%; Nasal: headache 9%, rhinitis 6%, respiratory congestion 5%. Not active vs. enterococci or gm-neg bacteria. Summary of resistance: *JAC 70:2681, 2015.* If large amounts used in azotemic pts, can accumulate polyethylene glycol *(CID 49:1541, 2009)*.
Polymyxin B—Bacitracin (Polysporin)	5000 units/gm; 400 units/gm. Apply 1-4x/day	Polymyxin active vs. some gm-neg bacteria but not Proteus sp., Serratia sp. or gm-pos bacteria. *See Bacitracin comment above.* Available without prescription.
Polymyxin B—Bacitracin—Neomycin (Neosporin, triple antibiotic ointment (TAO))	5000 units/gm; 400 units/gm; 3.5 mg/gm. Apply 1-3x/day.	*See Bacitracin and polymyxin B comments above.* Neomycin active vs. gm-neg bacteria and staphylococci; not active vs. streptococci. Contact dermatitis incidence 1%; risk of nephro- & oto-toxicity if absorbed. TAO spectrum broader than mupirocin and active mupirocin-resistant strains *(DMID 54:63, 2006)*. Available without prescription.

*NOTE: all dosage recommendations are for adults (unless otherwise indicated) & assume normal renal function.

TABLE 10A (15)

CLASS, AGENT, GENERIC NAME (TRADE NAME)	USUAL ADULT DOSAGE*	ADVERSE REACTIONS, COMMENTS
MISCELLANEOUS AGENTS/Topical Antimicrobial Agents Active vs. S. aureus & Strep. pyogenes *(continued)*		
Retapamulin (Altabax)	1% ointment; apply bid. 5, 10 & 15 gm tubes.	Microbiologic success in 90% S. aureus infections and 97% of S. pyogenes infections *(J Am Acd Derm 55:1003, 2006)*. Package insert says **for MSSA only** (not enough MRSA pts in clinical trials). Active vs. some mupirocin-resistant S. aureus strains. Resistance can occur *(see Clin Microbiol Rev 30: 827, 2017)*.
Silver sulfadiazine	1% cream, apply once or twice daily.	A sulfonamide but the active ingredient is released silver ions. Activity vs. gram-pos & gram-neg bacteria (including P. aeruginosa). Often used to prevent infection in pts with 2nd/3rd degree burns. Rarely, may stain into the skin.

*NOTE: all dosage recommendations are for adults (unless otherwise indicated) & assume normal renal function.

TABLE 10B – ANTIMICROBIAL AGENTS ASSOCIATED WITH PHOTOSENSITIVITY

Photosensitivity is classified as either photoallergic (type IV hypersensitivity) or phototoxic (direct tissue injury). Phototoxic reactions are much more common than photoallergic reactions.
UVA radiation is most commonly implicated.
The following drugs (listed alphabetically) are known to cause photosensitivity in some individuals. Note that photosensitivity lasts for several days after the last dose of the drug, at least for tetracyclines.
There is no intent to indicate relative frequency or severity of reactions. *Drug Saf 2019, 42:827.*

DRUG OR CLASS	COMMENT
Antiparasitic drugs	Pyrimethamine (one report), Quinine (may cross-react with quinidine). Rare reports with Chloroquine. Recent report of phototoxicity with Atovaquone-Proguanil, confirmed by photopatch testing.
Azole antifungals	Voriconazole, Itraconazole, Ketoconazole, (but not Fluconazole). One report of solar urticaria in a patient receiving Terbinafine.
Cefotaxime	Manifested as photodistributed telangiectasia *(Br J Dermatol 2000;143:674).*
Ceftazidime	Increased susceptibility to sunburn observed *(Lancet 1993;341(8854):1221).*
Dapsone	Rare, onset slow (weeks to months). Case report and literature review: *Photodermatol Photoimmunol Photomed 2023;39:407.*
Efavirenz	Three reports.
Flucytosine	Two reports.
Fluoroquinolones	The worst offenders have a halogen atom at C-8 of the quinolone nucleus (Lomefloxacin, Sparfloxacin). Recent data suggest that certain other molecular features, such as a large polar group at N-1, can mitigate the effect of the C-8 halogen; thus Delafloxacin seems to be relatively non-phototoxic despite having a chlorine at C-8. After Sparfloxacin, the rank of phototoxic potential among other FQs is Ciprofloxacin>Gemifloxacin>Levofloxacin>Norfloxacin>Ofloxacin. Gatifloxacin and Moxifloxacin have not been linked to phototoxic events to date *(Photochem Photobiol Sci 2018;17:773).*
Griseofulvin	Not thought to be a potent photosensitizer, although a few old reports exist.
Isoniazid	Confirmed both by rechallenge and photopatch testing.
Pyrazinamide	Confirmed by rechallenge.
Rezafungin	Listed in manufacturer's prescribing information.
Saquinavir	One report.
Tenofovir disoproxil fumarate	One report, confirmed by histopathology and photopatch testing.
Tetracyclines	Reported with Tetracycline and Doxycycline. Uncommon with Minocycline. Photosensitivity possibly more likely with Sarecycline than with other tetracyclines *(J Am Acad Dermatol 2022;87:1150).*
Tigecycline	No reports.
Trimethoprim	Alone and in combination with Sulfamethoxazole.

TABLE 10C – AMINOGLYCOSIDE ONCE DAILY AND MULTIPLE DAILY DOSING REGIMENS

(If estimated CrCl <90 mL/min or if on dialysis, *see Table 17A, page 288*)

- General Note: dosages are given as **once daily dose (OD)** and **multiple daily doses (MDD).**
- For **calculation of dosing weight in non-obese patients** use **Ideal Body Weight (IBW):**

  Female: 45.5 kg + 2.3 kg per inch over 60 inch height = dosing weight in kg;

  Male: 50 kg + 2.3 kg per inch over 60 inch height = dosing weight in kg.

- **Adjustment for calculation of dosing weight in obese patients** (actual body weight (ABW) is ≥ 30% above IBW): IBW + 0.4 (ABW minus IBW) = adjusted weight *(Pharmacotherapy 27:1081, 2007; CID 25:112, 1997).*
- **If estimated CrCl >90 mL/min, use doses in this table. If CrCl <90 mL/min or if on dialysis, use doses in *Table 17A, page 288.***

DRUG	MDD AND OD IV REGIMENS/ TARGETED PEAK (P) AND TROUGH (T) SERUM LEVELS	COMMENTS For more data on once-daily dosing, *see AAC 55:2528, 2011 and Table 17A, page 288*
Gentamicin (Garamycin), **Tobramycin** (Nebcin)	MDD: 2 mg per kg load, then 1.7 mg per kg q8h P 4–10 mcg/mL, T 1–2 mcg per mL	**All aminoglycosides have potential to cause tubular necrosis and renal failure, deafness due to cochlear toxicity, vertigo due to damage to vestibular organs, and rarely neuromuscular blockade.** Risk minimal with oral or topical application due to small % absorption unless tissues altered by disease.
	OD: 5.1 (7 if critically ill) mg per kg q24h P 16–24 mcg per mL, T <1 mcg per mL	
Kanamycin (Kantrex), **Amikacin** (Amikin), **Streptomycin**	MDD: 7.5 mg per kg q12h P 15–30 mcg per mL, T 5–10 mcg per mL	Risk of nephrotoxicity ↑ with concomitant administration of cyclosporine, vancomycin, ampho B, radiocontrast.
	OD: 15 mg per kg q24h P 56–64 mcg per mL, T <1 mcg per mL	Risk of nephrotoxicity ↓ by once-daily dosing method (especially if baseline renal function normal).
Netilmicin*	MDD: 2 mg per kg q8h P 4–10 mcg per mL, T 1–2 mcg per mL	In general, same factors influence risk of ototoxicity.
	OD: 6.5 mg per kg q24h P 22–30 mcg per mL, T <1 mcg per mL	**NOTE: There is no known method to eliminate risk of aminoglycoside nephro/ototoxicity. Proper rx attempts to ↓ the % risk.**
Plazomicin (Zemdri)	OD: 15 mg per kg q24h P: 74 mcg per mL, T: <1 mcg per mL	The clinical trial data of OD aminoglycosides have been reviewed extensively by meta-analysis *(CID 24:816, 1997).*
Isepamicin*	Only OD: Severe infections 15 mg per kg q24h, less severe 8 mg per kg q24h	**Serum levels:** Collect peak serum level (PSL) exactly 1 hr after the start of the infusion of the 3rd dose. In critically ill pts, PSL after the 1st dose as volume of distribution and renal function may change rapidly.
Spectinomycin (Trobicin)*	2 gm IM times 1–gonococcal infections	
Neomycin–oral	Prophylaxis GI surgery: 1 gm po times 3 with erythro, *see Table 15B, page 262* For hepatic coma: 4–12 gm per day po	One in 500 patients (Europe) have mitochondrial mutation that predicts cochlear toxicity *(NEJM 360:640 & 642, 2009).* Aspirin supplement (3 gm/day) attenuated risk of cochlear injury from gentamicin *(NEJM 354:1856, 2006).* Vestibular injury usually bilateral & hence no vertigo but imbalance & oscillopsia *(Med J Aust 196:701, 2012).*
Tobramycin—inhaled (Tobi): *See Cystic fibrosis, Table 1, page 48 & Table 10E, page 169.* Adverse effects few: transient voice alteration (13%) and transient tinnitus (3%).		
Paromomycin—oral: *See Entamoeba and Cryptosporidia, Table 13A, page 201.*		

* where available

TABLE 10D – PROLONGED OR CONTINUOUS INFUSION DOSING OF SELECTED ANTIBIOTICS

Prolonged or continuous infusion of beta-lactams is at least as successful as intermittent dosing. Hence, this approach can be part of stewardship programs as supported by recent publications.

Antibiotic stability is a concern. Factors influencing stability include drug concentration, IV infusion diluent *(e.g., NS vs. D5W)*, type of infusion device, and storage temperature *(Ref: P&T 36:723, 2011)*. Portable pumps worn close to the body expose antibiotics to temperatures closer to body temperature (37°C) than to room temperature (around 25°C). Carbapenems are particularly unstable and may require wrapping of infusion pumps in cold packs or frequent changes of infusion bags or cartridges.

A meta-analysis of observational studies found reduced mortality among patients treated with extended or continuous infusion of carbapenems or piperacillin-tazobactam (pooled data) as compared to standard intermittent regimens. The results were similar for extended and continuous regimens when considered separately. There was a mortality benefit with piperacillin-tazobactam but not carbapenems *(CID 56:272, 2013)*. The lower mortality could, at least in part, be due to closer professional supervision engendered by a study environment. On the other hand, a small prospective randomized controlled study of continuous vs. intermittent Pip-Tazo, and meropenem found a higher clinical cure rate and a trend toward lower mortality in the continuous infusion patients *(CID 56:236, 2013)*.

DRUG/METHOD	MINIMUM STABILITY	RECOMMENDED DOSE	COMMENTS
Ampicillin-sulbactam (Prolonged)	@ 37°C: In NS at 24 hr amp 77%, sulb 93% *(IJAA 6:S31, 1996)* @ 25°C: 8 hr (NS)* @ 4°C: 48 hr (NS)* *(amp/sulb conc ≤ 30 mg/15 mg per mL)	9 gm (6 gm amp + 3 gm sulb) IV over 4 hours q8h	For VAP due to Acinetobacter. High dose safe and effective *(Scand J ID 39:38, 2007; J Infect 56:432, 2008)*. High-dose prolonged-infusion sulbactam is supported by computer simulation studies *(Eur J Pharm Sci 136:104940, 2019)*. Recommended dose is for patients with normal renal function.
Cefazolin (Continuous)	Infusor LV elastomeric device, 3 gm or 6 gm of cefazolin in 250 mL D5W or NS. Antibiotic-filled device was stored in the refrigerator, removed immediately before use and worn in a pouch close to the body, then put it on a bedside table at night *(Clin Ther 2018;40:664)*: @ 4°C: 72 hr @ 35°C: 12 hr, then @ 25°C: 12 hr Easypump LT elastomeric device, 6 gm of cefazolin in 250 mL. Cefazolin shown to be stable for 24 hours under "real-life" conditions *(JAC 2017;72:1462)*.	30 mg/kg IV over 1 hr (initial dose), then 80-100 mg/kg (over 24 hours) daily. Dosing in renal impairment: *see comments*.	Dosing nomogram for a target steady-state plasma concentration of 40, 60, or 80 µg/mL according to eGFR, derived using data from 162 patients treated with continuous infusion cefazolin for bacteremia or endocarditis: *AAC 2019;63:e00806-19*.
Cefepime (Continuous)	@ 37°C: 8 hours @ 25°C: 24 hours @ 4°C: ≥24 hours	Initial dose: 15 mg/kg over 30 min, then immediately begin: • If CrCl >60: 6 gm (over 24 hr) daily • If CrCl 30-60: 4 gm (over 24 hr) daily • If CrCl 11-29: 2 gm (over 24 hr) daily	CrCl adjustments extrapolated from prescribing information, not clinical data *(JAC 57:1017, 2006; Am J Health Syst Pharm 68:319, 2011)*. One report of mortality benefit from extending infusion time from 30 minutes to 4 hours in patients with Pseudomonas pneumonia and/or bacteremia: *AAC 57:2907, 2013*.
Cefiderocol (Prolonged)	@ 25°C: 4 hr	2 gm IV over 3h q8h	For VAP, ventilated hospital-acquired bacterial pneumonia, including carbapenem-resistant Gram-negatives *(Lancet Infect Dis 2021; 21:226 and Lancet Infect Dis 2021;21:213)*.
Ceftazidime (Continuous)	@ 37°C: 8 hours @ 25°C: 24 hours @ 4°C: ≥24 hours	Initial dose: 15 mg/kg over 30 min, then immediately begin: • If CrCl >50: 6 gm (over 24 hr) daily • If CrCl 31-50: 4 gm (over 24 hr) daily • If CrCl 10-30: 2 gm (over 24 hr) daily	CrCl adjustments extrapolated from prescribing information, not clinical data. Refs: *Br J Clin Pharmacol 50:184, 2000; IJAA 17:497, 2001; AAC 49:3550, 2005; Infect 37: 418, 2009; JAC 68:900, 2013.* Pyridine, a byproduct of ceftazidime degradation, is a theoretic toxicity concern; minimize risk by limiting daily dose to 6 gm, using NS as the infusion vehicle, keeping ceftazidime concentration ≤3 gm per 100 mL if possible, and maintaining infusion device temperature between 15-22 °C *(AJHP 2019;76:200)*.

TABLE 10D (2)

DRUG/METHOD	MINIMUM STABILITY	RECOMMENDED DOSE	COMMENTS
Doripenem (Prolonged)	@ 37°C: 8 hours (in NS) @ 25°C: 24 hours (in NS) @ 4°C: 24 hours (in NS)	• If CrCl ≥50: 500 mg (over 4 hr) q8h • If CrCl 30-49: 250 mg (over 4 hr) q8h • If CrCl 10-29: 250 mg (over 4 hr) q12h	Based on a single study *(Crit Care Med 36:1089, 2008)*.
Meropenem (Prolonged)	@ 37°C: <4 hours @ 25°C: 4 hours @ 4°C: 24 hours	• If CrCl ≥50: 2 gm (over 3 hr) q8h • If CrCl 30-49: 1 gm (over 3 hr) q8h • If CrCl 10-29: 1 gm (over 3 hr) q12h	Initial 1 gm dose reasonable but not used by most investigators. Ref: *Intens Care Med 37:632, 2011.*
Pip-tazo (Prolonged)	@ 37°C: 24 hours @ 25°C: 24 hours @ 4°C: no data	• If CrCl ≥20: 4.5 gm (over 4 hr) q8h • If CrCl <20: 4.5 gm (over 4 hr) q12h	Refs: *CID 44:357, 2007; AAC 54:460, 2010.* *See CID 56:236, 245 & 272, 2013.* Suggested dosing in obesity particularly for critically ill patients, if MIC is ≥8 μg/mL, or CrCl >100 mL/min: 4.5 gm IV (over 4 hr) q6-8h *(Pharmacotherapy 2023;43:226)*.
Temocillin	@ 37°C: 24 hours @ 25°C: 24 hours These apply to Temocillin 4 gm/48 mL dilution *(JAC 61:382, 2008)*	Initial dose: 2 gm over 30 min, then immediately begin: • If CrCl >50: 6 gm (over 24 hr) daily • If CrCl 31-50: 3 gm (over 24 hr) daily • If CrCl 10-30: 1.5 gm (over 24 hr) daily • If CrCl <10: 750 mg (over 24 hr) daily CVVH: 750 mg (over 24 hr) daily	Offers higher probability of reaching desired PK/PD target than conventional q8h dosing. This study not designed to assess clinical efficacy *(JAC 70:891, 2015)*.
Vancomycin (Continuous)	@ 37°C: 48 hours @ 25°C: 48 hours @ 4°C: 58 days (at conc 10 μg/mL)	Initial dose 15-20 mg/kg (rate 10-15 mg/min), then 30-40 mg/kg (max 60 mg/kg) over 24 hours daily.	Vancomycin administration by continuous infusion is gaining acceptance as a treatment option. Target concentrations are more rapidly achieved with less variability, and the risk of nephrotoxicity appears to be similar to or lower than intermittent infusion *(Am J Health Syst Pharm 2020;77:835)*. Adjust dose to target steady-state concentration of 20-25 μg/mL. Higher concentrations (30-40 μg/mL) achieved with more aggressive dosing increase the risk of nephrotoxicity *(Clin Micro Inf 19:E98, 2013)*. Calculate AUC_{24} by multiplying the steady-state concentration by 24. A concentration of 20-25 μg/mL equates to an AUC_{24} of 480-600 μg/mL x hr. Because of incompatibilities with other drugs used in critically ill patients, it will be necessary to use multiple IV lines when vancomycin is administered by continuous infusion.

TABLE 10E – INHALATION ANTIBIOTICS

There are many reasons to consider inhaled antibiotics as an adjunct to parenteral therapy: • spectrum of activity that includes MDR GNB • documented high drug concentration in lung epithelial alveolar lining fluid • benefit in animal models of pneumonia • improved drug delivery (nebulizer) systems • Low risk of serious AEs. Refs: *Adv Drug Del Rev 2015,85-65* (review); *Chest 2017, 151:737* (clinical debate). The 2016 IDSA HAP/VAP guidelines suggest augmenting parenteral therapy with inhaled antibiotics, especially for highly resistant bacteria *(CID 2016;63:e61)*.

INHALED DRUG	DELIVERY SYSTEM	DOSE	COMMENT
Aztreonam (Cayston)	Altera vibrating mesh nebulizer	75 mg tid x 28 days (every other month)	Improves pulmonary function, reduces bacterial load, reduces frequency of exacerbations, and improves symptoms in **cystic fibrosis (CF)** pts *(Exp Opin Pharmacother 14:2115, 2013)*. Cost per treatment cycle about $6070.
Colistin (colistimethate) dry powder (EMA approved) Note: Polymyxin B is not used for inhalation due to toxicity to lung epithelial cells *(AAC 2017,61:e02690-16)*	Various *(see Comments)*	Most commonly used: 50-75 mg CBA in 3-4 mL NS via vibrating mesh nebulizer 2-3 times/day	Much variability and confusion in dosing. Nebulized colistimethate (CMS) 1-2 million IU (33-66 mg CBA) effective in **cystic fibrosis** *(Exp Opin Drug Deliv 9:333, 2012)*. Recent review is encouraging *(Expert Rev Anti Infect Ther 13:1237, 2015)*. In-depth PK study in 6 CF patients supportive in that nebulization of colistimethate achieved sputum colistimethate and colistin concentrations higher than those achieved from IV administration *(AAC 58:2570, 2014)*.
Fosfomycin + Tobramycin (FTI) 4:1 wt/wt	eFlow vibrating mesh nebulizer	FTI 160/40 or 80/20 bid x 28 days	Both doses maintained improvements in FEV1 following a 28-day inhaled aztreonam run-in (vs. placebo) in **CF patients** with *P. aeruginosa*; FTI 80/20 better tolerated than 160/40 *(AJRCCM 185:171, 2012)*.
Levofloxacin	eFlow vibrating mesh nebulizer	240 mg bid x 28 days	Reduced sputum density of *P. aeruginosa*, need for other antibiotics, and improved pulmonary function compared to placebo in **CF pts** *(AJRCCM 183:1510, 2011)*.
Liposomal Amikacin (Arikayce)	eFlow vibrating mesh nebulizer (Lamira, PARI Pharma)	590 mg (8.4 mL) once daily	For use as part of a combination regimen for **refractory MAC** in patients with limited or no alternative treatment options. Black box warning: associated with an increased risk of respiratory adverse reactions including hypersensitivity pneumonitis, hemoptysis, bronchospasm, and exacerbation of underlying pulmonary disease.
Tobramycin (TOBI, Bethkis)	PARI LC PLUS jet nebulizer	300 mg bid x 28 days (every other month)	Cost (generic): about $5769 for one treatment cycle.
Tobramycin (TOBI Podhaler)	28 mg dry powder caps	4 caps (112 mg) bid x 28 days (every other month)	Improvement in FEV1 similar to Tobra inhaled solution in **CF patients** with chronic *P. aeruginosa* but more airway irritation with the powder. Cost of one month treatment cycle about $6700 *(Med Lett 56:51, 2014)*.

TABLE 10F – ECMO DRUG DOSING ADJUSTMENT

- Extracorporeal membrane oxygenation (ECMO) in critically ill patients can alter the pharmacokinetics and pharmacodynamics of drugs, including antibiotics. Our understanding of these alterations is evolving.
- **Circuit Sequestration (CS)** of a drug may significantly alter a patient's dosing requirements.
  - The type of tubing, the oxygenator and pump, and the composition of priming solution all influence the degree of CS.
  - CS is more likely with lipophilic and/or highly protein bound drugs.
- **Increased volume of distribution (Vd)** is typically observed with hydrophilic drugs (hemodilution). CS also increases the Vd.
- **Altered drug clearance (CL)** may also be observed. Increased clearance results from increased cardiac output, fluid resuscitation, and inotropic support, whereas decreased clearance results from renal dysfunction (many ECMO patients require renal replacement therapy).
- PK parameters similar to patients not on ECMO.
- Good references: *Ann Pharmacother 2023;57:706; Clin Pharmacokinet 2023;62:931.*

Drug or class	Effect of ECMO	Dosing adjustment	Comments, references
Aminoglycosides	Minimal CS, ↑Vd, ↓CL	**Insufficient data** for a recommendation	TDM-guided dosing recommended.
Amphotericin B	Minimal CS (deoxycholate); moderate CS (liposomal)	**Insufficient data** for a recommendation	2x the standard dose of liposomal required in one case report *(Pharmacotherapy 2020;40:89)*. Liposomal data conflict, consider changing to deoxycholate *(Clin Pharmacokinet 2023;62:931)*.
Ampicillin	No significant effect on serum conc	**No dose adjustment** appears necessary	First in vivo report, data from two patients *(Pharmacotherapy 2023;43:864)*.
Anidulafungin	Moderate CS	**No dose adjustment** may be necessary	Data from a single case report *(Clin Pharmacokinet 2023;62:931)*.
Caspofungin	Moderate CS	**No dose adjustment** may be necessary	Contradictory data *(Clin Pharmacokinet 2023;62:931)*.
Cefazolin	Minimal effect on cefazolin PK	**No dosing adjustment** required	Case report *(Chemotherapy 2019;64:115)*.
Cefepime	Minimal CS, ↓CL	Consider dose adjustment, TDM	Minimal interaction with the ECMO circuit. PK data show ↓ clearance and ↑ probability of toxicity, especially with ↓ pt weight. Consider modified dosage regimens. TDM likely beneficial *(J Extra Corpor Technol 2022;54:212; IJAA 2021;58:106466)*.
Cefiderocol	No significant effect on cefiderocol PK	**No dose adjustment** appears necessary	Data from a single case report, so caution advised *(Perfusion 2023;38(1 suppl):40)*.
Cefpirome	↑Vcentral, ↑CL	**Increased dosing** suggested: 2 gm IV (bolus) q8h, or 2 gm IV (over 4 hr) q12h	Prospective PK study in 15 patients *(Antimicrob Agents Chemother 2020;64:e00249-20)*.
Ceftazidime-avibactam	Cmin target values above predefined cutoff values	No dose adjustment appears necessary	Data from 14 patients. Increased renal clearance (CrCl >130) was main factor associated with underdosing *(JAC 2024;79:1182)*.
Ceftobiprole	No significant effect on ceftobiprole PK	**No dose adjustment** likely required	Retrospective study, 28 pts on ECMO *(IJAA 2023;61:106765)*.
Ceftolozane- tazobactam	Minimal CS, ↑CL	**No dosing adjustment** suggested	Data from an ex vivo and in vivo model, requires confirmation *(J Transl Med 2020;18:123)*.
Ceftriaxone	No significant effect on unbound ceftriaxone PK or target attainment	**No dosing adjustment** appears necessary	Limited data from 2 patients *(IJAA 2021;57:106326)*. Similar conclusions from a PK study in 14 critically ill pts *(Clin Pharmacokinet 2022;61:847)*.
Ciprofloxacin	Simulations suggest recommended dosing regimens provide adequate drug exposure	**No dosing adjustment** appears necessary	PK data from 8 critically ill pts *(Anaesth Crit Care Pain Med 2022;41:101080)*.
Colistin	Target colistin conc achieved with standard dosing	**No dose adjustment** appears necessary	Data from only 2 pts, caution advised *(JAC 2022;77:2298)*.

TABLE 10F (2)

Drug or class	Effect of ECMO	Dosing adjustment	Comments, references
Fluconazole	Minimal CS, ↑Vd	**Insufficient data** for a recommendation	Consider increased loading dose *(Clin Pharmacokinet 2023;62:931)*.
Ganciclovir	Reduced ganciclovir AUC_{24} observed	**Increased dosing** may be required (based on one case report)	10 mg/kg q12h required to achieve AUC targets in a 6-yo not on CRRT *(J Clin Pharm Ther 2020;45:218)*.
Imipenem-cilastatin	↑CL	**Increased dosing** suggested	750-1000 mg q6h in ICU patients suggested based on PK modeling, not clinical data; much variability in the PK data *(Antimicrob Agents Chemother 2020;64:e00385-20)*.
Imipenem-cilastatin-relebactam	PK parameters similar to patients not on ECMO	**No dose adjustment** appears necessary	Data from seven critically ill patients supported by ECMO *(JAC 2024;79:1118)*.
Isavuconazole	Moderate to significant CS	**Increased dosing may be required,** but data conflict	TDM-guided dosing suggested *(Clin Pharmacokinet 2023;62:931)*.
Linezolid	↑Vd, ↑CL ???	**Increased dosing** may be required	Data from three patients: standard dosing may be insufficient if MRSA MIC >1 µg/mL *(Am J Health Syst Pharm 2020;77:877; IJAA 2013;41:590)*.
Meropenem	Minimal CS	**No dosing adjustment** required	Data from a matched cohort study *(Microorganisms 2021;9:1310)*.
Micafungin	Moderate CS	**No dose adjustment** may be necessary	Data conflict *(Clin Pharmacokinet 2023;62:931)*.
Peramivir	Insignificant drug loss with ECMO circuit	**No dosing adjustment** suggested	Preliminary data from a small ex vivo single-dose observational study *(Perfusion 2023;38:501)*.
Piperacillin- tazobactam	No significant effect on Vd or piperacillin exposure	**No dosing adjustment** required	Prospective data, 21 critically ill adult ECMO patients matched to controls. Much interpatient variability observed, consider TDM- guided dosing if available. Note: tazobactam PK not assessed *(J Antimicrob Chemother 2021;76:1242)*.
Polymyxin B	Overall impact probably minimal	**No dosing adjustment** suggested	Two PK studies *(JAC 2022; 77:1379; J Clin Pharm Ther 2022; 47:1608)*.
Posaconazole	Moderate to significant CS	**No dose adjustment** may be necessary	PK study data in six critically ill hematology patients receiving IV posaconazole. TDM recommended *(JAC 2021;76:1234)*.
Teicoplanin	Effect on Vd and Cl difficult to assess	**Insufficient data** for a recommendation	Sparse data. Need for ↑ dosing suggested in one PK study, n=10 *(AAC 2017;61:e01015-17)*. Adequate troughs achieved after recommended loading doses in a second study *(J Formos Med Assoc 2020;119:1086)*.
TMP-SMX	No effect observed	**No dosing adjustment** suggested	Case report, requires confirmation *(Pharmacotherapy 2020;40:713)*.
Vancomycin	Minimal CS; ↑Vd?, ↓CL?	**No dosing adjustment** required	The effects of ECMO on vancomycin PK parameters are conflicting and poorly understood. Changes may be minimal, and no standard dosage adjustment seems reasonable. However, aggressive TDM is recommended to achieve efficacy and safety targets. Continuous infusion may lessen PK changes. Refs: *Antimicrob Agents Chemother 2021;65:e02408-20; J Clin Pharm Ther 2020;45:1066; Clin Pharmacokinet 2020;59:1575*
Voriconazole	Moderate to significant CS	**No dose adjustment** may be necessary, but data conflict	TDM-guided dosing suggested *(Clin Pharmacokinet 2023;62:931)*.

- Suggested dosing relative to critically ill patients not on ECMO support
- CS=circuit sequestration, Vd = volume of distribution, CL = drug clearance, TDM = therapeutic drug monitoring, Cmax = maximum serum concentration, Cmin = minimum serum concentration

TABLE 10G – QTc PROLONGATION

Below is a list of antimicrobials with the potential to prolong the QTc interval. Concomitant risk factors: female gender, bradycardia, PVCs, CHF, older age, hypokalemia, hypomagnesemia, positive family history of arrhythmia/sudden death, use of stimulant drugs (dopamine, epinephrine, albuterol), use of drugs that delay repolarization (e.g., class Ia/III antiarrhythmics).

CredibleMeds, maintained by AZCERT, is a comprehensive resource for other drugs that prolong the QT interval.

Review of antimicrobials and QT prolongation: *J Antimicrob Chemother 2017;72:1272*

Antibacterials	Antifungals*	Antimycobacterials	Antiparasitics	Antiretrovirals	Antivirals
Azithromycin	Fluconazole	Azithromycin	Artemether-Lumefantrine	Atazanavir	Peramivir?
Ciprofloxacin	Itraconazole	Bedaquiline	Chloroquine	Cabenuva	
Clarithromycin	Posaconazole	Clarithromycin	DHA-PPQ	Efavirenz	
Erythromycin	Voriconazole	Clofazimine	Fexinidazole	Fostemsavir	
Gatifloxacin		Delamanid	Halofantrine	Lopinavir/RTV	
Gemifloxacin		Levofloxacin	Hydroxychloroquine	Rilpivirine	
Lefamulin		Moxifloxacin	Mefloquine	Saquinavir	
Levofloxacin		Pretomanid	Pentamidine		
Moxifloxacin			Pentavalent antimony		
Norfloxacin			Quinine		
Ofloxacin			Spiramycin		
Prulifloxacin			Triclabendazole		
Telavancin					
Telithromycin					

*Isavuconazole shortens the QT-interval

Management
Suggested management when using antibiotics known to prolong the QTc:
- Avoid use of drugs known to prolong QTc if other efficacious options available.
- Take family history; any sudden death episodes suspected due to cardiac arrhythmia?
- Pre-therapy measure QTc on 12-lead EKG.
- If baseline QTc borderline or prolonged, check for hypokalemia, hypomagnesemia, presence of another drug known to prolong the QTc, and subtle congestive heart failure.
- If QT-prolonging antibiotic prescribed, monitor QTc; reduce dose or discontinue suspect drug(s) if QTc increases by >60 ms or exceeds 500 ms.

TABLE 11A – TREATMENT OF FUNGAL INFECTIONS

For Antifungal Activity Spectra, *see Table 4B, page 84*

TYPE OF INFECTION/ORGANISM/ SITE OF INFECTION	ANTIMICROBIAL AGENTS OF CHOICE		COMMENTS
	PRIMARY	ALTERNATIVE	
Aspergillosis (A. fumigatus most common, also A. flavus and others) *(See NEJM 360:1870, 2009; Chest 146:1358, 2014)*. Diagnosis: *Chest 156:834, 2019.*			
Allergic bronchopulmonary aspergillosis (ABPA) Clinical manifestations: wheezing, pulmonary infiltrates, bronchiectasis & fibrosis. Airway colonization assoc. with ↑ blood eosinophils, ↑ serum IgE, ↑ specific serum antibodies.	Acute asthma attacks associated with ABPA: **Corticosteroids**	Rx of ABPA: **Itra** oral sol'n 200 mg po bid times 16 wks or longer	Itra decreases number of exacerbations requiring corticosteroids with improved immunological markers, improved lung function & exercise tolerance *(CID 63:433, 2016).*
Allergic fungal sinusitis: relapsing chronic sinusitis; nasal polyps without bony invasion; asthma, eczema or allergic rhinitis; ↑ IgE levels and isolation of Aspergillus sp. or other dematiaceous sp. (Alternaria, Cladosporium, etc.)	**Rx controversial:** systemic corticosteroids + surgical debridement (relapse common).	For failures try **Itra** 200 mg po bid times 12 mos or **Flu** nasal spray.	Controversial area.
Aspergilloma (fungus ball)	No therapy or surgical resection. Efficacy of antifungal agents not proven.		Aspergillus may complicate pulmonary sequestration.
Invasive, pulmonary (IPA) or extrapulmonary: Post-transplantation and post-chemotherapy in neutropenic pts (PMN <500 per mm³) but may also present with neutrophil recovery. Common pneumonia in transplant recipients. Usually a late (≥100 days) complication in allogeneic bone marrow & liver transplantation: High mortality *(CID 44:531, 2007).* **Typical x-ray/CT lung lesions** (halo sign, cavitation, or macronodules) *(CID 44:373, 2007).* **Galactomannan antigen immunoassay:** Detects aspergillus cell wall polysaccharide. Adjunct to diagnosis in neutropenic pts. Serum sens/spec. varies from 21-86% sens/80-92% spec. BAL fluid 60-100% sens/68-100% spec. False neg. if receiving antifungals. False pos. if colonized by aspergillus or infected by Fusarium, histo or blasto *(JAMA 2017;318:1175).* **Better diagnostic strategy:** combination of serum galactomannan & aspergillus PCR (not routinely available) *(LnID 13:519, 2013).* **Beta D-Glucan:** in fungal cell wall. Can detect with immunoassay. Many false positives + low sensitivity *(JCM 51:3478, 2013).*	**Primary therapy** *(See CID 63:433, 2016):* **Isavuconazonium sulfate** loading dose of 372 mg (equivalent to isavuconazole 200 mg) IV/po q8 x 6 doses then 372 mg IV/po daily OR **Vori** 6 mg/kg IV q12h on day 1; then either (4 mg/kg IV q12h) or (200 mg po q12h for body weight ≥40 kg, but 100 mg po q12h for body weight <40 kg) (use actual wt). Goal trough (day 4): 1.0–5.5 mg/L associated with improved response rates and reduced adverse effects *(Clin Infect Dis 55:1080, 2012).* Verify in vitro susceptibility *(CID 68:1463, 2019).* **Alternative therapies:** **Liposomal Ampho B (LAB)** (L-AmB) 3-5 mg/kg/day IV; OR **Ampho B lipid complex** (ABLC) 5 mg/kg/d IV; OR **Caspo** 70 mg/day then 50 mg/day thereafter; OR **Mica**[NAI] 100 mg bid *(JAC 64:840, 2009– based on PK/PD study);* OR **Posaconazole** (NOTE: different dosing delayed release tabs/IV vs. suspension, better levels achieved with delayed-release tabs): Delayed-release tabs 300 mg po bid x 2 doses and then 300 mg po daily or Suspension 200 mg qid, then 400 mg po bid after stabilization of disease or Posaconazole IV 300 mg IV over 90 minutes bid x 1 day, then 300 mg IV daily. Not FDA approved for this indication, but RCT supporting it as effective as Vori. In documented azole-resistant invasive aspergillosis, most experts suggest change to either **Liposomal Ampho B** or combination of **Vori + echinocandin** *(JID 2017;216(S3):S436)*		**Voriconazole** more effective than Ampho B. Vori, both a substrate and an inhibitor of CYP2C19, CYP2C9, and CYP3A4, has potential for deleterious drug interactions (e.g., with protease inhibitors). Review concomitant medications. Measure serum level with prolonged therapy or for patients with possible drug-drug interactions. In patients with CrCl <50 mL/min, po may be preferred due to concerns for nephrotoxicity of IV vehicle in renal dysfunction. *(Clin Infect Dis 54:913, 2012)* **Isavuconazole:** (prodrug isavuconazonium sulfate): A randomized control trial of Isavuconazole vs. Voriconazole for invasive aspergillosis demonstrated that Isavuconazole is non-inferior to voriconazole for the treatment of invasive aspergillosis *(Ln 2016;387:760).* **Posaconazole:** A randomized control trial of Posaconazole vs. Voriconazole for invasive aspergillosis demonstrated that Posaconazole is non-inferior to Voriconazole for the treatment of invasive aspergillosis. However, Posaconazole was associated with fewer treatment-related side effects overall *(Lancet 397:499 2021).* **Ampho B: not recommended except as a lipid formulation,** either L-AMB or ABLC. 10 mg/kg and 3 mg/kg doses of L-AMB are equally efficacious with greater toxicity of higher dose *(CID 2007; 44:1289–97).* One comparative trial found greater toxicity with ABLC than with L-AMB: 34.6% vs 9.4% adverse events and 21.2% vs 2.8% nephrotoxicity *(Cancer 112:1282, 2008).* Vori preferred as primary therapy. **Caspofungin:** ~50% response rate in IPA. Licensed for salvage therapy. **Micafungin:** Favorable responses to micafungin as a single agent in 6/12 patients in primary therapy group and 9/22 in the salvage therapy group *(J Infect 53: 337, 2006).* **Combination therapy:** A RCT of Voriconazole plus Anidulafungin vs. Voriconazole alone showed a trend towards reduced mortality in all patients with invasive aspergillosis in the combination therapy arm *(Ann Intern Med 162:81, 2015).* Combination therapy should be strongly considered although further data is needed to determine which patients would benefit the most. Some experts would recommend addition of echinocandin to amphotericin-based regimen or other azoles as well.

See page 2 for abbreviations. All dosage recommendations are for adults (unless otherwise indicated) and assume normal renal function.

TABLE 11A (2)

TYPE OF INFECTION/ORGANISM/ SITE OF INFECTION	ANTIMICROBIAL AGENTS OF CHOICE		COMMENTS
	PRIMARY	ALTERNATIVE	
Blastomycosis *(CID 46: 1801, 2008)* *(Blastomyces dermatitidis)* Cutaneous, pulmonary or extrapulmonary.	**LAB,** 3-5 mg/kg per day; OR **Ampho B,** 0.7-1 mg/kg per day, for 1-2 weeks, **then Itra** oral sol'n 200 mg tid for 3 days followed by Itra 200 mg bid for 6 -12 months	**Itra** oral sol'n 200 mg tid for 3 days then once or twice per day for 6-12 months for mild to moderate disease; OR **Flu** 400-800 mg per day for those intolerant to Itra	Serum levels of **Itra** should be determined after 2 weeks to ensure adequate drug exposure. Flu less effective than Itra; role of Vori or Posa unclear but active in vitro. Can look for Blastomyces in antigen in urine as aid to diagnosis.
Blastomycosis: CNS disease *(CID 50:797, 2010)*	**LAB** 5 mg/kg per day for 4–6 weeks, followed by **Flu** 800 mg per day	**Itra** oral sol'n 200 mg bid or tid; OR **Vori** 200-400 mg q12h	Flu and Vori have excellent CNS penetration, to counterbalance their slightly reduced activity compared to Itra. Treat for at least 12 months and until CSF has normalized. Monitor serum Itra levels to assure adequate drug concentrations. More favorable outcome with Voriconazole *(CID 50:797, 2010)*.
Candidiasis: Candida is a common cause of nosocomial bloodstream infection. *C. albicans* & non-albicans species show ↓ susceptibility to antifungal agents (esp. fluconazole). In immunocompromised pts where antifungal prophylaxis (esp. fluconazole) is widely used. Oral, esophageal, or vaginal candidiasis is a major manifestation of advanced HIV & represents common AIDS-defining diagnosis. *See CID 62:e1, 2016 for updated IDSA Guidelines.*			
Candidiasis: Bloodstream infection *(C. albicans & C. glabrata).* Diagnosis: *Chest 156:834, 2019.*			
Bloodstream: non-neutropenic patient Remove all intravascular catheters if possible; replace catheters at a new site (not over a wire). Higher mortality associated with delay in therapy *(CID 43:25, 2006)*. ***Candida auris:*** This is an emerging **multi-drug resistant** Candida species able to cause a wide-range of infections. It can be misidentified as *Candida haemulonii* or *Saccharomyces cerevisiae*. Molecular methods are needed to confirm species. Often resistant to azoles and amphotericin, some are also echinocandin resistant *(CID 2018,66:306)*. Multi-drug resistant Candida species *(JID 2017;216(S3):S445)*.	**Caspo** 70 mg IV loading dose, then 50 mg IV daily; OR **Mica** 100 mg IV daily; OR **Anidula** 200 mg IV loading dose then 100 mg IV daily OR **Rezafungin** 400 mg IV loading dose, then 200 mg IV once weekly. Note: Reduce **Caspo** dose for renal impairment **Funduscopic examination** within first week of therapy to exclude ophthalmic involvement. Ocular disease present in ~15% of patients with candidemia, but endophthalmitis is uncommon (~2%) *(CID 53:262, 2011)*. Intraocular injections of Ampho B required for endophthalmitis as echinocandins have poor penetration into the eye. For **septic thrombophlebitis,** catheter removal and incision and drainage and resection of the vein, as needed, are recommended; duration of therapy at least 2 weeks after last positive blood culture.	**Flu** 800 mg (12 mg/kg) loading dose, then 400 mg daily IV OR **Lipid-based Ampho B** 3-5 mg/kg IV daily; OR **Ampho B** 0.7 mg/kg IV daily; OR **Vori** 400 mg (6 mg/kg) IV twice daily for 2 doses then 200 mg q12h.	**Echinocandin** is recommended for empiric therapy, particularly for patients with recent azole exposure or with moderately severe or severe illness, hemodynamic instability. **An echinocandin should be used for treatment of *Candida glabrata* unless susceptibility to fluconazole or voriconazole has been confirmed.** Echinocandin preferred empiric therapy in centers with high prevalence of non-albicans candida species. Echinocandin vs. polyenes or azole associated with better survival *(Clin Infect Dis 54:1110, 2012)*. A double-blind randomized trial of anidulafungin (n=127) and fluconazole (n=118) showed an 88% microbiologic response rate (119/135 candida species) with anidulafungin vs a 76% (99/130 candida species) with fluconazole (p=0.02) *(NEJM 356: 2472, 2007)*. **Fluconazole** is not recommended for empiric therapy but could be considered recommended for patients with mild-to-moderate illness, hemodynamically stable, with no recent azole exposure. **Fluconazole not recommended for treatment of documented *C. krusei*: use an echinocandin or voriconazole or posaconazole (note: echinocandins have better in vitro activity than either Vori or Posa against *C. glabrata*).** **Fluconazole recommended for treatment of *Candida parapsilosis*** because of reduced susceptibility of this species to echinocandins. Transition from echinocandin to fluconazole for stable patients with *Candida albicans* or other azole-susceptible species. **Voriconazole** with little advantage over fluconazole (more drug-drug interactions) except for oral step-down therapy of *Candida krusei* or voriconazole-susceptible *Candida glabrata*. Recommended **duration of therapy** is 14 days after last positive blood culture. Duration of systemic therapy should be extended to 4-6 weeks for eye involvement.

TABLE 11A (3)

TYPE OF INFECTION/ORGANISM/ SITE OF INFECTION	ANTIMICROBIAL AGENTS OF CHOICE		COMMENTS
	PRIMARY	ALTERNATIVE	
Candidiasis: Bloodstream infection *(continued)*			
Bloodstream: neutropenic patient Remove all intravascular catheters if possible; replace catheters at a new site (not over a wire).	**Caspo** 70 mg IV loading dose, then 50 mg IV daily, 35 mg for moderate hepatic insufficiency; OR **Mica** 100 mg IV daily; OR **Anidula** 200 mg IV loading dose then 100 mg IV daily; OR **Lipid-based Ampho B** 3-5 mg/kg IV daily.	**Flu** 800 mg (12 mg/kg) loading dose, then 400 mg daily IV or po; OR **Vori** 400 mg (6 mg/kg) IV twice daily for 2 doses then 200 mg (3 mg/kg) IV q12h. Another alternative: **Rezafungin** 400 mg IV loading dose, then 200 mg IV once weekly.	**Duration of therapy** in absence of metastatic complications is for 2 weeks after last positive blood culture, resolution of signs, and resolution of neutropenia. Perform funduscopic examination after recovery of white count as signs of ophthalmic involvement may not be seen during neutropenia. *See comments above for recommendations concerning choice of specific agents.*
Candidiasis: Bone and joint infections			
Osteomyelitis	**Flu** 400 mg (6 mg/kg) daily IV or po; OR **Lipid-based Ampho B** 3–5 mg/kg daily x several weeks, then oral fluconazole.	**Caspo**, **Mica** or **Anidula** or **Ampho B** 0.5–1 mg/kg IV daily x several weeks then oral **Flu**. Another alternative: **Rezafungin** 400 mg IV loading dose, then 200 mg IV once weekly.	Treat for a total of 6-12 months. **Surgical debridement** often necessary; **remove hardware** whenever possible.
Septic arthritis	**Flu** 400 mg (6 mg/kg) daily IV or po; OR **Lipid-based Ampho B** 3–5 mg/kg IV daily x several weeks, then oral fluconazole.	**Caspo**, **Mica** or **Anidula** or **Ampho B** 0.5–1 mg/kg IV daily for several weeks then oral **Flu**. Another alternative: **Rezafungin** 400 mg IV loading dose, then 200 mg IV once weekly.	**Surgical debridement** in all cases; removal of prosthetic joints whenever possible. Treat for at least 6 weeks and indefinitely if retained hardware.
Candidiasis: Cardiovascular infections			
Endocarditis, Myocarditis, Pericarditis *(See Eur J Clin Microbiol Infect Dis 27:519, 2008)*	**Caspo** 50–150 mg/day IV; OR **Mica** 100–150 mg/day IV; OR **Anidula** 100–200 mg/day IV; OR **Lipid-based Ampho B** 3–5 mg/kg IV daily + **Flucytosine** 25 mg/kg po qid.	**Ampho B** 0.6–1 mg/kg IV daily + **Flucytosine** 25 mg/kg po qid OR **Rezafungin** 400 mg IV loading dose, then 200 mg IV once weekly.	Consider use of higher doses of echinocandins for endocarditis or other endovascular infections. Can switch to **Fluconazole 400-800 mg orally in stable patients** with negative blood cultures and fluconazole susceptible organism. *See Med 90:237, 2011.* Valve replacement strongly recommended, particularly if prosthetic valve endocarditis. Duration of therapy not well defined, but treat for at least 6 weeks after valve replacement and longer in those with complications (e.g., perivalvular or myocardial abscess, extensive disease, delayed resolution of candidemia). Pericarditis: Pericardial window or pericardiectomy is also recommended. Long-term (life-long?) suppression with Fluconazole 400-800 mg daily for native valve endocarditis and no valve replacement; life-long suppression for prosthetic valve endocarditis if no valve replacement.

See page 2 for abbreviations. All dosage recommendations are for adults (unless otherwise indicated) and assume normal renal function.

TABLE 11A (4)

TYPE OF INFECTION/ORGANISM/ SITE OF INFECTION	ANTIMICROBIAL AGENTS OF CHOICE		COMMENTS
	PRIMARY	ALTERNATIVE	
Candidiasis: Mucosal, esophageal, and oropharyngeal			
Candida esophagitis Primarily encountered in HIV-positive patients Dysphagia or odynophagia predictive of esophageal candidiasis.	**Flu** 200-400 (3-6 mg/kg) mg IV/po daily; OR (**Caspo** 50 mg IV daily; OR **Mica** 150 mg IV daily; OR **Anidula** 200 mg IV loading dose then 100 mg IV daily); OR **Ampho B** 0.5 mg/kg IV daily.	An azole (**Itra** solution 200 mg daily; or **Posa** delayed release tabs/IV loading dose of 300 mg q12h x 2 doses then 300 mg daily (posaconazole oral suspension 200 mg po qid) or **Vori** IV/po 200 mg q12h. Another alternative: **Rezafungin** 400 mg IV loading dose, then 200 mg IV once weekly.	**Duration of therapy** 14-21 days. IV Echinocandin or Ampho B for patients unable to tolerate oral therapy. For Fluconazole refractory disease, Itra (80% will respond), Posa, Vori, an Echinocandin, or Ampho B. Echinocandins associated with higher relapse rate than fluconazole. ART recommended. Suppressive therapy with fluconazole 200 mg po 3x/wk until CD4 >200/mm³.
Oropharyngeal candidiasis			
Non-AIDS patient	**Clotrimazole troches** 10 mg 5 x daily; OR **Nystatin suspension** or pastilles po qid; OR **Flu** 100-200 mg daily.	**Itra** solution 200 mg daily; OR **Posa** delayed release tabs/IV loading dose of 300 mg q12h x 2 doses then 300 mg daily (posaconazole oral suspension 200 mg po qid); or **Vori** 200 mg q12h; OR (**Caspo** 70 mg loading dose then 50 mg IV daily; or **Mica** 100 mg IV daily; or **Anidula** 200 mg IV loading dose then 100 mg IV daily); OR **Ampho B** 0.3 mg/kg daily.	**Duration of therapy** 7-14 days. Clotrimazole or nystatin recommended for mild disease; Fluconazole preferred for moderate-to-severe disease. Alternative agents reserved for refractory disease.
AIDS patient	**Flu** 100-200 mg po daily x 7-14 days.	Same as for non-AIDS patient x 7-14 days.	ART in HIV-positive patients. Suppressive therapy until CD4 >200/mm³, but if required fluconazole 100 mg po thrice weekly. Oral Itra, Posa, or Vori for 28 days for Fluconazole-refractory disease. IV echinocardin also an option. Dysphagia or odynophagia predictive of esophageal candidiasis.
Vulvovaginitis			
Non-AIDS Patient	**Topical azole therapy: Butoconazole 2% cream** (5 gm) q24h at bedtime x 3 days or 2% cream SR 5 gm x 1; OR **Clotrimazole 100 mg vaginal tabs** (2 at bedtime x 3 days) or 1% cream (5 gm) at bedtime times 7 days (14 days may ↑ cure rate) or 100 mg vaginal tab x 7 days or 500 mg vaginal tab x 1; OR **Miconazole 200 mg vaginal suppos** (1 at bedtime x 3 days) or 100 mg vaginal suppos. q24h x 7 days or 2% cream (5 gm) at bedtime x 7 days; OR **Terconazole 80 mg vaginal tab** (1 at bedtime x 3 days) or 0.4% cream (5 gm) at bedtime x 7 days or 0.8% cream 5 gm intravaginal q24h x 3 days; or **Tioconazole** 6.5% vag. ointment x 1 dose. **Oral therapy:** **Flu** 150 mg po x 1; OR If severe, **Flu** 150 mg q72h x 3 OR **Itra** 200 mg po bid x 1 day OR **Ibrexafungerp** 300 mg (2 tablets 150 mg each) po, with or without food, q12h x 2 doses for one day		**Recurrent vulvovaginal candidiasis: Fluconazole** 150 mg weekly for 6 months. If severe can induce with Flu 150 mg q10-14 days, then weekly.
AIDS Patient	Topical **azoles** (clotrimazole, buto, mico, tico, or tercon) x3-7d; OR Topical **Nystatin** 100,000 units/day as vaginal tablet x14d; OR **Flu** 150 mg po x1 dose.		For recurrent disease 10-14 days of topical azole or oral Flu 150 mg, then **Flu** 150 mg po weekly for 6 mos.

See page 2 for abbreviations. All dosage recommendations are for adults (unless otherwise indicated) and assume normal renal function.

TABLE 11A (5)

TYPE OF INFECTION/ORGANISM/ SITE OF INFECTION	ANTIMICROBIAL AGENTS OF CHOICE		COMMENTS
	PRIMARY	ALTERNATIVE	
Candidiasis: Other infections			
CNS Infection	**Lipid-based Ampho B** 3–5 mg/kg IV daily + 5-FC 25 mg/kg po qid.	**Flu** 400–800 mg (6-12 mg/kg) IV or po.	Removal of **intraventricular devices** recommended. Flu 400-800 mg as step-down therapy in the stable patient and in patient intolerant of Ampho B. Experience too limited to recommend echinocandins at this time. **Treatment duration** for several weeks until resolution of CSF, radiographic, and clinical abnormalities.
Cutaneous *(including paronychia, Table 1, page 30)*	Apply topical **Ampho B, Clotrimazole, Econazole, Miconazole, or Nystatin** 3-4 x daily for 7–14 days or ketoconazole 400 mg po once daily x 14 days. Ciclopirox olamine 1% cream/lotion; apply topically bid x 7–14 days.		
Endophthalmitis /Chorioretinitis • Occurs in 10% of candidemia, thus ophthalmological consult for all pts • Diagnosis: typical white exudates on retinal exam and/or positive vitrectomy culture • Chorioretinitis accounts for 85% of ocular disease while endophthalmitis occurs in only 15% *(Clin Infect Dis 53:262, 2011)*.	Chorioretinitis or Endophthalmitis: Lipid-based **Ampho B** 3-5 mg/kg daily + **Flucytosine** 25 mg/kg qid OR **Vori** 6 mg/kg po/IV q12 x 2 doses and then 4 mg/kg po/IV q12. Consider intravitreal **Ampho B** 5–10 mcg in 0.1 mL or intravitreal **Vori** 100 mcg in 0.1 mL for sight threatening disease.	Chorioretinitis or Endophthalmitis: **Flu** 6-12 mg/kg IV daily (poor activity against C. glabrata or C. krusei) and consider intravitreal **Ampho B** 5-10 mcg in 0.1 mL for sight-threatening disease. Consider vitrectomy in advanced disease. *Clin Infect Dis. 52:648, 2011.*	**Duration of therapy:** 4-6 weeks or longer, based on resolution determined by repeated examinations. Vitrectomy may be necessary for those with vitritis or endophthalmitis *(Br J Ophthalmol 92:466, 2008; Pharmacotherapy 27:1711, 2007)*.
Neonatal candidiasis	**Ampho B** 1 mg/kg IV daily; OR **Flu** 12 mg/kg IV daily.	**Lipid-based Ampho B** 3-5 mg/kg IV daily.	**Lumbar puncture** to rule out CNS disease, **dilated retinal examination,** abdominal ultrasound and **intravascular catheter removal** strongly recommended. Lipid-based Ampho B used only if there is no renal involvement. Echinocandins considered 3rd line therapy but appear non-inferior in recent trials *(Pediatr Infect Dis J 38:42,2018)*. **Duration of therapy is at least 3 weeks.**
Peritonitis (Chronic Ambulatory Peritoneal Dialysis) *See Table 19, page 325.*	**Flu** 400 mg po q24h x 2–3 wks; or **Caspo** 70 mg IV on day 1 followed by 50 mg IV q24h x 14 days; or **Mica** 100 mg IV q24h x 14 days.	**Ampho B,** continuous intraperitoneal dosing at 1.5 mg/L of dialysis fluid x 4–6 wks.	Remove cath immediately or if no clinical improvement in 4–7 days.
Candidiasis: Urinary tract infections			
Cystitis **Asymptomatic** *See CID 52:s427, 2011; CID 52:s452, 2011.*	**If possible, remove catheter or stent.** No therapy indicated except in patients at high risk for dissemination or undergoing a urologic procedure.		**High risk patients** (neonates and neutropenic patients) should be managed as outlined for treatment of bloodstream infection. For patients undergoing urologic procedures, Flu 200 mg (3 mg/kg) IV/po daily or Ampho B 0.5 mg/kg IV daily (for flu-resistant organisms) for several days pre- and post-procedure.
Symptomatic	**Flu** 200 mg (3 mg/kg) IV/po daily x 14 days.	**Ampho B** 0.5 mg/kg IV daily (for fluconazole resistant organisms) x 7-10 days.	Concentration of echinocandins is low; case reports of efficacy versus azole resistant organisms *(Can J Infect Dis Med Microbiol 18:149, 2007; CID 44:e46, 2007)*. Persistent candiduria in immunocompromised pt warrants ultrasound or CT of kidneys to rule out fungus ball.
Pyelonephritis	**Flu** 200–400 mg (3–6 mg/kg) po once daily.	**Ampho B** 0.5 mg/kg daily IV + 5-FC 25 mg/kg po qid.	**Treat for 2 weeks.** For suspected disseminated disease treat as if bloodstream infection is present.
Chromoblastomycosis *(Clin Exp Dermatol, 34:849, 2009)*. (Cladophialophora, Phialophora, or Fonsecaea); Cutaneous (usually feet, legs): raised scaly lesions, most common in tropical areas	If lesions small & few, **surgical excision or cryosurgery with liquid nitrogen.** If lesions chronic, extensive, burrowing: **Itraconazole.**	**Itra:** 200-400 mg oral sol'n q24h or 400 mg pulse therapy once daily for 1 week of each month x 6-12 months (or until response)[NAI].	**Terbinafine**[NAI] 500-1000 mg once daily alone or in combination with **Itra** 200-400 oral sol'n mg; or **Posa** (800 mg/d) po may be effective. Anecdotal report of efficacy of topical imiquimod 5%: 5x/wk *(CID 58:1734, 2014)*.

See page 2 for abbreviations. All dosage recommendations are for adults (unless otherwise indicated) and assume normal renal function.

TABLE 11A (6)

TYPE OF INFECTION/ORGANISM/ SITE OF INFECTION	ANTIMICROBIAL AGENTS OF CHOICE		COMMENTS
	PRIMARY	ALTERNATIVE	
Coccidioidomycosis *(Coccidioides immitis) (IDSA Guidelines: CID 63: e112, 2016; see also Mayo Clin Proc 83:343, 2008)*			
Primary pulmonary (San Joaquin or Valley Fever): **For pts at low risk of persistence/complication**	**Antifungal rx not generally recommended.** Treat if fever, wt loss and/or fatigue that does not resolve within 4-8 wks		Uncomplicated pulmonary in normal host common in endemic areas *(Emerg Infect Dis 12:958, 2006)* Influenza-like illness of 1–2 wks duration.
Primary pulmonary in pts with ↑ risk for complications or dissemination. Rx indicated: • Immunosuppressive disease, post-transplantation, hematological malignancies or therapies (steroids, TNF-α antagonists) • Pregnancy in 3rd trimester. • Diabetes • CF antibody >1:16 • Pulmonary Infiltrates • Dissemination (identification of spherules or culture of organism from ulcer, joint effusion, pus from subcutaneous abscess or bone biopsy, etc.)	**Mild to moderate severity** *(EID 20:983, 2014)*: **Itra** solution 200 mg po or IV bid; OR **Flu** 400 mg po q24h x 3–12 mos **Locally severe or disseminated disease** **Ampho B** 0.6–1 mg/kg per day x 7 days then 0.8 mg/kg every other day or **liposomal Ampho B** 3-5 mg/kg/d IV or **ABLC** 5 mg/kg/d IV, until clinical improvement (usually several wks or longer in disseminated disease), followed by **Itra** or **Flu** for at least 1 year. Some use combination of Ampho B & Flu for progressive severe disease; controlled series lacking. **Consultation with specialist recommended:** surgery may be required. Suppression in HIV+ patients until CD4 >250 & infection controlled: **Flu** 200 mg po q24h or Itra oral sol'n 200 mg po bid *(Mycosis 46:42, 2003)*.		**Ampho B cure rate 50–70%. Responses to azoles are similar. Itra** may have slight advantage esp. in soft tissue infection. Relapse rates after rx 40%: Relapse rate ↑ if ↑ CF titer ≥1:256. Following CF titers after completion of rx important; rising titers warrant retreatment. **Posaconazole** reported successful in 73% of pts with refractory non-meningeal cocci *(Chest 132:952, 2007)*. Not frontline therapy. Treatment of pediatric cocci to include salvage therapy with Vori & Caspo *(CID 56:1573, 1579 & 1587, 2013)*. Can detect delayed hypersensitivity with skin test antigen called Spherusol; helpful if history of Valley Fever.
Meningitis: occurs in 1/3 to 1/2 of pts with disseminated coccidioidomycosis			
Adult *(CID 42:103, 2006)*	**Flu** 400–1,000 mg po q24h indefinitely	**Ampho B** IV as for pulmonary *(above)* + 0.1–0.3 mg daily intra-thecal (intraventricular) via reservoir device. **OR Itra** oral sol'n 400–800 mg q24h **OR Vori** *(See Comment)*	**80% relapse rate, continue flucon indefinitely,** **Voriconazole** successful in high doses (6 mg/kg IV q12h) followed by oral suppression (200 mg po q12h). For practical spects of intrathecal ampho B, see *CID 2017,64:519*. Small retrospective study suggests benefit from adjunctive corticosteroids *(CID 2017,65:338)*.
Child *(Cryptococcus neoformans, C. gattii)*	**Flu** (Pediatric dose not established, 6 mg per kg po q24h used)		
Cryptococcosis *IDSA Guideline: CID 50:291, 2010.*			
Non-meningeal (non-AIDS) Risk 57% in organ transplant & those receiving other forms of immunosuppressive agents *(EID 13:953, 2007)*.	**Flu** 400 mg/day IV or po x 8 wks to 6 mos **For more severe disease:** **Ampho B** 0.5–0.8 mg/kg per day IV till response then change to **Flu** 400 mg po q24h x 8–10 wks course	**Itra** 200-400 mg solution q24h x 6-12 mos OR (**Ampho B** 0.3 mg/kg per day IV + **Flucytosine** 37.5 mg/kg po qid) x 6 wks (use ideal body wt)	**Flu alone 90% effective for meningeal and non-meningeal forms.** Fluconazole as effective as Ampho B. Addition of **interferon-g** (IFN-γ-lb 50 mcg per M² subcut. 3x per wk x 9 wks) to liposomal Ampho B assoc. with response in pt failing antifungal rx *(CID 38: 910, 2004)*. Posaconazole 400-800 mg also effective in a small series of patients *(CID 45:562, 2007; Chest 132:952, 2007)*

Meningitis (non-AIDS) IDSA Guidelines: *CID 50:291, 2010.*	• Induction phase: (**Liposomal Ampho B** 3-4 mg/kg IV q24h or **Ampho B lipid complex** 5 mg/kg IV q24h) + **Flucytosine** 25 mg/kg po q6h
	  ○ Duration: Minimum 2 weeks for transplant recipients and minimum 4 weeks in non-immunocompromised patients. Treat until patient is afebrile and cultures are negative.
	  ○ Need to monitor intracranial pressure; If over 25 cm, need to remove CSF. *See comment*.
	• Consolidation phase: **Flu** 400-800 mg po daily x 8 weeks
	• Maintenance phase: **Flu** 200 mg po daily x 6-12 months
			If CSF opening pressure >25 cm H_2O, repeat LP to drain fluid to control pressure.
			C. gattii meningitis reported in the Pacific Northwest *(EID 13:42, 2007)*; severity of disease and prognosis appear to be worse than with C. neoformans; initial therapy with **Ampho B + Flucytosine** recommended. C. gattii less susceptible to flucon than C. neoformans *(Clin Microbiol Inf 14:727, 2008)*.
			Outcomes in both AIDS and non-AIDS cryptococcal meningitis improved with Ampho B + 5-FC induction therapy for 14 days in those with neurological abnormalities or high organism burden *(PLoS ONE 3:e2870, 2008)*.

TABLE 11A (7)

TYPE OF INFECTION/ORGANISM/ SITE OF INFECTION	ANTIMICROBIAL AGENTS OF CHOICE		COMMENTS
	PRIMARY	ALTERNATIVE	
Cryptococcosis *(continued)*			
HIV+/AIDS: Cryptococcemia and/or Meningitis			
Treatment *See Clin Infect Dis 50:291, 2010 (IDSA Guidelines).* ↓ with ARV but still common presenting OI in newly diagnosed AIDS pts. Cryptococcal infection may be manifested by positive blood culture or positive serum cryptococcal antigen (CRAG: >95% sens). CRAG no help in monitoring response to therapy. With ARV, symptoms of acute meningitis may return: immune reconstitution inflammatory syndrome (IRIS). ↑ CSF pressure **(>250 mm H2O)** associated with high mortality: lower with CSF removal. If frequent LPs not possible, ventriculoperitoneal shunts an option *(Surg Neurol 63:529 & 531, 2005).*	**Ampho B** 0.7 mg/kg IV q24H or Liposomal **Ampho B** 3-4 mg/kg IV q24 or **Ampho B** lipid complex 5 mg/kg IV q24 + **Flucytosine** 25 mg/kg po q6h for at least two weeks or longer until CSF is sterilized. *See Comment.* **Then** **Consolidation therapy: Flu** 400-800 mg po q24h to complete a 10-wks course then suppression *(see below).*	**If 5-FC not possible:** Ampho B product + Fluc 800-1200 mg/day IV/po x 2 weeks **If Ampho B product not possible:** Fluc 800-1200 mg/day IV/po + 5-FC 25 mg/kg po q6h x 4–6 weeks **If Ampho B nor 5-FC possible:** Fluc 1200-2000 mg po daily x 10-12 weeks **Liposomal Ampho B** 10 mg/kg IV x1 + (**flucytosine** 100 mg/kg q24h + **fluconazole** 1200 mg po q24h x 14 days)	• Outcome of treatment: treatment failure associated with dissemination of infection & high serum antigen titer, indicative of high burden of organisms and lack of 5FC use during inductive Rx, abnormal neurological evaluation & underlying hematological malignancy. Mortality rates still high, particularly in those with concomitant pneumonia *(Postgrad Med 121:107, 2009).* Early Dx essential for improved outcome *(PLOS Medicine 4:e47, 2007).* • Ampho B + 5FC treatment ↓ crypto CFUs more rapidly than ampho + Flu or Ampho + 5FC + Flu. Ampho B 1 mg/kg/d alone much more rapidly fungicidal in vivo than Flu 400 mg/d *(CID 45:76&81, 2007).* Use of lipid-based Ampho B associated with lower mortality compared to Ampho B deoxycholate in solid organ transplant recipients *(CID 48:1566, 2009).* • Monitor 5-FC levels: peak 70-80 mg/L, trough 30-40 mg/L. Higher levels assoc. with bone marrow toxicity. No difference in outcome if given IV or po *(AAC 51:1038, 2007).* • 5-FC is renally cleared therefore if renal failure occurs during treatment with Ampho B, 5-FC dose needs adjustment. • Trend toward improved outcomes with fluconazole 400-800 mg combined with Ampho B versus Ampho B alone in AIDS patients *(CID 48:1775, 2009).* Role of other azoles uncertain: successful outcomes were observed in 14/29 (48%) subjects with cryptococcal meningitis treated with posaconazole *(JAC 56:745, 2005).* Voriconazole also may be effective. • **When to initiate antiretroviral therapy (ART)?** Defer ART to allow for 2-4 weeks of anti-fungal treatment. When ART was started 1-2 weeks after diagnosis of cryptococcal meningitis mortality was increased when compared to later initiation of ART *(NEJM 370:2487, 2014)* in Africa. Cohort study in US and Europe showed no harm in earlier initiation of ARV Rx *(CID 77(1):64-73, 2023)*
Suppression (chronic maintenance therapy) Discontinuation of antifungal rx can be considered among pts who remain asymptomatic, with CD4 >100/mm³ for ≥3 months. Some perform a lumbar puncture before discontinuation of maintenance rx. Reappearance of pos. serum CRAG may predict relapse	**Flu** 200 mg/day po [If CD4 count rises to >100/mm³ with effective antiretroviral rx, some authorities recommend dc suppressive rx. *See www.hivatis.org.* Authors would only dc if CSF culture negative.]	**Itra** 200 mg po q12h if Flu intolerant or failure. No data on Vori for maintenance.	Itraconazole less effective than fluconazole & not recommended because of higher relapse rate (23% vs 4%). Recurrence rate of 0.4 to 3.9 per 100 patient-years with discontinuation of suppressive therapy in 100 patients on ARV with CD4 >100 cells/mm³.

See page 2 for abbreviations. *All dosage recommendations are for adults (unless otherwise indicated) and assume normal renal function.*

TABLE 11A (8)

TYPE OF INFECTION/ORGANISM/ SITE OF INFECTION	ANTIMICROBIAL AGENTS OF CHOICE		COMMENTS
	PRIMARY	ALTERNATIVE	
Dermatophytosis			
Onychomycosis *(Tinea unguium)* (primarily cosmetic) **Laser rx FDA approved:** modestly effective, expensive *(Med Lett 55:15, 2013)*. Review: *JAMA 2018,319:397.*	**Fingernail Rx Options:** **Terbinafine**[1] 250 mg po q24h [children <20 kg: 62.5 mg/day, 20–40 kg: 125 mg/day, >40 kg: 250 mg/day] x 6 wks (79% effective) OR **Itra**[2] 200 mg po q24h x 3 mos.[NAI] OR **Itra** 200 mg po bid x 1 wk/mo x 2 mos OR **Flu** 150–300 mg po q wk x 3-6 mos.[NAI] Note: Cure rates for all options are low.		**Toenail Rx Options:** **Terbinafine**[1] 250 mg po q24h [children <20 kg: 62.5 mg/day, 20–40 kg: 125 mg/day, >40 kg: 250 mg/day] x 12 wks (76% effective) OR **Itra** 200 mg po q24h x 3 mos (59% effective) OR **Efinaconazole** 10% solution applied to nail once daily for 48 wks OR **Itra** 200 mg bid x 1 wk/mo. x 3–4 mos (63% effective)[NAI] OR **Flu** 150–300 mg po q wk x 6–12 mos (48% effective)[NAI] OR topical **Tavaborole** (Kerydin) or topical **Efinaconazole** (Jublia).
Tinea capitis ("ringworm") *(Trichophyton tonsurans, Microsporum canis*, N. America; other sp. elsewhere) *(PIDJ 18:191, 1999)* Emerging pathogen: *Trichophyton indotineae (See comment)*	**Terbinafine**[1] 250 mg po q 24h x 2-4 wks (adults); 4-6 mg/kg/day (children) 10-20 kg: 62.5 mg q24h x2 weeks 20-40 kg: 125 mg q24h x2 weeks >40 kg: 250 mg q24h x2 weeks	**Itra**[2] 5 mg/kg per day x 4 wks.[NFDA] **Flu** 6 mg/kg q wk x 8-12 wks.[NAI] Cap at 150 mg po q wk for adults **Griseo:** adults 500 mg po q24h x 6-8 wks; children age >2 years: Micro susp: 20-25 mg/kg/day; Ultramicro tabs: 10-15 mg/kg/day Dur: at least 6 wks, continue until clear	Durations of therapy are for T. tonsurans; treat for approx. twice as long for M. canis. All agents with similar cure rates (60-100%) in clinical studies. Addition of topical ketoconazole or selenium sulfate shampoo reduces transmissibility *(Int J Dermatol 39:261, 2000)*. Terbinafine-resistant *Trichophyton indotineae (JAMA 2024, 332:859)*.
Tinea corporis, cruris, or pedis *(Trichophyton rubrum, T. mentagrophytes, Epidermophyton floccosum)* "Athlete's foot, jock itch", and ringworm	**Topical rx:** Generally applied 2x/day. Available as creams, ointments, sprays, by prescription & "over the counter". Apply 2x/day for 2–3 wks. Recommend: Lotrimin Ultra or Lamisil AT; contain butenafine & terbinafine—both are fungicidal	**Terbinafine** 250 mg po q24h x 2 wks[NAI] OR **Keto** 200 mg po q24h x 4 wks OR **Flu** 150 mg po 1x/wk for 2–4 wks[NAI] **Griseo:** adults 500 mg po q24h times 4–6 wks, children 10–20 mg/kg per day. Duration: 2-4 wks for corporis, 4-8 wks for pedis.	**Keto** po often effective in severe recalcitrant infection. Follow for hepatotoxicity; many drug-drug interactions.
Tinea versicolor *(Malassezia furfur or Pityrosporum orbiculare)* Rule out erythrasma—*see Table 1, page 61*	**Keto** (400 mg po single dose)[NAI] or (200 mg q24h x 7 days) or (2% cream 1x q24h x 2 wks)	**Flu** 400 mg po single dose or **Itra** 400 mg po q24h x 3–7 days	**Keto** (po) times 1 dose was 97% effective in 1 study. Another alternative: **Selenium sulfide** (Selsun), 2.5% lotion, apply as lather, leave on 10 min then wash off, 1/day x 7 day or 3–5/wk times 2–4 wks.
Fusariosis			
Third most common cause of invasive mold infections, after *Aspergillus* and *Mucorales* and related molds, in patients with hematologic malignancies *(Mycoses 52:197, 2009)*. Pneumonia, skin infections, bone and joint infections, and disseminated disease occur in severely immunocompromised patients. In contrast to other molds, blood cultures are frequently positive. *Fusarium solani, F. oxysporum, F. verticillioides* and *F. moniliforme* account for approx. 90% of isolates *(Clin Micro Rev 20: 695, 2007)* Frequently fatal, outcome depends on decreasing the level of immunosuppression.	**Lipid-based Ampho B** 5-10 mg/kg/d IV; OR **Ampho B** 1-1.5 mg/kg/d IV PLUS **Vori** 6 mg/kg po/IV q12 x 2 doses and then 4 mg/kg po/IV q12, while awaiting speciation and susceptibilities	**Posa** delayed release tabs/IV loading dose of 300 mg q12h x 2 doses then 300 mg daily (posaconazole oral suspension 200 mg po qid); OR **Vori** IV: 6 mg per kg q12h times 1 day, then 4 mg per kg q12h; po: 400 mg q12h, then 200 mg q12h. *See comments.*	**Surgical debridement** for localized disease. *Fusarium* spp. resistance to most antifungal agents, including echinocandins. *F. solani* and *F. verticillioides* typically are resistant to azoles. *F. oxysporum* and *F. moniliforme* may be susceptible to voriconazole and posaconazole. Role of combination therapy not well defined but case reports of response *(Mycoses 50: 227, 2007)*. Given variability in susceptibilities can consider combination therapy with Vori and Ampho B awaiting speciation. Outcome dependent on reduction or discontinuation of immunosuppression. Duration of therapy depends on response; long-term suppressive therapy for patients remaining on immunosuppressive therapy.

[1] **Serious but rare cases of hepatic failure** have been reported in pts receiving Terbinafine & should not be used in those with chronic or active liver disease *(see Table 11B, page 187)*.
[2] Use of Itraconazole has been associated with myocardial dysfunction and with onset of congestive heart failure.
See page 2 for abbreviations. All dosage recommendations are for adults (unless otherwise indicated) and assume normal renal function.

TABLE 11A (9)

TYPE OF INFECTION/ORGANISM/ SITE OF INFECTION	ANTIMICROBIAL AGENTS OF CHOICE		COMMENTS
	PRIMARY	ALTERNATIVE	
Histoplasmosis *(Histoplasma capsulatum)*: See *IDSA Guideline: CID 45:807, 2007.* Best diagnostic test is urinary, serum, or CSF histoplasma antigen: MiraVista Diagnostics (1-866-647-2847)			
Acute pulmonary histoplasmosis	**Mild to moderate disease, symptoms <4 wks:** No rx; If symptoms last over one month: **Itra** oral sol'n 200 mg po tid for 3 days then once or twice daily for 6-12 wks. **Moderately severe or severe: Liposomal Ampho B,** 3-5 mg/kg/d IV or **ABLC** 5 mg/kg/d IV or Ampho B 0.7-1.0 mg/kg/d for 1-2 wks, then Itra 200 mg tid for 3 days, then bid for 12 wks. + **methylprednisolone** 0.5-1 mg/kg/d for 1-2 wks.		Ampho B for patients at low risk of nephrotoxicity. Check for Itra drug-drug interactions.
Chronic cavitary pulmonary histoplasmosis	**Itra** oral sol'n 200 mg po tid for 3 days then once or twice daily for at least 12 mos (some prefer 18-24 mos).		Document therapeutic itraconazole blood levels at 2 wks. Relapses occur in 9-15% of patients.
Mediastinal lymphadenitis, mediastinal granuloma, pericarditis; and rheumatologic syndromes	**Mild cases:** Antifungal therapy not indicated. Nonsteroidal anti-inflammatory drug for pericarditis or rheumatologic syndromes. If no response to non-steroidals, **Prednisone** 0.5-1 mg/kg/d tapered over 1-2 weeks for 1) pericarditis with hemodynamic compromise, 2) lymphadenitis with obstruction or compression syndromes, or 3) severe rheumatologic syndromes. **Itra** 200 oral sol'n mg po once or twice daily for 6-12 wks for moderately severe to severe cases, or if prednisone is administered.		Check Itra blood levels to document therapeutic concentrations. Check for Itra drug-drug interactions.
Progressive disseminated histoplasmosis	**Mild to moderate disease: Itra** 200 mg po tid for 3 days then bid for at least 12 mos. **Moderately severe to severe disease: Liposomal Ampho B,** 3 mg/kg/d or **ABLC** 5 mg/kg/d for 1-2 weeks then **Itra** 200 mg tid for 3 days, then bid for at least 12 mos.		**Ampho B** 0.7-1.0 mg/kg/d may be used for patients at low risk of nephrotoxicity. Confirm therapeutic Itra blood levels. Azoles are teratogenic; Itra should be avoided in pregnancy; use a lipid ampho formulation. Urinary antigen levels useful for monitoring response to therapy and relapse.
CNS histoplasmosis	**Liposomal Ampho B,** 5 mg/kg/d, for a total of 175 mg/kg over 4-6 wks, then **Itra** 200 mg 2-3x a day for at least 12 mos. Vori likely effective for CNS disease or Itra failures. *(Arch Neurology 65: 666, 2008; J Antimicro Chemo 57:1235, 2006).*		Monitor CNS histo antigen, monitor Itra blood levels. PCR may be better for Dx than histo antigen. Absorption of Itra (check levels) and CNS penetration may be an issue; case reports of success with Fluconazole *(Braz J Infect Dis 12:555, 2008)* and Posaconazole *(Drugs 65:1553, 2005)* following Ampho B therapy.
Prophylaxis (immunocompromised patients)	**Itra** 200 mg po daily. Check for Itra drug-drug interactions.		Consider primary **prophylaxis in HIV-infected** patients with <150 CD4 cells/mm³ in high prevalence areas. Secondary prophylaxis (i.e., suppressive therapy) indicated in HIV-infected patients with <150 CD4 cells/mm³ and other immunocompromised patients in who immunosuppression cannot be reversed

See page 2 for abbreviations. All dosage recommendations are for adults (unless otherwise indicated) and assume normal renal function.

TABLE 11A (10)

TYPE OF INFECTION/ORGANISM/ SITE OF INFECTION	ANTIMICROBIAL AGENTS OF CHOICE		COMMENTS
	PRIMARY	ALTERNATIVE	
Madura foot *(See Nocardia & Scedosporium)*			
Mucormycosis & other related species—*Rhizopus, Rhizomucor, Lichtheimia (CID 54:1629, 2012).* Rhinocerebral, pulmonary due to angioinvasion with tissue necrosis.	**Liposomal Ampho B** 5-10 mg/kg/day; OR **Ampho B** 1-1.5 mg/kg/day.	**Posaconazole** delayed-release tabs/ IV loading dose of 300 mg q12 x 2 doses then 300 mg daily (posaconazole oral suspension 200 mg po QID) **Isavuconazonium sulfate** loading dose of 372 mg (equivalent to isavuconazole 200 mg) IV/po q8 x 6 doses then 372 mg IV/po daily Recommend checking MICs to above agents prior to use	**Ampho B** (ABLC) monotherapy relatively ineffective with 20% success rate vs 69% for other polyenes *(CID 47:364, 2008)*. Complete or partial response rates of 60-80% in **Posa** salvage protocols *(JAC 61, Suppl 1, i35, 2008)*. **Isavuconazole:** Approved for treatment of invasive mucor infection based on historical controls *(Ln 2016;387:760)* **Combination therapy:** Adjunctive echinocandin to liposomal Amphotericin B is promising given safety profile, synergy in murine models, and observational clinical data *(Clin Infect Dis 54(S1):S73, 2012)*. Resistant to **Vori:** prolonged use of voriconazole prophylaxis predisposes to mucormycosis infections. Total duration of therapy based on response: continue therapy until 1) resolution of clinical signs and symptoms of infection, 2) resolution or stabilization of radiographic abnormalities; and 3) resolution of underlying immunosuppression. Posaconazole for secondary prophylaxis for those on immunosuppressive therapy *(CID 48:1743, 2009)*.
Paracoccidioidomycosis (South American blastomycosis) *P. brasiliensis*	Mild-moderate disease: **Itra** 200 mg po daily for 6-9 months for mild and x 12-18 months for moderate disease. Severe disease: **Ampho B** 0.7-1 mg/kg IV daily to a cumulative total of 30 mg/kg followed by **Itra** 200 mg po daily for at least 12 months	**Keto** 200-400 mg daily x 6-18 months; OR **Ampho B** total dose >30 mg/kg OR **TMP/SMX** 800/160 mg bid-tid x 30 days, then 400/80 mg/day indefinitely (up to 3-5 years)	Improvement in >90% pts on Itra or Keto.[NAI] **Ampho B** reserved for severe cases and for those intolerant to other agents. TMP-SMX suppression life-long in HIV+. Check for Itra or Keto drug-drug interactions.
Lobomycosis (keloidal blastomycosis)/ P. loboi	**Surgical excision**, **clofazimine** or **itra**.		
Penicilliosis (***Talaromyces marneffei***, *formerly Penicillium marneffei)*: Common disseminated fungal infection in AIDS pts in SE Asia (esp. Thailand & Vietnam).	**Ampho B** 0.5–1 mg/kg per day times 2 wks followed by **Itra** 400 mg/day x 10 wks followed by 200 mg/day po **indefinitely for HIV-infected pts.**	For less sick patients **Itra** oral sol'n 200 mg po tid x 3 days, then 200 mg po bid x 12 wks, then 200 mg po q24h. (IV if unable to take po) (Oral sol'n better absorbed)	3rd most common OI in AIDS pts in SE Asia following TBc and cryptococcal meningitis. Prolonged fever, lymphadenopathy, hepatomegaly. Skin nodules are umbilicated (mimic cryptococcal infection or molluscum contagiosum). Preliminary data suggests Vori effective: *CID 43:1060, 2006*.
Phaeohyphomycosis, Black molds, Dematiaceous fungi *(See Clin Microbiol Rev 27:527, 2014)* Most clinically relevant species are within the genera of *Exophiala, Cladophialophora, Coniosporium, Cyphellophora, Fonsecaea, Phialophora*, and *Rhinocladiella*.	**Surgery + Itra** oral sol'n 400 mg/day po, duration not defined, probably 6 mo[NAI]	Voriconazole 6 mg/kg po bid x 1 day and then 4 mg/kg po bid or Posaconazole (suspension) 400 mg po bid	Both Vori and Posa have demonstrated efficacy *(Med Mycol 48:769, 2010; Med Mycol 43:91, 2005)* often in addition to surgical therapy. Consider obtaining anti-fungal susceptibility testing.

TABLE 11A (11)

TYPE OF INFECTION/ORGANISM/ SITE OF INFECTION	ANTIMICROBIAL AGENTS OF CHOICE		COMMENTS
	PRIMARY	ALTERNATIVE	
Pneumocystis pneumonia (PJP) caused by ***Pneumocystis jirovecii***. Ref: *JAMA 301:2578, 2009.*			
Not acutely ill, able to take po meds. PaO_2 >70 mmHg Diagnosis: sputum PCR. Serum Beta-D Glucan may help; reasonable sensitivity & specificity, but also many false positives *(JCM 51:3478, 2013).*	(**TMP-SMX-DS**, 2 tabs po q8h x 21 days) OR (**Dapsone** 100 mg po q24h + **TMP** 5 mg/kg po tid x 21 days)	[**Clinda** 300–450 mg po q6h + **Primaquine** 15 mg base po q24h] x 21 days OR **Atovaquone** suspension 750 mg po bid with food x 21 days	Mutations in gene of the enzyme target (dihydropteroate synthetase) of sulfamethoxazole identified. Unclear whether mutations result in resist to TMP-SMX or dapsone + TMP *(EID 10:1721, 2004).* Dapsone ref.: *CID 27:191, 1998.* **After 21 days, chronic suppression in AIDS pts *(see below—post-treatment suppression).***
	NOTE: Concomitant use of corticosteroids usually reserved for sicker pts with PaO_2 <70 *(see below)*		
Acutely ill, po rx not possible. PaO_2 <70 mmHg. Still unclear whether antiretroviral therapy (ART) should be started during treatment of PCP *(CID 46: 634, 2008).*	[**Prednisone** (15–30 min. before **TMP-SMX**): 40 mg po bid times 5 days, then 40 mg q24h times 5 days, then 20 mg po q24h times 11 days] + [**TMP-SMX** (15 mg of TMP component per kg per day) IV div. q6–8h times 21 days]	**Prednisone** as in primary rx + [(**Clinda** 600 mg IV q8h) + (**Primaquine** 30 mg base po q24h)] times 21 days OR **Pentamidine** 4 mg per kg per day IV times 21 days. **Caspo** active in animal models: *CID 36:1445, 2003*	**After 21 days, chronic suppression in AIDS pts** *(see post-treatment suppression).* **PJP can occur in absence of HIV infection & steroids** *(CID 25:215 & 219, 1997).* Wait 4–8 days before declaring treatment failure& switching to clinda + primaquine or pentamidine *(JAIDS 48:63, 2008),* or adding caspofungin *(Transplant 84:685, 2007).*
	Can substitute IV prednisolone (reduce dose 25%) for po prednisone		
Primary prophylaxis and post-treatment suppression	(**TMP-SMX-DS or -SS**, 1 tab po q24h or 1 DS 3x/wk) OR (**Dapsone** 100 mg po q24h). DC when CD4 >200 x/3 mos *(NEJM 344:159, 2001).*	(**Pentamidine** 300 mg in 6 mL sterile water by aerosol q4 wks) OR (**Dapsone** 200 mg po + **Pyrimethamine** 75 mg po + **folinic acid** 25 mg po —**all once a week**) or **Atovaquone** 1500 mg po q24h with food.	TMP-SMX-DS regimen provides cross-protection vs Toxo and other bacterial infections. Dapsone + pyrimethamine protects vs Toxo. Atovaquone suspension 1500 mg once daily as effective as daily dapsone *(NEJM 339:1889, 1998)* or inhaled pentamidine *(JID 180:369, 1999).*
Lomentospora prolificans (formerly Scedosporium prolificans)	Surgical debridement and reduction of immunosuppression, consider addition of **Vori** although usually resistant.	Newer, non-FDA approved antifungal are promising	
Scedosporium apiospermum	**Vori** 6 mg/kg IV/po q12h on day 1, then 4 mg/kg IV/po q12h.	**Posa** delayed release tabs/IV loading dose of 300 mg q12h x 2 doses then 300 mg daily (posaconazole oral suspension 200 mg po qid)	

See page 2 for abbreviations. All dosage recommendations are for adults (unless otherwise indicated) and assume normal renal function.

TABLE 11A (12)

TYPE OF INFECTION/ORGANISM/ SITE OF INFECTION	ANTIMICROBIAL AGENTS OF CHOICE		COMMENTS
	PRIMARY	ALTERNATIVE	
Sporotrichosis *IDSA Guideline: CID 45:1255, 2007.*			
Cutaneous/Lymphocutaneous	**Itra** oral sol'n po 200 mg/day for 2-4 wks after all lesions resolved, usually 3-6 mos.	If no response, **Itra** 200 mg po bid or **Terbinafine** 500 mg po bid or **SSKI** 5 drops (eye drops) tid & increase to 40-50 drops tid	**Flu** 400-800 mg daily only if no response to primary or alternative suggestions. Pregnancy or nursing: local hyperthermia *(see below)*.
Osteoarticular	**Itra** oral sol'n 200 mg po bid x 12 mos.	**Liposomal Ampho B** 3-5 mg/kg/d IV or **ABLC** 5 mg/kg/d IV or **Ampho B Deoxycholate** 0.7-1 mg/kg IV daily; if response, change to **Itra** oral sol'n 200 mg po bid x total 12 mos.	After 2 wks of therapy, document adequate serum levels of itraconazole.
Pulmonary	If severe, **Lipid Ampho B** 3-5 mg/kg IV or **standard Ampho B** 0.7-1 mg/kg IV once daily until response, then **Itra** 200 mg po bid. Total of 12 mos.	Less severe: **Itra** 200 mg po bid x 12 mos.	After 2 weeks of therapy document adequate serum levels of Itra. Surgical resection plus Ampho B for localized pulmonary disease.
Meningeal or Disseminated	**Lipid Ampho B** 5 mg/kg IV once daily x 4-6 wks, then—if better—**Itra** 200 mg po bid for total of 12 mos.	AIDS/Other immunosuppressed pts: chronic therapy with **Itra** oral sol'n 200 mg po once daily.	After 2 weeks, document adequate serum levels of Itra.
Pregnancy and children	**Pregnancy:** Cutaneous—local hyperthermia. Severe: **Lipid Ampho B** 3-5 mg/kg IV once daily. **Avoid Itra.**	**Children:** Cutaneous: **Itra** 6-10 mg/kg (max of 400 mg) daily. Alternative is **SSKI** 1 drop tid increasing to max of 1 drop/kg or 40-50 drops tid/day, whichever is lowest.	For children with disseminated sporotrichosis: Standard **Ampho B** 0.7 mg/kg IV once daily & after response, Itra 6-10 mg/kg (max 400 mg) once daily.

TABLE 11B – ANTIFUNGAL DRUGS: DOSAGE, ADVERSE EFFECTS, COMMENTS

DRUG NAME, GENERIC (TRADE)/ USUAL DOSAGE	ADVERSE EFFECTS/COMMENTS
Non-lipid Amphotericin B deoxycholate (Fungizone): 0.5-0.7 mg/kg IV per day as single infusion **Ampho B predictably not active vs. Scedosporium, Candida lusitaniae & Aspergillus terreus**	**Admin:** Ampho B is a colloidal suspension that must be prepared in electrolyte-free D5W at 0.1 mg/mL to avoid precipitation. No need to protect suspensions from light. Infusions cause chills/fever, myalgia, anorexia, nausea, rarely hemodynamic collapse/hypotension. Postulated due to proinflammatory cytokines, doesn't appear to be histamine release *(Pharmacol 23:966, 2003)*. **Infusion duration usu. 4+ hrs.** No difference found in 1 vs 4 hr infus. except chills/fever occurred sooner with 1 hr infus. Febrile reactions ↓ with repeat doses. Rare pulmonary reactions (severe dyspnea & focal infiltrates suggest pulmonary edema) assoc with rapid infus. **Severe rigors respond to meperidine (25–50 mg IV).** Premedication with acetaminophen, diphenhydramine, hydrocortisone (25–50 mg) and heparin (1000 units) had no influence on rigors/fever. If cytokine postulate correct, NSAIDs or high-dose steroids may prove efficacious but their use may risk worsening infection under rx or increased risk of **nephrotoxicity** (i.e., NSAIDs). Clinical side effects ↓ with ↑ age. **Toxicity:** Major concern is nephrotoxicity. Manifest initially by kaliuresis and **hypokalemia**, then fall in serum bicarbonate (may proceed to renal tubular acidosis), ↓ in renal erythropoietin and anemia, and rising BUN/serum creatinine. Hypomagnesemia may occur. Can reduce risk of renal injury by **(a) pre- & post-infusion hydration with 500 mL saline (if clinical status allows salt load), (b)** avoidance of other nephrotoxins, eg, radiocontrast, aminoglycosides, cis-platinum, **(c)** use of lipid prep of Ampho B.
Lipid-based Ampho B products[1]**: Amphotericin B lipid complex (ABLC)** (Abelcet)**:** 5 mg/kg per day as single infusion	**Admin:** Consists of Ampho B complexed with 2 lipid bilayer ribbons. Compared to standard Ampho B, larger volume of distribution, rapid blood clearance and high tissue concentrations (liver, spleen, lung). Dosage: **5 mg/kg once daily;** infuse at 2.5 mg/kg per hr; adult and ped. dose the same. Saline pre- and post-dose lessens toxicity. Do NOT use an in-line filter. Do not dilute with saline or mix with other drugs or electrolytes.[2] **Toxicity:** Fever and chills 14–18%; nausea 9%, vomiting 8%; serum creatinine ↑ in 11%; renal failure 5%; anemia 4%; ↓ K 5%; rash 4%. A fatal fat embolism following ABLC infusion *(Exp Mol Path 177:246, 2004)*. Majority of pts intolerant of liposomal Ampho B can tolerate ABLC *(CID 56:701, 2013)*.
Liposomal Amphotericin B (**LAB,** AmBisome)**:** 3–5 mg/kg IV per day as single infusion. If intolerant, majority OK with lipid form *(CID 56:701, 2013)*.	**Admin:** Consists of vesicular bilayer liposome with Ampho B intercalated within the membrane. Dosage: **3–5 mg/kg per day** IV as single dose infused over a period of approx. 120 min. If tolerated, infusion time reduced to 60 min. *(See footnote*[2]*)*. Saline pre- and post-dose lessens toxicity. **Major toxicity:** Gen less than Ampho B. Nephrotoxicity 18.7% vs 33.7% for Ampho B, chills 47% vs 75%, nausea 39.7% vs 38.7%, vomiting 31.8% vs 43.9%, rash 24% for both, ↓ Ca 18.4% vs 20.9%, ↓ K 20.4% vs 25.6%, ↓ mg 20.4% vs 25.6%. Acute reactions common with liposomal Ampho B, 20– 40%. 86% occur within 5 min of infusion, incl chest pain, dyspnea, hypoxia or severe abdom, flank or leg pain; 14% dev flushing & urticaria near end of 4 hr infusion. All responded to diphenhydramine (1 mg/kg) & interruption of infusion. Reactions may be due to complement activation by liposome *(CID 36:1213, 2003)*.
Caspofungin (Cancidas) 70 mg IV on day 1 followed by 50 mg IV q24h (reduce to 35 mg IV q24h with moderate hepatic insufficiency)	An echinocandin which inhibits synthesis of β-(1,3)-D-glucan. Fungicidal against candida (MIC <2 mcg/mL) including those resistant to other antifungals & active against aspergillus (MIC 0.4–2.7 mcg/mL). Approved indications: empirical rx for febrile, neutropenic pts; rx of candidemia, candida intraabdominal abscesses, peritonitis, & pleural space infections; esophageal candidiasis; & invasive aspergillosis in pts refractory to or intolerant of other therapies. Serum levels on rec. dosages = peak 12, trough 1.3 (24 hrs) mcg/mL. **Toxicity:** remarkably non-toxic. Most common adverse effect: pruritus at infusion site & headache, fever, chills, vomiting, & diarrhea assoc with infusion. ↑ serum creatinine in 8% on caspo vs 21% short-course Ampho B in 422 pts with candidemia *(Ln, Oct. 12, 2005, online)*. Drug metab in liver & dosage ↓ to 35 mg in moderate to severe hepatic failure. Class C for preg (embryotoxic in rats & rabbits). Reversible thrombocytopenia reported *(Pharmacother 24:1408, 2004)*. **No drug in CSF, urine or vitreous humor of the eye.**
Micafungin (Mycamine) 50 mg IV q24h for prophylaxis post-bone marrow stem cell trans; 100 mg IV q24h candidemia, 150 mg IV q24h candida esophagitis.	Approved for rx of esophageal candidiasis & prophylaxis against candida infections in HSCT[3] recipients. Active against most strains of candida sp. & aspergillus sp. incl those resist to fluconazole such as C. glabrata & C. krusei. No antagonism seen when combo with other antifungal drugs. No dosage adjust for severe renal failure or moderate hepatic impairment. Watch for drug-drug interactions with sirolimus or nifedipine. Micafungin well tolerated & common adverse events incl nausea 2.8%, vomiting 2.4%, & headache 2.4%. Transient ↑ LFTs, BUN, creatinine reported; rare cases of significant hepatitis & renal insufficiency. *See CID 42:1171, 2006.* **No drug in CSF or urine**. ECMO: 200 mg IV qd *(Crit Care 22:289, 2018)*.

[1] Published data from patients intolerant of or refractory to conventional Ampho B deoxycholate. **None of the lipid Ampho B preps has shown superior efficacy compared to Ampho B in prospective trials (except liposomal Ampho B was more effective vs Ampho B in rx of disseminated histoplasmosis at 2 wks). Dosage equivalency has not been established** *(CID 36:1500, 2003)*. Nephrotoxicity ↓ with all lipid Ampho B preps.

[2] Comparisons between Abelcet & AmBisome suggest higher infusion-assoc. toxicity (rigors) & febrile episodes with Abelcet (70% vs 36%) but higher frequency of mild hepatic toxicity with AmBisome (59% vs 38%, p=0.05). Mild elevations in serum creatinine were observed in 1/3 of both *(BJ Hemat 103:198, 1998; Focus on Fungal Inf #9, 1999; Bone Marrow Tx 20:39, 1997; CID 26:1383, 1998)*.

[3] HSCT = hematopoietic stem cell transplant.

See page 2 for abbreviations. *All dosage recommendations are for adults (unless otherwise indicated) and assume normal renal function.*

TABLE 11B (2)

DRUG NAME, GENERIC (TRADE)/ USUAL DOSAGE	ADVERSE EFFECTS/COMMENTS
Anidulafungin (Eraxis) For Candidemia; 200 mg IV on day 1 followed by 100 mg/day IV). Esophageal candida: 100 mg IV x 1, then 50 mg IV once/d.	An echinocandin with antifungal activity (cidal) against candida sp. & aspergillus sp. including Ampho B- & triazole-resistant strains. FDA approved for treatment of esophageal candidiasis (EC), candidemia, and other complicated Candida infections. Effective in clinical trials of esophageal candidiasis & in 1 trial was superior to fluconazole in rx of invasive candidiasis/candidemia in 245 pts (75.6% vs 60.2%). Like other echinocandins, remarkably non-toxic; most common side-effects: nausea, vomiting, ↓ mg, ↓ K & headache in 11–13% of pts. No dose adjustments for renal or hepatic insufficiency. *See CID 43:215, 2006.* **No drug in CSF or urine**.
Fluconazole (Diflucan) 100 mg tabs 150 mg tabs 200 mg tabs 400 mg IV Oral suspension: 50 mg per 5 mL.	IV=oral dose because of excellent bioavailability. **Pharmacology:** absorbed po, water solubility enables IV. For peak serum levels *(see Table 9A, page 119)*. T½ 30hr (range 20–50 hr). 12% protein bound. **CSF levels 50–90% of serum in normals,** ↑ in meningitis. No effect on mammalian steroid metabolism. **Drug-drug interactions common**. Side-effects overall 16% [more common in HIV+ pts (21%)]. Nausea 3.7%, headache 1.9%, skin rash 1.8%, abdominal pain 1.7%, vomiting 1.7%, diarrhea 1.5%, ↑ SGOT 20%. Alopecia (scalp, pubic crest) in 12–20% pts on ≥400 mg po q24h after median of 3 mos (reversible in approx. 6mo). Rare: severe hepatotoxicity *(CID 41:301, 2005)*, exfoliative dermatitis. **Note: Candida krusei and Candida glabrata resistant to Flu.**
Flucytosine (Ancobon, 5-FC) 500 mg cap **Expensive:** $11,000 for 100 capsules (Sep 2015 US price)	AEs: Overall 30%. GI 6% (diarrhea, anorexia, nausea, vomiting); hematologic 22% [leukopenia, thrombocytopenia, when serum level >100 mcg/mL (esp. in azotemic pts)]; hepatotoxicity (asymptomatic ↑ SGOT, reversible); skin rash 7%; aplastic anemia (rare—2 or 3 cases). False ↑ in serum creatinine on EKTACHEM analyzer. Bioavailability 100%. Good levels in CSF, eye & urine.
Griseofulvin (Fulvicin, Grifulvin, Grisactin) 500 mg, susp 125 mg/mL.	Photosensitivity, urticaria, GI upset, fatigue, leukopenia (rare). Interferes with warfarin drugs. Increases blood and urine porphyrins, should not be used in patients with porphyria. Minor disulfiram-like reactions. Exacerbation of systemic lupus erythematosus.
Ibrexafungerp (Brexafemme) 150 mg tabs. Usual dose: 300 mg po bid x2 doses, with or without food	Triterpenoid antifungal indicated for the treatment of vulvovaginal candidiasis in adults and post-menarchal pediatric females. Inhibits the biosynthesis of β-(1,3)-D-glucan, like echinocandins (targets are different, so limited cross-resistance expected). **Contraindicated in pregnancy.** May cause fetal harm, based on animal studies. Before beginning treatment, verify pregnancy status in females of reproductive potential. Effective contraception should be used during treatment and for four days after second (final) dose. Adverse effects: GI, dizziness.
Imidazoles, topical For vaginal and/or skin use	Not recommended in 1st trimester of pregnancy. Local reactions: 0.5-1.5%: dyspareunia, mild vaginal or vulvar erythema, burning, pruritus, urticaria, rash. Rarely similar symptoms in sexual partner.
Isavuconazonium sulfate (prodrug Isavuconazole) (Cresemba) po: 186 mg caps IV: 372 mg vials No drug in CSF. Ref: *Med Lett 2016,58:33*	An azole antifungal agent for treatment of invasive aspergillosis and invasive mucormycosis in adults. **Contraindications:** Coadministration with strong CYP3A4 inhibitors, e.g., Ketoconazole or high-dose Ritonavir, or strong CYP3A4 inducers, e.g., Rifampin, carbamazepine, St. John's wort, or long-acting barbiturates is contraindicated. Do not use in patients with shortened QT interval. **Dosing: Isavuconazonium sulfate** loading dose of 372 mg (equivalent to isavuconazole 200 mg) IV/po q8 x 6 doses then 372 mg IV/po daily. **AEs:** Most common: nausea, vomiting, diarrhea, headache, elevated liver chemistry tests, hypokalemia, constipation, dyspnea, cough, peripheral edema, and back pain. Hepatic: increased ALT, AST. **Teratogenic.**
Itraconazole (Sporanox) 100 mg cap 10 mg/mL oral solution IV usual dose 200 mg bid x 4 doses followed by 200 mg q24h for a max of 14 days	**Itraconazole tablet & solution forms not interchangeable, solution preferred.** Many authorities recommend measuring drug serum concentration after 2 wks to ensure satisfactory absorption. To obtain highest plasma concentration, tablet is given with food & acidic drinks (e.g., cola) while solution is taken in fasted state; under these conditions, the peak conc. of capsule is approx. 3 mcg/mL & of solution 5.4 mcg/mL. Peak levels reached faster (2.2 vs 5 hrs) with solution. **Peak plasma concentrations after IV injection (200 mg) compared to oral capsule (200 mg): 2.8 mcg/mL (on day 7 of rx) vs 2 mcg/mL (on day 36 of rx).** Protein-binding for both preparations is over 99%, which explains virtual absence of penetration into CSF **(do not use to treat meningitis).** Adverse effects: dose-related nausea 10%, diarrhea 8%, vomiting 6%, & abdominal discomfort 5.7%. Allergic rash 8.6%, ↑ bilirubin 6%, edema 3.5%, & hepatitis 2.7% reported. ↑ doses may produce hypokalemia 8% & ↑ blood pressure 3.2%. Delirium, peripheral neuropathy & tremor reported *(J Neur Neurosurg Psych 81:327, 2010)*. **Reported to produce impairment in cardiac function.** Severe liver failure req transplant in pts receiving pulse rx for onychomycosis: FDA reports 24 cases with 11 deaths out of 50 mill people who received the drug prior to 2001. Other concern, as with fluconazole and ketoconazole, is **drug-drug interactions**. Some can be life-threatening.

TABLE 11B (3)

DRUG NAME, GENERIC (TRADE)/ USUAL DOSAGE	ADVERSE EFFECTS/COMMENTS
Ketoconazole (Nizoral) 200 mg tab	**Gastric acid required for absorption**—cimetidine, omeprazole, antacids block absorption. In achlorhydria, dissolve tablet in 4 mL 0.2N HCl, drink with a straw. Coca-Cola ↑ absorption by 65%. CSF levels "none". **Drug-drug interactions important. Some interactions can be life-threatening.** **Dose- dependent nausea and vomiting.** Liver toxicity of hepatocellular type reported in about 1:10,000 exposed pts—usually after several days to weeks of exposure. At doses of ≥800 mg per day serum testosterone and plasma cortisol levels fall. With high doses, adrenal (Addisonian) crisis reported.
Miconazole (Monistat IV) 200 mg—*not available in U.S.*	IV miconazole indicated in patient critically ill with Scedosporium (Pseudallescheria boydii) infection. Very toxic due to vehicle needed to get drug into solution.
Nystatin (Mycostatin) 30 gm cream 500,000 units oral tab	Topical: virtually no adverse effects. Less effective than imidazoles and triazoles. po: large doses give occasional GI distress and diarrhea.
Posaconazole (Noxafil) **Suspension** (40 mg/mL): 400 mg po bid with meals (if not taking meals, 200 mg qid). 200 mg po tid (with food) for prophylaxis. **Delayed-release tabs** (100 mg): 300 mg bid x 1 day and then 300 mg daily for prophylaxis. **Intravenous formulation:** 300 mg IV bid x 1 day the 300 mg daily (prophylaxis). **Takes 7-10 days to achieve steady state.**	**Suspension is dosed differently than delayed-release tablets (not interchangeable) – check dose carefully.** An oral triazole with activity against a wide range of fungi refractory to other antifungal rx including: aspergillosis, mucormycosis (variability by species), fusariosis, Scedosporium (Pseudallescheria), phaeohyphomycosis, histoplasmosis, refractory candidiasis, refractory coccidioidomycosis, refractory cryptococcosis, & refractory chromoblastomycosis. **Should be taken with high fat meal for maximum absorption.** Approved for treatment of invasive aspergillosis and prophylaxis of invasive aspergillus and candidiasis. Clinical response in 75% of 176 AIDS pts with azole-refractory oral/esophageal candidiasis. Posaconazole has similar toxicities as other triazoles: nausea 9%, vomiting 6%, abd. pain 5%, headache 5%, diarrhea, ↑ ALT, AST, & rash (3% each). In pts rx for >6 mos., serious side-effects have included adrenal insufficiency, nephrotoxicity, & QTc interval prolongation. Significant drug-drug interactions; inhibits CYP3A4. Consider monitoring serum concentrations *(AAC 53:24, 2009)*. **100 mg delayed-release tablets:** loading dose of 300 mg (three 100 mg delayed-release tablets) twice daily on the first day, followed by a once-daily maintenance dose of 300 mg (three 100 mg delayed-release tablets) starting on the second day of therapy. Approved for prophylaxis only and not treatment. Tablets allow patients to achieve better levels than the suspension. Treatment dose unknown but prophylactic dose often achieves therapeutic levels. **The tablet and solution are not interchangeable.** Intravenous formulation approved for prophylaxis at 300 mg IV daily after a loading dose of 300 mg bid x 1 day. Consider therapeutic drug monitoring with a goal trough of >0.7 for prophylaxis and >1.0 *for treatment. JAC 69:1162, 2014.*
Rezafungin (Rezzayo) 400 mg IV loading dose, then 200 mg IV once weekly	An echinocandin antifungal that is FDA-approved (Mar 2023) for treatment of candidemia and invasive candidiasis in persons age ≥18 years
Terbinafine (Lamisil) 250 mg tab Discontinued in U.S. in May 2017.	In pts given terbinafine for onychomycosis, rare cases (8) of idiosyncratic & symptomatic hepatic injury & more rarely liver failure leading to death or liver transplant. The drug is **not recommended** for pts with **chronic or active liver disease;** hepatotoxicity may occur in pts with or without pre-existing disease. Pretreatment serum transaminases (ALT & AST) advised & alternate rx used for those with abnormal levels. Pts started on terbinafine should be warned about symptoms suggesting liver dysfunction (persistent nausea, anorexia, fatigue, vomiting, RUQ pain, jaundice, dark urine or pale stools). If symptoms develop, drug should be discontinued & liver function immediately evaluated. In controlled trials, changes in ocular lens and retina reported—clinical significance unknown. Major drug-drug interaction is 100% ↑ in rate of clearance by rifampin. **AEs:** usually mild, transient and rarely caused discontinuation of rx. % with AE, terbinafine vs placebo: nausea/diarrhea 2.6–5.6 vs 2.9; rash 5.6 vs 2.2; taste abnormality 2.8 vs 0.7. Inhibits CYP2D6 enzymes. An acute generalized exanthematous pustulosis and subacute cutaneous lupus erythematosus reported.

TABLE 11B (4)

DRUG NAME, GENERIC (TRADE)/ USUAL DOSAGE	ADVERSE EFFECTS/COMMENTS
Voriconazole (Vfend) **IV: Loading dose 6 mg per kg q12h times 1 day, then 4 mg per kg q12h IV** for invasive aspergillus & serious mold infections; **3 mg per kg IV q12h** for serious candida infections. **Oral: >40 kg body weight:** 400 mg po q12h, then 200 mg po q12h. **<40 kg body weight:** 200 mg po q12h, then 100 mg po q12h **Take oral dose 1 hour before or 1 hour after eating.** Oral suspension (40 mg per mL). Oral suspension dosing: Same as for oral tabs. Reduce to ½ maintenance dose for moderate hepatic insufficiency	A triazole with activity against Aspergillus sp., **including Ampho resistant strains of A. terreus.** Active vs Candida sp. (including krusei), Fusarium sp., & various molds. Steady state serum levels reach 2.5–4 mcg per mL. Up to 20% of patients with subtherapeutic levels with oral administration: check levels for suspected treatment failure, life threatening infections. 300 mg bid oral dose or 8 mg/kg/d IV dose may be required to achieve target steady-state drug concentrations of 1-6 mcg/mL. **Toxicity** similar to other azoles/triazoles including uncommon serious hepatic toxicity (hepatitis, cholestasis & fulminant hepatic failure. Liver function tests should be monitored during rx & drug dc'd if abnormalities develop. **Photosensitivity is common and can be severe.** Many reports of associated skin cancers. Strongly recommend sun protective measures. *CID 58:997, 2014* & hallucinations & anaphylactoid infusion reactions with fever and hypertension. 1 case of QT prolongation with ventricular tachycardia in a 15 y/o pt with ALL reported. **Approx. 21% experience a transient visual disturbance** following IV or po ("altered/enhanced visual perception", blurred or colored visual change or photophobia) within 30–60 minutes. Visual changes resolve within 30–60 min. after administration & are attenuated with repeated doses **(do not drive at night for outpatient rx)**. Persistent visual changes occur rarely. Cause unknown. In patients with ClCr <50 mL per min., the intravenous vehicle (SBECD-sulfobutylether-B cyclodextrin) may accumulate but not obviously toxic *(CID 54:913, 2012)*. Hallucinations, hypoglycemia, electrolyte disturbance & pneumonitis attributed to ↑ drug concentrations. Potential for drug-drug interactions high. **With prolonged use, fluoride in drug can cause a painful periostitis.** *(CID 59:1237, 2014)* **NOTE: Not in urine in active form. No activity vs. mucormycosis.**

TABLE 12A – TREATMENT OF MYCOBACTERIAL INFECTIONS*

Diagnosis of M. tuberculosis, Updated Guidelines *(IDSA, ATS, CDC): CID 64:e1, 2017.*

Tuberculin skin test (TST). Same as PPD *[Chest 138:1456, 2010].* Criteria for positive TST after 5 tuberculin units (intermediate PPD) read at 48–72 hours:

- ≥5 mm induration: + HIV, immunosuppressed, ≥15 mg prednisone per day, healed TBc on chest x-ray, recent close contact
- ≥10 mm induration: foreign-born, countries with high prevalence; IVD Users; low income; NH residents; chronic illness; silicosis
- ≥15 mm induration: otherwise healthy

Two-stage to detect sluggish positivity: If 1st PPD + but <10 mm, repeat intermediate PPD in 1 wk. Response to 2rd PPD can also happen if pt received BCG in childhood.

BCG vaccine as child: If ≥10 mm induration and from country with TB, should be attributed to MTB. Prior BCG may result in booster effect in 2-stage TST. Routine anergy testing not recommended.

Interferon Gamma Release Assays (IGRAs): IGRAs detect sensitivities to MTB by measuring IFN-γ release in response to MTB antigens (for review see *JAMA 308:241, 2012* and *MMWR 59 (RR-5):1, 2010)*:

- Approved tests: T-SPOT.TB (Oxford Immunotec) and QuantiFERON-TB Gold and QuantiFERON-TB Gold Plus (Qiagen).
- May be used in place of TST in all situations in which TST is indicated.
- CDC recommends IGRA over TST in most circumstances the exception being children age < 5 years (although some experts recommend an age < 3 years.

IGRAs are relatively specific for MTB and do not cross-react with BCG or most nontuberculous mycobacteria. CDC recommends IGRA over TST for persons unlikely to return for reading TST & for persons who have received BCG. IGRA or TST may be used without preference for recent contacts of TB with special utility for follow-up testing since IGRAs do not produce "booster effect".

- May also be used without preference over TBc for occupational exposures.
- As with TST, testing with IGRAs in low prevalence populations will result in false-positive results *(CID 53:234, 2011).*
- Manufacturer's IFN-gamma cutoff ≥0.35 IU/mL for QFT-GIT may be too low for low prevalence settings, inflating positivity and conversion rates, and a higher cut-off may be more appropriate *(Am J Respir Crit Care Med 188:1005, 2013).* For detailed discussion of IGRAs, *see MMWR 59 (RR-5), 2010 and JAMA 308:241, 2012.* False positive IGRA *(JCM 54:845, 2016).*

Rapid (24-hr or less) diagnostic tests for MTB: (1) the Amplified Mycobacterium tuberculosis Direct Test amplifies and detects MTB ribosomal RNA; (2) the AMPLICOR Mycobacterium tuberculosis Test amplifies and detects MTB DNA. Both tests have sensitivities & specificities >95% in sputum samples that are AFB-positive. In negative smears, specificity remains >95% but sensitivity is 40–77% *(MMWR 58:7, 2009; CID 49:46, 2009)* to 60-90% *(see: http://www.cdc.gov/tb/publications/guidelines/amplification_tests/default.htm (3)* COBAS TaqMan MTB Test: real-time PCR test for detection of M. tuberculosis in respiratory specimens (not available in the U.S.) with performance characteristics similar to other rapid tests *(J Clin Microbiol 51:3225, 2013).*

Xpert MTB/RIF is a rapid test (2 hrs) for MTB in sputum samples which also detects RIF resistance with specificity of 99.2% and sensitivity of 72.5% in smear negative patients *(NEJM 363:1005, 2010).* Current antibody-based and ELISA-based rapid tests for TBc not recommended by WHO because they are less accurate than microscopy ± culture *(Lancet ID 11:736, 2011).*

Xpert MTB/RIF Ultra (Xpert Ultra) (not yet available in the US) *(Lancet Infect Dis 018 Jan;18(1):76-84)*: Higher sensitivity than Xpert MTB/RIF for detection of M. tuberculosis in smear-negative specimens, pediatric patients, HIV-infected patients, and in extra-pulmonary disease; slightly lower specificity than Xpert MTB/RIF. Recommended by WHO as initial diagnostic test for suspected tuberculous meningitis *(Lancet Infect Dis. 2018 Jan;18(1):68-75.)*

CAUSATIVE AGENT/ DISEASE	MODIFYING CIRCUMSTANCES	SUGGESTED REGIMENS	
		INITIAL THERAPY	CONTINUATION PHASE OF THERAPY
I. Mycobacterium tuberculosis exposure baseline TST/IGRA negative (household members & other close contacts of potentially infectious cases)	Neonate- Rx essential NOTE: If fever, abnormal CXR (pleural effusion, hilar adenopathy, infiltrate) at baseline, treat for active TBc and not with INH alone.	**INH** (10 mg/kg/ day for 8-10 wks) **RIF** 10-20 mg/kg/d also an option *(NEJM 379:454, 2018)*	Repeat tuberculin skin test (TST) in 8-12 wks: if TST neg & CXR normal & infant age at exposure >6 mos., stop INH, if TST (≥5 mm) or age ≤ 6 mos, treat with INH for total of 9 mos (4 mos if RIF used). If follow-up CXR abnormal, treat for active TB.
	Children <5 years of age—Rx indicated	As for neonate for 1st 8-10 wks.	If repeat TST at 8-10 wks is negative, stop. If repeat TST ≥5 mm, continue INH for total of 9 mos. If INH not given initially, repeat TST at 3 mos, if TST is positive, treat with INH for 9 mos. *(see Category II below).*
	Older children & adults— Risk 2-4% 1st yr		Pts at high risk of progression (e.g., HIV+, immunosuppressed or on immunosuppressive therapy) and no evidence of active infection should be treated for LTBI *(see below).* For others repeat TST/IGRA at 8-10 wks: no rx if repeat TST/IGRA neg.

See page 2 for abbreviations

* Dosages are for adults (unless otherwise indicated) and assume normal renal function

† **DOT** = directly observed therapy; **SAT** = self-administered therapy

TABLE 12A (2)

CAUSATIVE AGENT/ DISEASE	MODIFYING CIRCUMSTANCES	SUGGESTED REGIMENS	
		INITIAL THERAPY	ALTERNATIVE
II. Tuberculosis (LTBI, positive TST or IGRA as above, active TB ruled out) CDC recommended regimens: *https://www.cdc.gov/tb/topic/treatment/ltbi.htm* CDC guidance document: *MMWR Recommendations and Reports / February 14, 2020 / 69(1);1–11*	Choice of regimen is determined by 1) susceptibility to isoniazid and/or rifampin of isolate of index case, if known; 2) age; 3) pregnancy All persons with LTBI should be offered therapy regardless of age. If pre-anti-TNF therapy, recommend at least one month of treatment for LBTI prior to start of anti-TNF therapy *(Arth Care & Res 64:625, 2012)*. Short-course rifamycin-based regimens preferred over INH because of favorable toxicity profile and improved compliance. For patients on Isoniazid (INH) educate and monitor clinically for signs and symptoms of hepatitis. Baseline lab testing of liver function at start of therapy not routinely indicated but is indicated for patients with HIV infection, pregnant women, and women within 3 mo of delivery, persons with a history of chronic liver disease, persons who use alcohol regularly, and persons at risk for chronic liver disease. Lab monitoring of liver function during therapy is indicated if baseline liver function tests are abnormal, if risk factors for hepatic disease are present, or to evaluate for possible adverse effects. Co-administer pyridoxine (adult dose 50 mg, infant 6.25 mg, toddler 12.5 mg, school-aged child 25 mg) with dose of INH, if used.	3HP: a 12 dose once weekly 3-month regimen of INH + Rifapentine (RFP) • INH adult dose: adult 15 mg/kg po once weekly (max dose 900 mg); child 25 mg/kg po once weekly (max dose 900 mg) • RFP po (wt-based dose): 10-14 kg: 300 mg; 14.1-25 kg: 450 mg; 25.1-32 kg: 600 mg; 32.1-49.9 kg: 750 mg; 50 kg: 900 mg. Recommended for treatment of LTBI 1) in adults; 2) in persons with LTBI aged 2–17 years; 3) in persons with LTBI who have HIV infection, including AIDS, and are taking antiretroviral medications with acceptable drug-drug interactions with rifapentine; and 4) by DOT† or SAT† in persons aged ≥2 years *(MMWR 67:723, 2018)*. Not recommended for children age <2 yrs or in pregnancy.	**RIF** once daily po (adult: 10 mg/kg/day, max dose 600 mg/day; child: 15-20 mg/kg/day, max dose 600 mg/day) for 4 mos *(NEJM 379:440, 454, 2018)*. **INH + RIF** once daily x 3 mos *(AnIM 2017;167:248)*. **INH** po once daily (adult: 5 mg/kg/day, max 300 mg/day; child: 10-15 mg/kg/day not to exceed 300 mg/day) x 9 mos. For current recommendations for monitoring hepatotoxicity on INH see *MMWR 59:227, 2010*. Less desirable, but a consideration for those unable to comply with a 9-month regimen: INH 300 mg once daily for 6 mo (but slightly less effective than 9 mos.; not recommended in children, HIV+ persons, or those with fibrotic lesions on chest film). **INH** 2x/wk (adult: 15 mg/kg, max 900 mg; child: 20-30 mg/kg, max dose 900 mg) x 9 mo.
	Pregnancy	**RIF** once daily x 4 months or **INH** + **RIF** once daily x 3 months. Once active disease is excluded may delay initiation of therapy until after delivery unless patient is recent contact to an active case, HIV+. Supplemental pyridoxine 50 mg/d if INH used	**INH** po once daily 300 mg/day + pyridoxine 50 mg once daily
LTBI, suspected INH-resistant organism		**RIF** once daily po (adult: 10 mg/kg/day, max dose 600 mg/day; child: 15-20 mg/kg/day, max dose 600 mg/day) for 4 mos.	**RFB** 300 mg once daily po may be substituted for RIF (in HIV+ patient on anti-retrovirals, dose may need to be adjusted for drug interactions).
LTBI, suspected INH and RIF resistant organism	Pregnancy: expert consultation advised	**Moxi** 400 mg ± **EMB** 15 mg/kg once daily x 12 months	**Levo** 500 mg once daily + (**EMB** 15 mg/kg or **PZA** 25 mg/kg) once daily x 12 months. **NOTE:** PZA combo regimen, although perhaps most efficacious, poorly tolerated and may be overall less effective than FQ + EMB *(CID 64:1670, 2017)*

See page 2 for abbreviations

* Dosages are for adults (unless otherwise indicated) and assume normal renal function

† **DOT** = directly observed therapy; **SAT** = self-administered therapy

TABLE 12A (3)

CAUSATIVE AGENT/ DISEASE	MODIFYING CIRCUM-STANCES	SUGGESTED REGIMENS: INITIAL THERAPY			CONTINUATION PHASE OF THERAPY (in vitro susceptibility known)			
		SEE COMMENTS FOR DOSAGE AND DIRECTLY OBSERVED THERAPY (DOT) REGIMENS						
		Regimen: in order of preference	**Drugs**	**Interval/Doses (min. duration)**	**Regimen**	**Drugs**	**Interval/Doses (min. duration)**	**Range of Total Doses (min. duration)**
III. Mycobacterium tuberculosis **A. Pulmonary TB** **General reference on rx in adults & children:** *MMWR 52 (RR-11):1, 2003.* **In pts with newly diagnosed HIV and TB, Rx for both should be started as soon as possible** *(NEJM 362:697, 2010).* **Isolation essential!** Hospitalized pts with suspected or documented active TB should be isolated in single rooms using airborne precautions until deemed non-infectious. DC isolation if 3 negative AFB smears or 1-2 neg NAAT (Xpert MTB/RIF) *(CID 59:1353 & 1361, 2014).*	Rate of INH resistance known to be **<4%** (drug-susceptible organisms)	1	**INH RIF PZA EMB**	7 days per wk times 56 doses (8 wks) or 5 days per wk (DOT) times 40 doses (8 wks) If cavitary disease, treat for 9 mos. Fixed dose combination of INH, RIF, PZA & EMB currently being evaluated *(JAMA 305:1415, 2011).*	1a	**INH/ RIF**[9]	7 days per wk times 126 doses (18 wks) or 5 days per wk (DOT) times 90 doses (18 wks). If cavitary disease, treat for 9 mos.	182–130 (26 wks)
					1b	**INH/ RIF**	2 times per wk times 36 doses (18 wks)	92–76 (26 wks) (Not AIDS pts)
					1c	**INH/ RFP**	1 time per wk times 18 doses (18 wks) (only if HIV-neg)	74–58 (26 wks)
		2	**INH RIF PZA EMB**	7 days per wk times 14 doses (2 wks), then 2 times per wk times 12 doses (6 wks) or 5 days per wk (DOT) times 10 doses (2 wks) then 2 times per wk times 12 doses (6 wks)	2a	**INH/ RIF**	2 times per wk times 36 doses (18 wks)	62–58 (26 wks) (Not AIDS pts)
					2b[5]	**INH/ RFP**	1 time per wk times 18 doses (18 wks) (only if HIV-neg)	44–40 (26 wks)
		3	**INH RIF PZA EMB**	3 times per wk times 24 doses (8 wks)	3a	**INH/ RIF**	3 times per wk times 54 doses (18 wks)	78 (26 wks)
USE DOT REGIMENS IF POSSIBLE		4	**INH RIF EMB**	7 days per wk times 56 doses (8 wks) or 5 days per wk (DOT) times 40 doses (8 wks)	4a	**INH/ RIF**	7 days per wk times 217 doses (31 wks) or 5 days per wk (DOT) times 155 doses (31 wks)	273–195 (39 wks)
					4b	**INH/ RIF**	2 times per wk times 62 doses (31 wks)	118–102 (39 wks)

COMMENTS

Regimen*	Dose in mg per kg (max. q24h dose): INH	RIF	PZA	EMB	SM	RFB
Q24h:						
Child	10-20 (300)	10-20 (600)	15-30 (2000)	15-25	20-40 (1000)	10-20 (300)
Adult	5 (300)	10 (600)	15-30 (2000)	15-25	15 (1000)	5 (300)
2 times per wk (DOT):						
Child	20-40 (900)	10-20 (600)	50-70 (4000)	50	25-30 (1500)	10-20 (300)
Adult	15 (900)	10 (600)	50-70 (3000)	50	25-30 (1500)	5 (300)
3 times per wk (DOT):						
Child	20-40 (900)	10-20 (600)	50-70 (3000)	25-30	25-30 (1500)	NA
Adult	15 (900)	10 (600)	50-70 (3000)	25-30	25-30 (1500)	NA

Second-line anti-TB agents can be dosed as follows to facilitate DOT: Cycloserine 500–750 mg po q24h (5 times per wk)
Ethionamide 500–750 mg po q24h (5 times per wk)
Kanamycin or capreomycin 15 mg per kg IM/IV q24h (3–5 times per wk)
Ciprofloxacin 750 mg po q24h (5 times per wk)
Ofloxacin 600–800 mg po q24h (5 times per wk)
Levofloxacin 750 mg po q24h (5 times per wk)
(CID 21:1245, 1995)

Risk factors for drug-resistant (MDR) TB: Recent immigration from Latin America or Asia or living in area of ↑ resistance (≥4%) or previous rx without RIF; exposure to known MDR TB. Incidence of MDR TB in **US steady** at 0.7%. Incidence of primary drug resistance is particularly high (>25%) in parts of China, Thailand, Russia, Estonia & Latvia; ~80% of US MDR cases in foreign born.

NOTE: Thrice weekly therapy for both the initial and continuation phase and twice weekly therapy in the continuation phase have higher rates of relapse and microbiological failure, acquired drug resistance compared to daily therapy *(CID 64:1211, 2017).*

(Continued on next page)

* Dosages are for adults (unless otherwise indicated) and assume normal renal function

† **DOT** = directly observed therapy; **SAT** = self-administered therapy

TABLE 12A (4)

CAUSATIVE AGENT/ DISEASE	MODIFYING CIRCUM-STANCES	SUGGESTED REGIMEN[8]	DURATION OF TREATMENT (mos.)[8]	SPECIFIC COMMENTS[8]	COMMENTS
III. Mycobacterium tuberculosis **A. Pulmonary TB** *(continued from previous page)*	**INH resistance**	**RIF, PZA, EMB** (a **FQ** may strengthen the regimen for pts with extensive disease).	6	INH should be stopped in cases of INH resistance. Outcome similar for drug susceptible and INH-mono-resistant strains *(CID 48:179, 2009)*.	*(continued from previous page)* Mono-rifampin resistance is rare; resistance to rifampin is a marker for MDR, which should be assumed pending documentation of susceptibility to INH.
Multidrug-Resistant Tuberculosis (MDR TB): Defined as resistant to at least 2 drugs including INH & RIF. Pt clusters with high mortality *(NEJM 363:1050, 2010)*. **Extensively Drug-Resistant TB** (XDR-TB): Defined as resistant to INH & RIF plus any FQ and at least 1 of the 3 second-line drugs: capreomycin, kanamycin or amikacin *(MMWR 56:250, 2007; CID 51:379, 2010)*.	**Rifampin mono-resistance** (rare) or **resistance to INH and RIF** (MDR)	**Bedaquiline** 400 mg po once daily x 2 wks, then 200 mg 3 times per week, for 24 wks for a total of 26 weeks + **Pretomanid** 200 mg po once daily for 26 weeks + **Linezolid** 600 mg po once daily for 26 weeks. Administer with food.	6	Recently FDA-approved all oral treatment for MDR TB *(see Comments)* Bedaquiline can also be dosed at 200 mg daily for 8 weeks, then 100 mg daily for 18 weeks. Consider adding Levo or Moxifloxacin if active. QTc prolongation may occur: monitor ECGs frequently.	**Expert consultation strongly recommended for MDR and XDR cases.** Pretomanid FDA approved for use in combination with bedaquiline and linezolid for treatment of MDR or XDR TB based on 90% success rate in an open-label trial of 109 patients, 56 of whom were HIV-infected *(NEJM 2020; 382: 893)*. The 1200 mg dose of linezolid in that trial was associated with a high rate of adverse events. A follow-up study found that the 600 mg dose of linezolid was better tolerated and similarly efficacious *(NEJM 2022; 387: 810)*. This 3-drug oral regimen is a major advance over WHO recommended multi-drug regimen (5 preferred, but at least 4 active agents) of levofloxacin (or moxifloxacin) + bedaquiline + linezolid + clofazimine + cycloserine + other agents (e.g., amikacin, ethionamide, delamanid) as needed to construct an active multi-drug regimen administered for 18-24 months.
	XDR-TB	Expert consultation strongly advised. *See comments*	Duration dependent on regimen	Traditional approach has been to treat with 4-6 active drugs for 18-24 months. Above regimen may also be effective, but limited data.	

CAUSATIVE AGENT/DISEASE; MODIFYING CIRCUMSTANCES	SUGGESTED REGIMENS: INITIAL THERAPY	SUGGESTED REGIMENS: CONTINUATION PHASE OF THERAPY (in vitro susceptibility known)	COMMENTS
III. Mycobacterium tuberculosis *(continued)*			
B. Extrapulmonary TB Steroids: *see Comment*	**INH** + **RIF** (or **RFB**) + **PZA** + **EMB** q24h x 2 months	**INH** + **RIF** (or **RFB**)	IDSA recommends 6 mos for lymph node, pleural, pericarditis, disseminated disease, genitourinary & peritoneal TBc; 6–9 mos for bone & joint; 9-12 mos for CNS (including meningeal) TBc. **Corticosteroids** "strongly rec" only for meningeal TBc *[MMWR 52(RR-11):1, 2003]*. Steroids not recommended for pericarditis *(NEJM 371:1121 & 1155, 2014)*.
	Some add **pyridoxine** 25–50 mg po q24h to regimens that include INH.		

 * Dosages are for adults (unless otherwise indicated) and assume normal renal function † **DOT** = directly observed therapy; **SAT** = self-administered therapy

TABLE 12A (5)

CAUSATIVE AGENT/DISEASE; MODIFYING CIRCUMSTANCES	SUGGESTED REGIMENS: INITIAL THERAPY	SUGGESTED REGIMENS: CONTINUATION PHASE OF THERAPY (in vitro susceptibility known)	COMMENTS
III. Mycobacterium tuberculosis *(continued)*			
C. Tuberculous meningitis Excellent summary of clinical aspects and therapy in *CID 2016;63:e147*	**(INH** + **RIF** + **EMB** + **PZA)** + *see Comments*	May omit **EMB** when susceptibility to **INH** and **RIF** established. Can D/C PZA after 2 months. Treat for total of 12 months. *See Table 9, page 101,* for CSF drug penetration. For patients with severe infection (e.g., altered mental status, focal neurological deficits): consider pushing rifampin dose to 20 mg/kg/d and if available, use intravenous medications until clinical improvement.	Adjunctive corticosteroids improve survival *(Cochrane Database Syst Rev, Apr 28;4:CD002244, 2016)* and strongly recommended; Adult - dexamethasone 0.4 mg/kg/day week 1, 0.3 mg/kg/day week 2, 0.2 mg/kg/day week 3, 0.1 mg/kg/day week 4, then tapered to stop over 3-4 weeks; Child - dexamethasone 0.6 mg/kg/day or prednisolone 4 mg/kg/day for 4 weeks then tapered to stop over 4 weeks. Aspirin (dose range 75-81 mg once daily up to 100 mg/kg/d in 3 divided doses, typically for 1-2 months), may lower mortality and reduce risk of stroke in adults with tuberculous meningitis *(Curr Treat Options Neurol. 2018; 20:5; Neurol India. 2019; 67:993; Acta Neurologica Belgica. 2021;121:11)*; benefit in children not established.
D. Tuberculosis during pregnancy	**INH** + **RIF** + **EMB** x 9 mos	SM should not be substituted for EMB due to toxicity. AMK, capreomycin, kanamycin, FQs also contraindicated. PZA is recommended for routine use in pregnant women by the WHO but has not been recommended for general use in U.S. due to lack of safety data, although PZA has been used in some US health jurisdictions without reported adverse events. Breast-feeding should not be discouraged. If PZA is not included in the initial treatment regimen, the minimum duration of therapy is 9 months. Pyridoxine, 25 mg/ day, should be administered.	
E. Treatment failure or relapse Usually due to poor compliance or resistant organisms, or subtherapeutic drug levels *(CID 55:169, 2012).*	Directly observed therapy (DOT). Check susceptibilities. *(See section III. A, page 191 & above)*	Pts whose sputum is culture-positive after 5–6 mos. = treatment failures. Failures may be due to non-compliance or resistant organisms. Confirm susceptibilities of original isolates and obtain susceptibility to first and second line agents on current isolates. Non-compliance common, therefore institute DOT. If isolates show resistance, modify regimen to include at least 2 (preferably 3) new active agents, ones that the patient has not previously received if at all possible.	
F. HIV infection or AIDS—pulmonary or extrapulmonary All HIV infected patients with TB should be treated with ARVs. If CD4 <50, initiation of ARVs within 2 weeks of starting TB meds associated with improved survival *(Ann Intern Med 163:32, 2015).*	**INH** + **RIF** (or **RFB**) + **PZA** q24h x 2 mos.	**INH** + **RIF** (or **RFB**) q24h x 4 months (total 6 mos.). Treat up to 9 mos. in pts with delayed response, cavitary disease.	1. RIF may be coadministered with efavirenz 600 mg; nucleoside reverse transcriptase inhibitors. Co-administration of RIF with raltegravir best avoided (use RFB instead) but if necessary increase raltegravir dose to 800 mg q12h: RIF + dolutegravir OK at 50 mg bid of latter. 2. Because of possibility of developing resistance to RIF or RFB in pts with low CD4 cell counts who receive wkly or 2x/wk therapy, daily dosing (preferred), or at a minimum 3x/wk dosing (failure rate likely higher) recommended for initial or continuation phase of rx. 3. Clinical & microbiologic response similar to that of HIV-neg patient. 4. Post-treatment suppression not necessary for drug-susceptible strains. 5. In RCT, prednisone reduced IRIS from 47% to 33% *(NEJM 2018,379:1915).*
	Add pyridoxine 50 mg po q24h to regimens that include INH **Note the following drug-drug interactions with antiretrovirals (ARVs)** -**Rifampin** not recommended for use with the following: bictegravir, doravirine, cabotegravir/rilpivirine (IM/PO), elvitegravir/cobicistat, efavirenz 400 mg, etravirine, fostemsavir, lenacapavir (SC/PO), maraviroc, nevirapine, protease inhibitors (PIs), raltegravir (daily), rilpivirine (PO) -**Rifabutin** not recommended for use with the following: bictegravir, cabotegravir/rilpivirine (IM/PO), elvitegravir/cobicistat, etravirine with boosted PIs, lenacapavir (SC/PO), PIs with cobicistat -**Rifapentine** recommended for use only with efavirenz and nucleoside reverse transcriptase inhibitors; all other ARVs are not recommended		
Concomitant protease inhibitor (PI) therapy	**INH** 300 mg q24h + **RFB** (150 mg q24h or 300 mg tiw) + **EMB** 15 mg/kg q24h + **PZA** 25 mg/kg q24h x 2 mos.; then INH + RFB x 4 mos. (up to 7 mos.)	**INH** + **RFB** x 4 mos. (7 mos. in slow responders, cavitary disease)	Rifamycins induce cytochrome CYP450 enzymes (RIF > RFP > RFB) & reduce serum levels of concomitantly administered PIs. Conversely, PIs inhibit CYP450 & cause ↑ serum levels of RFP & RFB. If dose of RFB is not reduced, toxicity ↑.

* Dosages are for adults (unless otherwise indicated) and assume normal renal function

† **DOT** = directly observed therapy; **SAT** = self-administered therapy

TABLE 12A (6)

CAUSATIVE AGENT/DISEASE	MODIFYING CIRCUMSTANCES	SUGGESTED REGIMENS PRIMARY/ALTERNATIVE		COMMENTS
IV. Mycobacterium bovis		**INH + RIF + EMB** x 2 months then INH + RIF x 7 months		The M. tuberculosis complex includes M. bovis and regimens effective for MTB (except PZA based) also likely to be effective for M. bovis. **All isolates resistant to PZA**. Isolation not required. Increased prevalence of extrapulmonary disease in U.S. born Hispanic populations and elsewhere *(CID 47:168, 2008; EID 14:909, 2008; EID 17:457, 2011)*.
V. Bacillus Calmette-Guerin (BCG) (derived from M. bovis)	Only fever (>38.5°C) for 12–24 hrs	**INH** 300 mg q24h times 3 months		Intravesical BCG effective in superficial bladder tumors and carcinoma in situ. With sepsis, consider initial adjunctive prednisolone. Also susceptible to RFB, CIP, oflox, levo, moxi, streptomycin, amikacin, capreomycin. BCG may cause regional adenitis or pulmonary disease in HIV-infected children. **Resistant to PZA**.
	Systemic illness or sepsis	Same as for M. bovis.		
VI. Nontuberculous mycobacteria (NTM)				
Mycobacterium avium-intracellulare complex (MAC) ATS/ERS/ESCMID/IDSA Clinical Practice Guidelines: *Clin Infect Dis 2020; 71:e1; See http://aidsinfo.nih.gov/guidelines/html/4/adult-and-adolescent-oi-prevention-and-treatment-guidelines/0 for updated CDC recommendations for AIDS patients*.	**Immunocompetent patients**			Intermittent (tiw) therapy not recommended for patients with cavitary disease, patients who have been previously treated or patients with moderate of severe disease. Treat for 12 months after sputum converts to negative. Clari 500 mg bid can substitute for Azithro. Rifabutin 300 mg (150 mg if used daily and with Clari) can substitute for RIF. May also be associated with interferon gamma deficiency *(AJM 113:756, 2002)*. For cervicofacial lymphadenitis (localized) in immunocompetent children, surgical excision is as effective as chemotherapy *(CID 44:1057, 2007)*.
	Nodular/Bronchiectatic disease	**Azithro** 500 mg tiw + **EMB** 25 mg/kg tiw + **RIF** 600 mg tiw		
	Cavitary disease or severe nodular/bronchiectatic disease	(**Azithro** 250-500 mg/day + **EMB** 15 mg/kg/day + **RIF** 600 mg) 3x weekly + **AMK** 15-25 mg/kg IV or IM 3x weekly for first 2-3 months.		
		If sputum does not convert to culture-negative by 6 months, add Amikacin liposome inhalation suspension		
	HIV infection: **Primary prophylaxis—NO LONGER RECOMMENDED IF PATIENT IS ON EFFECTIVE ART**			
	Treatment Either presumptive dx or after + culture of blood, bone marrow, or usually, sterile body fluids, eg liver. Complete **<u>at least</u>** 12 mo therapy + no signs and symptoms of MAC disease + sustained (>6 months) CD4 count >100 cells/mm³ in response to ART	(**Clarithro** 500 mg po bid + **EMB** 15 mg/kg/day ± **RFB** 300 mg po q24h (adjust dose)	**Azithro** 500 mg po/day + **EMB** 15 mg/kg/day +/- **RFB** 300-450 mg po/day	Adjust RFB dose as needed for drug-drug interactions. Addition of a third or fourth drug should be considered for patients with advanced immunosuppression (CD4+ count <50 cells/µL), high mycobacterial loads (>2 log CFU/mL of blood), or in the absence of effective ART: AMK 10–15 mg/kg IV daily; Strep 1 gm IV or IM daily; CIP 500-750 mg po bid; Levo 500 mg po daily; Moxi 400 mg po daily. Testing of susceptibility to clarithromycin and azithromycin is recommended.
	Chronic post-treatment suppression—secondary prophylaxis	**Always necessary.** [**Clarithro** or azithro] + **EMB** 15 mg/kg/day *(dosage above)*	**Clarithro** or **Azithro** or **RFB** *(dosage above)*	Recurrences almost universal without chronic suppression. Can discontinue if no signs and symptoms of MAC disease and sustained (>6 months) CD4 count >100 cells/µL in response to ART.

* Dosages are for adults (unless otherwise indicated) and assume normal renal function

† **DOT** = directly observed therapy; **SAT** = self-administered therapy

TABLE 12A (7)

CAUSATIVE AGENT/DISEASE	MODIFYING CIRCUMSTANCES	SUGGESTED REGIMENS PRIMARY/ALTERNATIVE	COMMENTS
VI. Nontuberculous Mycobacteria (NTM) *(continued)*			
Mycobacterium celatum	Treatment; optimal regimen no defined	May be susceptible to **clarithro**, **FQ** Treat as if MAC.	Isolated from pulmonary lesions and blood in AIDS patients. Easily confused with M. xenopi (and MAC).
Mycobacterium abscessus **See:** *ATS/ERS/ESCMID/ IDSA Clinical Practice Guidelines: Clin Infect Dis 2020; 71:e1*	Treatment; Surgical excision may facilitate healing of subcutaneous abscess and is important adjunct to rx *(see CID 52:565, 2011).*	**Pulmonary or disseminated disease:** - Intensive phase, treat for 2-3 months No inducible and no constitutive/ mutational macrolide resistance 1-2 parenteral agents + 2-3 oral or inhaled agents, at least 3 drugs total **Parenteral agents: IMP** 1000 mg IV q12 h or Cefoxitin 8-12 gm/day IV in 2-3 divided doses; **AMK** 10-15 mg/kg IV once daily or 15-25 mg/kg IV thrice weekly; Tigecycline 100 mg loading dose then 50 mg q12h IV **Oral or inhaled agents: Azithro** 250-500 mg once daily; **Clofazimine** 100-200 mg once daily; Linezolid 600 mg once daily; Amikacin liposome inhalation suspension Any macrolide resistance, inducible or constitutive/mutational 2-3 parenteral agents + 2-3 oral or inhaled medications as above. NOTE: Azithromycin as above for its potential immunomodulatory effect but should not count as an active oral medication - Continuation phase: optimal duration of therapy not well defined, but 12 months after sputum cultures convert to negative is reasonable. No inducible or constitutive/mutational macrolide resistance Choose 2-3 oral or inhaled agents from those listed above Any macrolide resistance, inducible or constitutive Choose 2-3 oral or inhaled agents from those listed above. **Cutaneous infection:** Surgical debridement + at least 2 active agents from among those listed above; 4-6 months of Rx is sufficient in most cases, although deeper or more extensive infections may require longer	- M. abscesses is a complex of 3 subspecies: *M. abscessus, M. massiliense, M. bolletii.* - Test for susceptibility to Amikacin, Cefoxitin, Imipenem, Clarithromycin, Linezolid, Tigecycline, and Moxifloxacin. - **Resistance to macrolides** is either constitutive resistance due to a mutation(s) in rrl, which encodes 23S ribosomal RNA or inducible resistance due to a functional ribosomal methylase, encoded by erm(41) (not present in *M. massiliense*). Constitutive/mutational resistance is detected phenotypically in vitro by growth in the presence of macrolide (clarithromycin) after a 3-5 day incubation or molecularly by detection of resistance mutations. Inducible resistance is detected phenotypically in vitro by growth after a 14 day incubation or molecularly by detection of functional gene sequence. - Amikacin 10-15 mg/kg IV once daily: adjust dose to obtain a peak serum concentration of 35-45 μg/mL in a sample drawn 30 min after a 30 min infusion and a trough of < 5 μg/mL); 15-25 mg/kg IV thrice weekly (adjust dose to obtain a peak serum concentration of 65-80 μg/mL in a sample drawn 30 min after a 30 min infusion and a trough of < 5 μg/mL) - **Consultation with an expert** in the treatment and management of M. abscessus pulmonary infection is strongly recommended to design the antimicrobial regimen and assist with determination of duration of therapy.

TABLE 12A (8)

CAUSATIVE AGENT/DISEASE	MODIFYING CIRCUMSTANCES	SUGGESTED REGIMENS PRIMARY/ALTERNATIVE	COMMENTS
VI. Nontuberculous Mycobacteria (NTM) *(continued)*			
Mycobacterium chelonae	Rapid grower assoc. with skin, wound, soft tissue infection; rarely disseminated/pulmonary	Skin: **Clarithro** 500 mg po bid + one other active agent x 4-6 months; More serious infection: **Clarithro** 500 mg po bid + **Tobra** 5 mg/kg IV once daily + one additional active agent x 2-8 wk then **Clarithro** 500 mg po bid plus one additional active agent for up to 12 mo.	*M. chelonae* susceptible to AMK (80%), clarithro (92-100%), azithro, tobramycin (100%), IMP (8-50%), moxifloxacin (0-50%), Doxy (25%), linezolid (50-100%), omadacycline (MIC90 = 0.25 µg/mL), tigecycline (MIC90 = 0.125 µg/mL). Resistant to cefoxitin. Tigecycline successfully used as salvage in combination regimens *(J Antimicrob Chemother 69:1945, 2014)*.
Mycobacterium fortuitum	Treatment; optimal regimen not defined. Surgical excision of infected areas.	**AMK** + **Cefoxitin** + **Probenecid** 2–6 wks, then po **TMP- SMX**, or **doxy** 2–6 mos. Usually responds to 6–12 mos of oral rx with 2 drugs to which it is susceptible.	**Resistant to all standard anti-TBc drugs.** Sensitive in vitro to doxycycline, minocycline, cefoxitin, IMP, AMK, TMP-SMX, CIP, oflox, azithro, clarithro, linezolid, tigecycline, but some strains resistant to azithromycin, rifabutin. For M. fortuitum pulmonary disease treat with at least 2 agents active in vitro until sputum cultures negative for 12 months *(AJRCCM 175:367, 2007)*. Disseminated disease associated with auto-antibodies to *interferon-γ (Intern Med 53:1361, 2014)*.
Mycobacterium haemophilum	Combination of **CIP** + **RFB** + **Clarithro** *(EID 2019, 25:1648)*. Surgical debridement may be necessary.		Ulcerative skin lesions, tenosynovitis, osteomyelitis, lymphadenitis, pulmonary infection, disseminated infection usually in immunocompromised host. Lab: Requires supplemented media to isolate.
Mycobacterium genavense	2 or more drugs: **Clarithro**, **EMB**, **RFB**; **CLO**, **Amikacin**, Moxifloxacin as alternatives.		Seen in AIDS patients with CD4 <50 and in non-HIV severely immunocompromised hosts. *For review see Clin Microbiol Infect 19:432, 2013.*
Mycobacterium gordonae	Rarely a true pathogen.		Frequent colonizer, not associated with disease. In vitro: sensitive to EMB, RIF, AMK, CIP, clarithro, linezolid. Resistant to INH. Surgical excision.
Mycobacterium kansasii	[(**Azithro** 500 mg or **Clarithro** 500 mg bid) + **RIF** 600 mg + **EMB** 15 mg/kg] po q24h	**INH** 300 mg + **Pyridoxine** 50 mg + **RIF** 600 mg + **EMB** 15 mg/kg po q24h **For rifampin resistant organism: EMB** 15 mg/kg + **Moxi** 400 mg + **Azithro** 250-500 mg po q24h	**All isolates are resistant to PZA.** Treat until sputum cultures have been negative for 12 mo. For HIV+ patients on a protease inhibitor, substitute Rifabutin (150 mg/day) for Rifampin. For details see **ATS/ERS/ESCMID/IDSA Guidelines: *Clin Infect Dis 2020;71:e1.***
Mycobacterium marinum	Two active agents for 1-2 months after surgical incision: **Clarithro** 500 mg bid + **EMB** 25 mg/kg q24h or **RIF** 600 mg q24h + **EMB** 25 mg/kg q24h Surgical excision.		For deep tissue involvement a three drug combination therapy with Rifampin 600 mg q24h + [Minocycline 100–200 mg q24h or Doxycycline 100–200 mg q24h] + Clarithromycin 500 mg bid.
Mycobacterium scrofulaceum	Surgical excision. Chemotherapy seldom indicated. Although regimens not defined, **Clarithro** + **CLO** with or **without EMB. INH**, **RIF**, **strep** + **cycloserine** have also been used.		In vitro resistant to INH, RIF, EMB, PZA, AMK, CIP. Susceptible to clarithro, strep, erythromycin.
Mycobacterium simiae	Regimen(s) not defined. Start 4 drugs as for disseminated MAC		Most isolates resistant to all 1st-line anti-TBc drugs. Isolates often not clinically significant.
Mycobacterium ulcerans (Buruli ulcer)	**RIF** 600 mg po q24h + **Clarithro** 500 mg po bid or 15 mg/kg extended release once daily x 8-12 wk *(see Lancet. 2020; 395: 1259)*		Surgery not required for cure and reserved for those declining or intolerant of antibiotic, debridement of necrotic tissue, large defects.
Mycobacterium xenopi ATS/ERS/ESCMID/IDSA Guidelines: *Clin Infect Dis 2020;71:e1.*	**Azithro** 250-500 mg + **RIF** 600 mg + **EMB** 15 mg/kg each once daily.		Consider adding AMK 15-25 mg/kg IV thrice weekly for cavitary or advanced/severe bronchiectatic disease. Treat for 12 mo. after cultures convert to negative. See *Clin Infect Dis 2020;71:e1* for details.

* Dosages are for adults (unless otherwise indicated) and assume normal renal function

† **DOT** = directly observed therapy; **SAT** = self-administered therapy

TABLE 12A (9)

CAUSATIVE AGENT/DISEASE	MODIFYING CIRCUMSTANCES	SUGGESTED REGIMENS PRIMARY/ALTERNATIVE	COMMENTS
VII. Mycobacterium leprae			
Mycobacterium lepromatosis (leprosy): There are 2 sets of therapeutic recommendations here: one from USA *(National Hansen's Disease Program [NHDP], Baton Rouge, LA)* and one from WHO. Both are based on expert recommendations and neither has been subjected to controlled clinical trial.			
Paucibacillary Forms: (Intermediate, Tuberculoid, Borderline tuberculoid)	(**Dapsone** 100 mg/day + **RIF** 600 mg po/day) for 12 months	(**Dapsone** 100 mg/day (unsupervised) + **RIF** 600 mg 1x/mo (supervised)) x 12 mos, use for patients on prednisone	Side effects overall 0.4%
Multibacillary forms: **Borderline** **Borderline-lepromatous** **Lepromatous** *See Comment for erythema nodosum leprosum (ENL)* Rev.: *Lancet 363:1209, 2004*	(**Dapsone** 100 mg/day + **CLO** 50 mg/day + **RIF** 600 mg/day) for 24 mos **Alternative regimen:** (**Dapsone** 100 mg/day + **RIF** 600 mg/day + **Minocycline** 100 mg/day) for 24 mos if **CLO** is refused or unavailable.	(**Dapsone** 100 mg/day + **CLO** 50 mg/day (both unsupervised) + **RIF** 600 mg once monthly (supervised)). Continue regimen for 24 months.	Side-effects overall 5.1%. For **erythema nodosum leprosum:** prednisone 60–80 mg/day or thalidomide 100-400 mg/day. Thalidomide available in US at 1-800-4-CELGENE. Altho thalidomide effective, WHO no longer rec because of potential toxicity however the majority of leprosy experts feel thalidomide remains drug of choice for ENL under strict supervision. **CLO (Clofazimine)** available from NHDP under IND protocol; contact at 1-800-642-2477. **Ethionamide** (250 mg q24h) or prothionamide (375 mg q24h) may be subbed for CLO. Etanercept effective in one case refractory to above standard therapy *(CID 52:e133, 2011)*. Regimens incorporating clarithro, minocycline, dapsone monotherapy have been abandoned due to emergence of resistance *(CID 52:e127, 2011)*, but older patients previously treated with dapsone monotherapy may remain on lifelong maintenance therapy. Moxi highly active in vitro and produces rapid clinical response *(AAC 52:3113, 2008)*.

* Dosages are for adults (unless otherwise indicated) and assume normal renal function

† **DOT** = directly observed therapy; **SAT** = self-administered therapy

TABLE 12B – DOSAGE AND ADVERSE EFFECTS OF ANTIMYCOBACTERIAL DRUGS

AGENT (TRADE NAME)[1]	USUAL DOSAGE*	ROUTE/1º DRUG RESISTANCE (RES) US[2,§]	SIDE-EFFECTS, TOXICITY AND PRECAUTIONS	SURVEILLANCE
FIRST LINE DRUGS				
Ethambutol (Myambutol) (100, 400 mg tab)	25 mg/kg/day for 2 mos then 15 mg/ kg/day q24h as 1 dose (<10% protein binding) [Bacteriostatic to both extra-cellular & intracellular organisms]	RES: 0.3% (0–0.7%) po 400 mg tab	**Optic neuritis** with decreased visual acuity, central scotomata, and loss of green and red perception; peripheral neuropathy and headache (~1%), rashes (rare), arthralgia (rare), hyperuricemia (rare). Anaphylactoid reaction (rare).	Monthly visual acuity & red/ green with dose >15 mg/kg/ day. ≥10% loss considered significant. Usually reversible if drug discontinued.
Isoniazid (INH) (Nydrazid, Laniazid, Teebaconin) (50, 100, 300 mg tab)	Q24h dose: 5–10 mg/kg/day up to 300 mg/day as 1 dose. 2x/wk dose: 15 mg/kg (900 mg max dose) (<10% protein binding) [Bactericidal to both extracellular and intracellular organisms] Add pyridoxine in alcoholic, pregnant, or malnourished pts.	RES: 4.1% (2.6–8.5%) po 300 mg tab IM 100 mg/mL in 10 mL (IV route not FDA-approved but has been used, esp. in AIDS)	Overall ~1%. Liver: **Hep** (children 10% mild ↑ SGOT, normalizes with continued rx, age <20 yrs rare, 20–34 yrs 1.2%, ≥50 yrs 2.3%) [also ↑ with q24h alcohol & previous exposure to Hep C (usually asymptomatic—*CID 36:293, 2003*)]. May be fatal. With prodromal sx, dark urine do LFTs; discontinue if SGOT >3–5x normal. **Peripheral neuropathy** (17% on 6 mg/kg per day, less on 300 mg, incidence ↑ in slow acetylators); **pyridoxine 10 mg q24h will decrease incidence;** other neurologic sequelae, convulsions, optic neuritis, toxic encephalopathy, psychosis, muscle twitching, dizziness, coma (all rare); allergic skin rashes, fever, minor disulfiram-like reaction, flushing after Swiss cheese; blood dyscrasias (rare); + antinuclear (20%). **Drug-drug interactions** common.	Pre-rx liver functions. Repeat if symptoms (fatigue, weakness, malaise, anorexia, nausea or vomiting) >3 days (*AJRCCM 152: 1705, 1995*). Some recommend SGOT at 2, 4, 6 mos esp. if age >50 yrs. Clinical evaluation every mo.
Pyrazinamide (500 mg tab)	25 mg per kg per day (maximum 2.5 gm per day) q24h as 1 dose [Bactericidal for intracellular organisms]	po 500 mg tab	**Arthralgia; hyperuricemia** (with or without symptoms); hepatitis (not over 2% if recommended dose not exceeded); gastric irritation; photosensitivity (rare).	Pre-rx liver functions. Monthly SGOT, uric acid. Measure serum uric acid if symptomatic gouty attack occurs.
Rifamate®— combination tablet	2 tablets single dose q24h	po (1 hr before meal)	1 tablet contains 150 mg INH, 300 mg RIF	As with individual drugs
Rifampin (Rifadin, Rimactane, Rifocin) (100, 300, 450, 600 mg cap)	10.0 mg per kg per day up to 600 mg per day q24h as 1 dose (60–90% protein binding) [Bactericidal to all populations of organisms]	RES: 0.2% (0–0.3%) po 300 mg cap (IV available, Merrell-Dow)	INH/RIF dc'd in ~3% for toxicity; gastrointestinal irritation, antibiotic-associated colitis, drug fever (1%), pruritus with or without skin rash (1%), anaphylactoid reactions in HIV+ pts, mental confusion, thrombocytopenia (1%), leukopenia (1%), hemolytic anemia, transient **abnormalities in liver function. "Flu syndrome"** (fever, chills, headache, bone pain, shortness of breath) seen if RIF taken irregularly or if q24h dose restarted after an interval of no rx. **Discolors urine, tears, sweat, contact lens an orange-brownish color.** May cause drug-induced lupus erythematosus *(Ln 349: 1521, 1977)*.	Pre-rx liver function. Repeat if symptoms. **Multiple significant drug-drug interactions**.
Rifater®— combination tablet *(See Side-Effects)*	Wt ≥55 kg, 6 tablets single dose q24h	po (1 hr before meal)	1 tablet contains 50 mg INH, 120 mg RIF, 300 mg PZA. Used in 1st 2 months of rx (PZA 25 mg per kg). Purpose is convenience in dosing, ↑ compliance *(AnIM 122: 951, 1995)* but cost 1.58 more. Side-effects = individual drugs.	As with individual drugs, PZA 25 mg per kg
Streptomycin (IV/IM sol'n)	15 mg per kg IM q24h, 0.75–1.0 gm per day initially for 60–90 days, then 1.0 gm 2–3 times per week (15 mg per kg per day) q24h as 1 dose	RES: 3.9% (2.7–7.6%) IM (or IV)	Overall 8%. **Ototoxicity:** vestibular dysfunction (vertigo); paresthesias; dizziness & nausea (all less in pts receiving 2–3 doses per week); tinnitus and high frequency loss (1%); nephrotoxicity (rare); peripheral neuropathy (rare); allergic skin rashes (4–5%); drug fever. Available from X-Gen Pharmaceuticals, 607-732-4411. Ref. re: IV—*CID 19:1150, 1994*. Toxicity similar with qd vs tid dosing *(CID 38:1538, 2004)*.	Monthly audiogram. In older pts, serum creatinine or BUN at start of rx and weekly if pt stable

[1] Note: Malabsorption of antimycobacterial drugs may occur in patients with AIDS enteropathy. For review of adverse effects, see *AJRCCM 167:1472, 2003*.
[2] **RES** = % resistance of M. tuberculosis

See page 2 for abbreviations

* Dosages are for adults (unless otherwise indicated) and assume normal renal function

† **DOT** = directly observed therapy; **SAT** = self-administered therapy

§ Mean (range) (higher in Hispanics, Asians, and patients <10 years old)

TABLE 12B (2)

AGENT (TRADE NAME)[1]	USUAL DOSAGE*	ROUTE/1º DRUG RESISTANCE (RES) US[2,§]	SIDE-EFFECTS, TOXICITY AND PRECAUTIONS	SURVEILLANCE
SECOND LINE DRUGS (more difficult to use and/or less effective than first line drugs)				
Amikacin (Amikin) (IV sol'n)	7.5–10.0 mg per kg q24h [Bactericidal for extracellular organisms]	RES: (est. 0.1%) IM/IV 500 mg vial	*See Table 10C, page 166* Toxicity similar with qd vs tid dosing *(CID 38:1538, 2004)*.	Monthly audiogram. Serum creatinine or BUN weekly if pt stable
Amikacin liposomal suspension (for inhalation)	One daily oral inhalation	Via inhalation	Risk of respiratory AEs: hypersensitivity, pneumonitis, hemoptysis, bronchospasm.	
Bedaquiline (Sirturo) (100 mg tab) Ref: *JAC 69:2310, 2014; NEJM 371:723, 2014; CID 60:188, 2015.*	Directly observed therapy (DOT): 400 mg once daily for 2 weeks, then 200 mg 3 times weekly for 22 weeks, taken with food and always used in combination with other anti-TB medications.	Does not exhibit cross-resistance to other TB drugs; always use in combination with other TB drugs to prevent selection of resistant mutants	Most common: nausea, vomiting, arthralgia, headache, hyperuricemia. Elevated transaminases. Bedaquiline in clinical trials was administered as one component of a multiple drug regimen, so side-effects were common, yet difficult to assign to a particular drug. Resistance reported: *CID 2018,66:1625.*	Moderate QTc increases (average of 10-16 ms over the 24 weeks of therapy. Potential risks of pancreatitis, myopathy, myocardial injury, severe hepatotoxicity.
Capreomycin sulfate (Capastat sulfate)	1 gm per day (15 mg per kg per day) q24h as 1 dose	RES: 0.1% (0–0.9%) IM/IV	Nephrotoxicity (36%), ototoxicity (auditory 11%), eosinophilia, leukopenia, skin rash, fever, hypokalemia, neuromuscular blockade.	Monthly audiogram, biweekly serum creatinine or BUN
Ciprofloxacin (Cipro) (250, 500, 750 mg tab)	750 mg bid	500 mg or 750 mg po IV 200-400 mg vial	TB not an FDA-approved indication for CIP. Desired CIP serum levels 4–6 mcg per mL. *See Table 10A, page 159 for adverse effects.*	None
Clofazimine (Lamprene) (50, 100 mg cap)	50 mg per day (unsupervised) + 300 mg 1 time per month supervised or 100 mg per day	50 mg (with meals)	Skin: **pigmentation (pink-brownish black)** 75–100%, dryness 20%, pruritus 5%. GI: abdominal pain 50% (rarely severe leading to exploratory laparoscopy), splenic infarction (VR), bowel obstruction (VR), GI bleeding (VR). Eye: conjunctival irritation, retinal crystal deposits. Potential to prolong QTc interval.	None
Cycloserine (Seromycin) (250 mg tab)	750–1000 mg per day (15 mg per kg per day) 2–4 doses per day [Bacteriostatic for both extra-cellular & intracellular organisms]	RES: 0.1% (0–0.3%) 250 mg cap	Convulsions, **psychoses** (5–10% of those receiving 1.0 gm per day); headache; somnolence; hyperreflexia; increased CSF protein and pressure, **peripheral neuropathy.** 100 mg pyridoxine (or more) q24h should be given concomitantly. Contraindicated in epileptics.	None
Dapsone (25, 100 mg tab)	100 mg per day	100 mg tab	Blood: ↓ hemoglobin (1–2 gm) & ↑ retics (2–12%), in most pts. Hemolysis in G6PD deficiency. ↑ hemolysis due to concomitant atazanavir *(AAC 56:1081, 2012).* **Methemoglobinemia.** CNS: peripheral neuropathy (rare). GI: nausea, vomiting. Renal: albuminuria, nephrotic syndrome. Erythema nodosum leprosum in pts rx for leprosy (½ pts 1st year). Hypersensitivity syndrome in 0.5-3.6% *(See Surveillance)*.	Hypersensitivity syndrome: fever, rash, eosinophilia, lymphadenopathy, hepatitis, pneumonitis. Genetic marker identified *(NEJM 369:1620, 2013)*.
Ethionamide (Trecator-SC) (120, 250 mg tab)	500–1000 mg per day (15–20 mg per kg per day) divided 1–3 doses per day [Bacteriostatic for extracellular organisms only]	RES: 0.8% (0–1.5%) 250 mg tab	**Gastrointestinal irritation** (up to 50% on large dose); goiter; peripheral neuropathy (rare); convulsions (rare); changes in affect (rare); difficulty in diabetes control; rashes; hepatitis; purpura; stomatitis; gynecomastia; menstrual irregularity. Give drug with meals or antacids; 50–100 mg pyridoxine per day concomitantly; SGOT monthly. Possibly teratogenic.	

See page 2 for abbreviations

* Dosages are for adults (unless otherwise indicated) and assume normal renal function

§ Mean (range) (higher in Hispanics, Asians, and patients <10 years old)

† **DOT** = directly observed therapy; **SAT** = self-administered therapy

TABLE 12B (3)

AGENT (TRADE NAME)[1]	USUAL DOSAGE*	ROUTE/1º DRUG RESISTANCE (RES) US[2, §]	SIDE-EFFECTS, TOXICITY AND PRECAUTIONS	SURVEILLANCE
SECOND LINE DRUGS *(continued)*				
Levofloxacin (Levaquin) (250, 500, 750 mg tab)	250-750 mg q24h	PO or IV	Not FDA-approved indication. Overall adverse effects 11%, 4% discontinued due to side-effects. GI: nausea 3%, diarrhea 1%. CNS: insomnia 3%, headache 1%, dizziness 1%. Potential for QTc prolongation. Rare: tendinitis, tendon rupture is, tendon rupture.	None
Linezolid (Zyvox) (600 mg tab, oral suspension 100 mg/mL)	600 mg once daily	PO or IV	Not FDA-approved indication. High rate of adverse events (>80% with 4 months or longer of therapy: myelosuppression, peripheral neuropathy, optic neuropathy. Avoid tyramine-containing foods, soy products, adrenergic agents (e.g., pseudoephedrine, phenylpropanolamine) MOA inhibitors, SSRIs. 600 mg >300 mg dose for toxicity; consider reducing dose to 300 mg for toxicity or after 4 mos of therapy or culture-conversion to reduce toxicity.	Baseline and monthly complete blood count, visual acuity checks, screen for symptoms of peripheral neuropathy, neurologic examination.
Moxifloxacin (Avelox) (400 mg tab)	400 mg qd	400 mg cap	Not FDA-approved indication. Most common reactions (3% or greater): nausea, diarrhea, headache, and dizziness. Potential for QTc prolongation. Rare: tendinitis, tendon rupture.	None
Para-aminosalicylic acid (PAS, Paser) (Na^+ or K^+ salt) (4 gm cap)	4–6 gm bid (200 mg per kg per day) [Bacteriostatic for extracellular organisms only]	RES: 0.8% (0–1.5%) 450 mg tab *(see Comment)*	**Gastrointestinal irritation** (10–15%); goitrogenic action (rare); depressed prothrombin activity (rare); G6PD-mediated hemolytic anemia (rare), drug fever, rashes, hepatitis, myalgia, arthralgia. Retards hepatic enzyme induction, may ↓ INH hepatotoxicity. Available from CDC, (404) 639-3670, Jacobus Pharm. Co. (609) 921-7447.	None
Pretomanid (Pretomanid) (200 mg tab)	200 mg orally qd for 26 weeks in combination with bedaquiline and linezolid	200 mg tab	Adverse effects reported with the combination of pretomanid, bedaquiline, and linezolid include gastrointestinal effects (nausea, vomiting, abdominal pain, diarrhea), hepatotoxicity, increased transaminases, lactic acidosis, myelosuppression, peripheral and/or optic neuropathy, QT-interval prolongation, rash. Avoid co-administration with strong or moderate CYP3A4 inducers such as rifampin or efavirenz.	Monitor liver-related laboratory tests, complete blood counts, visual function and ECGs for QTcF interval prolongation. If pretomanid is co-administered with OAT3 substrate drugs (e.g., methotrexate), monitor for OAT3 substrate drug-related adverse reactions.
Rifabutin (Mycobutin) (150 mg cap)	300 mg per day (prophylaxis or treatment)	150 mg tab	Polymyalgia, polyarthralgia, granulocytopenia. Uveitis rare with 300 mg/day but increases to 8-38% if higher dose or combined with clarithro, PI or azole antifungal. Reddish urine, orange skin (pseudojaundice). *See Comment*	Clinical pharmacology *(see OFID doi:10.1093/ofid/ofa 460)*
Rifapentine (Priftin) (150 mg tab)	600 mg twice weekly for 1st 2 mos., then 600 mg q week	150 mg tab	Similar to other rifabutins. *(See RIF, RFB)*. Hyperuricemia seen in 21%. Causes red-orange discoloration of body fluids. Flu-like illness in pts given weekly Rifapentine + INH for latent MTB *(CID 61:527, 2015)*.	None
Thalidomide (Thalomid) (50, 100, 200 mg cap)	100–300 mg po q24h (may use up to 400 mg po q24h for severe erythema nodosum leprosum)	50 mg tab	**Contraindicated in pregnancy. Causes severe life-threatening birth defects. Both male and female patients must use barrier contraceptive methods (Pregnancy Category X).** Frequently causes drowsiness or somnolence. May cause peripheral neuropathy. *(AJM 108:487, 2000)* For review, *see Ln 363:1803, 2004*.	In US: contact Celgene (800-4-CELGENE)

See page 2 for abbreviations

* Dosages are for adults (unless otherwise indicated) and assume normal renal function

§ Mean (range) (higher in Hispanics, Asians, and patients <10 years old)

† **DOT** = directly observed therapy; **SAT** = self-administered therapy

TABLE 13A – TREATMENT OF PARASITIC INFECTIONS

- ***See Table 13D* for sources for antiparasitic drugs not otherwise commercially available.**
- The following resources are available through the Centers for Disease Control and Prevention (CDC) in Atlanta. Website is www.cdc.gov. General advice for parasitic diseases other than malaria: (+1) (404) 718-4745 (day), (+1) (770) 488-7100 (after hours). For CDC Drug Service 8:00 a.m. – 4:30 p.m. EST: (+1) (404) 639-3670; fax: (+1) (404) 639-3717. *See www.cdc.gov/laboratory/drugservice/index.html* For malaria: Prophylaxis advice (+1) (770) 488-7788; treatment (+1) (770) 488-7788; or after hours (+1) (770) 488-7100; toll-free (US) 1-855-856-4713; website: *www.cdc.gov/malaria*
- **NOTE: All dosage regimens are for adults with normal renal function unless otherwise stated.** Many of the suggested regimens are not FDA approved.
- For licensed drugs, suggest checking package inserts to verify dosage and side-effects. Occasionally, post-licensure data may alter dosage as compared to package inserts.

INFECTING ORGANISM	SUGGESTED REGIMENS		COMMENTS
	PRIMARY	ALTERNATIVE	
PROTOZOA—INTESTINAL (non-pathogenic: E. bangladeshi, E. hartmanni, E. dispar, E. moshkovskii, E. coli, Iodamoeba bütschlii, Endolimax nana, Chilomastix mesnili)			
Balantioides coli Review: *Acta Trop 2021 Jul 31;223:106069.*	**Tetracycline** 500 mg po qid x 10 days	**Metronidazole** 750 mg po tid x 5 days	Another alternative: Iodoquinol 650 mg po tid x 20 days.
Blastocystis hominis RCT showing no treatment benefit *(J Travel Med 2023 Feb 18;30(1):taac143)*	**Metronidazole** 1.5 gm po 1x/day x 10 days or 750 mg po tid x 10 days (need to treat is dubious).	**Alternatives: Iodoquinol*** 650 mg po tid x 20 days or **TMP-SMX-DS,** one bid x 7 days or **Nitazoxanide** 500 mg po bid x 3 days	Recent paradigm shift *(Trends Parasitol 2024 Sep;40(9):775)*, metagenomic proof of non-pathogenicity.
Cryptosporidium parvum & hominis Treatment is unsatisfactory Ref.: *Ln ID 15:85, 2015*	**Immunocompetent—No HIV: Nitazoxanide** 500 mg po bid x 3 days (expensive)	**HIV with immunodeficiency:** Effective antiretroviral therapy best therapy. **Nitazoxanide** no clinical or parasite response compared to placebo.	**Nitazoxanide:** Approved in liquid formulation for rx of children & 500 mg tabs for adults who are immunocompetent. Ref.: *CID 40:1173, 2005.* **C. hominis** assoc. with ↑ in post-infection eye & joint pain, recurrent headache, & dizzy spells *(CID 39:504, 2004).*
Cyclospora cayetanensis; cyclosporiasis Ref: *Ln ID 19:e226, 2019*	**Immunocompetent pts: TMP-SMX-DS** tab 1 po bid x 7–10 days. Other options: *see Comments.*	**AIDS pts: TMP-SMX-DS** tab 1 po qid for up to 3-4 wks. Immunocompromised pts: may require suppressive rx with **TMP-SMX** DS 1 tab 3x/wk	If sulfa-allergic: **CIP** 500 mg po bid x 7 days but results inconsistent. Biliary disease described in HIV pts.
Dientamoeba fragilis Ref: *Clin Micro Rev 54:2243, 2017; J Clin Microbiol pii: JCM.00400-16, 2016*	**Iodoquinol*** 650 mg po tid x 20 days or **Paromomycin*** 25-35 mg/kg/day po in 3 div doses x 7 days or **Metronidazole** 750 mg tid x 10 days.	For treatment failures: **Tetracycline** 500 mg po qid x 10 days + **Iodoquinol*** 650 mg po tid x 10 days OR (**Iodoquinol*** + **Paromomycin***) May try second course of Iodoquinol	**Metronidazole** failed in prospective random placebo-control DB study *(CID 58:1692, 2014). In vitro tinidazole, metronidazole most active. AAC 56:487, 2012*
Entamoeba histolytica; amebiasis. If available, use stool PCR for diagnosis. E. histolytica, E. dispar, E. moshkovskii, are microscopically identical; antigen testing needed to distinguish.			
Asymptomatic cyst passer	**Paromomycin*** 25-35 mg/kg/day po in 3 divided doses x 7 days OR **Iodoquinol*** 650 mg po tid x 20 days	**Diloxanide furoate*** (Furamide) 500 mg po tid x 10 days.	
Patient with diarrhea/dysentery; mild/moderate disease. Oral therapy possible	**Metronidazole** 500–750 mg po tid x 7-10 days or **Tinidazole** 2 gm po daily x 3 days, followed by: Either [**Paromomycin*** 25-35 mg/kg/day po divided in 3 doses x 7 days] or [**Iodoquinol*** 650 mg po tid x 20 days] to clear intestinal cysts. *See comment.*		General review: *Open Forum Infect Dise 2018, 5:ofy161.* Colitis can mimic ulcerative colitis; ameboma can mimic adenocarcinoma of colon. **Nitazoxanide** 500 mg po bid x 3 days may be effective *(JID 184:381, 2001 & Tran R Soc Trop Med & Hyg 101:1025, 2007)*
Severe or extraintestinal infection, e.g., hepatic abscess	(**Metronidazole** 750 mg **IV to po** tid x 10 days or **Tinidazole** 2 gm 1x/day x 5 days) followed by **Paromomycin*** 25-35 mg/kg/day po divided in 3 doses x 7 days or **Iodoquinol*** 650 mg po tid x 20 days.		Serology positive (antibody present) with extraintestinal disease. Serology positive (antibody present) with extraintestinal disease only, may be negative in first wk. May remain positive for life post-1st infection.

* For source of drug, see *Table 13D, page 222.*

TABLE 13A (2)

INFECTING ORGANISM	SUGGESTED REGIMENS		COMMENTS
	PRIMARY	ALTERNATIVE	
PROTOZOA—INTESTINAL *(continued)*			
Giardia duodenalis also known as **Giardia lamblia, Giardia intestinalis.**	**Tinidazole** 2 gm po x 1	**Metronidazole** 250 mg po tid x 5 days; Nitazoxanide 500 mg po bid x 3 days; Albendazole 400 mg po once daily with food x 5 days.	**Refractory pts: Quinacrine** 100 mg po tid x 5 days or **(metro 750 mg po + quinacrine 100 mg po)** or (**Paromomycin** 10 mg/kg po) 3x/day x 3 wks giardia genetically heterogeneous *https://pubmed.ncbi.nlm.nih.gov/34715087/*. **Pregnancy: Paromomycin*** 25-35 mg/kg/day po in 3 divided doses x 5-10 days.
Cystoisospora belli (formerly Isospora belli) Diagnosis requires special order: AFB stain of stool or use multiplex PCR stool assay	**Immunocompetent: TMP-SMX-DS** tab 1 po bid x 7-10 days; **Immunocompromised: TMP-SMX-DS** qid for up to 4 wks. If CD4<200 may not respond; need ART.	**CIP** 500 mg po bid x 7 days is second-line alternative *(AnIM 132:885, 2000)* OR **Pyrimethamine** 50-75 mg/day + **Folinic acid** 10-25 mg/day (po).	**Chronic suppression in AIDS pts:** either **TMP-SMX-DS** 1 tab po 3x/wk OR tab 1 po daily OR (**Pyrimethamine** 25 mg/day po + **Folinic acid** 10 mg/day po) OR as 2nd-line alternative: **CIP** 500 mg po 3x/wk.
Microsporidiosis	For HIV pts: antiretroviral therapy key. *See 2023 NIH Guidelines at aidsinfo.nih.gov.* Rec to treat until CD4 >200		
Ocular: Encephalitozoon hellum or cuniculi, Vittaforma (Nosema) corneae, Nosema ocularum	**Albendazole** 400 mg po bid x 3 wks plus fumagillin eye drops *(see Comment)*.	In HIV+ pts, reports of response of E. hellum to **Fumagillin*** eyedrops *(see Comment)*. For V. corneae, may need keratoplasty.	No source for humans though veterinary preps available. Neutropenia & thrombocytopenia serious adverse events. Dx: Most labs use modified trichrome stain. Need electron micrographs for species identification. IFA and PCR methods in development. Peds dose ref.: *PIDJ 23:915, 2004*
Intestinal (diarrhea): Enterocytozoon bieneusi (HIV), Encephalitozoon (Septata) intestinalis	**Albendazole** 400 mg po bid x 3 wks; peds dose: 15 mg/kg per day div. into 2 daily doses x 7 days for **E. intestinalis.** Fumagillin equally effective. For HIV-associated, treat until CD4 >200 for 6 mos.	Oral **Fumagillin*** 20 mg po tid reported effective for **E. bieneusi** *(NEJM 346:1963, 2002)* (only effective treatment but currently not available). For HIV-associated, treat until CD4 >200 *(see Comment)*. Albendazole not effective.	
Disseminated: E. hellum, cuniculi or intestinalis; Pleistophora sp., *others in Comment. Ref: JCM 52:3839, 2014.*	**Albendazole** 400 mg po bid x 3 wks. Fumagillin 20 mg po tid (where available). For HIV-associated, treat until CD4 >200.	No established rx for Pleistophora sp.	For Trachipleistophora sp., try itraconazole + albendazole *(NEJM 351:42, 2004)*. Other pathogens: Brachiola vesicularum & algerae *(NEJM 351:42, 2004)*.
PROTOZOA—EXTRAINTESTINAL			
Amebic meningoencephalitis and keratitis	Review of US experience *(CID 68:1815, 2019)*. CDC no longer provides miltefosine. *See www.impavido.com*		
Acanthamoeba sp.— no proven rx Rev.: *FEMS Immunol Med Micro 50:1, 2007*	Adult IV therapy: [**Pentamidine + Fluconazole**] + **Miltefosine*** 50 mg po tid. May add **TMP-SMX**, **Metronidazole**, and **Azithromycin**		
Acanthamoeba keratitis	Topical 0.02%-0.2% biguanide chlorhexidine or 0.02%-0.06% Polyhexamethylene biguanide (PHMB) in combination with propamidine (0.1%) or hexamidine (0.1%). Start with lower dose of biguanides and titrate to clinical response. Initially, drops should be applied up to hourly day and night for the first 48 hours then hourly during the daytime for the first week, then with subsequent taper over 3-4 weeks. Debridement may also be warranted.	Uncontrolled reports of amebic eradication with oral miltefosine but post-miltefosine inflammatory response leads to corneal thinning and possible perforation. Steroid coverage has been proposed. See *https://pubmed.ncbi.nlm.nih.gov/32469616/*	Large case series *https://pubmed.ncbi.nlm.nih.gov/35198803/*

* For source of drug, see *Table 13D, page 222.*

TABLE 13A (3)

INFECTING ORGANISM	SUGGESTED REGIMENS		COMMENTS
	PRIMARY	ALTERNATIVE	
PROTOZOA—EXTRAINTESTINAL/Amebic meningoencephalitis and keratitis *(continued)*			
Balamuthia mandrillaris	**Albendazole** + (**Fluconazole** or **Itraconazole**) + **Miltefosine*** 50 mg po tid ± **pentamidine** (poorly tolerated)		Need brain tissue for dx. Dramatic recovery of single case of Balamuthia with nitroxoline *(Emerg Infect Dis 2023; 29:197)*.
Naegleria fowleri. >95% mortality. Ref. *MMWR 57:573, 2008.*	**Amphotericin** B 1.5 mg/kg/day ± intrathecal + **Rifampin** 10 mg/kg/day + **Fluconazole** 10 mg/kg/day IV/po + **Miltefosine*** 50 mg po tid + **Azithromycin** 500 mg IV/po. Duration of therapy is empiric as there are few survivors		
Babesia microti (US), **Babesia duncani** (US West Coast), and **Babesia divergens** (EU) Recent comprehensive review: *https://pubmed.ncbi.nlm.nih.gov/36116841/*. See IDSA Guidelines in *CID 72:185, 2021.*	**Adult mild/moderate disease** (outpatient, <4% parasitemia) [(**Atovaquone** 750 mg po q12h) + (**Azithromycin** 500 mg po on day 1, then 250 mg/day po)] for a total of 7-10 days. **Acute severe disease** (hospitalized) Adult: **Atovaquone** 750 mg po q12h + **Azithromycin** 500–1000 mg IV q24h until symptoms abate, then convert to all oral step-down therapy. Follow with step-down therapy: **Atovaquone** 750 mg po q12h + **Azithromycin** 250–500 (500-1000 if immunocompromised) mg po q24h to complete a total of 7-10 days.	**Mild/moderate: Clindamycin** 600 mg po q8h + **quinine sulfate** 542 mg base (which equals 650 mg salt) po q6h–8h x 7 to 10 days. **Acute Severe Hospitalized: Clindamycin** 600 mg IV q6h + **quinine sulfate** 542 mg base po q6h–8h until symptoms abate, then convert to all oral step-down therapy. Follow with step-down therapy: **Clindamycin** 600 mg po q8h + **quinine sulfate** 542 mg base po q6h–8h to complete a total of 7-10 days. Compelling in vivo data for tafenoquine *(JID 220:442, 2019)*. Clinda/quinine in pregnancy.	Highly Immunocompromised patients: Treat for 6 consecutive weeks with a regimen as per severe disease ensuring negative blood smears for the final 2 weeks. For treatment failures or relapses consider following combinations: Atovaquone + Azithromycin + Clindamycin; Atovaquone + Clindamycin; Atovaquone/proguanil + Azithromycin; Atovaquone + Azithromycin + Clindamycin + quinine. Use 500-1000 mg of Azithromycin. Triple therapy with tafenoquine-atovaquone-azithromycin for 10 days under investigation.
Leishmaniasis *(Suggest consultation – CDC (+1) 404-718-4745)*. Therapy needs individualization according to species and many options for each manifestation. **Note: Miltefosine available directly from Profounda, Inc. (+1 407-270-7790), www.impavido.com.** Definitive guidelines from IDSA/ASTMH *academic.oup.com/cid/article/63/12/e202/2645609* and include geographic distribution maps for each species. Diagnosis of cutaneous disease: Sample full depth punch biopsy from raised edge of ulcer. PCR mandatory to speciate; culture and histology also available. Rapid diagnosis often possible using needle aspirate, slit skin smear, brushings, or scraping of lesion edge with giemsa staining. Serology not useful. Miltefosine and pentavalent antimony no longer available from CDC drug service. Glucantime (Meglumine antimoniate) available only from Sanofi (no cost) after obtaining an individual IND from FDA (laborious).			
Cutaneous: Mild Disease 4 or less lesions (1 cm or more), none > or = to 5 cm in diameter; no lesions in cosmetically sensitive areas, no lesions over joints or genitalia; may observe. Otherwise, consider Complex Disease which includes failure of previous treatment, or substantial local or lymphatic nodules, or large regional lymphadenopathy.	**Mild Disease** in travelers frequently responds to observation or local therapy and is preferred approach if patient agrees **Paromomycin*** 15% paromomycin and 12% MBCL ointment bid x 10 days rest for 10 days and then 10 more days; **cryotherapy** (freeze up to 3 x with liquid nitrogen); intralesional **Antimony** up to 5 mL into lesions weekly x 8-10 wks with cryotherapy at end of each treatment. New data on IL dosing in old world CL *https://pubmed.ncbi.nlm.nih.gov/35802749/* **Alternative: Miltefosine** (w/food) 50 mg po bid (wt 30-44 kg); 50 mg tid (wt ≥45 kg). Treat for 28 days. Response in about 70% of pts. Short course miltefosine (14d.) for new world cutaneous leishmaniasis when combined with thermotherapy *PLOS Neglected Tropical Diseases 2022; 16(3):e0010238. doi: 10.1371/journal.pntd.0010238*	**Moderate Disease:** **Meglumine antimoniate** (Glucantime) 20 mg/kg/day Sb IV x 20 days. Dilute in 120 mL of D5W and infuse over 1-2 hrs OR Liposomal **Amphotericin B** (3 mg/kg IV once daily days 1-5 and 10. Alternatives: **Fluconazole** 200 mg po daily x 6 weeks (for *L. mexicana, L. panamensis, L. major*) or **Ketoconazole** 600 mg po daily x 30 days *(L. mexicana)* or **Miltefosine** (dose as for mild disease). Some experts use **Ampho B** 0.5-1 mg/kg IV daily or qod to total dose of 15-30 mg/kg *PAHO Guidelines https://iris.paho.org/handle/10665.2/56120* Review of short course liposomal Amphotericin B for cutaneous and mucosal Leishmaniasis. *Open Forum Infect Dis. 2023 Jul 11;10(7):ofad348.*	Observation, oral therapy, thermotherapy (www.thermosurgery.com), topical paromomycin* only when low potential for mucosal spread; never use for lesions of any severity which are or may be *L. brasiliensis, L. panamensis* or *L. guyanensis* which always require therapy as per mucosal leishmaniasis below. Generic pentavalent antimony varies in quality and safety. Mild disease in travelers frequently responds to observation and is acceptable per IDSA/ASTMH guidelines. Monitor for gradual healing. Miltefosine is preg cat D (do not use in pregnancy). Large European experience in travelers: *https://pubmed.ncbi.nlm.nih.gov/35086613/*

* For source of drug, see *Table 13D, page 222.*

TABLE 13A (4)

INFECTING ORGANISM	SUGGESTED REGIMENS		COMMENTS
	PRIMARY	ALTERNATIVE	
PROTOZOA—EXTRAINTESTINAL *(continued)*			
Leishmaniasis, Mucosal (Espundia) All cutaneous lesions due to *L. brasiliensis*, *L. guyanensis*, or *L. panamensis* is proven or possible.	• **Cutaneous *L. braziliensis* of any severity:** ○ [**Sodium Stibogluconate** (Pentostam) or **Meglumine antimoniate** (Glucantime)] 20 mg/kg/day IV/IM x 20 days ○ **Liposomal Ampho B** (3 mg/kg IV once daily days 1-5 and days 14, 21 or days 1-5 and 10. • **Mucosal: Pentavalent antimony (Sb)*** 20 mg/kg/day Sb IV x 28 days for mucosal disease, or **Liposomal Amphotericin B** (regimens vary) with total cumulative dose of 20-60 mg/kg or **Amphotericin B** 0.5-1 mg/kg IV daily or qod to total dose of 20 45 mg/kg.	**Miltefosine*** (w/food) 50 mg po bid (wt 30-44 kg); 50 mg tid (wt ≥45 kg). Treat for 28 days. Complete resolution in 62% of pts.	*See Table 13D for contact information and drug availability.* Miltefosine has variable activity against mucosal disease according to geographic location. Expert consultation needed.
Visceral leishmaniasis (Kala-Azar) *New World & Old World* *L. donovani: India, Africa* *L. infantum: Mediterranean* *L. chagasi: New World (identical to L. infantum)*	*Immunocompetent:* **Liposomal Ampho B** 3 mg/kg once daily days 1-5 & days 14, 21 (increase to 40 mg/kg total dose for East African VL) *HIV/AIDS:* ***L. donovani:*** **Liposomal Amphotericin B** (up to 30 mg/kg cumulative, at 5 mg/kg on days 1, 3, 5, 7, 9, 11) + **Miltefosine** (100 mg/day po X 14 days in Asia and most places and 28d for East Africa) ***L. infantum/chagasi:*** **Liposomal Amphotericin B** (total dose of 20–60 mg/kg via either 3–5 mg/kg IV daily, or Interrupted schedule, such as 4 mg/kg IV on Days 1–5, 10, 17, 24, 31. This schedule (no miltefosine) is an alternate for *L. Donovani*	**Standard Ampho B** 1 mg/kg IV daily x 15-20 days or qod x 8 wks (to total of 15-20 mg/kg) OR **pentavalent antimony*** 20 mg/kg/day IV x 28 days OR **Miltefosine*** (w/food) 50 mg po bid (wt 30-44 kg); 50 mg tid (wt ≥45 kg). Do not use miltefosine in HIV pts.	**Secondary prophylaxis** (CD4 <200) with Liposomal Amphotericin B (3-5 mg/kg) or Amphotericin B (1 mg/kg) q2-4 wks until CD4 >350. Consider stopping secondary prophylaxis when the CD4 count is >350 cells/mm, viral load undetectable for 6 months, and asymptomatic. **Alternate Therapy:** Amphotericin B lipid complex 3 mg/kg every 21 days, or Pentavalent antimony (meglumine antimoniate) 20 mg/kg IV or IM every 4 weeks or Pentamidine isethionate 4 mg/kg (maximum of 300 mg) IV every 2–4 week. Reference: *WHO Guideline 7 Jun 2022 and NIH Guidelines for HIV OIs.*
Malaria (Plasmodia species) —NOTE: *CDC Malaria info— prophylaxis/treatment (770) 488-7788. After hours: 770-488-7100. US toll-free 1-855-856-4713. CDC offers species confirmation and drug resistance testing.* See: *www.cdc.gov/malaria*			
Prophylaxis—Drugs plus personal protection: screens, nets, 30–35% DEET skin repellent (avoid >50% DEET) permethrin spray on clothing and mosquito nets. Country risk: *see CDC malaria guidance (cdc.gov); https://wwwnc.cdc.gov/travel/destinations/list*			
For areas free of chloroquine (CQ)-resistant P. falciparum: Central America (west of Panama Canal), Caribbean, Korea, Middle East (most)	**CQ** phosphate 500 mg (300 mg base) po per wk starting 1–2 wks before travel, during travel, & 4 wks post-travel **or Atovaquone-Proguanil (AP)** 1 adult tab per day (1 day prior to, during, & 7 days post-travel) or **Tafenoquine** 200 mg once daily x3 days (starting 3 days before travel) then 200 mg once weekly (starting 7 days after last loading regimen dose) then a 200 mg one-time dose (7 days after last dose in malaria area in non-pregnant G6PD-normal travelers. Note: **CQ** may exacerbate psoriasis.	**CQ Peds dose:** 8.3 mg/kg (5 mg/kg of base) po 1x/wk up to 300 mg (base) max. dose **or AP** by weight (peds tabs): 5-8 kg 1/2 tab, 9-10 kg 3/4 tab, 11–20 kg, 1 tab; 21–30 kg, 2 tabs; 31–40 kg, 3 tabs; >40 kg, 1 adult tab per day. **Adults: Doxy** or **MQ** as below.	AP must be taken with food for adequate absorption. CQ safe during pregnancy. **The areas free of CQ-resistant falciparum malaria continue to shrink:** *See CDC or WHO maps for most current information on CQ resistance.* **Doxy AEs:** photosensitivity, candida vaginitis, gastritis. For Tafenoquine must document on at least 1 occasion during life a quantitative level of >70% normal level of G6PD activity before use. Do not use screening or qualitative G6PD tests.

* For source of drug, see *Table 13D, page 222.*

TABLE 13A (5)

INFECTING ORGANISM	SUGGESTED REGIMENS		COMMENTS
	PRIMARY	ALTERNATIVE	
PROTOZOA—EXTRAINTESTINAL/Malaria (Plasmodia species)/Prophylaxis *(continued)*			
For areas with CQ-resistant P. falciparum Details on considerations for malaria prophylaxis: *N Engl J Med. 2016; 375:247.*	**Atovaquone** 250 mg—**Proguanil** 100 mg **(Malarone)** comb. tablet, 1 per day with food 1–2 days prior to, during, & 7 days post-travel. Not FDA approved or yet recommended in pregnancy but safety data at *J Travel Med 2020 Jul 14;27(4):taaa074* and *(Trav Med ID 27:20, 2019)*. Malarone preferred for trips of a week or less; expense may preclude use for longer trips.	**Doxycycline** 100 mg po daily for adults & children >8 yrs of age. Take 1-2 days before, during & for 4 wks after travel **OR TQ** 200 mg once daily x3 days (starting 3 days before travel) then 200 mg once weekly (starting 7 days after last loading regimen dose) then a 200 mg one-time dose (7 days after last dose in malaria area) **OR Mefloquine (MQ)** 250 mg (228 mg base) po once per wk, 1-2 wks before, during, & for 4 wks after travel *(see Comment)*. **Doxy:** 2.2 mg/kg po per day,(max 100 mg/day) **MFQ:** ≤ 9 kg: 5 mg/kg weekly (4.6 mg/kg base) 10-19 kg: ¼ adult tab weekly 20-30 kg: ½ tab weekly 31-45 kg: ¾ tab weekly > 45 kg: 1 tab weekly **Doxy AEs:** photosensitivity, candida vaginitis, gastritis.	**Pregnancy: MQ current best option. Avoid doxycycline and tafenoquine.** **Tafenoquine** (TQ), **Primaquine: Can cause hemolytic anemia if G6PD deficiency present. For TQ must test for G6PD (as above). TQ causes benign vortex keratopathy in 21% after 6 months use.** **MQ not recommended** if cardiac conduction abnormalities, seizures, or psychiatric disorders, e.g., depression, psychosis. If used, can start 3 wks before travel to assure tolerability. Children: Weekly dosing may make MFQ preferable; TQ not licensed in children. If 8 yr or older doxycycline liquid is available. For children under 10 kg. MFQ needs to be compounded but AP pediatric tablets can be cut. TQ good option when weekly dosing preferable such as for long-stay trips. TQ not approved for use for >6 months consecutively; use 3-month washout.
Treatment of Malaria. Diagnosis is by microscopy. Alternative: rapid antigen detection test *(Binax NOW)*: detects 96-100% of P. falciparum and 50% of other plasmodia. Need microscopy or PCR to speciate or detect low level infection. Can stay positive for over a month after successful treatment. A negative RDT *(US: Binax; HRP based)* no longer reliably rules out P. falciparum infection due to the increasing global prevalence of HRP2/3 deletion mutants.			
Uncomplicated P. falciparum (or species unidentified). Real-time updated WHO Treatment guidelines see *https://app.magicapp.org/#/guideline/7661.* Use ACT as first line for all malaria species including in all pregnancy trimesters (use Artemether-lumefantrine in non-endemic countries). No obesity adjustment but close follow-up needed.			
Acquired in Cen. Amer., west of Panama Canal; Haiti, Dom. Repub., & most of Mid-East **CQ sensitive**	**Adults: CQ phosphate** 1 gm salt (600 mg base) po, then 0.5 gm in 6 hrs, then 0.5 gm daily x 2 days. Total: 2500 mg salt	**Peds: CQ** 10 mg/kg of base po; then 5 mg/kg of base at 6, 24, & 48 hrs. Total: 25 mg/kg base	Other chloroquine salts available in some countries, total dose may differ **Peds dose should never exceed adult dose. CQ + MQ prolong QTc. Doses >2x recommended may be fatal.**

* For source of drug, see *Table 13D, page 222.*

TABLE 13A (6)

INFECTING ORGANISM	SUGGESTED REGIMENS		COMMENTS
	PRIMARY	ALTERNATIVE	
PROTOZOA—EXTRAINTESTINAL/Malaria (Plasmodia species)/Treatment of Malaria *(continued)*			
Uncomplicated P. falciparum or species unknown / CQ-resistant or unknown resistance Note: If >4% parasitemia or Hb <7, treat as severe malaria regardless of clinical findings or lack thereof. CDC guidelines for IV artesunate requires >5% parasitemia if no other severe malaria criteria met. Note to reader re dosing: For Peds, developing world drugs are listed under Primary; drugs of choice are listed under Alternative; Pregnancy alternatives are listed under Comments.	**Adults: Atovaquone-Proguanil** 1 gm–400 mg (4 adult tabs) po 1x/day x 3 days w/ food OR [**QS** 650 mg po tid x 3 days (7 days if SE Asia)] + [(**Doxy** 100 mg po bid) or (**Tetra** 250 mg po qid) or **Clinda** 20 mg/kg/d divided tid) x 7 days] OR **Artemether-Lumefantrine*** tabs 20/120 mg: 4 tabs po (at 0, 8 hrs) then bid x 2 days (total 6 doses); take with food OR a less desirable adult alternative, **Mefloquine** 750 mg po x 1 dose, then 500 mg po x 1 dose 6-12 hr later. **MQ** is 2nd line alternative due to neuropsychiatric reaction and cannot use in SE Asia due to resistance. Clinda or Tetra only if doxy not available. Other options: Available in Europe and endemic countries, WHO pre-qualified and EMA approved is **Dihydroartemisinin-piperaquine**. Available as PPQ 320 mg/DHA 40 mg (adult tabs) and PPQ 160 mg/DHA 20 mg (pediatric tabs). 5 to <7 kg PPQ 80 mg/DHA 10 mg po q24h x3 days 7 to <13 kg PPQ 160 mg/DHA 20 mg po q24h x3 days 13 to <24 kg PPQ 320 mg/DHA 40 mg po q24h x3 days 24 to <36 kg PPQ 640 mg/DHA 80 mg po q24h x3 days 36 to <75 kg PPQ 960 mg/DHA 120 mg po q24h x3 days 75 to 100 kg PPQ 1280 mg/DHA 160 mg po q24h x3 days >100 kg no data Available in many endemic countries and WHO pre-qualified and EMA approved ACT is **Pyronaridine/ Artesunate** 2 tablets (180 mg/60 mg) as a single dose each day for 3 days for 24 to >45 kg or 1 tablet if 20 to <24 kg. Pediatric granule formulation for oral suspension (60 mg/20 mg) • 5 - <8 kg 1 sachet Daily for 3 days • 8 - <15 kg 2 sachets Daily for 3 days • 15 - <20 kg 3 sachets Daily for 3 days	**Peds (drugs of choice): QS** 10 mg/kg po tid x 3 days + **Doxy** 2.2 mg/kg/ bid up to 100 mg per dose both x 7 days. AAP now recommends that doxy can safely be administered for durations ≤21 days regardless of age. OR **Atovaquone-Proguanil** (all once daily x 3 d) by weight: • 5-8 kg: 2 peds tabs; • 9-10 kg: 3 peds tabs; • 11-20 kg: 1 adult tab; • 21-30 kg: 2 adult tabs; • 31-40 kg: 3 adult tabs; • >40 kg: 4 adult tabs. OR **MQ Salt:** 15 mg/kg x 1, then 6-12 hrs later, 10 mg/kg ALL po. OR **Artemether-Lumefantrine*** • 5 kg to <15 kg: 1 tablet (20 mg/ 120 mg) as a single dose, then 1 tablet again after 8 hours, then 1 tablet every 12 hours for 2 days • 15 kg to <25 kg: 2 tablets (40 mg/ 240 mg) as a single dose, then 2 tablets again after 8 hours, then 2 tablets every 12 hours for 2 days • 25 kg to <35 kg: 3 tablets (60 mg/ 360 mg) as a single dose, then 3 tablets again after 8 hours, then 3 tablets every 12 hours for 2 days • ≥35 kg: as per adult dose	**Pregnancy:** • Use ACT as first line for all malaria species including in all pregnancy trimesters. Use Artemether-lumefantrine in non-endemic countries) in usual doses. If ACT not available use, Quinine sulfate. • **Quinine sulfate** 10 mg/kg po tid x 3 days (7 days if SE Asia)) + Clindamycin 20 mg/kg/day divided tid x 7 days • Do not delay therapy if quinine available and Artemether-Lumefantrine is not In U.S., QS is only available as quinine 324 mg capsule, thus hard to use to treat children. **Note: Oral Artemether-Lumefantrine tabs FDA-approved but not widely stocked.** Call 1-800-COARTEM to obtain.

* For source of drug, see *Table 13D, page 222*.

TABLE 13A (7)

INFECTING ORGANISM	SUGGESTED REGIMENS		COMMENTS
	PRIMARY	ALTERNATIVE	
PROTOZOA—EXTRAINTESTINAL/Malaria (Plasmodia species)/Treatment of Malaria *(continued)*			
Uncomplicated/P. malariae or P. knowlesi All regions **– always CQ-sensitive**	**CQ** as above: adults & peds. In South Pacific, beware of P. knowlesi: looks like P. malariae, but behaves like P. falciparum.	**Artemether-Lumefantrine*** (20/120 mg tab) 4 tabs po x 1 dose, repeat in 8 hrs, then repeat q12h x 2 days (take with food) OR **Atovaquone-Proguanil** (250/100 mg tab) 4 adult tabs po daily x 3 days or **DHA-PPQ** or **Pyronaridine-artesunate**	
Uncomplicated/P. vivax or P. ovale **CQ-sensitive** (except Papua New Guinea, Indonesia which are CQ-resistant-*see below)*	**Adults: CQ** as above + **PQ/TQ** base. PQ/TQ to start or be given on day 1 or 2 of appropriate blood-stage therapy with CQ (or alternative drug). For PQ 30 mg po once daily x 14 days Each primaquine phosphate tab is 26.3 mg of salt and 15 mg of base. 30 mg of base = 2 x 26.3 mg tabs prim. phos. Where available Tafenoquine (TQ) 300 mg single dose preferable to PQ. **Peds:** CQ as above + PQ base 0.5 mg po once daily x 14 days.	**Artemether-Lumefantrine** or **DHA-PPQ** or **Pyronaridine-artesunate** as above + **PQ base** 0.5 mg po once daily x 14 days. TQ cannot be used if CQ is not the primary drug. Relapse rates: following TQ, *Cochrane Database Syst Rev 2020 9: CD010458, 2029*; Supportive evidence for efficacy of primaquine use in P. ovale remains limited. *Clin Infect Dis 2021 Jul 3:ciab610. doi: 10.1093/cid/ciab610.*	TQ/PQ added to eradicate latent parasites in liver. **Screen for G6PD def.** (must have 70% normal G6PD activity to use TQ) **before starting PQ or TQ;** if mildly G6PD deficient dose PQ as 45 mg po once weekly x 8 wks (cannot use TQ). **Note: rare severe reactions.** CQ safe in pregnancy. Avoid PQ in pregnancy. If P. vivax or P. ovale during pregnancy, after pregnancy check for G6PD deficiency & give PQ 30 mg po daily x 14 days or TQ x 300 mg.
Uncomplicated/P. vivax **CQ-resistant:** Papua, New Guinea & Indonesia	**Adults/Peds:** [**QS** + (**doxy** or **tetra**) + **PQ**] as above or **Artemether-Lumefantrine** or DHA-PPQ (same dose as for P. falciparum) + **PQ**	**Adults: MQ** + **PQ** as above.	Rarely acute. Lung injury and other serious complications. If pregnant treat as for uncomplicated P. falciparum in pregnancy. AAP now recommends that doxy can safely be administered for ≤21 days regardless of age.

* For source of drug, see *Table 13D, page 222.*

TABLE 13A (8)

INFECTING ORGANISM	SUGGESTED REGIMENS		COMMENTS
	PRIMARY	ALTERNATIVE	
PROTOZOA—EXTRAINTESTINAL/Malaria (Plasmodia species)/Treatment of Malaria *(continued)*			
Severe malaria, i.e., impaired consciousness, severe anemia, renal failure, pulmonary edema, ARDS, DIC, jaundice, acidosis, seizures, parasitemia ≥2%. One or more of latter. **Almost always P. falciparum.** Note: FDA approved IV Artesunate (Amivas), is now commercially available through major distributors (Cardinal Health, Americsource Bergen, and McKesson). See *https://ivartesunate.com* for distributors' 24/7 emergency numbers; all voice messages will receive a response in <30 minutes. CDC no longer distributes no-cost antimalarial drugs.	**Adult** (preferred regimen) **Artesunate** 2.4 mg/kg IV per dose at 0, 12, and 24 hours (total 3 doses) THEN After 24h, if parasitemia >1% give 2.4 mg/kg IV qday until the day when parasitemia <1%, then continue with a full course of oral therapy (see below) starting at least 4 hours after the last dose of artesunate. Artesunate IV should not be given for more than 7 days total. After 24h if parasitemia <1%, then continue with a full course of oral therapy (see below) starting at least 4 hours after the last dose of artesunate. If oral meds not tolerated at time for switch may continue artesunate 2.4 mg/kg IV qday or switch to IV Doxycycline 100 mg bid until oral meds tolerated. PLUS Oral Therapy (complete the full course no matter how many days IV artesunate used) **Atovaquone-proguanil** 4 adult tabs (250 mg/100 mg tabs) po in a single dose daily x 3 days (take with food; repeat dose if patient vomits within 30 minutes) OR **Artemether-lumefantrine** 4 tablets (20 mg/120 mg tabs) as a single dose, then 4 tablets again after 8 hours, then 4 tablets every 12 hours for 2 days (take with food) OR **Dihydroartemisinin/piperaquine** x 3 days **Pregnancy:** Use IV **Artesunate** in all trimesters then follow with oral **Quinine** x 3 days + **Clindamycin** 20 mg/kg/day divided tid x 7 days. Note: **Doxycycline** likely safe in 1st 15 weeks of pregnancy (prior to tooth/bone formation).	**Pediatric** (preferred regimen) **Artesunate** 2.4 mg/kg IV at 0, 12, and 24 hours Follow parenteral therapy exactly as with adults above with a complete oral course of anti-malarials (see pediatric dosing: **Atovaquone-proguanil**, **Artemether-lumefantrine**). WHO recommends to continue IV artesunate q24h if unable to take oral medication if <20 kg **Doxy** 2.2 mg/kg po/iv q12h x 7 days (less preferred regimen) if wt <45 kg. Adult dose for wt >45 kg. American Academy of Pediatrics now permits <21 days of doxy for any acute infection for children of all ages. - - - - - - - - - - IV **quinine dihydrochloride** still available in many endemic countries but second line only to be used if no IV **artemisinin** derivative is available.	Exchange transfusion no longer recommended. **Steroids not recommended for cerebral malaria.** IV Artesunate cause non-life threatening, but transfusion requiring, hemolytic anemia up to 15 days post-therapy *(AnIM 163:498, 2015)*. If needed, give interim po treatment until IV artesunate arrives (if oral medications are not tolerated, consider administration via nasogastric tube or after an antiemetic): Artemether-lumefantrine, Atovaquone proguanil, Quinine sulfate Dosing as above.
Malaria—self-initiated treatment: Only for people at high risk. Carry a reliable supply of recommended treatment (to avoid counterfeit meds). Use only if malaria is lab-diagnosed and no available reliable meds.	**Artemether-Lumefantrine** (20/120 mg tab) 4 tabs po x 1 dose, repeat in 8 hrs, then repeat q12h x 2 days (take with food) OR **Atovaquone-Proguanil (AP)** 4 adult tabs (1 gm/400 mg) po daily x 3 days	**Peds:** Using adult **AP** tabs for 3 consecutive days: 11-20 kg, 1 tab; 21–30 kg, 2 tabs; 31–40 kg, 3 tabs; >41 kg, 4 tabs. For Peds dosing of Artemether-Lumefantrine, *see Uncomplicated/P. falciparum, page 205.*	Do not use for renal insufficiency pts. Do not use if weight <11 kg, pregnant, or breast-feeding. **Artemether-Lumefantrine:** sold as Riamet (EU) and Coartem (US & elsewhere).

* For source of drug, see *Table 13D, page 222.*

TABLE 13A (9)

INFECTING ORGANISM	SUGGESTED REGIMENS: PRIMARY	SUGGESTED REGIMENS: ALTERNATIVE	COMMENTS
PROTOZOA—EXTRAINTESTINAL *(continued)*			
Toxoplasma gondii (Toxoplasmosis) Due to expense of pyrimethamine, TMP/SMX often used, but most experts favor pyrimethamine/sulfadiazine, if available.			
Immunologically normal patients *(For pediatric doses, see reference)*			
Acute illness w/ lymphadenopathy	No specific rx unless severe/persistent symptoms or evidence of vital organ damage		
Acq. via transfusion (lab accident)	Treat as for active chorioretinitis.		
Active chorioretinitis; meningitis; lowered resistance due to steroids or cytotoxic drugs	[**Pyrimethamine** (pyri) 200 mg po once on 1st day, then 50–75 mg q24h] + [**Sulfadiazine** *(see footnote[1])* S 1–1.5 gm po qid] + [**Leucovorin (folinic acid)** 5–20 mg 3x/wk]—*see Comment.* Treat 1–2 wks beyond resolution of signs/symptoms; continue leucovorin 1 wk after stopping pyri. For frequent recurrences, **TMP/SMX DS** 1 tab q12 x 45d then 1 DS tab qod x 311 d *Am J. Ophth 213:195 2020.*		For congenital Toxo, Toxo meningitis in adults, & chorioretinitis, **add prednisone 1 mg/kg/day in 2 div. doses** until CSF protein conc. falls or vision-threatening inflammation subsides. Adjust folinic acid dose by following CBC results.
Acute in pregnant women. Ref: *CID 47:554, 2008.*	**If <18 wks gestation at diagnosis: Spiramycin*** 1 gm po q8h until 16-18 wks; dc if amniotic fluid PCR is negative. Positive PCR: treat as below. **If >18 wks gestation & documented fetal infection by positive amniotic fluid PCR: (Pyrimethamine** 50 mg po q12h x 2 days, then 50 mg/day + **Sulfadiazine** 75 mg/kg po x 1 dose, then 50 mg/kg q12h (max 4 gm/day) + **Folinic acid** 10-20 mg po daily) for minimum of 4 wks or for duration of pregnancy.		Screen patients with IgG/IgM serology at commercial lab. IgG+ /IgM neg = remote past infection; IgM+ possible seroconversion. For Spiramycin, consult with Remington Toxoplasma Serology Lab: 650-853-4828 or remingtonlab@sutterhealth.org
Fetal/congenital	Mgmt complex. Combo rx with pyrimethamine + sulfadiazine + leucovorin—*see Comment*		Details in *Ln 363:1965, 2004.* **Consultation advisable.** 312 513 6365 or rmcleod@bsd.uchicago.edu
AIDS			
Cerebral toxoplasmosis Ref: *MMWR 58(RR-4) 1, 2009.*	[**Pyrimethamine** (pyri) 200 mg x 1 po, then 75 mg/day po] + (**Sulfadiazine** [Wt based dose: 1 gm if <60 kg, 1.5 gm if ≥60 kg] po q6h) + (**Folinic acid** 10–25 mg/day po) for minimum of 6 wks after resolution of signs/ symptoms, and then suppressive rx *(see below)* OR **TMP-SMX** 10/50 mg/kg per day po or IV div. q12h x 30 days *(AAC 42:1346, 1998)*	[**Pyri** + **Folinic acid** (as in primary regimen)] + 1 of the following: (1) **Clinda** 600 mg po/IV q6h or (2) **TMP-SMX** 5/25 mg/kg/day po or IV bid or (3) **Atovaquone** 750 mg po q6h. Treat 4–6 wks after resolution of signs/symptoms, then suppression.	Use alternative regimen for pts with severe sulfa allergy. If multiple ring-enhancing brain lesions (CT or MRI), >85% of pts respond to 7–10 days of empiric rx; if no response, suggest brain biopsy. Pyri penetrates brain even if no inflammation; folinic acid prevents pyrimethamine hematologic toxicity.
Primary prophylaxis, AIDS pts—IgG Toxo antibody + CD4 count <100 per mcL	(**TMP-SMX-DS**, 1 tab po q24h or 3x/wk) or (**TMP-SMX-SS**, 1 tab po q24h)	[(**Dapsone** 50 mg po q24h) + (**Pyri** 50 mg po q wk) + (**Folinic acid** 25 mg po q wk)] OR **Atovaquone** 1500 mg po q24h	Prophylaxis for pneumocystis also effective vs Toxo. Ref: *MMWR 58(RR-4):1, 2009.* **Another alternative:** (Dapsone 200 mg po + pyrimethamine 75 mg po + folinic acid 25 mg po) once weekly.
Suppression after rx of cerebral Toxo	(**Sulfadiazine** 2-4 gm po divided in 2-4 doses/day) + (**Pyri** 25–50 mg po q24h) + (**Folinic acid** 10–25 mg po q24h). DC if CD4 count >200 x 3 mos	[(**Clinda** 600 mg po q8h) + (**Pyri** 25–50 mg po q24h) + (**Folinic acid** 10–25 mg po q24h)] OR **Atovaquone** 750 mg po q6–12h. **TMP-SMX** 1DS bid or qd becoming standard due to difficulty obtaining Pyri.	(Pyri + sulfa or TMP-SMX) prevents PCP and Toxo; (clinda + pyri) prevents Toxo only. Additional drug needed to prevent PCP.
Trichomonas vaginalis	*See Vaginitis, Table 1, page 29.*		

[1] Sulfonamides for Toxo. Sulfadiazine now commercially available. Sulfisoxazole much less effective.

* For source of drug, see *Table 13D, page 222.*

TABLE 13A (10)

INFECTING ORGANISM	SUGGESTED REGIMENS		COMMENTS
	PRIMARY	ALTERNATIVE	
PROTOZOA—EXTRAINTESTINAL *(continued)*			
Trypanosomiasis. As of 2024 oral Fexinidazole is first line for almost all patients with both species of African trypanosomiasis is available from Sanofi in the US. Older, now second line, drugs are still available from the CDC. See *Table 13D, page 222*, for source information. Nifurtimox is now commercially available in US (*www.lampit.com*). Detailed WHO Guidelines *https://iris.who.int/bitstream/handle/10665/378083/9789240096035-eng.pdf?sequence=1*			
West African sleeping sickness (T. brucei gambiense)			
Stage 1: Blood/lymphatic parasites only. Clinical series in travelers *Int J Infect Dis (2018); https://doi.org/10.1016/j.ijid.2018.08.012* **Stage 2:** CNS disease. CSF with ≥5 WBC or parasite DNA by PCR Encephalitis	**Stage 1 or Stage 2** patients who are ≥6 yrs and body weight ≥20 kg presenting with <100 WBC/μL in CSF: Fexinidazole o Wt ≥35 kg: Loading dose 1800 mg (3 tablets) once/day for 4 days then 1200 mg (2 tablets) once/day for 6 days o Wt ≥20 and <35 kg: Loading dose 1200 mg (2 tablets) once/day for 4 days then 600 mg (1 tablet) once/day for 6 days **Severe Stage 2 patients with more than 100 WBC/μL in CSF** o Eflornithine 400 mg/kg/day IV divided q12h x 7 days + Nifurtimox 15 mg/kg/day po, divided q8h x 10 days (abbreviated NECT) non-inferior to 14-day standard Eflornithine therapy *(Lancet 374:56, 2009; Clin Infect Dis 56:195, 2013)*. **Children aged < 6 years or body weight < 20 kg** o **Stage 1:** Pentamidine 4 mg/kg IV X 7 days o **Stage 2:** NECT (as above)	Age ≥6 yrs and body weight ≥20 kg o Stage 1: Pentamidine 4 mg/kg IV X 7 days o Stage 2 (<100 WBC CSF): Pentamidine or NECT o Stage 2 (>100 WBC CSF): Fexinidazole as above Age <6 yrs or <20 kg: o Stage 1: NECT o Stage 2: Eflornithine 400 mg/kg/day IV divided q12h x 7 days	If CSF cell number not known do not use fexinidazole. Avoid Fexinidazole if eGFR <30 mL/min. Pregnancy: can use fexinidazole in 2nd and 3rd trimester. MUST complete full 10-days of fexinidazole. NECT may be preferred if: unable to swallow, fexinidazole contraindication, persistent vomiting, or questionable oral absorption.
East African sleeping sickness (T. brucei rhodesiense)			
Stage 1: Blood/lymphatic parasites only. Clinical series in travelers *Int J Infect Dis (2018); https://doi.org/10.1016/j.ijid.2018.08.012* **Stage 2:** CNS disease. CSF with ≥5 WBC or parasite DNA by PCR Encephalitis	Fexinidazole **Stage 1 and Stage 2** for persons who are ≥6 yrs and body weight ≥20 kg: o Wt ≥35 kg: Loading dose 1800 mg (3 tablets) once/day x 4 days then 1200 mg (2 tablets) once/day x 6 days o Wt ≥20 and <35 kg: Loading dose 1200 mg (2 tablets) once/day x 4 days then 600 mg (1 tablet) once/day x 6 days **Children aged < 6 years or body weight < 20 kg** o **Stage 1:** Suramin 5 mg/kg IV (test dose), then 20 mg/kg up to 1 gm (2 mg/kg test dose in children) on days 1, 3, 7, 14 and 21 o **Stage 2:** Melarsoprol 2.2 mg/kg/day IV x 10 days; non-inferior to long-standing standard regimen	≥6 yrs and body weight ≥20 kg. Stage 1 suramin (or pentamidine 4 mg/kg/day IM or IV) and add for Stage 2 add melarsoprol as shown adjacent for young children. Stage 1 who are <6 yrs and <20 kg: Pentamidine [4 mg/kg/day IM or IV] . Change to primary drugs immediately when available.	Stage 2: Melarsoprol IV may be preferred if: unable to swallow fexinidazole or questionable oral absorption. MUST complete full 10-days of fexinidazole. Pregnancy: Fexinidazole and pentamidine are preferred initially, can use fexinidazole in 2nd and 3rd trimesters.

* For source of drug, see *Table 13D, page 222*.

TABLE 13A (11)

INFECTING ORGANISM	SUGGESTED REGIMENS		COMMENTS
	PRIMARY	ALTERNATIVE	
PROTOZOA—EXTRAINTESTINAL/Trypanosomiasis *(continued)*			
T. cruzi infection (American trypanosomiasis) See *JAMA 2024 Jun 18;331(23):2037* for indications for treatment or non-treatment according to clinical stage of acute or chronic infection. Benznidazole *(www.benznidazole.com)*. Commercially available in the US see *www.benznidazole.com*. Use off-label for ages outside 2-12 year FDA range and use Nifurtimox off-label in children <q18 yrs. PAHO treatment guidelines: *https://iris.paho.org/bitstream/handle/10665.2/49653/9789275120439_eng.pdf*	*Adult (Age ≥12 years):* **Benznidazole*** 5-7 mg kg/day po in 2 doses (q12h) x 60 days *Pediatric (Age <12 years):* **Benznidazole*** 7.5 mg/kg/day po in 2 doses (q12h) x 60 days. **Benznidazole** 12.5 & 100 mg approved tabs for 2-12 yr olds. Preliminary trials on shorter duration Benznidazole regimens encouraging. • Phase 3 trials of 2 or 4 wks of 100 mg po tid are about to start.	Adult: **Nifurtimox** 8–10 mg/kg/day po divided 4x/day x 90-120 days Pediatric: **Nifurtimox** • >41 kg 8 to 10 mg/kg/day po divided 4x/day x 90-120 days • <41 kg 10 to 20 mg/kg/day Adverse effects: *Clin Infect Dis 2016, 63:1056*. **Diagnosis:** Two separate confirmatory serological tests based on different antigens and/or techniques (EIA and immunoblot (TESA)) needed to make diagnosis in those who screen positive in blood bank testing (Ortho EIA kit). **Non-blood bank screening:** EIA (Wiener kit) plus confirmatory TESA/IFA; all available via CDC Many US commercial labs use Hemagen or Inbios EIA kits which appear to have high false-positive rates in Central American populations. Positive commercial EIA tests should be confirmed at CDC before any treatment.	Due to adverse effects may give Benznidazole 300 mg per day for 60 days, regardless of body weight OR give 300 mg per day but prolong treatment to complete the total dose corresponding to 5 mg/kg per day for 60 days. *N Engl J Med 373:456, 2015*. Immunosuppression for heart transplant can reactivate chronic Chagas disease. Can transmit by organ/transfusions. Do not use benznidazole in pregnancy. To decrease adverse effects, shorter duration regimens under investigation.
NEMATODES—INTESTINAL (Roundworms). Eosinophilia? Think Strongyloides, toxocariasis and filariasis: *See Table 13C.*			
Anisakis simplex (**anisakiasis**) Anisakiasis differentiated from Anisakidosis. Other: A. pegreffii, A. physeteris, Pseudoterranova decipiens.	Physical removal: endoscope or surgery. IgE antibody test vs *A. simplex* may help diagnosis. No antimicrobial therapy.	Anecdotal reports of possible treatment benefit from albendazole	Anisakiasis acquired by eating raw fish: herring, salmon, mackerel, cod, squid. Similar illness due to Pseudoterranova species acquired from cod, halibut, red snapper.
Ascaris lumbricoides (**ascariasis**) *Ln 367:1521, 2006*	**Albendazole** 400 mg po x 1 dose OR **Mebendazole** 100 mg po bid X 3 days or 500 mg po x 1 dose	**Ivermectin** 150–200 mcg/kg po x 1 dose	Review of efficacy of single dose: Mebendazole 500 mg tabs not widely available.
Capillaria philippinensis (**capillariasis**)	**Albendazole** 400 mg po bid x 10 days	**Mebendazole** 500 mg po daily x 20 days	
Enterobius vermicularis (**pinworm**)	**Mebendazole** 500 mg po x 1 dose, repeat in 2 weeks OR **Pyrantel pamoate** 11 mg/kg base (to max. dose of 1 gm) po x 1 dose; repeat in 2 wks	**Albendazole** 400 mg po x 1 dose, repeat in 2 wks	*Side-effects in Table 13B, page 220.* Treat whole household.
Gongylonemiasis (adult worms in oral mucosa)	Surgical removal	**Albendazole** 400 mg/day po x 3 days	Ref: *CID 32:1378, 2001; J Helminth 80:425, 2006.*
Hookworm (Necator americanus and Ancylostoma duodenale)	**Albendazole** 400 mg po daily x 3 days	**Mebendazole** 500 mg po daily x 3 days OR **Pyrantel pamoate** 11 mg/kg (to max. dose of 1 gm) po daily x 3 days	**NOTE:** Ivermectin not effective. Single dose therapy as used in public health programs has lower cure rates and 3-day albendazole superior to 3-day mebendazole, *PLoS One 6:e25003, 2011.*

* For source of drug, see *Table 13D, page 222.*

TABLE 13A (12)

INFECTING ORGANISM	SUGGESTED REGIMENS		COMMENTS
	PRIMARY	ALTERNATIVE	
NEMATODES—INTESTINAL (Roundworms) *(continued)*			
Strongyloides stercoralis (**strongyloidiasis**) *(Hyperinfection, See Comment)*	**Ivermectin** 200 mcg/kg per day po x 2 days	**Albendazole** 400 mg po bid x 7 days; less effective **Moxidectin** (not commercially available yet) showed 88% cure in Phase 2 trial (n=785). *Lancet Infect Dis 21:1151, 2021*	For disseminated disease with larvae in stool and sputum, repeat treatment every 15 days while stools positive and then 1 more treatment cycle. For hyperinfection with sepsis, treat daily for at least 10 days or until larvae undetectable. For hyperinfection: veterinary ivermectin given subcutaneously or rectally *(CID 49:1411, 2009)*.
Trichostrongylus orientalis, T. colubriformis	**Pyrantel pamoate** 11 mg/kg (maximum 1 gm) po x 1 dose OR **Albendazole** 400 mg po daily x 10 doses OR **Mebendazole** 500 mg po qd x 10 days	**Albendazole** 400 mg po x 1 dose	
Trichuris trichiura (**whipworm**)	**Mebendazole** 100 mg po twice daily x 3 days. Low cure rates with either mebendazole or albendazole	**Albendazole** 400 mg po qd x 3 days or **Ivermectin** 200 mcg/kg po qd x 3 days	Mebendazole clearly superior for trichuris *(PLoS One.6:e25003, 2011; N Engl J Med 370:610, 2014)*. Single dose Mebendazole 500 mg tab significantly less effective than 3 days.
NEMATODES—EXTRAINTESTINAL (Roundworms)			
Ancylostoma braziliense & caninum: causes **cutaneous larva migrans**	**Albendazole** 400 mg po bid x 3-7 days *(Ln ID 8:302, 2008)*.	**Ivermectin** 200 mcg/kg po x 1 dose/day x 1–2 days (not in children wt <15 kg)	Also called "creeping eruption", dog and cat hookworm. Ivermectin cure rate 81-100% (1 dose) to 97% (2–3 doses) *(CID 31:493, 2000)*.
Angiostrongylus cantonensis (Angiostrongyliasis); causes eosinophilic meningitis. Pros/cons of antiparasitic drugs: *https://pubmed.ncbi.nlm.nih.gov/32729438/*	Mild/moderate disease: Analgesics, serial LPs (if necessary). Prednisone 60 mg/day x 14 days reduces headache & need for LPs.	Adding **Albendazole** 15 mg/kg/day to prednisone 60 mg/day both for 14 days may reduce duration of headaches and need for repeat LPs.	**Do not use Albendazole without prednisone,** *see TRSMH 102:990, 2008*. Gnathostoma and Baylisascaris also cause eosinophilic meningitis.
Baylisascariasis (Raccoon roundworm); eosinophilic meningitis	No drug proven efficacious. Try po **Albendazole,** Peds: 25–50 mg/kg/day po; Adults: 400 mg po bid with corticosteroids. Treat for one month.		*Clin Microbiol Rev. 29:375, 2016*. Other causes of eosinophilic meningitis: Gnathostoma & Angiostrongylus.
Dracunculus medinensis: **Guinea worm** Dog reservoir found in 3 countries hampering eradication.	Slow extraction of pre-emergent worm over several days	No drugs effective. Oral analgesics, anti-inflammatory drugs, topical antiseptics/antibiotic ointments to alleviate symptoms and facilitate worm removal by gentle manual traction over several days.	
Filariasis: Determine if co-infection with either Loa loa or Onchocerca			
Lymphatic filariasis (**Elephantiasis**): Etiologies: Wuchereria bancrofti Brugia malayi, Brugia timori	*Mono-infection:* **Diethylcarbamazine[2] (DEC)*** 6 mg/kg/day po in 3 divided doses x 12 days + **Doxy** 200 mg/day po x 6 wks	*Dual infection with Onchocerciasis:* Treat Onchocerciasis first: **Ivermectin** 150 mcg/kg po x 1 dose, wait 1 month, then start **DEC** as for mono-infection *Dual infection with Loa Loa:* DEC drug of choice for both but can cause severe encephalopathy if >2500 Loa Loa microfilaria/mL in blood. Refer to expert center for apheresis pre-DEC or prednisone + small doses of DEC. If <2500 microfilaria/mL, start regular dose of **DEC**	Doxy x 6 wks may improve mild/moderate lymphedema independent of parasite infection *(CID 55:621, 2012)*. **Note: DEC can cause irreversible eye damage if concomitant Onchocerciasis.**

[2] May need antihistamine or corticosteroid for allergic reaction from disintegrating organisms.

* For source of drug, see *Table 13D, page 222*.

TABLE 13A (13)

INFECTING ORGANISM	SUGGESTED REGIMENS		COMMENTS
	PRIMARY	ALTERNATIVE	
NEMATODES—EXTRAINTESTINAL (Roundworms)/Filariasis *(continued)*			
Loiasis, Loa loa, eye worm disease: **Look for dual infection with either Onchocerciasis or Lymphatic filariasis.** Moxidectin pivotal study *Lancet. 2018 Jan 17. pii: S0140-6736(17)32844-1*			
Large clinical experience with Loa and onchocerciasis. *Clin Infect Dis 2021 Aug 31;ciab751. doi: 10.1093/cid/ciab751*	*Mono-infection with <2500 L. loa microfilaria/mL:* **DEC** 8-10 mg/kg/day po in 3 divided doses x 21 days *Mono-infection with >2500 L. loa microfilaria/mL:* Refer to expert center for apheresis prior to **DEC** therapy; alternatively: **Albendazole** 200 mg po bid x 21 days	*Dual infection with Lymphatic filariasis:* See Lymphatic filariasis, above *Dual infection with Onchocerciasis:* Treat Onchocerciasis first with **Ivermectin**, then treat L. loa with **DEC**	If >5000 L. loa microfilaria/mL in blood & given Ivermectin for Onchocerciasis, can facilitate entry of L. loa into CNS with severe encephalopathy. May require multiple 21 day courses of DEC to clear mono-infection
Onchocerca volvulus (Onchocerciasis), river blindness: **Look for dual infection with either Loa loa or Lymphatic filariasis**			
	Mono-infection: **Ivermectin** 150 mcg/kg x 1 dose, then repeat every 3-6 months until asymptomatic + **Doxy** 200 mg/day x 6 wks. No accepted alternative therapy. **Moxidectin** 8 mg po (age 12 or over) to be used instead of Ivermectin but not widely available	*Dual infection with Lymphatic filariasis:* See Lymphatic filariasis, above *Dual infection with L. loa:* Treat Onchocerciasis first with **Ivermectin**, then treat L. loa with **DEC**. If >5000 L. Loa microfilaria/mL in blood. Refer to expert center for apheresis before starting DEC	Onchocerciasis and Loa loa are mildly co-endemic in West and Central Africa.
Body cavity			
Mansonella perstans	In randomized trial, **Doxy** 200 mg po once daily x 6 weeks cleared microfilaria from blood in 67 of 69 patients *(NEJM 361:1448, 2009)*. Doxy may not work outside Mali and Cameroon due to strain variation.	**Albendazole** in high dose x 3 weeks.	Efficacy of doxy believed to be due to inhibition of endosymbiont wolbachia; Ivermectin has no activity.
Mansonella streptocerca	**Ivermectin** 150 µg/kg x 1 dose.	**Diethylcarbamazine** 6 mg/kg x 12 days kills microfilaria in adults but causes transient exacerbation of clinical symptoms and may cause vision loss and hypotension if co-infected with O. volvulus.	May need antihistamine or corticosteroid for allergic reaction from disintegrating organisms. Chronic pruritic hypopigmented lesions that may be confused with leprosy. Can be asymptomatic.
Mansonella ozzardi	**Ivermectin** 200 µ/kg x 1 dose likely effective. *Am J Trop Med Hyg. 2018, 98: 786*	Usually asymptomatic. Articular pain, pruritus, lymphadenopathy reported. May have allergic reaction from dying organisms.	
Dirofilariasis: **Heartworms**			
D. immitis, dog heartworm	No effective drugs; surgical removal only option		Can lodge in pulmonary artery → coin lesion. Eosinophilia rare.
D. tenuis (raccoon), D. ursi (bear), D. repens (dogs, cats)	No effective drugs	Worms migrate to conjunctivae, subcutaneous tissue including face, scrotum, breasts, extremities. D. repens emerging throughout Europe *Clin Microbiol Rev 25:507, 2012*	
Gnathostoma spinigerum			
Cutaneous larva migrans	**Albendazole** 400 mg po q24h or bid times 21 days	**Ivermectin** 200 µg/kg/day po x 2 days.	*Other etiology of larva migrans: Ancylostoma sp., see page 212*
Eosinophilic meningitis	Supportive care; monitor for cerebral hemorrhage	Case reports of steroid use: both benefit and harm from Albendazole or ivermectin *(EIN 17:1174, 2011)*.	Other causes of eosinophilic meningitis: **Angiostrongylus** *(see page 212)* & **Baylisascaris** *(see page 212)*

* For source of drug, see *Table 13D, page 222*.

TABLE 13A (14)

INFECTING ORGANISM	SUGGESTED REGIMENS		COMMENTS
	PRIMARY	ALTERNATIVE	
NEMATODES—EXTRAINTESTINAL (Roundworms) *(continued)*			
Toxocariasis *(Lancet Infect Dis. 2018; 18:e14)*	**Rx directed at relief of symptoms as infection self-limited, e.g., steroids & antihistamines; use of anthelmintics controversial.**		
Visceral larval migrans	**Albendazole** 400 mg po bid x 5 days ± **Prednisone** 60 mg/day	**Mebendazole** 100–200 mg po bid times 5 days	Severe lung, heart or CNS disease may warrant steroids. Differential dx of larval migrans syndromes: Toxocara canis & catis, Ancylostoma spp., Gnathostoma spp., Spirometra spp.
Ocular larval migrans	First 4 wks of illness: (Oral **Prednisone** 30–60 mg po q24h + subtenon **Triamcinolone** 40 mg/wk) x 2 wks (Surgery is sometimes necessary)		No added benefit of anthelmintic drugs. Rx of little effect after 4 wks. Some use steroids *(Clin Micro Rev 16:265, 2003)*.
Trichinella spiralis (**Trichinellosis**) — muscle infection *(Review: Clin Micro Rev 22:127, 2009)*.	**Albendazole** 400 mg po bid x 8–14 days	**Mebendazole** 500 mg po tid x 10 days (still with concomitant prednisone)	Use albendazole/mebendazole with caution during pregnancy. ↑ IgE, ↑ CPK, ESR 0, massive eosinophilia: >5000/μL.
	Concomitant **prednisone** 40–60 mg po q24h		
TREMATODES (Flukes) – Liver, Lung, Intestinal. All flukes have snail intermediate hosts; transmitted by ingestion of metacercariae on plants, fish or crustaceans.			
Liver flukes: Clonorchis sinensis, Metorchis conjunctus, Opisthorchis viverrini	**Praziquantel** 25 mg/kg po tid x 2 days	**Albendazole** 10 mg/kg per day po x 7 days	Same dose in children
Fasciola hepatica (sheep liver fluke), Fasciola gigantica	**Triclabendazole*** single dose 10 mg/kg po; if severe infection, repeat in 12-24 hrs. Treatment failure: single dose 20 mg/kg po *(NEJM 382:1844, 2020)*		**Fasciola resistance:** *Emerg Infect Dis 27:1850, 2021*. Consider multiple triclabendazole courses for treatment failures. *J Glob Antimicrob Resist 25:264, 2021*.
Intestinal flukes: Fasciola buski Heterophyes heterophyes; Metagonimus yokogawai. Nanophyetus salmincola	**Praziquantel** 25 mg/kg po tid x 1 days		Same dose in children
Lung fluke: Paragonimus sp.	**Praziquantel** 25 mg/kg po tid x 2 days	**Triclabendazole*** 10 mg/kg po x 2 doses over 12-24 hrs.	Same dose in children
Schistosoma sp. No clinically important PZQ resistance anywhere *PLoS Negl Trop Dis 15:e0009189, 2021*.	• Travelers and temporary residents lightly infected with no chronic disease. o Light infection detected by serology, eggs not usually present in stool or urine. o Uncommon CNS involvement including spinal cord. o Almost all travel related cases are from Africa.		
Schistosoma haematobium; GU bilharziasis.	**Praziquantel** 40 mg/kg po on the same day (one dose of 40 mg/kg or two doses of 20 mg/kg)		Same dose in children. (this applies to all schisto species) Some clinicians use 60 mg/kg praziquantel for all species for travelers and temporary residents not expecting re-exposure.
Schistosoma intercalatum	**Praziquantel** 20 mg/kg po on the same day in 1 or 2 doses		Same dose in children
Schistosoma japonicum; Oriental schisto.	**Praziquantel** 60 mg/kg po on the same day (3 doses of 20 mg/kg)		Same dose in children. Cures 60–90% pts.
Schistosoma mansoni (intestinal bilharziasis)	**Praziquantel** 40 mg/kg po on the same day in (one dose of 40 mg/kg or two doses of 20 mg/kg)		Praziquantel: Same dose for children and adults. Cures 60–90% pts. No advantage to splitting dose in 2 Cochrane Database Syst Rev. *8:CD000053, 2014*
Schistosoma mekongi	**Praziquantel** 60 mg per kg po on the same day (3 doses of 20 mg/kg)		Same dose for children

* For source of drug, see *Table 13D, page 222*.

TABLE 13A (15)

INFECTING ORGANISM	SUGGESTED REGIMENS		COMMENTS
	PRIMARY	ALTERNATIVE	
TREMATODES (Flukes) *(continued)*			
Toxemic schisto; Katayama fever	**Praziquantel** 20 mg per kg po bid with short course of high dose prednisone. Repeat Praziquantel in 4-6 wks *(Clin Micro Rev 16:225, 2010).*		Reaction to onset of egg laying 4-6 wks after infection exposure in fresh water.
CESTODES (Tapeworms)			
Echinococcus granulosus (hydatid disease) *(Curr Opin Infect Dis 31:383,2018; LnID 12:871, 2012; BMC Infect Dis 2018, 18:306).* Dead or calcified cysts as determined by experienced radiologist require no therapy. Watch and wait for asymptomatic or non-compromising cysts.	**Liver cysts:** Image-based (U/S not CT/MRI) staging first. <5 cm CE1, CE3a cysts and possibly <5 cm CE2, CE3b cysts consider trial of albendazole 400 mg po bid for 3-6 months and assess response; 30-50% response rate. Uncomplicated 5-10 cm CE1 and CE3a cysts: Percutaneous aspiration-injection-reaspiration (PAIR) + Albendazole. Before & after drainage: **Albendazole** ≥60 kg, 400 mg po bid or <60 kg, 15 mg/kg/day divided bid, for a total of at least 30 days. Multivesicular or relapsing cysts may require longer therapy. Inject contrast after aspiration and before instilling scolocidal agent to ensure no biliary communication. Surgical resection (experienced surgeon only) with Albendazole starting 1 week pre-operatively and for 4 weeks post-operatively for CE2 and CE3b 5-10 cm and all viable cysts large than 10 cm. Complicated, multi vesicular, or infected cysts almost always require surgical intervention. Large hepatic cysts >7.5 cm likely to have biliary communication and require surgery. Laparoscopic and large bore non-surgical approaches being developed in endemic areas for CE2 and CE3b cysts have many compartments each one requiring individual puncture with usual PAIR; large bore catheter (can extract outer membranes) may be used with longer ABZ therapy but surgery preferable. Lung cysts Surgical resection. Avoid pre-operative Albendazole. May give Albendazole 400 mg po.		
Lung cysts	Surgical resection. Avoid pre-operative Albendazole. May give Albendazole 400 mg po bid x at least 28 days post-operatively. Ruptured or complicated cysts may require longer therapy. Never use PAIR for lung cysts. **Note:** Brain, cardiac, splenic, renal, bone locations uncommonly occur requiring surgical intervention. Metastatic spread into body cavities with spontaneous or iatrogenic (during surgery) cyst rupture require Albendazole 400 mg po bid indefinitely until clinical response with periodic surgical debulking if feasible.		
Echinococcus multilocularis (alveolar cyst disease) *(COID 16:437, 2003)*	**Albendazole** efficacy not clearly demonstrated, can try in dosages used for hydatid disease. Wide surgical resection only reliable rx; technique evolving. Post-surgical resection or if inoperable: Albendazole for several years *(Acta Tropic 114:1, 2010).* Mostly in Europe; rare but reported and may be emerging in US (Vermont; Alaska) and Canada: *Clin Infect Dis, 2021; 72:1124 and N Engl J Med 2019, 381:384.*		
Intestinal tapeworms			
Diphyllobothrium latum (fish), Dipylidium caninum (dog), Taenia saginata (beef), & Taenia solium (pork)	**Praziquantel** 5–10 mg/kg po x 1 dose for children and adults.	**Niclosamide*** 2 gm po x 1 dose	Niclosamide from Expert Compounding Pharm, *see Table 13D.*
Hymenolepis diminuta (rats) and H. nana (humans)	**Praziquantel** 25 mg/kg po x 1 dose for children and adults.	**Niclosamide*** 2 gm po daily x 7 days	
Neurocysticercosis (NCC) 2021 WHO Guidelines *https://www.who.int/publications/i/item/9789240032231.* Recent review: *https://pubmed.ncbi.nlm.nih.gov/35665719/* Larval form of T. solium IDSA treatment guidelines. *CID 2018,66:1159*	**NOTE: Treat concomitant T. solium intestinal tapeworms,** if present, with **praziquantel** 5-10 mg/kg po x 1 dose after starting steroid. Both CT and MRI should be performed. Immunoblot preferred; ELISA lacks specificity. Serology insensitive for single lesions, calcified lesions. For multiple parenchymal lesions, subarachnoid NCC, intraventricular NCC, serology almost 100% sensitive; CSF testing no advantage over serum testing. Parenchymal scolex on imaging is diagnostic, serology not necessary. In non-endemic areas, check stools of household contacts of confirmed cases for tapeworm eggs. **Anti-parasitic drugs are never urgent;** control seizures and intracranial pressure first. Levetiracetam better tolerated and preferable to phenytoin or carbamazepine.		

* For source of drug, see *Table 13D, page 222.*

TABLE 13A (16)

INFECTING ORGANISM	SUGGESTED REGIMENS		COMMENTS
	PRIMARY	ALTERNATIVE	
CESTODES (Tapeworms)/Neurocysticercosis (NCC) *(continued)*			
Parenchymal NCC 1-20 "Viable" or degenerating cysts by CT/MRI. Meta-analysis: Treatment assoc with cyst resolution, ↓ seizures, and ↓ seizure recurrence.	**Albendazole** 15 mg/kg/d po (max 800 mg/d) + **Praziquantel** 50 mg/kg/d po + **Dexamethasone** 0.1 mg/kg/d po. Start steroid 1 day before anti-parasitics. Treat for 10 days. Anti-seizure meds may be stopped after 6 mos with single lesion and 2 yrs with multiple lesions if seizures controlled. Slow steroid taper after 10 days increasing back if seizures develop. Albendazole alone adequate if only 1-2 cysts on an MRI.	**Albendazole** alone 800 mg per day plus **Dexamethasone** 0.1 mg/kg per day ± Anti-seizure medication). *See Comment*. Limited data indicates that increasing dexamethasone to 8 mg/day X 28 days with 2-week taper decreases seizures but prolongs steroid exposure. *Epilepsia 55:1452, 2014*	Retreat after 6 months if any viable cysts remain. Methotrexate at ≤20 mg/wk allows a reduction in steroid use *(CID 44:449, 2007)*. Some recommend longer courses of albendazole (even >30 days) if large number of parenchymal cysticerci.
Dead calcified cysts	**No treatment indicated**		
Subarachnoid NCC Review of newer approaches *Curr Opin Infect Dis 33; 339, 2020*	Albendazole 15 mg/kg per day (max. 1200 mg/day) + Dexamethasone (doses as above with very slow taper) + v-p shunt prior to therapy. 30 day course, may need to repeat multiple times or give continuously for months according to clinical and MRI evolution *(Expert Rev Anti Infect Ther 9:123, 2011)*; continue until radiologic resolution. Intracranial pressure must be monitored and managed by an experienced clinician. If diffuse cerebral edema or raised ICP, control with steroids or shunting prior to any anti-parasitic therapy.	Long courses of combination therapy with Albendazole/praziquantel combination therapy for refractory disease. Monitor according to clinical and MRI evolution *Curr Opin Infect Dis 33; 339, 2020*; continue therapy until radiologic resolution and resolution of antigen levels (if available) *Am J Trop Med Hyg. 102:78, 2020.*	
Intraventricular NCC	Neuroendoscopic removal is treatment of choice with or without obstruction. If surgery not possible, **Albendazole + Dexamethasone; observe closely for evidence of obstruction of flow of CSF.**	**Albendazole** + **Dexamethasone** (as above); place v-p shunt prior to therapy when no access to neuroendoscopy.	
Sparganosis (Spirometra mansonoides) Larval cysts; source—frogs/snakes	Surgical resection. No antiparasitic therapy. Can inject alcohol into subcutaneous masses.		

* For source of drug, see *Table 13D, page 222*.

TABLE 13A (17)

INFECTING ORGANISM		SUGGESTED REGIMENS		COMMENTS
		PRIMARY	ALTERNATIVE	
ECTOPARASITES. Ref.: *CID 36:1355, 2003; Ln 363:889, 2004.* **NOTE: Due to potential neurotoxicity and risk of aplastic anemia, lindane not recommended.**				
DISEASE	**INFECTING ORGANISM**			
Head lice *Med Lett 54:61, 2012.*	Pediculus humanus, var. capitis. Re-treatment often necessary as current drugs do not kill eggs.	**Permethrin** 1% lotion: Apply to shampooed dried hair for 10 min.; repeat in 9-10 days. **OR** **Malathion** 0.5% lotion (Ovide): Apply to dry hair for 8–12 hrs, then shampoo. 2 doses 7-9 days apart. **OR** **Spinosad** 0.9% suspension; wash off after 10 min (85% effective). Repeat in 7 days, if needed. Use nit comb initially & repeat in 7-10 days	**Ivermectin** 200-400 μg/kg po once; 3 doses at 7 day intervals effective in 95% *(JID 193:474, 2006)*. Topical ivermectin 0.5% lotion, 75% effective. **Malathion:** Report that 1–2 20-min. applications 98% effective *(Ped Derm 21:670, 2004)*. In alcohol—potentially flammable. **Benzyl alcohol:** 76% effective.	**Permethrin:** success in 78%. Resistance increasing. No advantage to 5% permethrin. **Spinosad** is effective, but expensive. Wash hats, scarves, coats & bedding in hot water, then dry in hot dryer for 20+ minutes.
Pubic lice (crabs)	Phthirus pubis	**Pubic hair: Permethrin** OR **Malathion** as for head lice. Shave pubic hair.	**Eyelids: Petroleum jelly** applied qid x 10 days OR **yellow oxide of mercury** 1% qid x 14 days	**Do not use lindane.** Treat sex partners of the last 30 days.
Body lice	Pediculus humanus, var. corporis	No drugs for the patient. Organism lives in & deposits eggs in seams of clothing. Discard clothing; if not possible, treat clothing with 1% malathion powder or 0.5% permethrin powder. Success with ivermectin in homeless shelter: 12 mg po on days 0, 7, & 14 *(JID 193:474, 2006)*		
Myiasis Due to larvae of flies		Usually cutaneous/subcutaneous nodule with central punctum. Treatment: Occlude punctum to prevent gas exchange with petrolatum, fingernail polish, makeup cream or bacon. When larva migrates, manually remove. Ref: *Clin Microbiol Rev 25:79, 2012.*		
Scabies	Sarcoptes scabiei			
Immunocompetent patients Refs: *MMWR 64(RR-3):1, 2015; NEJM 362:717, 2010.*		**Permethrin** 5% cream (ELIMITE) under nails (finger and toe). Apply entire skin from chin down to and including under fingernails and toenails. Leave on 8–14 hrs. Repeat in 1-2 wks. Safe for children age >2 mos.	**Ivermectin** 200 μg/kg po with food x 1, then second dose in 2 wks. **Less effective: Crotamiton** 10% cream, apply x 24 hr, rinse off, then reapply x 24 hr.	Trim fingernails. Reapply cream to hands after handwashing. Treat close contacts; wash and heat dry linens. Pruritus may persist times 2 wks after mites gone.
AIDS and HTLV-infected patients (CD4 <150 per mm³), debilitated or developmentally disabled patients (**Norwegian scabies**—*see Comments)*		For Norwegian crusted scabies: **Permethrin** 5% cream daily x 7 days, then twice weekly until cured. Add **Ivermectin** po (dose in Alternative)	**Ivermectin** 200 mcg/kg po on days 1, 2, 8, 9 & 15+ **Permethrin** cream. May need addt'l doses of Ivermectin on days 22 & 29.	**Norwegian scabies** in AIDS pts: Extensive, crusted. Can mimic psoriasis. Not pruritic. Highly contagious—isolate!

* For source of drug, see *Table 13D, page 222.*

TABLE 13B – DOSAGE AND SELECTED ADVERSE EFFECTS OF ANTIPARASITIC DRUGS

Doses vary with indication. For convenience, drugs divided by type of parasite; some drugs used for multiple types of parasites, e.g., albendazole.

CLASS, AGENT, GENERIC NAME (TRADE NAME)	USUAL ADULT DOSAGE	ADVERSE REACTIONS/COMMENTS
Antiprotozoan Drugs		
Intestinal Parasites		
Diloxanide furoate[NUS] (Furamide)	500 mg po tid x 10 days	Source: *See Table 13D, page 222.* Flatulence, N/V, diarrhea.
Iodoquinol (Yodoxin)	Adults: 650 mg po tid (or 30-40 mg/kg/day div. tid); children: 40 mg/kg per day div. tid.	Rarely causes nausea, abdominal cramps, rash, acne. **Contraindicated if iodine intolerance** (contains 64% bound iodine). Can cause iododerma (papular or pustular rash) and/or thyroid enlargement.
Metronidazole	Side-effects similar for all. *See metronidazole in Table 10A, page 162*	
Nitazoxanide (Alinia)	Adults: 500 mg po q12h. Children 4–11: 200 mg susp. po q12h. Take with food. Expensive.	Abdominal pain 7.8%, diarrhea 2.1%. Rev.: *CID 40:1173, 2005; Expert Opin Pharmacother 7:953, 2006.* Headaches; rarely yellow sclera (resolves after treatment).
Paromomycin (Humatin)	15-35 mg/kg/day po in 3 divided doses x 5-10 days (250 mg tabs). Source: *See Table 13D.*	**Aminoglycoside similar to neomycin;** if absorbed due to concomitant inflammatory bowel disease can result in oto/nephrotoxicity. Doses >3 gm daily are associated with nausea, abdominal cramps, diarrhea.
Quinacrine	100 mg po tid x 5 days. *See Table 13D.*	**Contraindicated for pts with history of psychosis or psoriasis. Yellow staining of skin.** Dizziness, headache, vomiting, toxic psychosis (1.5%), hemolytic anemia, leukopenia, thrombocytopenia, urticaria, rash, fever, minor disulfiram-like reactions.
Tinidazole (Tindamax)	250-500 mg tabs, with food. Regimen varies with indication.	**Chemical structure similar to metronidazole but better tolerated.** Seizures/peripheral neuropathy reported. **Adverse effects:** Metallic taste 4–6%, nausea 3–5%, anorexia 2–3%.
Antiprotozoan Drugs: Non-Intestinal Protozoa		
Extraintestinal Parasites		
Antimony compounds Meglumine antimonate (Glucantime)—French trade name	For IV use: vials with 100 mg antimony/mL. Dilute selected dose in 50 mL of D5W shortly before use. Infuse over at least 10 minutes. Intralesional injection preferred for mild uncomplicated cutaneous disease; 20 mg/kg qwk X 5-10 weeks.	**AEs in 1st 10 days:** headache, fatigue, elevated lipase/amylase, clinical pancreatitis. After 10 days: elevated AST/ALT/ALK/PHOS. CBC, biochemistry weekly, EKG q2 weeks if prolonged therapy. **NOTE: Reversible T wave changes in 30-60%. Risk of QTc prolongation. Renal excretion; modify dose if renal insufficiency. Metabolized in liver; lower dose if hepatic insufficiency. Generic drug may have increased toxicity due to antimony complex formation.**
Artemether-Lumefantrine, po (Coartem)	4 (20 mg Artemether and 120 mg Lumefantrine) combination tablets X 6 doses over 3 days for adults. Take with food. Can be crushed and mixed with a few teaspoons of water	**Can prolong QT_c:** avoid in patients with congenital long QT_c, family history of sudden death or long QT_c, or need for drugs known to prolong QT_c *(see list under fluoroquinolones, Table 10A, page 159).* Artemether induces CYP3A4 and both Artemether & Lumefantrine are metabolized by CYP3A4. Adverse effects experienced by >30% of adults: headache, anorexia, dizziness, arthralgia and myalgia. Non-life threatening, but transfusion requiring, hemolytic anemia can occur up to 15 days post-therapy *(AnIM 163:498, 2015).*
Artesunate, IV Ref: *NEJM 358:1829, 2008*	Now commercially available, discontinued by CDC. 2.4 mg/kg IV at 0, 12, 24, & 48 hrs for adults. Follow with 2nd drug po.	**More effective than quinine & safer than quinidine.** No dosage adjustment for hepatic or renal insufficiency. No known drug interactions. Delayed hemolysis, monitor CBC weekly x4.
Atovaquone (Mepron) Ref.: *AAC 46:1163, 2002*	Suspension: 1 tsp (750 mg) po bid 750 mg/5 mL.	No. pts stopping rx due to side-effects was 9%; rash 22%, GI 20%, headache 16%, insomnia 10%, fever 14%
Atovaquone and Proguanil (Malarone) For prophylaxis of P. falciparum; little data on P. vivax. Generic available in US.	**Prophylaxis:** 1 tab po (250 mg + 100 mg) q24h with food **Treatment:** 4 tabs po (1000 mg + 400 mg) once daily with food x 3 days. Adult tab: 250/100 mg; Peds tab 62.5/25 mg. *Treatment see comment, page 206.*	Adverse effects in rx trials: Adults—abd. pain 17%, N/V 12%, headache 10%, dizziness 5%. Rx stopped in 1%. Asymptomatic mild ↑ in ALT/AST. Children—cough, headache, anorexia, vomiting, abd. pain. Safe in G6PD-deficient pts. Can crush tabs for children and give with milk or other liquid nutrients. Renal insufficiency: contraindicated if CrCl <30 mL per min.

* For source of drug, see *Table 13D, page 222.*

TABLE 13B (2)

CLASS, AGENT, GENERIC NAME (TRADE NAME)	USUAL ADULT DOSAGE	ADVERSE REACTIONS/COMMENTS
Antiprotozoan Drugs: Non-Intestinal Protozoa/Extraintestinal Parasites *(continued)*		
Benznidazole* Benznidazole 12.5 & 100 mg approved tabs for 2-12 yr olds. CDC advocates off-label use in adults *(www.benznidazoletablets.com)*	5 mg/kg per day po. 100 mg tabs. May use 300 mg per day for 60 days, regardless of body weight OR give 300 mg per day but prolong treatment to complete the total dose corresponding to 5 mg/kg per day for 60 days.	**Photosensitivity in 50% of pts.** GI: abdominal pain, nausea/vomiting/anorexia. Dermatitis including Stevens-Johnson. CNS: disorientation, insomnia, twitching/seizures, paresthesias, polyneuritis. Discontinue if leucopenia or thrombocytopenia. **Contraindicated in pregnancy**. Recommended dose range 5-7.5 mg/kg/day but more than 5 mg/kg has unacceptable side effects in adults, higher doses better tolerated in children.
Chloroquine phosphate (Aralen)	Dose varies—*see Malaria Prophylaxis and rx, pages 204-205.*	Minor: anorexia/nausea/vomiting, headache, dizziness, blurred vision, pruritus in dark-skinned pts. Major: protracted rx in rheumatoid arthritis can lead to retinopathy. Can exacerbate psoriasis. Can block response to intradermally administered rabies vaccine. **Contraindicated in pts with epilepsy.**
Dapsone *See Comment re methemoglobinemia*	100 mg po q24h	Usually tolerated by pts with rash after TMP-SMX. **Dapsone is common etiology of acquired methemoglobinemia** *(NEJM 364:957, 2011)*. Metabolite of dapsone converts heme iron to + 3 charge (no O2 transport) from normal +2. Normal blood level 1%; cyanosis at 10%; headache, fatigue, tachycardia, dizziness at 30-40%, acidosis & coma at 60%, death at 70-80%. Low G6PD is a risk factor. Treatment: methylene blue 1-2 mg/kg IV over 5 min x 1 dose.
Eflornithine (Ornidyl) (WHO or CDC drug service)	400 mg/kg/day IV divided q12h x 7 days in combination with Nifurtimox for West African Trypanosomiasis	Diarrhea in ½ pts, vomiting, abdominal pain, anemia/leukopenia in ½ pts, seizures, alopecia, jaundice, ↓ hearing. Contraindicated in pregnancy.
Fexinidazole	Wt ≥ 35 kg: Loading dose 1800 mg (3 tablets) once/day for 4 days then 1200 mg (2 tablets) once/day for 6 days for Stage 1 or mild Stage 2 (<100 WBC in CSF)	Able to swallow the 600 mg tablets after food, be able to complete 10d Rx. FDA suggests avoiding use if eGFR < 30 mL/min. If CSF cell number not known do not use fexinidazole. **Contraindications:** Cirrhosis, jaundice or existing or risk of long QTFc interval >470 ms. Must obtain directly from Sanofi in US.
Fumagillin	Eyedrops or 20 mg po tid treatment of E. bieneusi, (no longer available from Sanofi; no human formulations though veterinary formulations still available)	Adverse events: Neutropenia & thrombocytopenia.
Mefloquine	One 250 mg tab/wk for **malaria prophylaxis**; for rx, 1250 mg x 1 or 750 mg & then 500 mg in 6–8 hrs. In U.S.: 250 mg tab = 228 mg base; outside U.S.: 275 mg tab = 250 mg base	Side-effects in roughly 3%. Minor: headache, irritability, insomnia, weakness, diarrhea. **Toxic psychosis, seizures can occur.** Do not use with quinine, quinidine, or halofantrine. Rare: Prolonged QT interval and toxic epidermal necrolysis *(Ln 349:101, 1997)*. **Not used for self-rx due to neuropsychiatric side-effects.** FDA black box for possible prolonged effects. Avoid if pre-existing overlay of depression or other psychiatric disorders.
Melarsoprol (Mel B, Arsobal) *(CDC)* High toxicity only use for Stage 2, T. rhodesiense when no Fexinidazole available	2.2 mg/kg/day IV x 10 days	**Post-rx encephalopathy (2-10%) with 50% mortality overall, risk of death 2° to rx 8-14%.** Prednisolone 1 mg per kg per day po may ↓ encephalopathy. Other: Heart damage, albuminuria, abdominal pain, vomiting, peripheral neuropathy, Herxheimer-like reaction, pruritus. o Prednisone may prevent/attenuate encephalopathy. o Pretreatment with Suramin (dose as above) is often used in late-stage East African trypanosomiasis to clear the hemolymphatic system of trypanosomes before administration of melarsoprol.
Miltefosine (Impavido) No longer available from CDC, purchase from *www.impavido.com*	50 mg po bid (wt 33-44 kg); 50 mg po tid (wt ≥45 kg) (max 150 mg/d). Treat for 28 days	**Pregnancy—No;** teratogenic. Side-effects vary: kala-azar pts, vomiting in up to 40%, diarrhea in 17%; "motion sickness", headache & increased creatinine. Metabolized by liver; virtually no urinary excretion.
Nifurtimox (Lampit) *(CDC)* (Manufactured in Germany by Bayer) FDA approved, commercially available from *lampit.com*	8–10 mg/kg per day po div. 4 x per day for 90-120 days for Chaga's. 15 mg/kg/day po, divided q8h x 10 days for West African trypanosomiasis	**Side-effects in 40–70% of pts.** GI: abdominal pain, nausea/vomiting. CNS: polyneuritis (1/3), disorientation, insomnia, twitching, seizures. Skin rash. Hemolysis with G6PD deficiency. Monitor CBC, biochemistry after 4-6 weeks. Monitor frequently for neuropathy. Ref: *https://www.cdc.gov/mmwr/volumes/71/wr/mm7110a2.htm*
Pentamidine	4 mg/kg IV or IM daily x 7-10 days for African Trypanosomiasis. 300 mg via aerosol q month.	Hypotension, hypocalcemia, hypoglycemia followed by hyperglycemia, pancreatitis. Neutropenia (15%), thrombocytopenia. Nephrotoxicity. Others: nausea/vomiting, ↑ liver tests, rash.

* For source of drug, see *Table 13D, page 222*.

TABLE 13B (3)

CLASS, AGENT, GENERIC NAME (TRADE NAME)	USUAL ADULT DOSAGE	ADVERSE REACTIONS/COMMENTS
Antiprotozoan Drugs: Non-Intestinal Protozoa/Extraintestinal Parasites *(continued)*		
Primaquine phosphate	26.3 mg (=15 mg base). Adult dose is 30 mg of base po daily.	**In G6PD def. pts, can cause hemolytic anemia with hemoglobinuria, esp. African, Asian peoples.** Methemoglobinemia. Rapid G6PD screening tests now available. Nausea/abdominal pain if pt. fasting. **Pregnancy: No.**
Pyrimethamine (Daraprim, Malocide) Also combined with Sulfadoxine as **Fansidar** (25–500 mg)	100 mg po, then 25 mg/day. **Very expensive:** Current sources include Daraprim Direct +1 844 267 3323 (Optime Care Pharmacy/Tilde Sciences) or Dr. Reddy's *https://www.drreddys.com/united-states/our-products/prescription*.	**Major problem is hematologic:** megaloblastic anemia, ↓ WBC, ↓ platelets. Can give 5 mg folinic acid per day. If high-dose pyrimethamine, ↑ folinic acid to 10–50 mg/day. Pyrimethamine + sulfadiazine can cause mental changes. Other: Rash, vomiting, diarrhea, xerostomia.
Quinine sulfate (Qualaquin)	324 mg tabs. No IV prep. in US. Oral rx of chloroquine-resistant falciparum malaria: 624 mg po tid x 3 days, then x 7 days	Cinchonism; tinnitus, headache, nausea, abdominal pain, blurred vision. Rarely: blood dyscrasias, drug fever, asthma, hypoglycemia. **Contraindicated if prolonged QTc, myasthenia gravis, optic neuritis or G6PD deficiency.**
Spiramycin (Rovamycin)	1 gm po q8h *(see Comment).*	GI and allergic reactions have occurred. Available at no cost after consultation with Remington Laboratory for Specialty Diagnostics (formerly Toxoplasma Serology Lab): 650-853-4828 or need to file IND with U.S. FDA 301-796-1600.
Sulfadiazine	1–1.5 gm po q6h.	*See Table 10A, page 163, for sulfonamide side-effects*
Sulfadoxine & Pyrimethamine combination (Fansidar)	Contains 500 mg Sulfadoxine & 25 mg Pyrimethamine	Long half-life of both drugs: Sulfadoxine 169 hrs, pyrimethamine 111 hrs allows weekly dosage. In African, used empirically in pregnancy for intermittent preventative treatment (ITPp) against malaria: dosing at 3 set times during pregnancy. Reduces material and fetal mortality if HIV+. **Fatalities reported due to Stevens-Johnson syndrome and toxic epidermal necrolysis.** Renal excretion—caution if renal impairment.
Tafenoquine (Arakoda, Krintafel) (for P. vivax malaria, age ≥ 16 yrs, ≥ 18 yrs for prophylaxis) Arakoda: 100 mg tab Krintafel: 150 mg tab	Radical cure (prevention of relapse): 300 mg single dose on day 1 or 2 of appropriate blood-stage therapy. Prophylaxis: 200 mg qd x 3 days (starting 3 days before travel), then 200 mg qwk maintenance starting 7 days after last loading dose, then after leaving endemic area, 200 mg once, 7 days after last maintenance dose	Test for G6PD deficiency before use. **Must have 70% normal G6PD activity on quantitative testing to use TQ;** do not use screening tests or qualitative tests. AEs: hemolytic anemia (G6PD deficiency), methemoglobinemia, psychiatric effects only if previous psychosis, hypersensitivity. For radical cure of P. vivax use TQ only combination with chloroquine, not other malaria treatment drugs.
DRUGS USED TO TREAT NEMATODES, TREMATODES, AND CESTODES		
Albendazole (Albenza) www.expertpharmacy.com compounded for $10/tab	Doses vary with indication. Take with food; fatty meal increases absorption. See *Table 13D* for US availability	FDA Pregnancy Category C due to lack of data but available evidence suggests no difference in congenital abnormalities. WHO allows use of albendazole in 2nd and 3rd trimesters. CDC suggests consideration in 3rd trimester if infection is compromising the pregnancy. Abdominal pain (with prolonged courses), nausea/vomiting, alopecia, ↑ serum transaminase. Rare leukopenia.
Diethylcarbamazine *(CDC)*	Dose varies with species of filaria.	Headache, dizziness, nausea, fever. In Onchocerciasis, host may experience inflammatory reaction to death of microfilariae: fever, urticaria, asthma, GI upset **(Mazzotti reaction). Pregnancy—No.**
Ivermectin (Stromectol, Ivermectina) (3 mg tab & topical 0.5% lotion for head lice). Take on empty stomach.	Strongyloidiasis dose: 200 µg/kg/day po x 2 days Onchocerciasis: 150 µg/kg x 1 po Scabies: 200 µg/kg po x 1; if AIDS, wait 14 days & repeat	Mild side-effects: fever, pruritus, rash. In rx of onchocerciasis, can *see tender lymphadenopathy,* headache, bone/joint pain.
Mebendazole (Vermox)	In developing world chewable tablet, 500 mg po once in public health campaigns. 100 mg po twice/day for 3 days is optimal for most intestinal nematodes. 100 mg single dose adequate for pinworm. See Table 13D for US availability	Rarely causes abdominal pain, nausea, diarrhea. FDA Pregnancy Category C due to lack of data but available evidence suggests no difference in congenital abnormalities. WHO allows use of mebendazole in 2nd and 3rd trimesters. CDC suggests consideration in 3rd trimester if infection is compromising the pregnancy.

* For source of drug, see *Table 13D, page 222.*

TABLE 13B (4)

CLASS, AGENT, GENERIC NAME (TRADE NAME)	USUAL ADULT DOSAGE	ADVERSE REACTIONS/COMMENTS
DRUGS USED TO TREAT NEMATODES, TREMATODES, AND CESTODES *(continued)*		
Praziquantel (Biltricide)	Doses vary with parasite; *see Table 13A*.	Mild: dizziness/drowsiness, N/V, rash, fever. **Only contraindication is ocular cysticercosis**. Potential exacerbation of neurocysticercosis. Metab.-induced by anticonvulsants and steroids; can negate effect with cimetidine 400 mg po tid. Reduce dose if advanced liver disease. Praziquantel is pregnancy category B. Available evidence suggests no difference in adverse birth outcomes. WHO encourages the use of praziquantel in any stage of pregnancy. CDC advises individual risk-benefit assessment according to clinical disease in the mother.
Pyrantel pamoate (over-the-counter)	Oral suspension. Dose for all ages: 11 mg/kg (to max. of 1 gm) x 1 dose	Rare GI upset, headache, dizziness, rash
Suramin (Germanin) *(CDC)*	Drug powder mixed to 10% solution with 5 mL water and used within 30 min. First give test dose of 0.1 gm IV. Try to avoid during pregnancy.	Does not cross blood-brain barrier; no effect on CNS infection. Side-effects: vomiting, pruritus, urticaria, fever, paresthesias, albuminuria (discontinue drug if casts appear). Do not use if renal/liver disease present. Deaths from vascular collapse reported.
Triclabendazole (Egaten) *(CDC)* Available at no charge from Novartis. *See Table 13D*	Used for fasciola hepatica liver fluke infection: 10 mg/kg po x 1 dose. May repeat in 12-24 hrs. 250 mg tabs	AEs ≥10%: sweating and abdominal pain. AEs 1-10%: weakness, chest pain, fever, anorexia, nausea, vomiting. **Note: use with caution if G6PD def. or impaired liver function.**

TABLE 13C – PARASITES THAT CAUSE EOSINOPHILIA (EOSINOPHILIA IN TRAVELERS)

Frequent and Intense (>5000 eos/mcL)	Moderate to Marked Early Infections	During Larval Migration; Absent or Mild During Chronic Infections	Other	
Strongyloides (absent in compromised hosts); Lymphatic Filariasis; Toxocara (cutaneous larva migrans); Trichinella; Angiostrongylus; Opisthorchis	Ascaris; Hookworm; Clonorchis; Paragonimus; Fasciola; Schistosomiasis	Opisthorchis; Baylisascaris	Schistosomiasis; Cysticercosis; Trichuris; Angiostrongylus; Onchocerciasis; echinococcus	Non-lymphatic filariasis; Gnathostoma; Capillaria; Trichostrongylus

* For source of drug, see *Table 13D, page 222*.

TABLE 13D – SOURCES FOR HARD-TO-FIND ANTIPARASITIC DRUGS

Source	Drugs Available	Contact Information
CDC Drug Service	Diethylcarbamazine (DEC), Eflornithine, Melarsoprol, Suramin.	www.cdc.gov/laboratory/drugservice/index.html (+1) 404-639-3670 or drugservice@cdc.gov
CDC Malaria Branch CDC no longer distributes no-cost antimalarial drugs.	FDA approved IV Artesunate (Amivas), now commercially available in the US through major distributors (Cardinal Health, Americsource Bergen, and McKesson). See *https://ivartesunate.com* for distributors' 24/7 emergency numbers; all voice messages will receive a response in <30 minutes. Wholesale cost is $5,000 USD per vial; the average 80 kg person requires 6 vials for the first day and then 2 vials per day for each subsequent day that parasitemia is greater than 1%.	Malaria treatment advice CDC Malaria Hotline (770-488-7788) from 9:00 am to 5:00 pm Eastern Time. After hours or on weekends and holidays, call the CDC Emergency Operation Center at 770-488-7100 and ask to page the person on call for the Malaria Branch
WHO	Drugs for treatment of African trypanosomiasis	priottog@who.int; (+41) 794-682-726; (+41) 227-911-345 francoj@who.int; (+41) 796-198-535; (+41) 227-913-313
Compounding Pharmacies, Specialty Distributors, Direct from Mfgr		
Amivas	IV artesunate for severe malaria	Amivas, 855-526-4827 See *amivas.com* for commercial distributors with 24/7 emergency supplies.
Bayer	Nifurtimox available through normal retail channels. Patient assistance program in place. Use off-label in adults.	www.lampit.com
Exeltis, Inc.	Benznidazole. Commercial FDA approved tab for child age 2-12 yrs, may use off-label in adults (www.benznidazoletablets.com)	+1 800-964-9650
Expert Compounding Pharmacy (intermittent availability for each drug)	Albendazole, Iodoquinol, Paromomycin (oral), Praziquantel, Pyrantel pamoate	www.expertpharmacy.org 1-800-247-9767; (+1) 818-988-7979
Novartis, Inc.	Triclabendazole. Available and shipped for free to any pharmacy having a valid prescription on hand. Novartis will request patient name, DOB, and pharmacy address/phone. Can also call if advice needed about general toxoplasmosis treatment or diagnostics	Tel: +1 888-669-6682.
Remington Toxoplasma Serology	Spiramycin (consultation required for release)	(+1) 650-853-4828; remingtonlab@sutterhealth.org
Profounda, Inc.	Miltefosine (leishmaniasis or free-living ameba)	www.impavido.com; +1 407-270-7790
Sanofi	Glucantime (Meglumine antimoniate) is available only from Sanofi (no cost) after obtaining an individual IND from FDA. Contact each simultaneously	**FDA:** druginfo@fda.hhs.gov; or 301-796-3400 during business hours. FDA form 3926 plus clinical info, plus local IRB is required. Sanofi: Will need to provide FDA IND# and extensive paperwork.
Sanofi	Fexinidazole tablets - fully FDA approved.	Contact Sanofi Medical Affairs at 1-800-372-6634 or customersupport@sanofi.com. and request for free. Contact CDC Drug Service to liaise with Sanofi to expedite.
Victoria Apotheke Zurich will ship worldwide if sent physicians prescription.	Paromomycin (oral and topical), Triclabendazole. Other hard to find anti-parasitic drugs	www.pharmaworld.com (+41) 43-344-6060
Waylis Therapeutics	Paromomycin sulfate capsules Labelled only for amebiasis and buyer must indicate confirmed diagnosis on the prescription	https://www.waylistherapeutics.com/products; 1 800 689 0255

Note: In the U.S. FDA-approved branded Albendazole (Albenza; produced by GSK Canada) and Mebendazole marketed by Amneal is very costly and is difficult for retail pharmacies to access. Vermox brand mebendazole 500 mg tablets is FDA-approved but for donation only and not sold in the U.S.

* For source of drug, see *Table 13D, page 222*.

TABLE 14A – ANTIVIRAL THERAPY*

For HIV, *see Table 14C*; for Hepatitis, *see Table 14E* and *Table 14F*.

VIRUS/DISEASE	DRUG/DOSAGE	SIDE EFFECTS/COMMENTS
Adenovirus: Cause of RTIs including fatal pneumonia in children & young adults and 60% mortality in transplant pts. Frequent cause of cystitis in transplant patients. **Findings include:** fever, ↑ liver enzymes, leukopenia, thrombocytopenia, diarrhea, pneumonia, or hemorrhagic cystitis. Encephalitis: *NEJM 381:1459, 2019.* Treatment Guidelines: https://doi.org/10.1111/ctr.13527	In severe cases of pneumonia or post HSCT[1]: **Cidofovir** • 5 mg/kg/wk x 2 wks, then q 2 wks + **Probenecid** 1.25 gm/M² given 3 hrs before cidofovir and 3 & 9 hrs after each infusion • Or 1 mg/kg IV 3x/wk. For adenovirus hemorrhagic cystitis: Intravesical **Cidofovir** (5 mg/kg in 100 mL saline instilled into bladder).	Routine monitoring with HAdV viral load recommended 1- 2 times/wk in high-risk patients: Allo-HSCT with haploidentical donor or unrelated cord blood graft; Severe GVHD; Severe lymphopenia; and/or Rx with alemtuzumab. Monitoring should continue until immune reconstitution. Those with at least 1 risk factor and viremia should be Rx'd with cidofovir. Ribavirin not recommended. Brincidofovir mixed results. Donor specific T-cells should be reserved for those who have failed antiviral therapy and administered as part of a clinical trial. A live, oral vaccine against adenovirus types 4 and 7 is approved by the U.S. Food and Drug Administration for U.S. military personnel ages 17 through 50 who may be at higher risk for infection.
Bunyaviridae: Severe fever with thrombocytopenia syndrome virus (SFTSV) Possibly transmitted by *Haemaphysalis longicomis* and *Amblyomma americanum (lone star)* ticks.	No therapy recommended. Ribavirin ineffective. Clinical symptoms: Fever, weakness, myalgias, GI symptoms	Lab: Elevated LDH (>1200) and CPK (>800) associated with higher mortality rates. Initially thought to be an anaplasma infection, but serology showed a new virus. Reservoir in animals (goats/cattle/dogs/cats)
Coronavirus— **MERS-CoV:** Middle East respiratory syndrome *(NEJM 2017,376:584)*	**MERS:** Increased 14 day survival with **Ribavirin** po + **PEG-IFN** 180 mcg/kg sc x 2 wks *(LnID 14:1090, 2014)*. Other therapies: *LnID 14:1136, 2014.*	**MERS:** Suspected reservoirs are camels and perhaps other animals. *Review: Clin Micro Rev. 28:465, 2015.*
SARS CoV-2 / COVID-19 **Primary Prevention:** 1) **Vaccination:** consult current national recommendations; 2) **PrEP Pemivibart** (Pemgarda), IV over 60 min q3 mo, is indicated in adults and adolescents (12 years of age ; > 40 kg,) who are not currently infected with SARS-CoV-2. **PEP:** No current PEP recommendations.	**The situation continues to evolve as this edition goes to press. See *http://web.sanfordguide.com* or Sanford Guide mobile app for continually updated information, treatment recommendations, vaccine developments and prevention measures.** See also *cdc.gov, nih.gov/coronavirus, fda.gov* and *who.int* for updates.	
Setting, disease severity, risk of progression	**Therapy (as of January 2025)**	**Comments**
Not hospitalized or hospitalized, asymptomatic	Rx those who are immunocompromised and those >65 years of age	Close clinical monitoring
Not hospitalized, mild-to-moderate disease, NOT at high risk of disease progression	Rx those who are immunocompromised and those >65 years of age	Close clinical monitoring

[1] HSCT = Hematopoietic stem cell transplant

** See page 2 for abbreviations. NOTE: All dosage recommendations are for adults (unless otherwise indicated) and assume normal renal function.*

TABLE 14A (2)

VIRUS/DISEASE	DRUG/DOSAGE	SIDE EFFECTS/COMMENTS
SARS CoV-2 / COVID-19 *(continued)*		
Setting, disease severity, risk of progression	**Therapy**	**Comments**
Not hospitalized, mild-to-severe disease, high risk of disease progression Activity against variants is a continually evolving situation! Check for latest recommendations	In order of preference (NIH Guidelines): **Paxlovid** 300/100 mg po bid x 5 days OR **Remdesivir** 200 mg day 1, then 100 mg days 2-3 OR **Molnupiravir** 800 mg po bid x 5 days	Antiviral therapy and/or monoclonal antibody should be administered as early as possible in the course of disease: Paxlovid: within 3-5 days Remdesivir within 7 days Molnupiravir within 5 days Dexamethasone / systemic steroids NOT recommended
Hospitalized, mild disease (no lower respiratory tract disease). Patient at high risk of disease progression	**Remdesivir** Prophylactic anticoagulation	Dexamethasone NOT recommended
Hospitalized, moderate disease (evidence of lower respiratory tract disease) with no supplemental O_2 requirement. Patient at high risk of disease progression.	**Remdesivir** Prophylactic anticoagulation	Dexamethasone NOT recommended
Hospitalized, severe disease (O_2 saturation <94% and/ or PaO2/FiO2 <300) requires supplemental O_2.	**Remdesivir** + **Dexamethasone** + **Tocilizumab** Consider therapeutic anticoagulation	In patients who are unable to receive dexamethasone, use as alternative **Baricitinib** (plus Remdesivir)
Hospitalized, critical disease -- requires mechanical ventilation or ECMO	**Dexamethasone** + **Remdesivir** + **Tocilizumab** Prophylactic anticoagulation	Benefit of Remdesivir unproven, but recommended by some authorities Consider IL-6 receptor blocker in the first 24 hours of ICU admission (ok to use with Remdesivir and dexamethasone, would not recommend in conjunction with Baricitinib) In patients who are unable to receive dexamethasone, consider **Baricitinib**. Consult Sanford Guide digital content (web or mobile app) for current recommendations

VIRUS/DISEASE	DRUG/DOSAGE	SIDE EFFECTS/COMMENTS
Enterovirus—Meningitis: most common cause of aseptic meningitis. Rapid CSF PCR test is accurate; reduces costs and hospital stay for infants	**No rx currently recommended.**	Up to 1/3rd of adults have neutrophilic pleocytosis in CSF. Reviewed *(J Clin Virology, 104, 56-60, 2018)*
Hemorrhagic Fever Virus Infections:		
Congo-Crimean Hemorrhagic Fever (HF) Tick-borne; symptoms include N/V, fever, headache, myalgias, & stupor (1/3). Signs: *conjunctival* injection, hepatomegaly, petechiae (1/3). Lab: ↓ platelets, ↓ WBC, ↑ ALT, AST, LDH & CPK (100%).	**RBV** 30 mg/kg/day po loading dose, then 15 mg/kg q6h x 4 days, then 7.5 mg/kg q8h x 6 days (WHO recommendation) *(see Comment)*.	(89%) with confirmed CCHF rx with ribavirin survived in Iran *(CID 36:1613, 2003)*. Suggested benefit from ribavirin & dexamethasone *(281 pts) (CID 57:1270, 2013)*. Treatment must be given early. Efficacy marginal. *(Nature Reviews Microbiology / 21 / July 2023 / 463–477)*

** See page 2 for abbreviations. NOTE: All dosage recommendations are for adults (unless otherwise indicated) and assume normal renal function.*

TABLE 14A (3)

VIRUS/DISEASE	DRUG/DOSAGE	SIDE EFFECTS/COMMENTS
Hemorrhagic Fever Virus Infections *(continued)*		
Ebola/Marburg HF (Central Africa) Diagnostic testing at U.S. CDC. Within a few days of symptom onset, diagnosis is most commonly made by antigen-capture enzyme linked immunosorbent assay (ELISA), IgM antibody ELISA, NAAT or viral culture *(NEJM 382:1832, 2020); (Journal of Infection and Public Health 15 (2022) 285–292).*	**Treatment: Inmazeb** (REGN-EB3: 3 fully human monoclonal antibodies - atoltivimab, maftivimab, odesivimab-ebgn) 50 mg/kg of each of the 3 mAbs (150 mg/kg total) IV as single infusion. **Ebanga** (ansuvimab-zyk Ab) 50 mg/kg IV as single infusion. **Prevention: Ervebo** (live recombinant VSV vector with ebola env glycoprotein insert) 1 ml IM (deltoid, in non-dominant arm)	**Abrupt onset of symptoms typically 8-10 days after exposure (range 2-21 days).** Nonspecific symptoms, which may include fever, chills, myalgias, and malaise. Fever, anorexia, asthenia / weakness are the most common signs and symptoms. Patients may develop a diffuse erythematous maculopapular rash (days 5-7) (usually involving the face, neck, trunk, and arms) that can desquamate. EVD can **often be confused with** other more common infectious diseases such as malaria, typhoid fever, meningococcemia, and other bacterial infections (e.g., pneumonia). **Gastrointestinal symptoms:** severe watery diarrhea, nausea, vomiting and abdominal pain. **Other:** chest pain, shortness of breath, headache or confusion, may also develop. Patients often have conjunctival injection. Hiccups reported. Seizures may occur, and cerebral edema reported. Bleeding is not universally present but can manifest later in the course as petechiae, ecchymosis/bruising, or oozing from venipuncture sites and mucosal hemorrhage. Frank hemorrhage is less common. Pregnant women may experience spontaneous miscarriages.
With pulmonary syndrome: Hantavirus pulmonary syndrome, "sin nombre virus"	**No Effective Treatment.** Early recognition of disease and supportive (usually ICU) care is key to successful outcome.	Acute onset of fever, headache, myalgias, non-productive cough, thrombocytopenia, increased PT and non-cardiogenic pulmonary edema with respiratory insufficiency following exposure to droppings of infected rodents.
With renal syndrome: Lassa, Venezuelan, Korean, HF, Sabia, Argentinian HF, Bolivian HF, Junin, Machupo (>90% occur in China *CID 59:1040, 2014*)	**RBV** 30 mg/kg/day po loading dose, then 15 mg/kg q6h x 4 days, then 7.5 mg/kg x 6 days (WHO recommendation) *(see Comment).*	Toxicity low, hemolysis reported but recovery when treatment stopped. *See CID 36:1254, 2003,* for management of contacts. ARF in Lassa associated with 15-fold higher mortality *(Lancet ID 18, (6): 684-695, 2018).*
Dengue and dengue hemorrhagic fever (DHF) *www.cdc.gov/ncidod/dvbid/dengue/dengue-hcp.htm* Think dengue in traveler to tropics or subtropics (incubation period usually 4-7 days) with fever, bleeding, thrombocytopenia, or hemoconcentration with shock. Dx by viral isolation or serology; serum to CDC (telephone 787-706-2399).	**No data on antiviral rx.** Fluid replacement with careful hemodynamic monitoring critical. Review of treatment: *Current Treatment Opinion ID 9:185-93, 2017.*	Diagnosis: Combination IgG, IgM, and NS1 antigen panel is preferred test (Quest Diagnostics). Should only be used in pts with symptoms c/w Dengue Fever. Many candidates' antiviral drugs in development; non effective yet. Rupatadine shortened symptoms and modestly reduced severity of illness in small clinical trial *(Scientific Reports 8: 3857, 2018).*
West Nile virus *(JAMA 310:308, 2013)* A flavivirus transmitted by mosquitoes, blood transfusions, transplanted organs & breast-feeding. Birds (>200 species) are main host with humans & horses incidental hosts.	**No proven rx**. Supportive care (See *www.cdc.gov/westnile/healthcareproviders*). RCT of IVIG of no benefit.	Usually nonspecific febrile disease but 1/150 cases develops meningoencephalitis, aseptic meningitis or polio-like paralysis. Long-term sequelae (neuromuscular weakness & psychiatric) common. Diagnosis: increased IgM antibody in serum & CSF or CSF PCR (contact State Health Dept./CDC). Blood supply now tested in U.S.
Yellow fever	**No data on antiviral rx** **Guidelines for use of preventative vaccine:** *(http://www.cdc.gov/mmwr/preview/mmwrhtml/mm6423a5.htm?s_cid=mm6423a5_w)*	Reemergence in Africa & S. Amer. due to urbanization of susceptible population *(https://www.nejm.org/doi/full/10.1056/NEJMp1702172).* Vaccination Diagnosis: increased IgM antibody safe and effective in HIV patients, especially in those with suppressed VL and higher CD4 counts *(CID 48:659, 2009).*
Chikungunya fever: brake bone fever A self-limited arbovirus illness spread by Aedes mosquito. High epidemic potential (Caribbean).	**No antiviral therapy.** Fluids, analgesics, anti-pyretics.	Clinical presentation: high fever, severe myalgias & headache, morbilliform rash with occ. thrombocytopenia. Rarely hemorrhagic complications. Dx mostly clinical; definitive diagnosis by PCR.
SFTSV (Severe fever with thrombocytopenia syndrome virus)	***See Bunyaviridae, page 223***	
Oropouche	**No Effective Rx** Supportive care only *(see Lancet ID 24: 935: 2024)*	Indigenous in Tropical Regions (Amazon Basin; Brazil; Central and South America). Disease similar to Dengue /Zika. Hemorrhagic fever (15%). Pregnant women risk of microcephaly in fetus.

TABLE 14A (4)

VIRUS/DISEASE	DRUG/DOSAGE	SIDE EFFECTS/COMMENTS
Hepatitis Viral Infections	*See Table 14E (Hepatitis A & B), Table 14F (Hepatitis C)*	
Herpesvirus Infections		
Cytomegalovirus (CMV) Solid Organ Treatment Guidelines *(Transplantation 102:900-31, 2018)* Review of anti-CMV drugs *(Curr Opin Organ Transplant 2019, 24:469)*	**Primary prophylaxis** recommended in certain transplant populations *(see Table 15E)*. When prophylaxis indicated, **Valganciclovir** 900 mg po q12h *(CID 32: 783, 2001)*. **Letermovir** 480 mg IV or po daily (Kidney Transplant)	Resistance demonstrated in 5% of transplant recipients receiving primary prophylaxis *(J Antimicrob Chemother 65:2628. 2010)*. Letermovir effective as primary preventative therapy in patients who have undergone stem cell transplant and high-risk for CMV disease. Duration of prophylaxis depends on donor/recipient status and type of transplant.
CMV: Colitis, Esophagitis, Gastritis Symptoms relate to site of disease	*Mild:* **Valganciclovir** 900 mg po bid with food x 14-21 days *Severe:* **Ganciclovir** 5 mg/kg IV q12h x 14-21 days OR **Foscarnet** (60 mg/kg IV q8h or 90 mg/kg q12h) x 14-21 days *Post-treatment suppression:* **Valganciclovir** 900 mg po once daily until CD4 >100 x 6 mos	Diagnosis: Elevated whole blood quantitative PCR & histopathology. Severe bouts of Inflammatory Bowel Disease (IBD) colitis may be complicated by CMV; Rx of CMV in this setting is recommended. Rx of CMV in less severe bouts of IBD colitis is unclear.
CMV: Neurologic disease, Encephalitis Myelitis, polyradiculopathy, peripheral neuropathy Symptoms relate to site of disease	Treat as for severe colitis, esophagitis, gastritis above	Diagnosis: Elevated whole blood and/or CSF quantitative PCR. Most experts would not delay start of ARV therapy for more than 1 week in those with HIV. Watch for IRIS and treat if it develops.
CMV: Pneumonitis At risk: 1st 6 months post-transplant & 3 months post-stopping prophylaxis Require evidence of invasive disease. Diagnosis: prefer whole blood quantitative PCR and/or positive lung biopsy histopathology	*Viremic but no/mild symptoms:* **Valganciclovir** 900 mg po bid. *Severe in lung transplant or AIDS pts (rare in HIV pts):* **Ganciclovir** 5 mg/kg IV q12h (adjust for renal insufficiency). Treat until clinical resolution & neg blood PCR; min duration: 2 wks, then transition to **Valganciclovir** 900 mg po bid (duration individualized). Reduce immunosuppression if possible.	*Post-treatment suppression:* Valganciclovir 900 mg po once daily x 1-3 months if high risk of relapse. Suspect resistant CMV if treatment failure or relapse. Do genotype resistance testing. *If Ganciclovir-resistant:* Foscarnet (60 mg/kg q8h or 90 mg/kg q12h) IV (adjust for renal insufficiency). NOTE: IVIG or CMV specific immunoglobulin did not improve overall or attributable mortality in retrospective study of 421 bone marrow transplant pts *(CID 61:31, 2015)*. Cidofovir is an alternative therapy.
CMV: Retinitis Most common ocular complication of HIV/AIDS. Rare in pts on ART with CD4 >200. If not on ART, do not delay ART for more than 2 wks of CMV therapy. Ref: *aidsinfo.nih.gov/guidelines* **CMV immune recovery retinitis:** new retinitis after starting ART. Do not stop ART or Valganciclovir. No steroids.	*Not sight-threatening:* **Valganciclovir** 900 mg po bid with food x 14-21 days, then 900 mg po once daily until CD4 >100 x 6 months. Sight-threatening *(see Comment):* **Valganciclovir** + intravitreal **Ganciclovir** 2 mg (1-4 doses over 7-10 days).	Sight-threatening: <1500 microns from fovea or next to head of optic nerve. If can't use Valganciclovir, Ganciclovir 5 mg/kg IV q12h x 14-21 days, then 5 mg/kg IV once daily. If suspect Ganciclovir resistance: Foscarnet (60 gm/kg q8h or 90 mg/kg q12h) x 14-21 days. Ganciclovir ocular implants no longer available.
CMV in Transplant patients: *See Table 15E for CMV prophylaxis.* CMV disease can manifest as CMV syndrome with or without end-organ disease. **Guidelines for CMV therapy**. **Ganciclovir** 5 mg/kg IV q12h OR **Valganciclovir** 900 mg po q12h are effective treatment options. Treatment duration should be individualized. Continue treatment until (1) CMV PCR is undetectable and, (2) clinical evidence of disease has resolved, and (3) at least 2-3 weeks of treatment. Secondary prophylaxis (**Valganciclovir** 900 mg daily) should be considered for 1-3 month course in patients recently treated with high-dose immunosuppression such as lymphocyte depleting antibodies, those with severe CMV disease, or those with >1 episode of CMV disease. In HSCT recipients, secondary prophylaxis should be considered in similar cases balancing the risk of recurrent infection with drug toxicity. Brincidofovir not effective against CMV in transplant patients. **Maribavir** 400 mg po bid is new option for refractory disease (adult and child age 12 or older (wt ≥ 35 kg).		
CMV in pregnancy: Hyperimmune globulin failed in large study *(NEJM 385:436, 2021)*		
CMV: Congenital/Neonatal Symptomatic	**Valganciclovir** 16 mg/kg po bid x 6 mos	Better outcome after 6 mos in symptomatic infants treated before 30 DOL compared to 6 wks with no difference in AEs. Monitor for neutropenia.

** See page 2 for abbreviations. NOTE: All dosage recommendations are for adults (unless otherwise indicated) and assume normal renal function.*

TABLE 14A (5)

VIRUS/DISEASE	DRUG/DOSAGE	SIDE EFFECTS/COMMENTS
Herpesvirus Infections *(continued)*		
Epstein Barr Virus (EBV) — Mononucleosis	**No treatment.** Corticosteroids for tonsillar obstruction, CNS complications, or threat of splenic rupture.	**Diff dx of atypical lymphocytes:** EBV, CMV, Hep A, Hep B, Toxo, measles, mumps, drugs, HHV6, HHV7, HIV & others.
EBV, chronic active disease	Bone Marrow Transplant is most commonly used Rx (Allo-HSCT	Dx base on > 3 months mononucleosis like symptoms; Elevated EBV genomic DNA in peripheral blood; EBV infection of T-cells or NK cells in tissue or peripheral blood; Exclusion of other causes of chronic disease. Most cases in Asia; more cases now identified world-wide. Review: *Front. Pediatr., 05 February 2019 (https://doi.org/10.3389/fped.2019.00014)*
HHV-6—Cause of roseola (exanthem subitum) & other febrile diseases of childhood. Fever & rash in transplant pts. Reactivation in 47% of 110 U.S. hematopoietic stem cell transplant pts. Associated with meningoencephalitis, infectious mono & DRESS syndrome in immunocompetent adults. Diagnosis made by pos. PCR in CSF & compatible clinical syndrome. CSF film array PCR, 15 pos. for HHV-5, only 1 of 15 with compatible clin. illness *(CID 67:1125, 2018)*. RX; **Ganciclovir** is primary regimen.		
HHV-7—Ubiquitous virus (>90% of the population is infected by age 3 yrs). No relationship to human disease. Infects CD4 lymphocytes via CD4 receptor; transmitted via saliva.		
HHV-8—The agent of Kaposi's sarcoma, Castleman's disease, & body cavity lymphoma. Associated with diabetes in sub-Saharan Africa.	**No antiviral treatment.** Effective anti-HIV therapy may help.	Localized lesions: radiotherapy, laser surgery or intralesional chemotherapy. Systemic: chemotherapy. Castleman's disease responded to steroids, chemotherapy, IL6 antagonists, rituximab.
Herpes simplex virus (HSV Types 1 & 2)		
Bell's palsy H. simplex most implicated etiology. Other etiologic considerations: VZV, HHV-6, Lyme disease.	As soon as possible after onset of palsy: **Valacyclovir** 500 mg bid x first 5 days + **Prednisone** 1 mg/kg po divided bid x 5 days then taper to 5 mg bid over the next 5 days (total of 10 days Prednisone).	Cochrane Review *(2015)(JAMA 2016,316:874)* "compared with oral corticosteroids alone, addition of valacyclovir or famciclovir associated with greater number of recoveries at 3-12 mos". Meta-analysis proves combination Rx (steroids plus antivirals) superior to either alone *Laryngoscope, 131:1615–1625, 2021*
Encephalitis HSV-1 is most common cause of sporadic encephalitis. Survival & recovery from neurological sequelae are related to mental status at time of initiation of rx. **Early dx and rx imperative**.	**Acyclovir** 10-12.5 mg/kg IV (infuse over 1 hr) q8h x 14-21 days. 20 mg/kg q8h in children <12 yrs. Dose calculation in obese patients uncertain. To lessen risk of nephrotoxicity with larger doses seems reasonable to infuse each dose over more than 1 hour. In morbid obesity, use "adjusted" body weight. Adjusted BW = ideal BW + 0.4 (actual BW-ideal BW).	Mortality rate reduced from >70% to 19% with acyclovir rx. PCR analysis of CSF for HSV-1 DNA is 100% specific & 75–98% sensitive. 8/33 (25%) CSF samples drawn before day 3 were neg. by PCR; neg. PCR assoc. with ↓ protein & <10 WBC per mm^3 in CSF. All were + after 3 days. Autoimmune encephalitis following successful Rx (via NMDA receptor antibodies). HSV DNA neg. Rx with steroids.
Genital Herpes: *Sexually Transmitted Treatment Guidelines MMWR 70(RR4):1, 2021.*		
Primary (initial episode)	**Acyclovir** (Zovirax or generic) 400 mg po tid x 7–10 days	↓ by 2 days, time to resolution of signs & symptoms, ↓ by 4 days, time to healing of lesions, ↓ by 7 days, duration of viral shedding. Does not prevent recurrences. For severe cases only: 5 mg per kg IV q8h times 5–7 days.
	Valacyclovir (Valtrex) 1000 mg po bid x 7-10 days	An ester of acyclovir, which is well absorbed, bioavailability 3–5 times greater than acyclovir.
	Famciclovir (Famvir) 250 mg po bid or tid x 7–10 days	Metabolized to penciclovir, which is active component. Side effects and activity similar to acyclovir. **Famciclovir** 250 mg po tid **equal to acyclovir** 200 mg 5 times per day.

** See page 2 for abbreviations. NOTE: All dosage recommendations are for adults (unless otherwise indicated) and assume normal renal function.*

TABLE 14A (6)

VIRUS/DISEASE	DRUG/DOSAGE	SIDE EFFECTS/COMMENTS
Herpesvirus Infections/Herpes simplex virus (HSV Types 1 & 2)/Genital Herpes *(continued)*		
Episodic recurrences	**Acyclovir** 800 mg po tid **x 2 days** or 400 mg po tid **x 5 days** or **Famciclovir** 1000 mg bid **x 1 day**, 250 mg bid x 2 days or 125 mg po bid x 5 days or **Valacyclovir** 500 mg po bid **x 3 days** or 1 gm po once daily **x 5 days** Valacyclovir more effective overall. For HIV patients, *see Comment*	For episodic recurrences in **HIV patients:** **Acyclovir** 400 mg po tid x 5-10 days or **Famciclovir** 500 mg po bid x 5-10 days or **Valacyclovir** 1 gm po bid x 5-10 days
Chronic daily suppression	Suppressive therapy reduces the frequency of genital herpes recurrences by 70–80% among pts who have frequent recurrences (i.e., >6 recurrences per yr) & many report no symptomatic outbreaks. **Acyclovir** 400 mg po bid, **or Famciclovir** 250 mg po bid, **or Valacyclovir** 1 gm po q24h; pts with <9 recurrences per yr could use 500 mg po q24h and then use **Valacyclovir** 1 gm po q24h if breakthrough for episodic therapy. For HIV patients, *see Comment.*	For chronic suppression in HIV patients: all regimens equally efficacious (Often not needed with current era ART) **Acyclovir** 400-800 mg po bid or tid or **Famciclovir** 500 mg po bid or **Valacyclovir** 500 mg po bid
Genital, immunocompetent		
Gingivostomatitis, primary (children)	**Acyclovir** 15 mg/kg po 5x/day x 7 days	Efficacy in randomized double-blind placebo-controlled trial *(BMJ 314:1800, 1997)*.
Keratoconjunctivitis and recurrent epithelial keratitis	**Trifluridine** (Viroptic), 1 drop 1% solution q2h (max. 9 drops per day) for max. of 21 days *(see Table 1, page 15)*	In controlled trials, response % > idoxuridine. Suppressive rx with acyclovir (400 mg bid) reduced recurrences of ocular HSV from 32% to 19% *(NEJM 339:300, 1998)*.
Mollaret's recurrent "aseptic" meningitis (usually HSV-2)	No controlled trials of antiviral rx & resolves spontaneously. If therapy is to be given, **Acyclovir** (15–30 mg/kg/day IV) or **Valacyclovir** 1-2 gm po qid should be used.	Pos. PCR for HSV in CSF confirms dx. No benefit from valacyclovir suppressive rx.
Mucocutaneous *(for Genital see page 227)*		
Oral labial, "fever blisters":		
Normal host	Start rx with prodrome symptoms (tingling/burning) before lesions show. Drug — Dose — Sx Decrease **Oral: Valacyclovir** — 2 gm po q12h x 1 day — ↓ 1 day **Famciclovir**[2] — 500 mg po bid x 7 days — ↓ 2 days **Acyclovir**[NFDA] — 400 mg po 5 x per day (q4h while awake) x 5 days) — ↓ ½ day **Topical:** **Penciclovir** 1% cream — q2h during day x 4 days — ↓ 1 day **Acyclovir** 5% cream[3] — 6x/day (q3h) x 7 days — ↓ ½ day	Oral therapy preferred over topical antiviral therapy.
Herpes Whitlow	*See Table 1, page 30*	

[2] FDA approved only for HIV pts
[3] Approved for immunocompromised pts

* *See page 2 for abbreviations. NOTE: All dosage recommendations are for adults (unless otherwise indicated) and assume normal renal function.*

TABLE 14A (7)

VIRUS/DISEASE	DRUG/DOSAGE	SIDE EFFECTS/COMMENTS
Herpesvirus Infections/Herpes simplex virus (HSV Types 1 & 2)/Mucocutaneous *(continued)*		
Oral labial or genital: Immunocompromised		
(includes pts with AIDS) and critically ill pts in ICU setting/large necrotic ulcers in perineum or face. *(See Comment)* Primary HSV in pregnancy: increased risk of dissemination, including severe hepatitis, Risk greatest in 3rd trimester.	**Acyclovir** 5 mg per kg IV (infused over 1 hr) q8h times 7 days (250 mg per M^2) or 400 mg po 5 times per day times 14-21 days *(see Comment if suspect acyclovir-resistant)* **OR** **Famciclovir:** In HIV infected, 500 mg po bid for 7 days for recurrent episodes of genital herpes **OR** **Valacyclovir**[NAI]**:** In HIV-infected, 500 mg po bid for 5–10 days for recurrent episodes of genital herpes or 500 mg po bid for chronic suppressive rx.	**Acyclovir-resistant HSV: IV foscarnet** 90 mg/kg IV q12h x 7 days. Suppressive therapy with famciclovir (500 mg po bid), valacyclovir (500 mg po bid) or acyclovir (400-800 mg po bid) reduces viral shedding and clinical recurrences.
Neonatal herpes. 3 distinct syndromes: **Skin, eye and mouth** (SEM): typically presents 9-11 days of life (range 4-14 days). **Disseminated**: presents with septic appearance, LFT abnormalities 9-11 days of life (range 4-14 days). **Central nervous system** (CNS): presents 16-17 days of life (range 10-21 days)	**Acyclovir** 60 mg/kg/d div q8h. Duration 14 days for SEM, 21 days for disseminated or CNS. For CNS, repeat HSV PCR of CSF before stopping. Continue 7 more days if PCR still positive.	Infants can progress from one syndrome to another. After treatment, suppressive therapy reduces recurrence, improves outcome. Acyclovir 900 mg/m²/day po divided 3 times daily x 6 months. For management of asymptomatic infant born to mother with active lesions see *Pediatrics. 2013 Feb;131(2):e635-4.*
Pregnancy and genital H. simplex	Acyclovir safe even in first trimester. No proof that acyclovir at delivery reduces risk/severity of neonatal Herpes. In contrast, C-section in women with active lesions reduces risk of transmission.	
Herpes simiae (Herpes B virus): **Monkey bite** Decision whether to initiate prophylaxis after exposure based on an algorithm: McGill Criteria. Algorithm and approach to assessment/wound management in this article *(Emerg Infect Dis. 2019 Sep; 25(9): e190045)*	**Postexposure prophylaxis: Valacyclovir** 1 gm po q8h times 14 days or acyclovir 800 mg po 5 times per day times 14 days. **Treatment of disease:** (1) CNS symptoms absent: **Acyclovir** 12.5–15 mg per kg IV q8h or ganciclovir 5 mg per kg IV q12h. (2) CNS symptoms present: **Ganciclovir** 5 mg per kg IV q12h.	Fatal human cases of myelitis and hemorrhagic encephalitis have been reported following bites, scratches, or eye inoculation of saliva from monkeys. Initial sx include fever, headache, myalgias and diffuse adenopathy, incubation period of 2–14 days.
Varicella-Zoster Virus (VZV)		
Varicella: Diagnosis *(JEADV 31:9, 2017)* and treatment *(JEADV 31:20, 2017)*. Immunization: *www.cdc.gov/vaccines/schedules/hcp/imz/child-adolescent* or *Med Lett 2018;60:73.* Therapy review: *Molecules 26: 1132, 2021.*		
Normal host (chickenpox)		
Child (2–12 years)	**In general, treatment not necessary.** Might use oral **acyclovir** or **valacyclovir** for healthy persons at ↑ risk for moderate to severe varicella, i.e., >12 yrs of age; chronic cutaneous or pulmonary diseases; chronic salicylate rx (↑ risk of Reye syndrome), **Acyclovir** dose: 20 mg/kg po qid x 5 days (start within 24 hrs of rash) or **Valacyclovir** 20 mg/kg tid x 5 days.	Acyclovir slowed development and ↓ number of new lesions and ↓ duration of disease in children: 9 to 7.6 days *(PIDJ 21:739, 2002)*. Oral dose of acyclovir in children should not exceed 80 mg per kg per day or 3200 mg per day.
Adolescents, young adults	Start within 24 hrs of rash: **Valacyclovir** 1000 mg po tid x 7 days or **Famciclovir** 500 mg po tid x 7 days (probably effective, but data lacking)	↓ duration of fever, time to healing, and symptoms.
Pneumonia or chickenpox in 3rd trimester of pregnancy	**Acyclovir** 800 mg po 5 times per day or 10 mg per kg IV q8h times 5 days. Risks and benefits to fetus and mother still unknown. Many experts recommend rx, especially in 3rd trimester. Some would add VZIG (varicella-zoster immune globulin).	Varicella pneumonia associated with 41% mortality in pregnancy Acyclovir ↓ incidence and severity *(JID 185:422, 2002)*. If varicella-susceptible mother exposed and respiratory symptoms develop within 10 days after exposure, start acyclovir

** See page 2 for abbreviations. NOTE: All dosage recommendations are for adults (unless otherwise indicated) and assume normal renal function.*

TABLE 14A (8)

VIRUS/DISEASE	DRUG/DOSAGE	SIDE EFFECTS/COMMENTS
Herpesvirus Infections/Varicella-Zoster Virus (VZV)/Varicella *(continued)*		
Immunocompromised host	**Acyclovir** 10–12 mg per kg (500 mg per M^2) IV (infused over 1 hr) q8h times 7 days	Disseminated 1º varicella infection reported during infliximab rx of rheumatoid arthritis.
Prevention—Postexposure prophylaxis Varicella deaths still occur in unvaccinated persons	**CDC Recommendations for Prevention:** Since <5% of cases of varicella but >50% of varicella-related deaths occur in adults >20 yrs of age, the CDC recommends a more aggressive approach in this age group: **1st, varicella-zoster immune globulin** (VZIG) (125 units/10 kg (22 lbs) body weight IM up to a max. of 625 units; minimum dose is 125 units) is recommended for postexposure prophylaxis in susceptible persons at greater risk for complications (immunocompromised such as HIV, malignancies, pregnancy, and steroid therapy) as soon as possible after exposure (<96 hrs). If varicella develops, initiate treatment quickly (<24 hrs of rash) with **Acyclovir** as below. Some would rx presumptively with acyclovir in high-risk pts. **2nd,** susceptible adults should be vaccinated. Check antibody in adults with negative or uncertain history of varicella (10–30% will be AB-neg.) and vaccinate those who are Ab-neg. **3rd,** susceptible children should receive vaccination. Recommended routinely before age 12–18 mos. but OK at any age.	
Herpes zoster (shingles)		
Normal host ▪ Effective therapy most evident in pts age >50 yrs. ▪ *(For treatment of post-herpetic neuralgia, see CID 36: 877, 2003; Ln 374:1252, 2009)* ▪ Herpes zoster subunit vaccine (Shingrix) preferred for immunocompetent adults age 50 yrs or older ▪ Analgesics for acute pain associated with Herpes zoster	**[NOTE: Trials showing benefit of therapy: only in pts treated within 3 days of onset of rash]** **Valacyclovir** 1000 mg po tid times 7 days (adjust dose for renal failure) *(See Table 17A)* **OR**	Increasing recognition of ↑risk of stroke during 6 mos after episode of Shingles. Oral antivirals during clinical H. zoster infection may have protective effect. VZV found in wall of cerebral and temporal arteries of pts with giant cell arteritis *(Neurology 84:1948, 2015; JID 51:537, 2015)*.
	Famciclovir 500 mg tid x 7 days. Adjust for renal failure *(see Table 17A)* **OR**	Time to healing more rapid. Reduced incidence of post-herpetic neuralgia (PHN) vs placebo in pts >50 yrs of age. Famciclovir similar to acyclovir in reduction of acute pain and incidence of PHN.
	Acyclovir 800 mg po 5 times per day times 7 days	
	Duloxetine (Cymbalta) reduced post-herpetic neuralgia using visual analog pain scale *(CID 78:880, 2024)*	
Immunocompromised host		
Not severe Guidelines: *Clinical Transplantation (June 2019) https://doi.org/10.1111/ctr.13622*	**Acyclovir** 800 mg po 5 times per day times 7 days. (**Options: Famciclovir** 750 mg po q24h or 500 mg bid or 250 mg 3 times per day times 7 days **OR Valacyclovir** 1000 mg po tid times 7 days, though both are not FDA-approved for this indication)	If progression, switch to IV. RA pts on TNF-alpha inhibitors at high risk for VZV. Zoster more severe, but less post-herpetic neuralgia.
Severe: >1 dermatome, trigeminal nerve or disseminated	**Acyclovir** 10-12.5 mg per kg IV (infusion over 1 hr) q8h times 7 days. In older pts, ↓ to 7.5 mg per kg. If nephrotoxicity and pt improving, ↓ to 5 mg per kg q8h.	Treatment must be initiated within 72 hr of onset of symptoms. A common manifestation of immune reconstitution following ART in HIV-infected children. For Acyclovir-resistant VZV in HIV+ pts previously treated with acyclovir: **Foscarnet** (40 mg per kg IV q8h for 14–26 days).

TABLE 14A (9)

VIRUS/DISEASE	DRUG/DOSAGE	SIDE EFFECTS/COMMENTS
Herpesvirus Infections/Varicella-Zoster Virus (VZV)/Herpes zoster (shingles)/Immunocompromised host *(continued)*		
Progressive Outer Retinal Necrosis (PORN)	**Ganciclovir** 5 mg/kg and/or **Foscarnet** 90 mg/kg IV q12h + **Ganciclovir** 2 mg/0.05 mL and/or **Foscarnet** 1.2 mg/0.05 mL intravitreal twice weekly.	Expert consultation with an ophthalmologist. NB: **Ganciclovir** ocular implants no longer manufactured. If HIV pt, optimize ARV therapy.
Human T-cell Leukotrophic Virus-1 (HTLV-1) Causes illness in only 5% of infected persons. Two are associated with HTLV-1: Adult T-cell leukemia/ lymphoma and HTLV-1-associated myelopathy (HAM), also known as tropical spastic paraparesis (TSP).	No proven therapy. Some nucleoside antiretroviral therapies used with limited success.	Laboratory diagnosis is by blood and CSF. Anti-HTLV-1 antibodies are detected by ELISA antibody testing; Western Blot is used for confirmation (Focus Diagnostics or Quest Diagnostics). HTLV DNA can be detected by PCR in circulating CD4 cells. One tube multiplex qPCR highly specific / sensitive.

Influenza, RSV and COVID-19: concurrently circulating respiratory viruses of particular concern in 2023-2024 season. See *https://web.sanfordguide.com* and mobile app for updated guidance on prevention and treatment.

Influenza A & B and novel influenza viruses. IDSA Influenza Guideline: *CID 68:895, 2019.*
See current CDC and ACIP recommendations for vaccination and prevention.

- **Oseltamivir, baloxavir and zanamivir are recommended drugs.** Amantadine and rimantidine should not be used because of widespread resistance.
- Novel H1N1 (referred to as pandemic H1N1, pH1N1, H1N1pdm and formerly swine flu) emerged in 2009 and now is the dominant H1N1 strain worldwide. Old distinction from seasonal H1N1 is still sometimes used but not relevant.
- Rapid influenza tests can be falsely negative in 20-50%. NAAT, including PCR is gold standard test. **Testing for both influenza and SARS-CoV-2 are essential in era of COVID-19; PCR tests are preferred.**
- Initiate therapy as close to the onset of symptoms as possible, and certainly within 48 hrs of onset of symptoms. Starting therapy after 48 hours of onset of symptoms is associated with reduced therapeutic benefit. However, starting therapy up to 5 days after onset in patients who are hospitalized is associated with improved survival.
- Empiric therapy should be started for all patients who are hospitalized, have severe or progressive influenza or are at higher risk of complications due to age or underlying medical conditions. It is not necessary to wait for test results.
- Look for concomitant bacterial pneumonia.

Virus/Disease	Susceptible to (Recommended Drug/Dosage):	Resistant to:	Alternatives/Side Effects/Comments
• **A/H1N1 (current seasonal resembles pandemic H1N1)** • Influenza B • Influenza A A(H1N1) pdm09, A(H3N2) for 2023-24 season	**Oseltamivir** Adult: Oseltamivir 75 mg po bid x 5 days Pediatric (child age 1-12 years): Infant 2 wks-11 months: 3 mg/kg bid x 5 days ≤15 kg: 30 mg bid x 5 days >15 kg to 23 kg: 45 mg bid x 5 days >23 kg to 40 kg: 60 mg bid x 5 days >40 kg: 75 mg bid x 5 days or **Zanamivir** 2 inhalations (5 mg each) bid x 5 days or **Baloxavir** 40 mg po single dose if >12 years (80 mg if > 80 kg) or **Peramivir** 600 mg IV once daily x 5-10 days For IV Zanamivir, *see Comment* **Laninamivir** (approved in Japan): Age < 10 yrs: 20 mg once daily by inhalation Age > 10 yrs: 40 mg once daily by inhalation	Amantadine and rimantidine (100%)	• **A/H1N1:** Higher dose (150 mg bid) **not** more effective for H1N1 • **Zanamivir** not recommended for children <7 years or those with reactive airway disease • **IV zanamivir**, approved in the UK, is not available in the U.S. • **Influenza B:** Baloxavir was more effective than oseltamivir in one trial *(IDWeek 20018 LB)*. • Association between corticosteroid rx & increased mortality *(JID 212:183, 2015)*. For now, avoid steroids unless indicated for another reason. • Oseltamivir and baloxavir active in vitro. Discuss treatment with CDC.
• Avian influenza (H5N1, H7N9)	**Oseltamivir** 75 mg po bid (post-exposure prophylaxis for 5-10 days)(CDC recommendation)		

* *See page 2 for abbreviations. NOTE: All dosage recommendations are for adults (unless otherwise indicated) and assume normal renal function.*

TABLE 14A (10)

VIRUS/DISEASE	DRUG/DOSAGE	SIDE EFFECTS/COMMENTS
Measles Increasing reports of measles in unvaccinated children and adults *(NEJM 391:349, 2019)*.		
Children	**Vitamin A:** 50,000 IU (age < 6 mos); 100,000 IU (age 6-11 mos); 200,000 IU (age > 12 mos)	Vitamin A may ↓ severity of measles.
Children & Adults	Post-exposure prophylaxis: Vaccine within 72 hrs of exposure or IVIG within 6 days of exposure (0.5 mL/kg up to wt 30 kg; wt > 30 kg: 400 mg). Need MMR vaccine within 6 mos of IVIG.	↓ severity of illness in adults.
Metapneumovirus (HMPV)		
A paramyxovirus isolated from pts of all ages, with mild bronchiolitis/bronchospasm to pneumonia.	**No proven antiviral therapy**	Human metapneumovirus isolated from 6-21% of children with RTIs. Dual infection with RSV assoc. with severe bronchiolitis. Aerosolized ribavirin not recommended.
Mpox (orthopox virus)		
2022 U.S. outbreak primarily among MSM. Vaccine available for PEP and PrEP (CDC limited availability).	**Tecovirimat** (Tpoxx) 600 mg (three 200 mg capsules) twice daily x 14 days (active in monkey models; likely effective in humans). (FDA EUA or refer to STOMP trial). Cidofovir is active in vitro & in mouse model.	Incubation period of 12 days, then fever, headache, cough, adenopathy, & a vesicular papular rash that pustulates, umbilicates, & crusts on the head, trunk, & extremities. Clade I mpox more severe; seen in Central Africa. No cases in US.
Norovirus (Norwalk-like virus, or NLV)		
Vast majority of outbreaks of non-bacterial gastroenteritis	**No antiviral therapy.** Replete volume. Transmission by contaminated food, fecal-oral contact with contaminated surfaces, or fomites.	Sudden onset of nausea, vomiting, and/or watery diarrhea lasting 12-60 hours. Ethanol-based hand rubs effective.
Papillomaviruses: Warts		
External Genital Warts Also look for warts in anal canal	**Patient applied:** **Podofilox** (0.5% solution or gel): apply 2x/day x 3 days, 4th day no therapy, repeat cycle 4x; OR **Imiquimod** 5% cream: apply once daily hs 3x/wk for up to 16 wks. **Sinecatechins:** Apply to external genital warts only 3x/day until effect or adverse effect **Provider administered:** Cryotherapy with liquid nitrogen; repeat q1-2 wks; OR **Trichloroacetic acid** (TCA): repeat weekly as needed; OR surgical removal.	**Podofilox:** Inexpensive and safe (pregnancy safety not established). Mild irritation after treatment. **Imiquimod:** Mild to moderate redness & irritation. Topical imiquimod effective for treatment of vulvar intraepithelial neoplasms. Safety in pregnancy not established. **Sinecatechins:** Local irritation, redness, pain, and itching **Cryotherapy:** Blistering and skin necrosis common. **Podophyllin resin:** No longer recommended as other less toxic regimens available. **TCA:** Caustic. Can cause severe pain on adjacent normal skin. Neutralize with soap or sodium bicarbonate.
Warts on cervix	Need evaluation for evolving neoplasia	Gynecological consult advised.
Vaginal warts	Cryotherapy with liquid nitrogen or **TCA**	
Urethral warts	Cryotherapy with liquid nitrogen	
Anal warts	Cryotherapy with liquid nitrogen or **TCA** or surgical removal	Advise anoscopy to look for rectal warts; check for rectal carcinoma.
Skin papillomas	**Topical α-lactalbumin. Oleic acid** (from human milk) applied 1x/day for 3 wks	↓ lesion size & recurrence vs placebo (p <0.001) *(NEJM 350:2663, 2004)*. Further studies warranted.

TABLE 14A (11)

VIRUS/DISEASE	DRUG/DOSAGE	SIDE EFFECTS/COMMENTS
Parvo B19 Virus (Erythrovirus B19). *Review: NEJM 350:586, 2004. Wide range of manifestation.* **Treatment options for common symptomatic infections:**		
Erythema infectiosum	Symptomatic treatment only	Diagnostic tools: IgM and IgG antibody titers. Perhaps better: blood parvovirus PCR. Dose of IVIG not standardized; suggest 400 mg/kg IV of commercial IVIG for 5 or 10 days or 1000 mg/kg IV for 3 days. Most dramatic anemias in pts with pre-existing hemolytic anemia. Bone marrow shows erythrocyte maturation arrest with giant pronormoblasts *(Rev Med Virol 25:224, 2015).*
Arthritis/arthralgia	Nonsteroidal anti-inflammatory drugs (NSAID)	
Transient aplastic crisis	Transfusions and oxygen	
Fetal hydrops	Intrauterine blood transfusion	
Chronic infection with anemia	**IVIG** and transfusion *(CID 56:968, 2013)* For dose, *see Comment*	
Chronic infection without anemia	Perhaps **IVIG**	
Papovavirus/Polyomavirus		
Progressive multifocal leukoencephalopathy (PML) Serious demyelinating disease due to JC virus in immunocompromised pts.	No specific therapy for JC virus. Two general approaches: 1. In HIV pts: ART essential. Cidofovir may be effective. 2. Stop or decrease immunosuppressive therapy: highest risk with natalizumab & rituximab.	Failure of treatment with interferon alfa-2b, cytarabine and topotecan. Biologics ref: *ID Clin N Am 34:359, 2020*. Mixed reports on **cidofovir.** Most likely effective in ART-experienced pts. **Watch for IRIS when starting ARV Rx.**
BK virus induced nephropathy in immunocompromised pts and hemorrhagic cystitis	Decrease immunosuppression if possible. Suggested antiviral therapy based on anecdotal data. If progressive renal dysfunction: 1. **Fluoroquinolone** first; 2. **IVIG** 500 mg/kg IV; 3. **Leflunomide** 100 mg po daily x 3 days, then 10-20 mg po daily; 4. **Cidofovir** only if refractory to all of the above *(see Table 14B for dose).*	Use PCR to monitor viral "load" in urine and/or plasma. Report of cidofovir as potentially effective for BK hemorrhagic cystitis *(CID 49:233, 2009).* Systemic review of treatment in *International Journal of Surgery 63: 34, 2019*; cidofovir promising.
Rabies *(see Table 20B, page 328; diagnosis and management: www.cdc.gov/rabies)*		
Rabid dogs account for 50,000 cases per yr worldwide. Most cases in the U.S. are cryptic, 70% assoc. with 2 rare bat species. An organ donor with early rabies infected 4 recipients (2 kidneys, liver & artery) all died avg. 13 days after transplant *(NEJM 352:1103, 2005).*	**Mortality 100% with only survivors those who receive rabies vaccine before the onset of illness/symptoms** *(CID 36:61, 2003).* PEP: thorough wound washing, passive neutralization of the virus with infiltration of human rabies immune globulin (HRIG) into and around the wound site, and a series of 4 doses of rabies vaccine given over a 2-week timeframe	Corticosteroids ↑ mortality rate and ↓ incubation time in mice. Therapies that have failed after symptoms develop include rabies vaccine, rabies immunoglobulin, rabies virus neutralizing antibody, ribavirin, alfa interferon, induced coma & ketamine. For post-exposure prophylaxis, *see Table 20B, page 328.*
Respiratory Syncytial Virus (RSV) Major cause of morbidity in neonates/infants. Major cause of hospitalization in older adults. Diagnosis: airway swab for RSV PCR Review: *Infect Dis Clin N Amer 2017;31:455.* **RSV, Influenza and COVID-19** concurrently circulating.	*All ages:* Hydration, O2 as needed. If wheezing, trial of beta-agonist. *Corticosteroids:* children-no; adults-maybe **Ribavirin** may be effective in immunocompromised adults (HSCT) *(CID 56:258, 2013).* Oral ribavirin as effective as aerosolized, and much less expensive, in immunocompromized patients *(Transplant ID 20:e12844, 2018).*	In adults, RSV accounted for 10.6% of hospitalizations for pneumonia, 11.4% of AECB, 7.2% for asthma & 5.4% for CHF in pts >65 yrs of age. RSV caused 11% of clinically important respiratory illnesses in military recruits *(CID 41:311, 2005).* In children RSV causes majority of bronchiolitis and 28% of hospitalizations for pneumonia *(NEJM 372:835 2015).* **RSV Vaccine recommended in Adults >60 yrs of age**
Prevention of RSV: Two options for all infants in first RSV season: 1) Maternal immunization with Pfizer RSVpre-F vaccine between 32 and 36 6/7 weeks 2) Nirsevimab for all infants in first RSV season. For certain very high risk infants in second RSV season: Severe lung disease of prematurity requiring treatment, immunocompromized, Alaska Native/American Indian children: Nirsevimab. Alternative in year 2, if Nirsevimab not available, Palivizumab.	**Nirsevimab** (Beyfortus) 50 mg IM once if <5 kg; 100 IM mg if >5 kgs Second RSV season if indicated: Nirsevimab 200 mg IM once Alternative: **Palivizumab** (Synagis) 15 mg per kg IM q month Nov-Apr or guided by local epidemiology (More expensive, requires monthly dosing).	Nirsevimab or maternal immunization preferred but shortages in 2023/24 season of 100 mg syringes. Expense and inconvenience of monthly palivizumab argue against its use if nirsevimab available. See *https://www.cdc.gov/vaccines/vpd/rsv/index.html.*

TABLE 14A (12)

VIRUS/DISEASE	DRUG/DOSAGE	SIDE EFFECTS/COMMENTS
Rhinovirus (Colds) Found in 27% of children hospitalized for pneumonia	No antiviral rx indicated. Symptomatic rx: • **Ipratropium bromide** nasal (2 sprays per nostril tid) • **Clemastine** 1.34 mg 1–2 tab po bid–tid (OTC). • Oral zinc preparations reduce duration of symptoms by ~ 1 day; does not reduce severity of symptoms Avoid intranasal zinc products *(see Comment)*.	Sx relief: ipratropium nasal spray ↓ rhinorrhea and sneezing vs placebo. Clemastine (an antihistamine) ↓ sneezing, rhinorrhea but associated with dry nose, mouth & throat in 6–19%. **Echinacea** *(CID 38:1367, 2004 & 40:807, 2005)*. Public health advisory advising that three over-the-counter cold remedy products containing **zinc** (e.g., Zicam) should not be used because of multiple reports of permanent anosmia *(www.fda.gov/Safety/MedWatch/SafetyInformation/SafetyAlertsforHumanMedicalProducts/ucm166996.htm)*.
Rotavirus: Leading recognized cause of diarrhea-related illness among infants and children world-wide and kills ½ million children annually.	**No antiviral rx available;** oral hydration life-saving.	**Two live-attenuated vaccines highly effective (85 and 98%)** and safe in preventing rotavirus diarrhea and hospitalization. ACIP recommends either of the two vaccines, RV1 or RV5, for infants.
SARS CoV-2 (COVID-19): see *Coronavirus*, page 223		
Smallpox	Smallpox vaccine (if within 4 days of exposure) + **Tecovirimat** (Tpoxx) 600 mg (three 200 mg capsules) po bid x 14 days OR **cidofovir** (dosage uncertain but likely similar to CMV) 5 mg/kg IV once weekly for 2 weeks followed by once weekly dosing. Must be used with hydration and Probenecid; *contact CDC: 770-488-7100)*.	
Contact vaccinia	From vaccination: Progressive vaccinia—vaccinia immune globulin may be of benefit. To obtain immune globulin, contact CDC: 770-488-7100.	
West Nile virus: *See page 225*		
Zika Virus: Mosquito (Aedes sp.) transmitted flavivirus CDC updates at: *http://www.cdc.gov/zika/index.html*	No treatment available. Symptomatic support (avoid aspirin, NSAIDs until Dengue ruled out. Most serious manifestation of infection is **congenital birth defect(s)**: microcephaly and fetal demise. Sexual transmission occurs. For preconception counseling and prevention.	3-7 day incubation. Asymptomatic infection most often; when symptoms occur, usually consists of low grade fever, arthralgias, morbiliform rash, and / or conjunctival redness (non-purulent conjunctivitis). Duration of symptoms ranges from a few days to one week. Rare Guillain-Barré syndrome. Hospitalization very infrequent, fatalities are very rare.

TABLE 14B – ANTIVIRAL DRUGS (NON-HIV)

DRUG NAME(S) GENERIC (TRADE)	DOSAGE/ROUTE IN ADULTS*	COMMENTS/ADVERSE EFFECTS
CMV		
Cidofovir (Vistide)	5 mg per kg IV once weekly for 2 weeks, then once every other week. **Properly timed IV prehydration with normal saline & Probenecid must be used with each cidofovir infusion:** **Probenecid** 2 gm po 3 hrs before each dose and further 1 gm doses 2 & 8 hrs after completion of the cidofovir infusion. Renal function (serum creatinine and urine protein) must be monitored prior to each dose *(see pkg insert for details)*. Contraindicated if creatinine >1.5 mg/dL, CrCl ≤55 mL/min or urine protein ≥100 mg/dL.	**Adverse effects: Nephrotoxicity;** dose-dependent proximal tubular injury (Fanconi-like syndrome): proteinuria, glycosuria, bicarbonaturia, phosphaturia, polyuria (nephrogenic diabetic insipidus, ↑ creatinine. Concomitant saline prehydration, probenecid, extended dosing intervals allow use but still highly nephrotoxic. Other major toxicities: neutropenia (give G-CSF as needed); eye: monthly intra-ocular pressure. Dc cidofovir if pressure decreases 50% or uveitis occurs. **Black Box warning.** Renal impairment can occur after ≤2 doses. Contraindicated in pts receiving concomitant nephrotoxic agents. Monitor for ↓ WBC. In animals, carcinogenic, teratogenic, causes ↓ sperm and ↓ fertility. FDA indication only CMV retinitis in HIV pts. **Comment:** Dose must be reduced or discontinued if changes in renal function occur during rx. For ↑ of 0.3-0.4 mg per dL in serum creatinine, cidofovir dose must be ↓ from 5 to 3 mg per kg; discontinue cidofovir if ↑ of 0.5 mg per dL above baseline or 3+ proteinuria develops (for 2+ proteinuria, observe pts carefully and consider discontinuation).
Foscarnet (Foscavir)	<u>Induction</u>: 90 mg per kg IV, over 1.5-2 hours, q12h **OR** 60 mg per kg, over 1 hour, q8h <u>Maintenance</u>: 90 –120 mg per kg IV, over 2 hours, q24h Dosage adjustment with renal dysfunction *(see Table 17A)*.	Use infusion pump to control rate of administration. **Adverse effects: Major toxicity is renal impairment (1/3 of patients).** Can cause infusion-related ionized hypocalcemia: manifests as arrhythmia, tetany, paresthesia, changes in mental status. Slow infusion rate and avoid drugs that lower Ca++, e.g., pentamidine. --↑ creatinine, proteinuria, nephrogenic diabetes insipidus, ↓K+, ↓Ca++, ↓ Mg++. Adequate hydration may ↓ toxicity. Other: headache, mild (100%); fatigue (100%), nausea (80%), fever (25%). CNS: seizures. Hematol: ↓ WBC, ↓ Hgb. Hepatic: liver function tests ↑. Neuropathy. Penile and oral ulcers.
Ganciclovir (Cytovene)	IV: 5 mg per kg q12h times 14 days (induction) 5 mg per kg IV q24h or 6 mg per kg 5 times per wk (maintenance) Dosage adjust. with renal dysfunction *(see Table 17A)*	**Adverse effects: Black Box warnings:** cytopenias, carcinogenicity/teratogenicity & aspermia in animals. Absolute neutrophil count dropped below 500 per mm³ in 15%, thrombocytopenia 21%, anemia 6%. Fever 48%. GI 50%: nausea, vomiting, diarrhea, abdominal pain 19%, rash 10%. Confusion, headache, psychiatric disturbances and seizures. Neutropenia may respond to granulocyte colony stimulating factor (G-CSF or GM-CSF). Severe myelosuppression may be ↑ with coadministration of zidovudine or azathioprine. 32% dc/interrupted rx, principally for neutropenia. Avoid extravasation.
Letermovir (Prevymis)	Indicated for prophylaxis of cytomegalovirus (CMV) infection and disease in seropositive recipients of an allogeneic hematopoietic stem cell transplant and high-risk renal transplant recipients 480 mg po/IV once daily starting between days 0-28 post-transplant & continuing to day 100	**Activity:** It does not have activity against HSV or VZV so prophylaxis against these viruses would need to be continued if indicated. **Adverse effects:** N/V, diarrhea, peripheral edema, cough, headache, abdominal pain **Drug interactions:** if concomitant cyclosporine, reduce dose to 240 mg once daily. Avoid if severe hepatic impairment.
Maribavir (Livtencity)	400 mg (two 200 mg tablets) po twice daily, with or without food	**Activity:** No activity against HSV or VZV so prophylaxis against these viruses would need to be continued if indicated. For treatment of adults and pediatric patients (≥12 years of age, weight ≥35 kg) with **post-transplant cytomegalovirus (CMV)** infection/disease that is refractory to treatment (with or without genotypic resistance) with ganciclovir, valganciclovir, cidofovir or foscarnet. Adverse effects: dysgeusia, GI, fatigue, neutropenia, AKI. Numerous DDI.
Valganciclovir (Valcyte)	450 mg tablets; take with food. Oral solution: 50 mg/mL. Adult does 900 mg. Treatment (induction): 900 mg po q12h with food; Prophylaxis (maintenance): 900 mg po q24h. Dosage adjustment for renal dysfunction *(See Table 17A)*.	A prodrug of ganciclovir with better bioavailability than oral ganciclovir: 60% with food. Preg cat: C (may be teratogenic, contraceptive precaution for females). **Adverse effects:** Similar to ganciclovir. May cause dose limiting neutropenia, anemia, thrombocytopenia. Acute renal failure may occur. Diarrhea (16-41%), nausea (8-30%), vomiting (3-21%). **CMV retinitis** (sight-threatening lesions): 900 mg po q12h + intravitreal Ganciclovir: 900 mg po q12h x 14-21 days, then 900 mg po q24h for maintenance.

* *See page 2 for abbreviations.* *NOTE: All dosage recommendations are for adults (unless otherwise indicated) and assume normal renal function.*

TABLE 14B (2)

DRUG NAME(S) GENERIC (TRADE)	DOSAGE/ROUTE IN ADULTS*	COMMENTS/ADVERSE EFFECTS
Coronavirus: SARS CoV-2 (COVID-19)		
Molnupiravir (Lagevrio)	Adult: 800 mg po q12h x 5 days	Take with or without food. Caps should not be opened, crushed or chewed. **AEs:** diarrhea, nausea, dizziness, headache, rash, urticaria
Nirmatrelvir/ritonavir (Paxlovid)	Age ≥12 yrs: Nirmatrelvir 300 mg po q12h + RTV 100 mg po q12h, both times 5 days	Take with or without food. Initiate treatment within 5 days of symptom onset (The earlier the better). **AEs:** dysgeusia, diarrhea, hypertension, myalgia, LFT elevations, clinical hepatitis, jaundice. Observe for **rebound**, use clinical judgment regarding retreatment. **CAUTION:** Numerous CYP450-mediated drug interactions. Check for DDI before prescribing.
Remdesivir See *https://web.sanfordguide.com* for complete coverage as the emergence of new variants affects recommendations	**Adult** (wt ≥40 kg): 200 mg IV loading dose, then 100 mg IV daily. Infuse each dose over 30-120 min. **Child** (age ≥12 years, weight ≥40 kg) 200 mg IV loading dose, then 100 mg IV daily; (<12 years, weight 3.5-40 kg) 5 mg/kg loading dose, then 2.5 mg/kg IV daily	**Duration:** 10 day course if on mech ventilation / ECMO; otherwise 5 days unless no clinical improvement, then 10 days. Outpatient duration of therapy 3 days. **Contraindications:** known hypersensitivity. **Warnings, AEs:** hypotension, nausea, vomiting, shivering, increased ALT, liver toxicity.
Herpesvirus		
Acyclovir (Zovirax or generic)	Doses: *see Table 14A for various indications* 400 mg or 800 mg tab 200 mg cap Suspension 200 mg per 5 mL Ointment or cream 5% IV injection Dosage adjustment for renal dysfunction *(See Table 17A)*.	**po:** Generally well-tolerated with occ. diarrhea, vertigo, arthralgia. Less frequent rash, fatigue, insomnia, fever, menstrual abnormalities, acne, sore throat, muscle cramps, lymphadenopathy. **IV:** Phlebitis, caustic with vesicular lesions with IV infiltration. **IV or po:** Renal (5%): ↑ creatinine, hematuria. With high doses may crystallize in renal tubules → obstructive uropathy (rapid infusion, dehydration, renal insufficiency and ↑ dose ↑ risk). Adequate pre-hydration may prevent such nephrotoxicity. Hepatic: ↑ ALT, AST. Uncommon: neutropenia, rash, diaphoresis, hypotension, headache, nausea. **Neurotoxicity:** hallucination, death delusions, involuntary movements. To avoid, lower dose if renal impairment.
Famciclovir (Famvir)	125 mg, 250 mg, 500 mg tabs Dosage depends on indication: *(see label and Table 14A)*.	Metabolized to penciclovir. **Adverse effects:** similar to acyclovir, included headache, nausea, diarrhea, and dizziness but incidence does not differ from placebo. May be taken without regard to meals. Dose should be reduced if CrCl <60 mL per min *(see package insert & Table 14A, page 227 & Table 17A, page 311)*. May be taken with or without food.
Penciclovir (Denavir)	Topical 1% cream	Apply to area of recurrence of herpes labialis with start of sx, then q2h while awake times 4 days. Well tolerated.
Trifluridine (Viroptic)	Topical 1% solution: 1 drop q2h (max. 9 drops/day) until corneal re-epithelialization, then dose is ↓ for 7 more days (one drop q4h for at least 5 drops/day), not to exceed 21 days total rx.	Mild burning (5%), palpebral edema (3%), punctate keratopathy, stromal edema. For HSV keratoconjunctivitis or recurrent epithelial keratitis.
Valacyclovir (Valtrex)	500 mg, 1 gm tabs Dosage depends on indication and renal function *(see label, Table 14A & Table 17A)*	An ester pro-drug of acyclovir that is well-absorbed, bioavailability 3–5 times greater than acyclovir. **Adverse effects** similar to acyclovir. Thrombotic thrombocytopenic purpura/hemolytic uremic syndrome reported in pts with advanced HIV disease and transplant recipients participating in clinical trials at doses of 8 gm per day. Death delusion with high serum levels.
Valganciclovir (Valcyte)	450 mg tablets; take with food. Oral solution: 50 mg/mL. Adult does 900 mg. Treatment (induction): 900 mg po q12h with food; Prophylaxis (maintenance): 900 mg po q24h. Dosage adjustment for renal dysfunction *(See Table 17A)*.	A prodrug of ganciclovir with better bioavailability than oral ganciclovir: 60% with food. Preg cat: C (may be teratogenic, contraceptive precaution for females). **Adverse effects:** Similar to ganciclovir. May cause dose limiting neutropenia, anemia, thrombocytopenia. Acute renal failure may occur. Diarrhea (16-41%), nausea (8-30%), vomiting (3-21%). **CMV retinitis** (sight-threatening lesions): 900 mg po q12h + intravitreal Ganciclovir: 900 mg po q12h x 14-21 days, then 900 mg po q24h for maintenance.

** See page 2 for abbreviations.   NOTE: All dosage recommendations are for adults (unless otherwise indicated) and assume normal renal function.*

TABLE 14B (3)

DRUG NAME(S) GENERIC (TRADE)	DOSAGE/ROUTE IN ADULTS*	COMMENTS/ADVERSE EFFECTS
Hepatitis B		
Adefovir dipivoxil (Hepsera)	10 mg po q24h (with normal CrCl) 10 mg tab	It is an acyclic nucleotide analog with activity against hepatitis B (HBV) at 0.2–2.5 mM (IC_{50}). *See Table 9A* for Cmax & T½. Active against lamivudine-resistant HBV strains and in vitro vs. entecavir- resistant strains. To minimize resistance, use in combination with lamivudine for lamivudine-resistant virus; consider alternative therapy if viral load remains >1,000 copies/mL with treatment. Primarily renal excretion—adjust dose. No food interactions. Generally few side effects, but **Black Box warning** regarding lactic acidosis/hepatic steatosis with nucleoside analogs. At 10 mg per day potential for delayed nephrotoxicity. Monitor renal function, esp. with pts with pre-existing or other risks for renal impairment. Pregnancy Category C. **Hepatitis may exacerbate when treatment discontinued;** Up to 25% of pts developed ALT ↑ 10 times normal within 12 wks; usually responds to re-treatment or self-limited, but hepatic decompensation has occurred. **Do not use adefovir in HIV infected patients.**
Entecavir (Baraclude)	0.5 mg q24h. If refractory or resistant to lamivudine or telbivudine: 1 mg per day Tabs: 0.5 mg & 1 mg. Oral solution: 0.05 mg/mL. Administer on an empty stomach.	A nucleoside analog active against HBV including lamivudine-resistant mutants. Minimal adverse effects reported: headache, fatigue, dizziness, & nausea reported in 22% of pts. Alopecia, anaphylactoid reactions reported. Potential for lactic acidosis and exacerbation of hepB at discontinuation (**Black Box warning**). Do not use as single anti-retroviral agent in HIV co-infected pts; M134 mutation can emerge. Adjust dosage in renal impairment *(see Table 17A, page 309)*.
Lamivudine (3TC) (Epivir-HBV)	**HBV** dose: 100 mg po q24h Dosage adjustment with renal dysfunction *(see label)*. Tabs 100 mg and oral solution 5 mg/mL.	**Black Box warnings:** caution, dose is lower than HIV dose, so must exclude co-infection with HIV before using this formulation; lactic acidosis/hepatic steatosis; severe exacerbation of liver disease can occur on dc. YMDD-mutants resistant to lamivudine may emerge on treatment. Do not use as monotherapy vs HBV. **Adverse effects:** *See Table 14D.*
Telbivudine (Tyzeka)	**HBV:** 600 mg orally q24h, without regard to food. Dosage adjustment with renal dysfunction, Ccr <50 mL/min *(see label)*. 600 mg tabs; 100 mg per 5 mL solution.	An oral nucleoside analog approved for Rx of Hep B. It has ↑ rates of response and superior viral suppression than lamivudine. **Black Box warnings** regarding lactic acidosis/hepatic steatosis with nucleosides and potential for severe exacerbation of HepB on dc. Generally well-tolerated with ↓ mitochondrial toxicity vs other nucleosides and no dose limiting toxicity observed. Myalgias, myopathy and rhabdomyolysis reported. Peripheral neuropathy. Genotypic resistance rate was 4.4% by one yr, ↑ to 21.5% by 2 yrs of rx of eAg+ pts. Selects for YMDD mutation like lamivudine. Combination with lamivudine was inferior to monotherapy *(Hepatology 45:507, 2007)*.
Tenofovir (TDF/TAF)	*See page 252*	
Hepatitis C - (For all HCV direct acting agents (DAA) a **Black Box warning** exists regarding potential flare of HBV when HCV is cured among those coinfected with HBV and HCV)		
Direct Acting Agents:		
Daclatasvir (Daklinza)	60 mg 1 tab po once daily (dose adjustment when used with CYP 3A4 inhibitors / inducers)	Contraindicated with strong CYP3A inducers, e.g., phenytoin, carbamazepine, Rifampin, St. John's wort. Most common AE: headache and fatigue. Bradycardia when administered in combination with Sofosbuvir and Amiodarone. **Co-administration with Amiodarone not recommended**. If used, cardiac monitoring advised.
Elbasvir + Grazoprevir (Zepatier)	Combination formulation (Elbasvir 50 mg + Grazoprevir 100 mg) 1 tab po once daily	NS5A and NS3-4a PI inhibitors with activity against genotypes 1 and 4. Contraindicated in patients with moderate or severe hepatic impairment (Child-Pugh Class B or C). Also contraindicated with concomitant use of organic ion transporter polypeptide 1B (OATP1B) inhibitors, strong inducers of cytochrome P450 3A (CYP3A), and efavirenz.
Glecaprevir + Pibrentasvir (Mavyret)	Combination formulation (Glecaprevir 100 mg + Pibrentasvir 40 mg) 3 tabs po once daily with food	Contraindicated if severe hepatic impairment (Child-Pugh C). **Do not co-administer with Atazanavir or Rifampin.** Most common AEs: headache and fatigue.

* *See page 2 for abbreviations.* *NOTE: All dosage recommendations are for adults (unless otherwise indicated) and assume normal renal function.*

TABLE 14B (4)

DRUG NAME(S) GENERIC (TRADE)	DOSAGE/ROUTE IN ADULTS*	COMMENTS/ADVERSE EFFECTS
Hepatitis C/Direct Acting Agents *(continued)*		
Ledipasvir + Sofosbuvir (Harvoni); **Velpatasvir + Sofosbuvir** (Epclusa); **Voxilaprevir + Velpatasvir + Sofosbuvir** (Vosevi)	Combination formulations: (Ledipasvir 90 mg + Sofosbuvir 400 mg) 1 tab po once daily; (Velpatasvir 100 mg + Sofosbuvir 400 mg) 1 tab po daily; Voxilaprevir 100 mg + Velpatasvir 100 mg + Sofosbuvir 400 mg) 1 tab po once daily with food	NS5A/NS5B inhibitors combination for Genotype 1 HCV. First agent for HCV treatment without Ribavirin or Interferon. No adjustment for mile/moderate renal or hepatic impairment. Most common AEs: fatigue (16%), headache (14%), nausea (7%), diarrhea (3%), insomnia (5%). Antacids and H2 blockers interfere with absorption of ledipasvir. The drug solubility decreases as pH increases. Recommended to separate administration of ledipasvir and antacid Rx by at least 4 hours.
Paritaprevir + Ritonavir + Ombitasvir + Dasabuvir (PrOD) (Viekira Pak); **Paritaprevir + Ritonavir + Ombitasvir** (Technivie)	Ombitasvir 12.5 mg, Paritaprevir 75 mg, and Ritonavir 50 mg co-packaged with tablets of Dasabuvir 250 mg (Viekira Pak); or without Dasabuvir (Technivie)	Do not co-administer with drugs that are highly dependent on CYP3A for clearance; strong inducers of CYP3A and CYP2C8; and strong inhibitors of CYP2C8. Do not use if known hypersensitivity to Ritonavir (e.g., toxic epidermal necrolysis, Stevens-Johnson syndrome). If used with Ribavirin: fatigue, nausea, pruritus, other skin reactions, insomnia and asthenia. When used without Ribavirin: nausea, pruritus and insomnia. **Warning: Hepatic decompensation and hepatic failure, including liver transplantation or fatal outcomes, have been reported mostly in patients with advanced cirrhosis.**
Simeprevir (Olysio)	150 mg 1 cap po once daily with food + both Ribavirin and Interferon	NS3/4A inhibitor. Need to screen patients with HCV genotype 1a for the Q80K polymorphism; if present consider alternative therapy. Contraindicated in pregnancy and in men whose female partners are pregnant (risk category C); concern is combination with ribavirin (risk category X). No dose adjustment required in patients with mild, moderate or severe renal impairment; no dose adjustment for mild hepatic impairment. Most common AEs (in combination with Ribavirin, Interferon): rash, pruritus, nausea. CYP3A inhibitors affect plasma concentration of Simeprevir.
Sofosbuvir (Sovaldi)	400 mg 1 tab po once daily with food + both Pegylated Interferon and Ribavirin. For combination formulation, *see Ledipasvir.*	NS5B inhibitor for Genotypes 1, 2, 3, 4 HCV. Efficacy established in patients awaiting liver transplant and in patients with HIV-1/HCV co-infection. No adjustment needed for mild to moderate renal impairment. No dose adjustment for mild, moderate, or severe hepatic impairment. Most common AEs (in combination with interferon and ribavirin): fatigue, headache, nausea, insomnia, anemia. Rifampin and St. John's wort may alter concentrations of Sofosbuvir.
Other:		
Interferon alfa is available as alfa-2a (Roferon-A), **alfa-2b** (Intron-A)	For HCV combination therapy, usual Roferon-A and Intron-A doses are 3 million international units 3x weekly subQ.	Depending on agent, available in pre-filled syringes, vials of solution, or powder. **Black Box warnings:** can cause/aggravate psychiatric illness, autoimmune disorders, ischemic events, infection. Withdraw therapy if any of these suspected. **Adverse effects: Flu-like syndrome** is common, esp. during 1st wk of rx: fever 98%, fatigue 89%, myalgia 73%, headache 71%. **GI:** anorexia 46%, diarrhea 29%. CNS: dizziness 21%. Hemorrhagic or ischemic stroke. Rash 18%, may progress to Stevens Johnson or exfoliative dermatitis. Alopecia. ↑ TSH, autoimmune thyroid disorders with ↓- or ↑- thyroidism. **Hematol:** ↓ WBC 49%, ↓ Hgb 27%, ↓ platelets 35%. Post-marketing reports of antibody-mediated pure red cell aplasia in patients receiving interferon/ribavirin with erythropoiesis-stimulating agents. Acute reversible hearing loss &/or tinnitus in up to 1/3 *(Ln 343:1134, 1994)*. Optic neuropathy (retinal hemorrhage, cotton wool spots, ↓ in color vision) reported *(AIDS 18:1805, 2004)*. Doses may require adjustment (or dc) based on individual response or adverse events, and can vary by product, indication (eg, HCV or HBV) and mode of use (mono- or combination-rx). (Refer to labels of individual products and to ribavirin if used in combination for details of use.)
PEG interferon alfa-2b (PEG-Intron)	0.5–1.5 mcg/kg subQ q wk	
Pegylated-40k interferon alfa-2a (Pegasys)	180 mcg subQ q wk	

* *See page 2 for abbreviations.* *NOTE: All dosage recommendations are for adults (unless otherwise indicated) and assume normal renal function.*

TABLE 14B (5)

DRUG NAME(S) GENERIC (TRADE)	DOSAGE/ROUTE IN ADULTS*	COMMENTS/ADVERSE EFFECTS
Hepatitis C/Other *(continued)*		
Ribavirin (Rebetol, Copegus)	For use with an interferon for hepatitis C. Available as 200 mg caps and 40 mg/mL oral solution (Rebetol) or 200 mg and 400 mg tabs (Copegus) *(See Comments regarding dosage).*	**Black Box warnings:** ribavirin monotherapy of HCV is ineffective; hemolytic anemia may precipitate cardiac events; teratogenic/ embryocidal (**Preg Category X**). Drug may persist for 6 mos, avoid pregnancy for at least 6 mos after end of rx of women *or their partners.* Only approved for pts with Ccr >50 mL/min. Do not use in pts with severe heart disease or hemoglobinopathies. ARDS reported *(Chest 124:406, 2003).* **Adverse effects:** hemolytic anemia (may require dose reduction or dc), dental/periodontal disorders, and all adverse effects of concomitant interferon used *(see above)*. Postmarketing: retinal detachment, ↓ hearing, hypersensitivity reactions. See *Table 14A* for specific regimens, but dosing depends on: interferon used, weight, presence of cirrhosis, and is modified (or dc) based on side effects (especially degree of hemolysis, with different criteria in those with/without cardiac disease). **Initial Rebetrol dose with Intron A (interferon alfa-2b) is wt-based:** 400 mg am & 600 mg pm for ≤75 kg, and 600 mg am & 600 mg pm for wt >75 kg, but with Pegintron approved dose is 400 mg am & 400 mg pm with meals.
Influenza A		
Amantadine (Symmetrel) or **Rimantadine** (Flumadine) Influenza B intrinsically resistant and most circulating Influenza A is resistant.	**Amantadine** 100 mg caps, tabs; 50 mg/mL oral solution & syrup. Treatment or prophylaxis: 100 mg bid; or 100 mg daily if age ≥65 y; dose reductions with CrCl starting at ≤50 mL/min. **Rimantadine** 100 mg tabs, 50 mg/5 mL syrup. Treatment or prophylaxis: 100 mg bid, or 100 mg daily in elderly nursing home pts, or severe hepatic disease, or CrCl ≤10 mL/min. For children, rimantadine only approved for prophylaxis.	**Side-effects/toxicity: CNS** (can be mild: nervousness, anxiety, difficulty concentrating, and lightheadedness). Serious: delirium, hallucinations, and seizures—are associated with high plasma drug levels resulting from renal insufficiency, esp. in older pts, those with prior seizure disorders, or psychiatric disorders.
Influenza A and B—For both drugs, initiate within 48 hrs of symptom onset		
Baloxavir marboxil (Xofluza) *CID 70:1790, 2020*	For age ≥12 yrs & within 48 hr of symptoms onset. Wt 40-80 kg: 40 mg po x 1 dose Wt ≥80 kg: 80 mg po x 1 dose	FDA indicated for uncomplicated influenza. One trial demonstrated efficacy in high risk patients with similar efficacy against flu A and superior activity against flu B. Active against oseltamivir-resistant influenza. Compared to oseltamivir, faster decrease in viral load in airway and, if Influenza B, faster clinical recovery. **AEs:** diarrhea (3%) headache (1%), nausea (1%) Distinct mechanism of action: inhibits viral endonuclease. Cost: $150 per dose compared to $50 for 5 days of oseltamivir.
Zanamivir (Relenza) For pts ≥ 7 yrs of age (treatment) or ≥5 yrs (prophylaxis)	Powder is inhaled by specially designed inhalation device. Each blister contains 5 mg zanamivir. **Treatment:** oral inhalation of 2 blisters (10 mg) bid for 5 days. **Prophylaxis:** oral inhalation of 2 blisters (10 mg) once daily for 10 days (household outbreak) to 28 days (community outbreak).	Active by inhalation against neuraminidase of both influenza A and B and inhibits release of virus from epithelial cells of respiratory tract. Approx. 4–17% of inhaled dose absorbed into plasma. Excreted by kidney but with low absorption, dose reduction not necessary in renal impairment. Minimal side-effects: <3% cough, sinusitis, diarrhea, nausea and vomiting. **Reports of respiratory adverse events in pts with or without h/o airways disease, should be avoided in pts with underlying respiratory disease.** Allergic reactions and neuropsychiatric events have been reported. **Caution: do not reconstitute zanamivir powder for use in nebulizers or mechanical ventilators** (MedWatch report of death). **Zanamivir for IV** administration is available for compassionate use through an emergency IND application. Contact GSK *(919-315-5215)* for forms, then contact FDA *(301-796-1500 or 301-796-9900).*

** See page 2 for abbreviations.* *NOTE: All dosage recommendations are for adults (unless otherwise indicated) and assume normal renal function.*

TABLE 14B (6)

DRUG NAME(S) GENERIC (TRADE)	DOSAGE/ROUTE IN ADULTS*	COMMENTS/ADVERSE EFFECTS
Influenza A and B *(continued)*		
Oseltamivir (Tamiflu) For pts ≥1 yr (treatment or prophylaxis)	For adults: **Treatment,** 75 mg po bid for 5 days; 150 mg po bid has been used for morbidly obese patients but this dose is not FDA-approved. **Prophylaxis,** 75 mg po once daily for 10 days to 6 wks. *(See label for pediatric weight-based dosing.)* Adjust doses for CrCl ≤30 mL/min. 30 mg, 45 mg, 75 mg caps; powder for oral suspension 75 mg bid if unsure of timing of exposure.	Well absorbed (80% bioavailable) from GI tract as ethyl ester of active compound GS 4071. T½ 6–10 hrs; excreted unchanged by kidney. Adverse effects include diarrhea, nausea, vomiting, headache. Nausea ↓ with food. Rarely, severe skin reactions (toxic epidermal necrolysis, Stevens-Johnson syndrome, erythema multiforme). **Delirium** & abnormal behavior reported *(CID 48:1003, 2009)*. No benefit from higher dose in non- critically ill; not recommended *(CID 57:1511, 2013)*.
Peramivir (Rapivab)	600 mg IV single dose (acute uncomplicated influenza)	FDA indication is for single dose use in acute uncomplicated influenza. No approved dose for hospitalized patients but 200-400 mg IV daily for 5 days used in trial. Not superior to oseltamivir in trials. Flu with H275Y oseltamivir resistance has moderate resistance to peramivir.
Pox viruses (Smallpox, Monkeypox)		
Brincidofovir (Tembexa)	Wt <10 kg: 6 mg/kg (susp) on days 1 & 8 Wt 10 to <48 kg: 4 mg/kg (susp) on days 1 & 8 Wt ≥48 kg: 200 mg (tabs, susp) on days 1 & 8	Lipid conjugate prodrug of cidofovir, then phosphorylated to cidofovir diphosphate (inhibitor of orthopoxvirus DNA polymerase). Indicated for human smallpox (variola) disease. **Black-box warning:** increased mortality in CMV prevention trial. May cause fetal harm; perform pregnancy testing before use, stress effective contraception x2-4 months after 2nd dose. Potential human carcinogen (avoid direct contact with drug). Adverse effects: increased LFTs, GI, decreased appetite, dysgeusia, muscle weakness, rash.
Tecovirimat (Tpoxx)	600 mg (three 200 mg caps) po bid x 14 days	Inhibitor of the orthopoxvirus VP37 envelope wrapping protein. **No Clinical Trial data in humans** (approval by FDA for smallpox based on animal treatment studies). Clinical trial (STOMP) underway (2024).
Respiratory Syncytial Virus (RSV) monoclonal antibody		
Nirsevimab (Beyfortus) Used for all children in 1st RSV season if mother did not receive RSV vaccine and in high risk infants in second year of life	50 mg IM once if wt <5 kg 100 mg IM once if wt >5 kg 200 mg IM once for infants qualifying in second RSV season	Monoclonal antibody modified for long half life, directed against neutralizing domain of pre-fusion conformation of F protein. In trials, only injection site reaction reported. Risk of anaphylaxis for all monoclonal Abs.
Palivizumab (Synagis) Used for prevention of RSV infection in high-risk children	15 mg per kg IM q month throughout RSV season Single dose 100 mg vial	A monoclonal antibody directed against the surface F glycoprotein; **AEs:** uncommon, occ. ↑ ALT. Anaphylaxis <1/10^5 pts; acute hypersensitivity reaction <1/1000. Postmarketing reports: URI, otitis media, fever, ↓ plts, injection site reactions.
Warts Regimens are from drug labels specific for external genital and/or perianal condylomata acuminata only *(see specific labels for indications, regimens, age limits)*.		
Interferon alfa-2b (IntronA)	Injection of 1 million international units into base of lesion, thrice weekly on alternate days for up to 3 wks. Maximum 5 lesions per course.	Interferons may cause "flu-like" illness and other systemic effects. 88% had at least one adverse effect. **Black box warning:** alpha interferons may cause or aggravate neuropsychiatric, autoimmune, ischemic or infectious disorders.
Interferon alfa-N3 (Alferon N)	Injection of 0.05 mL into base of each wart, up to 0.5 mL total per session, twice weekly for up to 8 weeks.	Flu-like syndrome and hypersensitivity reactions. Contraindicated with allergy to mouse IgG, egg proteins, or neomycin.
Imiquimod (Aldara)	5% cream. Thin layer applied at bedtime, washing off after 6-10 hr, thrice weekly to maximum of 16 wks; 3.75% cream apply qd.	Erythema, itching & burning, erosions. Flu-like syndrome, increased susceptibility to sunburn (avoid UV).
Podofilox (Condylox)	0.5% gel or solution twice daily for 3 days, no therapy for 4 days; can use up to 4 such cycles.	Local reactions—pain, burning, inflammation in 50%. Can ulcerate. Limit surface area treated as per label.
Sinecatechins (Veregen)	15% ointment. Apply 0.5 cm strand to each wart three times per day until healing but not more than 16 weeks.	Application site reactions, which may result in ulcerations, phimosis, meatal stenosis, superinfection.

* See page 2 for abbreviations. *NOTE: All dosage recommendations are for adults (unless otherwise indicated) and assume normal renal function.*

TABLE 14C – ANTIRETROVIRAL THERAPY (ART) IN TREATMENT-NAÏVE ADULTS (HIV/AIDS)

Overview

- Human immunodeficiency virus (HIV)
- Antiretroviral therapy (ART) in **treatment-naïve adults** *(aidsinfo.nih.gov/guidelines/html/1/adult-and-adolescent-treatment-guidelines/0)*
- Guidelines: *JAMA. doi:10.1001/jama.2024.24543, Published online December 1, 2024.* Also Commentary - *JAMA. Published online December 1, 2024. doi:10.1001/jama.2024.24027; www.aidsinfo.nih.gov*

When to Start ART

- **All patients with HIV regardless of CD4 count**
- Only exceptions are:
  - Patient is not ready to start (for personal reasons or lack of commitment to take medications)
  - Patient is an "Elite Controller", i.e., HIV RNA undetectable for extended period without ART. Controversy exists about treating such patients, though many experts suggest ART owing to inflammation resulting from ongoing de novo HIV replication.
  - Many clinics are adopting a 'treat now' policy whereby the ARV regimen is started on the first encounter with the clinic. In such instances, resistance tests and HBV panels are obtained and the regimen(s) adjusted as indicated once the resistance test data return.

What Regimen to Start

- Design a regimen consisting of:

Dual nucleoside / nucleotide reverse transcriptase inhibitor **(NRTI component) PLUS** a	Integrase strand-transfer inhibitor **(INSTI)**
Note: Prefer combination that includes Tenofovir-AF OR Tenofovir-DF; in selected patients, a combination of Dolutegravir + Lamivudine can be used *(see below)*	

NRTI: e.g., Tenofovir (TAF or TDF), Abacavir (ABC), Emtricitabine (FTC), or Lamivudine (3TC)
NNRTI: e.g., Efavirenz (EFV), Rilpivirine (RPV), Doravirine (DOR) or Etravirine (ETV)
PI: e.g., Darunavir (DRV) or Atazanavir (ATV) [both boosted with either Ritonavir (/r) or Cobicistat (Cobi)]
INSTI: e.g., Bictegravir (BIC), Dolutegravir (DTG), Elvitegravir (ETG) plus Cobi or Ritonavir, Cabotegravir or Raltegravir (RAL)
Capsid inhibitor: Lenacapavir (LEN)

- Selection of components is influenced by many factors, including:
  - Results of viral resistance testing
  - **Pregnancy:** DTG and TAF (plus FTC or 3TC) now recommended in pregnancy as drugs of choice. BIC+TAF+FTC acceptable regimen
  - Potential drug interactions or adverse drug effects; special focus on tolerability (even low grade side effects can profoundly affect adherence)
  - Co-morbidities (e.g., lipid effects of PIs, liver or renal disease, cardiovascular disease risk, chemical dependency, psychiatric disease)
  - Convenience of dosing. Co-formulations increase convenience, but sometimes prescribing the two constituents individually is preferred, as when dose-adjustments are needed for renal disease
  - HLA-B5701 testing required prior to using ABC
  - DTG/3TC used only in those with neg HBsAg, VL < 500,000 c/mL, and no evidence of 3TC resistance on genotype

TABLE 14C (2)

RECOMMENDED AND ALTERNATIVE TREATMENT REGIMENS FOR HIV INFECTED ADULTS				
	Frequency & Formulation	**Drug/Dose**	**Components**	**Comments**
Recommended	Once daily, single tablet	**Biktarvy** 1 tablet once daily	Bictegravir (BIC) + FTC + TAF	
		Dovato 1 tablet once daily	DTG + 3TC	Avoid when M184V or M184I resistance mutation present or in patients with HBV co-infection
	Once daily, separate tablets	**Descovy** + **Dolutegravir** 1 tablet each once daily	(FTC + TAF) + DTV	
Alternative	Once daily, single tablet combinations	**Atripla** 1 tablet once daily qhs	TDF + FTC + EFV	
		Complera/Eviplera 1 tablet once daily with food	FTC + TDF + RPV	Avoid when VL >100,000 cells/mL
		Delstrigo 1 tablet once daily	Doravirine (DOR) + 3TC + TDF	
		Genvoya 1 tablet once daily	EVG + Cobi + FTC + TAF	
		Odefsey 1 tablet once daily	FTC + TAF + RPV	
		Stribild 1 tablet once daily	EVG + Cobi + FTC + TDF	
		Symtuza 1 tablet once daily	DRV + Cobi + FTC + TAF	
		Triumeq 1 tablet once daily	ABC + 3TC + DTG	Only if HLA B*5701 neg *(See Warnings)*
Alternative	NNRTI-based, multi-tablet	**Efavirenz** (EFV) 1 tablet once daily + (**Descovy** or **Truvada** or **Epzicom/Kivexa**) 1 tablet once daily	**Descovy**: FTC + TAF; **Truvada**: FTC + TDF; **Epzicom/Kivexa**: ABC + 3TC; **Evotaz**: ATV + Cobi; **/r**: Ritonavir boosted; **Prezcobix**: DRV + Cobi	Epzicom/Kivexa: take qhs. Avoid when VL >100,000 cells/mL. Use only if HLA-B* 5701 neg; see Warnings. Rilpivirine-based regimens should not be used in patients with VL > 100,000 c/mL (except if RPV is used with DTG)
		Rilpivirine (RPV) 1 tablet once daily + (**Descovy** or **Truvada** or **Epzicom/Kivexa**) 1 tablet once daily		
		Doravirine 1 tablet once daily + (**Descovy** or **Truvada** or **Epzicom/Kivexa**) 1 tablet once daily		
	PI-based (boosted), multi-tablet	**Evotaz** 1 tablet once daily + (**Descovy** or **Truvada** or **Epzicom/Kivexa**) 1 tablet once daily		
		Atazanavir/r 1 tablet once daily + (**Descovy** or **Truvada** or **Epzicom/Kivexa**) 1 tablet once daily		
		Prezcobix 1 tablet once daily + (**Descovy** or **Truvada** or **Epzicom/Kivexa**) 1 tablet once daily		
		Darunavir/r 1 tablet once daily + (**Descovy** or **Truvada** or **Epzicom/Kivexa**) 1 tablet once daily		
	INSTI-based, multi-tablet	**Descovy** 1 tablet once daily + **Raltegravir** (RAL) 600 mg 2 tablets once daily		
		Truvada 1 tablet once daily + **RAL** 600 mg 2 tablets once daily		
		Truvada + **Dolutegravir** (DTG) 1 tablet each once daily		
		Epzicom/Kivexa + **DTG** 1 tablet each once daily		
	Dual therapy	**DTG** + (**3TC** or **FTC**) 1 tablet each once daily		
		DTG + **RPV** 1 tablet each once daily		
	Dual therapy (injectable)	**Cabenuva** 2 IM injections qMonthly x 2 mos., then every other month	Cabo + RPV	"Direct to inject". Need resistance testing showing no RAMs to DTG or RPV; No HBV co-infection

TABLE 14C (3)

Legend, Warnings and Notes Regarding Regimens

- Legend
  - **NNRTI** = Non-nucleoside reverse transcriptase inhibitor
  - **PI** = Protease inhibitor
  - **INSTI** = Integrase strand-transfer inhibitor
- Warnings
  - Epzicom/Kivexa (ABC/3TC) containing regimens: Use only in patients who are HLA-B5701 negative.
  - Use ABC with caution in those with HIV RNA > 100,000 c/mL at baseline (this does not apply when DTG is the anchor drug of the regimen).
- Notes
  - Co-formulations increase convenience, but sometimes prescribing the components individually is preferred, e.g., when dose adjustments are needed for renal impairment.
  - Rilpivirine (RPV) with 2 nucleosides should be used only in patients with a baseline HIV RNA level < 100,000 c/mL. However, RPV can be used in combination with DTG in those with > 100,000 c/mL. Avoid use of RPV when PPI used.
  - Higher rates of renal dysfunction occur when TDF is combined with boosted PIs; TAF is the preferred drug in this setting. Conversely, TDF does not have nearly as much renal toxicity when paired with non-boosted PI drugs.
  - RAL reformulated as 600 mg tablet. Preferred dose is 2 tablets (1200 mg) once daily.
  - Cabo + RPV injectable administered as cabotegravir 600 mg (3 mL) IM and rilpivirine 900 mg (3 mL) at initiation, same dosing 1 month later (month 2), then same dosing every other month (e.g., months 4, 6, 8, and so forth)

Other drugs that may be used in selected populations (typically not used as initial therapy)

- FDC DTG/RPV or DTG/3TC can be used to simplify 3-drug regimen to 2-drugs when initial regimen successful (< 50 c/mL for > 6 months), no baseline pre-Rx resistance mutations, and no virologic failure.
- ETV, DOR and RPV are options for some patients who have NNRTI resistance mutations, e.g., K103N, at baseline. Expert consultation is recommended.
- Boosted PIs can be administered once or twice daily.
- Both Ritonavir and Cobicistat are available as PI-boosting agents.
- Non-boosted PIs are no longer recommended.

Pregnancy Considerations

- Timing of initiation of therapy and drug choice must be individualized.
- Viral resistance testing should be performed.
- Long-term effects of agents are unknown.
- Efavirenz is alternative in pregnancy. DTG and TAF (plus either FTC or 3TC) preferred regimen in pregnancy; TDF (instead of TAF) ok as well.
- BIC/TAF/FTC an acceptable alternative in pregnancy. Most clinicians continue BIC/T/F if patient is on this regimen at the time of pregnancy.
- Cobi-based regimens should NOT be used in pregnancy until further data are available.
- If recommended drugs are not available, remember that certain drugs are contraindicated, e.g., Didanosine plus Stavudine.

Other Special Populations

- Primary (acute) HIV (INSTI preferred).
- Hepatitis B/C co-infection (See Table 14E & 14F) (Should always use a TDF or TAF-based regimen).
- Opportunistic infection (Treat early in course of Rx of OI; use DTG or BIC if possible owing to fewer drug-drug interactions).

Multidrug Resistance

- Treatment choices guided by resistance test results.
- Use of lenacapavir, fostemsavir, or ibalizumab in selected settings.
- Most often can identify a regimen with 2 or more active agents based on resistance test and clinical treatment history.

TABLE 14C (4)

Selected Characteristics of Antiretroviral Drugs (*CPE = CSF penetration effectiveness: 1-4)

1. **Selected Characteristics of Nucleoside or Nucleotide Reverse Transcriptase Inhibitors (NRTIs)**

All agents have Black Box warning: Risk of lactic acidosis/hepatic steatosis. Also, risk of fat redistribution/accumulation. For combinations, *see warnings for component agents.*

* **CPE (CNS Penetration Effectiveness) value:** 1= Low Penetration; 2 - 3 = Intermediate Penetration; 4 = Highest Penetration into CNS *(AIDS 25:357, 2011)*

Generic/ Trade Name	Pharmaceutical Prep.	Usual Adult Dosage & Food Effect	% Absorbed, po	Serum $T_{1/2}$, hrs	Intracellular $T_{1/2}$, hrs	CPE*	Elimination	Major Adverse Events/Comments *(See Table 14D)*
Abacavir (ABC; Ziagen)	300 mg tabs or 20 mg/mL oral solution	300 mg po bid or 600 mg po q24h. Food OK	83	1.5	20	1	Liver metab., renal excretion of metabolites, 82%	**Hypersensitivity reaction:** fever, rash, N/V, malaise, diarrhea, abdominal pain, respiratory symptoms. (Severe reactions may be ↑ with 600 mg dose.) **Do not rechallenge!** Report to 800-270-0425. **Test HLA-B*5701 before use.** ***See Comment Table 14D.*** Studies raise concerns re ABC/3TC regimens in pts with VL ≥ 100,000 *(www.niaid.nih.gov/news/newsreleases/2008/actg5202bulletin.htm).* Controversy re increased CV events with use of ABC. Large meta-analysis shows no increased risk *(JAIDS 61, 441, 2012)*
Abacavir (ABC)/lamivudine (Epzicom or Kivexa)	Film coated tabs ABC 600 mg + 3TC 300 mg	1 tab once daily (not recommended)	*(See individual components)*					*(See for individual components)* **Black Box warning**— limited data for VL >100,000 copies/mL. Not recommended as initial therapy because of inferior virologic efficacy.
Abacavir (ABC)/ lamivudine (3TC)/ dolutegravir (DTG) (Triumeq)	Film coated tabs: ABC 600 mg + 3TC 300 mg + DTG 50 mg	1 tab po once daily						
Abacavir (ABC)/ lamivudine (3TC)/ zidovudine (AZT) (Trizivir)	Film-coated tabs: ABC 300 mg + 3TC 150 mg + ZDV 300 mg	1 tab po bid (not recommended for wt <40 kg or CrCl <50 mL/min or impaired hepatic function)						
Dolutegravir (DTG)/ Rilpivirine (RPV) (Juluca)	Film-coated tabs: DTG 50 mg + RPV 25 mg	1 tab once daily with meal	*(See individual components)*					Contraindicated if prior hypersensitivity reaction to DTV or RPV; do not co-administer with dofetilide or with drugs that significantly decrease RPV plasma concentrations. Warnings: Severe skin and hypersensitivity reactions (rash) and sometimes liver injury reported with DTV and RPV. **Common AEs:** diarrhea and headache.
Cabotegravir (CAB)/Rilpivirine (RPV) (Cabenuva)	Injectable: CAB 200 mg/mL + RPV 300 mg/mL	ACB 600 mg (3 mL) IM + RPV 900 mg (3 mL) IM at initiation, same dosing 1 month later, then same dosing every other month (months 4, 6, 8 and beyond). Can start with po lead-in: CAB 30 mg po + RPV 25 mg po each once daily with food, then start injections as above.	ND	7 days	ND	4	UGT 1A1	Similar contraindications to components (RPV and DTG), which are similar to CAB.

TABLE 14C (5)

Selected Characteristics of Antiretroviral Drugs (*CPE = CSF penetration effectiveness: 1-4)

1. **Selected Characteristics of Nucleoside or Nucleotide Reverse Transcriptase Inhibitors (NRTIs)** *(continued)*

Generic/ Trade Name	Pharmaceutical Prep.	Usual Adult Dosage & Food Effect	% Absorbed, po	Serum $T_{1/2}$, hrs	Intracellular $T_{1/2}$, hrs	CPE*	Elimination	Major Adverse Events/Comments *(See Table 14D)*
Dolutegravir (DTG)/ Lamivudine (3TC) (Dovato)	Film-coated tabs: DTG 50 mg + 3TC 300 mg	1 tab once daily with or without food	*(See individual components)*					Do not use if baseline M184V or I mutation is present. Contraindicated in those with HIV-HBV co-infection unless other HBV specific agent is also administered.
Emtricitabine (FTC, Emtriva)	200 mg caps; 10 mg per mL oral solution.	200 mg po q24h. Food OK	93 (caps), 75 (oral sol'n)	Approx. 10	39	3	Renal excretion 86%	Well tolerated; headache, nausea, vomiting & diarrhea occasionally, skin rash rarely. Skin hyperpigmentation. Differs only slightly in structure from lamivudine (5-fluoro substitution). **Exacerbation of Hep B reported in pts after stopping FTC.** Monitor at least several months after stopping FTC in Hep B pts; some may need anti-HBV therapy.
Emtricitabine/ tenofovir disoproxil fumarate (Truvada)	Film-coated tabs: FTC 200 mg + TDF 300 mg	1 tab po q24h for CrCl ≥50 mL/min. Food OK	92/25	10/17	—	*(See individual components)*	Primarily renal/renal	*See Comments for individual agents* **Black Box warning—Exacerbation of HepB after stopping FTC;** but preferred therapy for those with Hep B/HIV co-infection.
Emtricitabine/ Tenofovir/Efavirenz (Atripla)	Film-coated tabs: FTC 200 mg + TDF 300 mg + Efavirenz 600 mg	1 tab po q24h on an empty stomach, preferably at bedtime. Do not use if CrCl <50 mL/min	*(See individual components)*					Not recommended for pts <18 yrs. *(See warnings for individual components).* **Exacerbation of Hep B** reported in pts discontinuing component drugs; some need anti-HBV therapy (tenofovir preferred). **Pregnancy category D-** Efavirenz may cause fetal harm. Avoid in pregnancy or in women who may become pregnant.
Emtricitabine/ Tenofovir/ Rilpivirine (Complera/Eviplera)	Film-coated tabs: FTC 200 mg + TDF 300 mg + RPL 25 mg	1 tab po q24h with food	*(See individual components)*					*See individual components.* Preferred use in pts with HIV RNA level <100,000 c/mL. Should not be used with PPI agents.
Lamivudine (3TC; Epivir)	150, 300 mg tabs; 10 mg/mL oral solution	150 mg po bid or 300 mg po q24h. Food OK	86	5–7	18	2	Renal excretion, minimal metabolism	**Use HIV dose, not Hep B dose.** Usually well-tolerated. **Risk of exacerbation of Hep B after stopping 3TC.** Monitor at least several months after stopping 3TC in Hep B pts; some may need anti-HBV therapy.
Lamivudine/ abacavir (Epzicom)	Film-coated tabs: 3TC 300 mg + abacavir 600 mg	1 tab po q24h. Food OK Not recommended for CrCl <50 mL/min or impaired hepatic function	86/86	5-7/1.5	16/20	*(See individual components)*	Primarily renal/ metabolism	*See Comments for individual agents.* **Note abacavir hypersensitivity Black Box warnings** (severe reactions may be somewhat more frequent with 600 mg dose) and 3TC Hep B warnings. Test HLA-B*5701 before use.

TABLE 14C (6)

Generic/ Trade Name	Pharmaceutical Prep.	Usual Adult Dosage & Food Effect	% Absorbed, po	Serum T½, hrs	Intracellular T½, hrs	CPE*	Elimination	Major Adverse Events/Comments *(See Table 14D)*
Selected Characteristics of Antiretroviral Drugs (*CPE = CSF penetration effectiveness: 1-4)								
1. **Selected Characteristics of Nucleoside or Nucleotide Reverse Transcriptase Inhibitors (NRTIs)** *(continued)*								
Lamivudine/ zidovudine (Combivir)	Film-coated tabs: 3TC 150 mg + ZDV 300 mg	1 tab po bid. Not recommended for CrCl <50 mL/min or impaired hepatic function Food OK	86/64	5-7/0.5-3	—	*(See individual components)*	Primarily renal/ metabolism with renal excretion of glucuronide	*See Comments for individual agents* **Black Box warning**—exacerbation of Hep B in pts stopping 3TC
Tenofovir alafenamide (TAF)	25 mg (10 mg when used with Cobi or RTV)	CrCl >30 mL/min Food OK; high-fat meal increases absorption						Headache, N/V. **Cases of renal dysfunction reported:** check renal function before using (dose reductions necessary if CrCl <50 cc/min); avoid concomitant nephrotoxic agents. One study found ↑ renal function at 48-wks in pts receiving TDF with a PI (mostly lopinavir/ritonavir) than with a NNRTI *(JID 197:102, 2008)*. Avoid concomitant ddI. Atazanavir & lopinavir/ritonavir ↑ tenofovir concentrations: monitor for adverse effects. **Black Box warning—exacerbations of Hep B reported after stopping tenofovir.** Monitor liver enzymes if TDF stopped on HBV pts.
Tenofovir disoproxil fumarate (TDF; Viread)—a nucleotide	300 mg tabs	CrCl ≥50 mL/min: 300 mg po q24h. Food OK; high-fat meal increases absorption	39 (with food) 25 (fasted)	17	>60	1	Renal excretion	
Zidovudine (ZDV, AZT; Retrovir)	100 mg caps, 300 mg tabs; 10 mg per mL IV solution; 10 mg/mL oral syrup	300 mg po q12h. Food OK	64	1.1	11	4	Metabolized to glucuronide & excreted in urine	Bone marrow suppression, GI intolerance, headache, insomnia, malaise, myopathy.
2. **Selected Characteristics of Non-Nucleoside Reverse Transcriptase Inhibitors (NNRTIs)**								
Doravirine (Pifeltro)	100 mg tabs	100 mg daily ± food	64	20	ND	ND	Metabolism; 6% excreted in urine unchanged	Nausea, dizziness, headache, fatigue; Co-administration with drugs that are strong CYP3A inducers significantly decreases Doravirine plasma concentrations
Efavirenz (Sustiva) OK for use in pregnancy (WHO and HHS Guidelines)	50, 100, 200 mg capsules; 600 mg tablet	600 mg po q24h at bedtime, without food. Food may ↑ serum conc., which can lead to ↑ in risk of adverse events.	42	40–55 *See Comment*	3		Cytochrome P450 2B6 (3A mixed inducer/ inhibitor). 14-34% excreted in urine as glucuronidated metabolites, 16–61% in feces	Severe rash in 1.7%. High frequency of CNS AEs: somnolence, dreams, confusion, agitation. Serious psychiatric symptoms. Certain CYP2B6 polymorphisms may predict exceptionally high plasma levels with standard doses *(CID 45:1230, 2007)*. False-pos. cannabinoid screen. Very long tissue T½. **If rx to be discontinued, stop Efavirenz 1–2 wks before stopping companion drugs.** Otherwise, risk of developing Efavirenz resistance, as after 1–2 days only Efavirenz in blood &/or tissue. Some bridge this gap by adding a PI to the NRTI backbone after Efavirenz is discontinued. *(CID 42:401, 2006)*

TABLE 14C (7)

Generic/ Trade Name	Pharmaceutical Prep.	Usual Adult Dosage & Food Effect	% Absorbed, po	Serum $T\frac{1}{2}$, hrs	Intracellular $T\frac{1}{2}$, hrs	CPE	Elimination	Major Adverse Events/Comments *(See Table 14D)*
Selected Characteristics of Antiretroviral Drugs (*CPE = CSF penetration effectiveness: 1-4)								
2. **Selected Characteristics of Non-Nucleoside Reverse Transcriptase Inhibitors (NNRTIs)** *(continued)*								
Etravirine (Intelence)	100 mg tabs 200 mg tabs	200 mg twice daily after a meal. May also be given as 400 mg once daily	Unknown (↓ systemic exposure if taken fasting)	41	2		Metabolized by CYP 3A4 (inducer) & 2C9, 2C19 (inhibitor). Fecal extraction.	For pts with HIV-1 resistant to NNRTIs & others. Active in vitro against most such isolates. Rash common, but rarely can be severe. Potential for multiple drug interactions. Generally, multiple mutations are required for high-level resistance. *See Table 14D, page 253 for specific mutations and effects.* Because of interactions, do not use with boosted atazanavir, boosted tipranavir, unboosted PIs, or other NNRTIs.
Nevirapine (Viramune) Viramune XR	200 mg tabs; 50 mg per 5 mL oral suspension; XR 400 mg tabs	200 mg po q24h x 14 days & then 200 mg po bid *(see comments & **Black Box warning**)* Food OK. **If using Viramune XR, Still need the lead in dosing of 200 mg q24h prior to using 400 mg/d**	>90	25–30	4		Cytochrome P450 (3A4, 2B6) inducer; 80% excreted in urine as glucuronidated metabolites, 10% in feces	**Black Box warning—fatal hepatotoxicity.** Women with CD4 >250 esp. vulnerable, inc. pregnant women. Avoid in this group unless benefits clearly > risks *(www.fda.gov/cderdrug/advisory/nevirapine.htm)*. Intensive monitoring for liver toxicity required. Men with CD4 >400 also at ↑ risk. Severe rash in 7%, **severe or life-threatening skin reactions** in 2%. Do not restart if any suspicion of such reactions. 2 wks dose escalation period may ↓ skin reactions. Because of long $T\frac{1}{2}$, consider continuing companion agents for several days if nevirapine is discontinued.
Rilpivirine (Edurant); also co-packaged with IM **cabotegravir** as Cabenuva	25 mg tabs; and injectable (300 mg/mL)	Cabenuva: *see page 244*	absolute bioavailability unknown; 40% lower Cmax in fasted state	50	unknown		Metabolized by Cyp3A4 in liver; 25% excreted unchanged in feces.	For oral formulation, QTc prolongation with doses higher than 50 mg per day. Common AEs: depression, insomnia, headache, and rash. Do not co-administer with carbamazepine, phenobarbitol, phenytoin, rifabutin, rifampin, rifapentine, proton pump inhibitors, or multiple doses of dexamethasone. A fixed dose combination of rilpivirine + TDF/FTC (Complera/Eviplera) is approved. **Needs stomach acid for absorption. Do not administer with PPI.**

TABLE 14C (8)

Generic/ Trade Name	Pharmaceutical Prep.	Usual Adult Dosage & Food Effect	% Absorbed, po	Serum T½, hrs	Intracellular T½, hrs	CPE	Elimination	Major Adverse Events/Comments *(See Table 14D)*

Selected Characteristics of Antiretroviral Drugs (*CPE = CSF penetration effectiveness: 1-4)

3. **Selected Characteristics of Protease Inhibitors (PIs)**

All PIs: Glucose metabolism: new diabetes mellitus or deterioration of glucose control; fat redistribution; possible hemophilia bleeding; hypertriglyceridemia or hypercholesterolemia. Exercise caution re: potential drug interactions & contraindications. QTc prolongation has been reported in a few pts taking PIs; some PIs can block HERG channels in vitro *(Lancet 365:682, 2005)*.

Generic/ Trade Name	Pharmaceutical Prep.	Usual Adult Dosage & Food Effect	% Absorbed, po	Serum T½, hrs	CPE*	Elimination	Major Adverse Events/Comments *(See Table 14D)*
Atazanavir (Reyataz)	100, 150, 200, 300 mg capsules	400 mg po q24h with food. Ritonavir-boosted dose (atazanavir 300 mg po q24h + ritonavir 100 mg po q24h), with food, is recommended for ART-experienced pts. Use boosted dose when combined with either Efavirenz 600 mg po q24h or TDF 300 mg po q24h. If used with buffered ddI, take with food 2 hrs pre or 1 hr post ddI.	Good oral bioavailability; food enhances bioavailability & ↓ pharmacokinetic variability. Absorption ↓ by antacids, H_2-blockers, proton pump inhibitors. Avoid unboosted drug with PPIs/H2-blockers. Boosted drug can be used with or >10 hr after H2-blockers or >12 hr after a PPI, if limited doses of the acid agents are used.	Approx. 7	2	Cytochrome P450 (3A4, 1A2 & 2C9 inhibitor) & UGT1A1 inhibitor, 13% excreted in urine (7% unchanged), 79% excreted in feces (20% unchanged)	Lower potential for ↑ lipids. Asymptomatic unconjugated hyperbilirubinemia common; jaundice especially likely in Gilbert's syndrome *(JID 192:1381, 2005)*. Headache, rash, GI symptoms. Prolongation of PR interval (1st degree AV block) reported. Caution in pre-existing conduction system disease. Efavirenz & Tenofovir ↓ atazanavir exposure: use atazanavir/ritonavir regimen; also, atazanavir ↑ tenofovir concentrations—watch for adverse events. In rx-experienced pts taking TDF and needing H2 blockers, atazanavir 400 mg with ritonavir 100 mg can be given; do not use PPIs. Rare reports of renal stones.
Darunavir (Prezista)	400 mg, 600 mg, 800 mg tablets	[600 mg darunavir + 100 mg ritonavir] po bid, with food or **[800 mg darunavir (two 400 mg tabs or one 800 mg tab) + 100 mg ritonavir] po once daily with food (Preferred regimen in ART naïve pts)**	82% absorbed (taken with ritonavir). Food ↑ absorption.	Approx 15 hr (with ritonavir)	3	Metabolized by CYP3A and is a CYP3A inhibitor	Contains sulfa moiety. Rash, nausea, headaches seen. Coadmin of certain drugs cleared by CYP3A is contraindicated *(see label)*. Use with caution in pts with hepatic dysfunction. (FDA warning about occasional hepatic dysfunction early in the course of treatment). Monitor carefully, esp. first several months and with pre-existing liver disease. May cause hormonal contraception failure.
Lopinavir + ritonavir (Kaletra)	(200 mg lopinavir + 50 mg ritonavir), and (100 mg lopinavir + 25 mg ritonavir) tablets. Tabs do not need refrigeration. Oral solution: (80 mg lopinavir + 20 mg ritonavir) per mL. Refrigerate, but can be kept at room temp. (≤77°F) x 2 mos.	(400 mg lopinavir + 100 mg ritonavir)—2 tabs po bid. Higher dose may be needed in non-rx-naïve pts when used with Efavirenz, nevirapine, or unboosted fosamprenavir. [Dose adjustment in concomitant drugs may be necessary.	No food effect with tablets.	5–6	3	Cytochrome P450 (3A4 inhibitor)	Nausea/vomiting/diarrhea (worse when administered with zidovudine), ↑ AST/ ALT, pancreatitis. Oral solution 42% alcohol. Lopinavir + ritonavir can be taken as a single daily dose of 4 tabs (total 800 mg lopinavir + 200 mg ritonavir), except in treatment-experienced pts or those taking concomitant Efavirenz, nevirapine, amprenavir, or nelfinavir. Possible PR and QT prolongation. Use with caution in those with cardiac conduction abnormalities or when used with drugs with similar effects.

TABLE 14C (9)

Generic/ Trade Name	Pharmaceutical Prep.	Usual Adult Dosage & Food Effect	% Absorbed, po	Serum $T\frac{1}{2}$, hrs	CPE*	Elimination	Major Adverse Events/Comments *(See Table 14D)*
Selected Characteristics of Antiretroviral Drugs (*CPE = CSF penetration effectiveness: 1-4)							
3. **Selected Characteristics of Protease Inhibitors (PIs)** *(continued)*							
Ritonavir (Norvir)	100 mg capsules; 600 mg per 7.5 mL solution. Refrigerate caps but not solution. Room temperature for 1 mo. is OK.	Full dose not recommended *(see comments)*. **With rare exceptions, used exclusively to enhance pharmacokinetics of other PIs, using lower ritonavir doses.**	Food ↑ absorption	3–5	1	Cytochrome P450. Potent 3A4 & 2 d6 inhibitor	Nausea/vomiting/diarrhea, extremity & circum-oral paresthesias, hepatitis, pancreatitis, taste perversion, ↑ CPK & uric acid. **Black Box warning—**potentially fatal drug interactions. Many drug interactions.

4. **Selected Characteristics of Fusion Inhibitors**

Generic/ Trade Name	Pharmaceutical Prep.	Usual Adult Dosage	% Absorbed	Serum $T\frac{1}{2}$, hrs	CPE*	Elimination	Major Adverse Events/Comments *(See Table 14D)*
Enfuvirtide (T20, Fuzeon)	Single-use vials of 90 mg/mL when reconstituted. Vials should be stored at room temperature. Reconstituted vials can be refrigerated for 24 hrs only.	90 mg (1 mL) subcut. bid. Rotate injection sites, avoiding those currently inflamed.	84	3.8	1	Catabolism to its constituent amino acids with subsequent recycling of the amino acids in the body pool. Elimination pathway(s) have not been performed in humans. Does not alter the metabolism of CYP3A4, CYP2 d6, CYP1A2, CYP2C19 or CYP2E1 substrates.	Local reaction site reactions 98%, 4% discontinue; erythema/induration ~80–90%, nodules/cysts ~80%. **Hypersensitivity reactions reported** (fever, rash, chills, N/V, ↓ BP, &/or ↑ AST/ALT)—do not restart if occur. Including background regimens, peripheral neuropathy 8.9%, insomnia 11.3%, ↓ appetite 6.3%, myalgia 5%, lymphadenopathy 2.3%, eosinophilia ~10%. ↑ incidence of bacterial pneumonias.
5. **Selected Characteristics of CCR-5 Co-receptor Antagonists**							
Maraviroc (Selzentry)	150 mg, 300 mg film-coated tabs	Without regard to food: - 150 mg bid if concomitant meds include CYP3A inhibitors including PIs - 300 mg bid without significantly interacting meds including NRTIs, neverapine - 600 mg bid if concomitant meds include CYP3A inducers, including Efavirenz (without strong CYP3A inhibitors)	Est. 33% with 300 mg dosage	14-18	3	CYP3A and P-glycoprotein substrate. Metabolites (via CYP3A) excreted feces > urine	**Black Box Warning-Hepatotoxicity,** may be preceded by rash, ↑ eos or IgE. NB: no hepatoxicity was noted in MVC trials. Black box inserted owing to concern about potential CCR5 class effect. Data lacking in hepatic/renal insufficiency; ↑ concern with either could ↑ risk of ↓BP. Currently for treatment-experienced patients with multi-resistant strains. **Document CCR-5-tropic virus before use, as treatment failures assoc. with appearance of CXCR-4 or mixed-tropic virus.**

TABLE 14C (10)

Generic/ Trade Name	Pharmaceutical Prep.	Usual Adult Dosage & Food Effect	% Absorbed	Serum $T_{1/2}$, hrs	CPE	Elimination	Major Adverse Events/Comments *(See Table 14D)*
Selected Characteristics of Antiretroviral Drugs (*CPE = CSF penetration effectiveness: 1-4)							
6. **Selected Characteristics of Integrase Strand Transfer Inhibitors (INSTI)**							
Bictegravir (part of Biktarvy)	50 mg (per Biktarvy tab)	50 mg once daily with or without food	No data	17.3	No data	Mainly metabolized by CYP3A enzymes; also glucuronidated by UGT1A1.	Indicated (as Biktarvy) for treatment naive pts and as replacement for prior or existing therapy. Generally well tolerated. Expect increased serum creatinine by 0.1-0.15 mg/dL due to inhibition of proximal tubular secretion; does not reflect a reduced GFR. **Black box warning: possible acute exacerbation of hep B** in co-infected patients who discontinue Biktarvy.
Cabotegravir (Vocabria). Also co-packaged with IM rilpivirine as Cabenuva	30 mg tablets, injectable (200 mg/mL)	Oral Lead-in dosing: 30 mg (+ RPV 25 mg) once daily x1 month, with food. After oral lead-in: 600 mg IM, then 400 mg IM monthly (with IM rilpivirine)	No data	41	No data	Metabolized mainly by UGT1A1, with some contribution from UGT1A9a	All <1%: headache, nausea, abnormal dreams, anxiety, insomnia. Others: hypersensitivity, hepatotoxicity, depressive disorders.
Dolutegravir (Tivicay)	50 mg	50 mg po once daily 50 mg po bid (if INSTI resistance present or if co-admin with EFV, FOS, TIP, or RIF	Unknown	14	4	Glucuronidation via UGT1A1 (therefore does not require ritonavir or cobicistat boosting)	Hypersensitivity (rare); Most common: insomnia (3%) headache (2%), N/V (1%), rash (<1%). Watch for IRIS; Watch for elevated LFTs in those with HCV. Similar increase in serum creatinine as described for bictegravir above.
Elvitegravir/ cobicistat (Stribild)	150 mg - 150 mg	150 mg-150 mg once daily with or without food	<10%	12.9 (Cobi), 3.5 (ELV)	Un-known	The majority of **elvitegravir** metabolism is mediated by CYP3A enzymes. Elvitegravir also undergoes glucuronidation via UGT1A1/3 enzymes. **Cobicistat** is metabolized by CYP3A and to a minor extent by CYP2D6	For both treatment naïve patients and treatment experienced pts with multiply-resistant virus. Generally well-tolerated. Use of cobicistat increases serum creatinine by ~ 0.1 mg/dl via inhibition of proximal tubular enzyme; this does not result in reduction in true GFR but will result in erroneous apparent reduction in eGFR by MDRD or Cockcroft Gault calculations. Usual AEs are similar to those observed with ritonavir (cobi) and tenofovir/FTC.
Raltegravir (Isentress)	600 mg film-coated tabs	600 mg po bid without regard to food	Unknown	~ 9	3	Glucuronidation via UGT1A1, with excretion into feces and urine. (Therefore does NOT require ritonavir boosting)	For naïve patients and treatment experienced pts with multiply-resistant virus. Well-tolerated. Nausea, diarrhea, headache, fever similar to placebo. CK↑ & rhabdomyolysis reported: unclear relationship. Increased depression in those with a history of depression. Low genetic barrier to resistance. Increase in CPK, myositis, rhabdomyolysis have been reported. Rare Stevens Johnson Syndrome. Better oral absorption if chewed *(CID 57:480, 2013)*.

TABLE 14C (11)

Generic/ Trade Name	Pharmaceutical Prep.	Usual Adult Dosage & Food Effect	% Absorbed	Serum $T_{1/2}$, hrs	CPE	Elimination	Major Adverse Events/Comments *(See Table 14D)*
7. Selected Characteristics of Attachment Inhibitors							
Fostemsavir (Rukobia)	600 mg ER tabs	600 mg bid, with or without food. Do not chew, crush, or split tablets.	26.9	11	No data	Metabolism (esterase-mediated hydrolysis, CYP450-mediated oxidation)	Most common AE: headache, rash, N/V, diarrhea, fatigue, lack of energy. Watch for IRIS, QT-prolongation, elevations in liver transaminases in pts co-infected with HBV or HCV. Potential for drug interactions.
Ibalizumab-uiyk (Trogarzo)	200 mg vials for injection	2 gm IV, then 800 mg IV q2-wks	N/A	2.7-64	No data	Non-linear, concentration-dependent	Most common AE: diarrhea, dizziness, nausea, rash. Watch for IRIS.
8. Selected Characteristics of Capsid Inhibitor							
Lenacapavir (Sunlenca)	Tab 300 mg, Injection for sc	*Option 1:* Day 1: 927 mg inject sc, 600 mg po Day 2: 600 mg po *Option 2:* Days 1, 2, 8: 600 mg po Day 15: 927 mg inject sc	6-10%	po 10-12 d, sc 8-12 wks	No data	Fecal, metabolism	See *Table 14 D*

Other Considerations in Selection of Therapy

Caution: Initiation of ART may result in immune reconstitution syndrome with significant clinical consequences.

1. Resistance testing: Given current rates of resistance, resistance testing is recommended in all patients prior to initiation of therapy, including those with acute infection syndrome (may initiate therapy while waiting for test results and adjusting Rx once results return), at time of change of therapy owing to antiretroviral failure, when suboptimal virologic response is observed, and in pregnant women. **Resistance testing NOT recommended if pt is off ART for >4 weeks or if HIV RNA is <500 c/mL.**
2. Drug-induced disturbances of glucose & lipid metabolism *(see Table 14D)*
3. Drug-induced lactic acidosis & other FDA "box warnings" *(see Table 14D)*
4. Drug-drug interactions
5. Risk in pregnancy *(see Table 8A)*
6. Use in women & children *(see Table 14C)*
7. Dosing in patients with renal or hepatic dysfunction *(see Table 17A & Table 17B)*

* **CPE (CNS Penetration Effectiveness) value:** 1= Low Penetration; 2 - 3 = Intermediate Penetration; 4 = Highest Penetration into CNS *(AIDS 25:357, 2011)*

TABLE 14D – ANTIRETROVIRAL DRUGS & ADVERSE EFFECTS
(www.aidsinfo.nih.gov)

DRUG NAME(S): GENERIC (TRADE)	MOST COMMON ADVERSE EFFECTS	MOST SIGNIFICANT ADVERSE EFFECTS
Nucleoside Reverse Transcriptase Inhibitors (NRTI) Black Box warning for all nucleoside/nucleotide RTIs: lactic acidosis/hepatic steatosis, potentially fatal. Also carry Warnings that fat redistribution and immune reconstitution syndromes (including autoimmune syndromes with delayed onset) have been observed		
Abacavir (Ziagen)	Headache 7–13%, nausea 7–19%, diarrhea 7%, malaise 7-12%	**Black Box warning-Hypersensitivity reaction (HR)** in 8% with malaise, fever, GI upset, rash, lethargy & respiratory symptoms most commonly reported; myalgia, arthralgia, edema, paresthesia less common. **Discontinue immediately if HR suspected. Rechallenge contraindicated; may be life-threatening.** Severe HR may be more common with once-daily dosing. **HLA-B*5701 allele** predicts ↑ risk of HR in Caucasian pop.; excluding pts with B*5701 markedly ↓'d HR incidence. DHHS guidelines recommend testing for B*5701 and use of abacavir-containing regimens only if HLA-B*5701 negative; Vigilance essential in all groups. Possible increased risk of MI with use of abacavir had been suggested. Other studies found no increased risk of MI. A meta-analysis of randomized trials by FDA also did not show increased risk of MI *(www.fda.gov/drugs/drugsafety/ucm245164.htm)*. Nevertheless, care is advised to optimize potentially modifiable risk factors when abacavir is used.
Emtricitabine (FTC) (Emtriva)	Well tolerated. Headache, diarrhea, nausea, rash, skin hyperpigmentation	Potential for lactic acidosis (as with other NRTIs). Also **in Black Box—severe exacerbation of hepatitis B on stopping drug reported—monitor clinical/labs for several months after stopping in pts with hepB.** Anti-HBV rx may be warranted if FTC stopped.
Lamivudine (3TC) (Epivir)	Well tolerated. Headache 35%, nausea 33%, diarrhea 18%, abdominal pain 9%, insomnia 11% (all in combination with ZDV). Pancreatitis more common in pediatrics.	**Black Box warning.** Make sure to use HIV dosage, not Hep B dosage. **Exacerbation of hepatitis B on stopping drug. Patients with hepB who stop lamivudine require close clinical/lab monitoring for several months.** Anti-HBV rx may be warranted if 3TC stopped.
Zidovudine (ZDV, AZT) (Retrovir)	Nausea 50%, anorexia 20%, vomiting 17%, **headache 62%.** Also reported: asthenia, insomnia, myalgias, nail pigmentation. Macrocytosis expected with all dosage regimens.	**Black Box warning—hematologic toxicity, myopathy. Anemia** (<8 gm, 1%), granulocytopenia (<750, 1.8%). Anemia may respond to epoetin alfa if endogenous serum erythropoietin levels are ≤500 milliUnits/mL. Possible ↑ toxicity if used with ribavirin. Co-administration with Ribavirin not advised. Hepatic decompensation may occur in HIV/HCV co-infected patients receiving zidovudine with interferon alfa ± ribavirin.
Tenofovir disoproxil fumarate (TDF) (Viread); Tenofovir alafenamide (TAF)	Diarrhea 11%, nausea 8%, vomiting 5%, flatulence 4% (generally well tolerated)	**Black Box Warning—Severe exacerbations of hepatitis B reported in pts who stop tenofovir.** Monitor carefully if drug is stopped; anti-HBV rx may be warranted if TDF stopped. Reports of renal injury from TDF, including Fanconi syndrome. Fanconi syndrome and diabetes insipidus reported with TDF + ddI. Modest decline in renal function appears greater with TDF than with NRTIs or TAF and may be greater in those receiving TDF with a PI instead of an NNRTI. Monitor Ccr, serum phosphate and urinalysis, especially carefully in those with pre-existing renal dysfunction or nephrotoxic medications. TDF, but not TAF, Tenofovir also appears to be associated with increased risk of bone loss.

TABLE 14D (2)

DRUG NAME(S): GENERIC (TRADE)	MOST COMMON ADVERSE EFFECTS	MOST SIGNIFICANT ADVERSE EFFECTS
Non-Nucleoside Reverse Transcriptase Inhibitors (NNRTI). Labels caution that fat redistribution and immune reconstitution can occur with ART.		
Doravirine (Pifeltro)	Nausea (5-7%), diarrhea (3-5%), abdominal pain (1-5%), headache (4-6%), fatigue (4-6%), rash (2%). Dizziness: 9% (37% with Atripla). Sleep disturbances: 12% (26% with Atripla). Better lipid profile than efavirenz- or PI-based regimens.	Co-administration with drugs that are strong CYP3A inducers will significantly decrease Doravirine plasma concentrations. Monitor for IRIS during initiation of therapy.
Efavirenz (Sustiva)	**CNS side effects 52%;** symptoms include dizziness, insomnia, somnolence, impaired concentration, psychiatric sx, & abnormal dreams; symptoms are worse after 1st or 2nd dose & improve over 2–4 weeks; discontinuation rate 2.6%. Rash 26% (vs. 17% in comparators); often improves with oral antihistamines; discontinuation rate 1.7%. Can cause false-positive urine test results for cannabinoid with CEDIA DAU multi-level THC assay. Metabolite can cause false-positive urine screening test for benzodiazepines.	**Caution:** CNS effects may impair driving and other hazardous activities. Serious neuropsychiatric symptoms reported, including severe depression (2.4%) & suicidal ideation (0.7%). Elevation in liver enzymes. Fulminant hepatic failure has been reported *(see FDA label)*. **OK for use in pregnancy as an alternative (WHO and HHS Guidelines).** NOTE: No single method of contraception is 100% reliable. Barrier + 2nd method of contraception advised, continued 12 weeks after stopping Efavirenz. Contraindicated with certain drugs metabolized by CYP3A4. Slow metabolism in those homozygous for the CYP-2B6 G516T allele can result in exaggerated toxicity and intolerance. This allele much more common in blacks and women. Stevens-Jonson syndrome and erythema multiforme reported in post-marketing surveillance.
Etravirine (Intelence)	Rash 9%, generally mild to moderate and spontaneously resolving; 2% dc clinical trials for rash. More common in women. Nausea 5%.	Severe rash (erythema multiforme, toxic epidermal necrolysis, Stevens-Johnson syndrome) has been reported. Hypersensitivity reactions can occur with rash, constitutional symptoms and organ dysfunction, including hepatic failure *(see FDA label)*. Potential for CYP450-mediated drug interactions. Rhabdomyolysis has been reported in post-marketing surveillance.
Nevirapine (Viramune)	**Rash 37%:** usually occurs during 1st 6 wks of therapy. Follow recommendations for 14-day lead-in period to ↓ risk of rash *(see Table 14C)*. Women experience 7-fold ↑ in risk of severe rash. 50% resolve within 2 wks of dc drug & 80% by 1 month. 6.7% discontinuation rate.	**Black Box warning—Severe life-threatening skin reactions reported:** Stevens-Johnson syndrome, toxic epidermal necrolysis, & hypersensitivity reaction or drug rash with eosinophilia & systemic symptoms (DRESS). For severe rashes, dc drug immediately & do not restart. In a clinical trial, the use of prednisone ↑ the risk of rash. **Black Box warning—Life-threatening hepatotoxicity reported,** 2/3 during the first 12 wks of rx. Overall 1% develops hepatitis. Pts with pre-existing ↑ in ALT or AST &/or history of chronic Hep B or C ↑ susceptible. Women with CD4 >250, including pregnant women, at ↑ risk. Avoid in this group unless no other option. Men with CD4 >400 also at ↑ risk. Monitor pts intensively (clinical & LFTs), esp. during the first 12 wks of rx. If clinical hepatotoxicity, severe skin or hypersensitivity reactions occur, dc drug & never rechallenge.
Rilpivirine (Edurant)	Headache (3%), rash (3%; led to discontinuation in 0.1%), insomnia (3%), depressive disorders (4%). Psychiatric disorders led to discontinuation in 1%. Increased liver enzymes observed.	Drugs that induce CYP3A or increase gastric pH may decrease plasma concentration of rilpivirine and co-administration with rilpivirine should be avoided. Among these are certain anticonvulsants, rifamycins, PPIs, dexamethasone and St. John's wort. At supra-therapeutic doses, rilpivirine can increase QTc interval; use with caution with other drugs known to increase QTc. May cause depressive disorder, including suicide attempts or suicidal ideation. Overall, appears to cause fewer neuropsychiatric side effects than Efavirenz.

TABLE 14D (3)

DRUG NAME(S): GENERIC (TRADE)	MOST COMMON ADVERSE EFFECTS	MOST SIGNIFICANT ADVERSE EFFECTS
Protease inhibitors (PI)		
Diarrhea is common AE (**crofelemer** 125 mg bid may help, but expensive). Abnormalities in glucose metabolism, dyslipidemias, fat redistribution syndromes are potential problems. Pts taking PI may be at increased risk for developing osteopenia/osteoporosis. Spontaneous bleeding episodes have been reported in HIV+ pts with hemophilia being treated with PI. Rheumatoid complications have been reported. Potential for QTc prolongation. **Caution for all PIs**—Coadministration with drugs dependent on CYP3A or other enzymes for elimination & for which ↑ levels can cause serious toxicity may be contraindicated. ART may result in immune reconstitution syndromes, which may include early or late presentations of autoimmune syndromes. Increased premature births among women receiving ritonavir-boosted PIs as compared with those receiving other antiretroviral therapy, even after accounting for other potential risk factors.		
Atazanavir (Reyataz)	Asymptomatic unconjugated hyperbilirubinemia in up to 60% of pts, jaundice in 7–9% (especially with Gilbert syndrome). Moderate to severe events: Diarrhea 1–3%, nausea 6–14%, abdominal pain 4%, headache 6%, rash 20%.	Prolongation of PR interval (1st degree AV block in 5-6%) reported; rarely 2° AV block. QTc increase and torsades reported. Acute interstitial nephritis and urolithiasis (atazanavir stones) reported. Potential ↑ transanimases in pts co-infected with HBV or HCV. Severe skin eruptions (Stevens-Johnson syndrome, erythema multiforme, and toxic eruptions, or DRESS syndrome) have been reported.
Darunavir (Prezista)	With background regimens, headache 15%, nausea 18%, diarrhea 20%, ↑ amylase 17%. Rash in 10% of treated; 0.5% discontinuation.	Hepatitis in 0.5%, some with fatal outcome. Use caution in pts with HBV or HCV co-infections or other hepatic dysfunction. Monitor for clinical symptoms and LFTs. Stevens-Johnson syndrome, toxic epidermal necrolysis, erythema multiforme. Contains sulfa moiety. Potential for major drug interactions. May cause failure of hormonal contraceptives.
Lopinavir/Ritonavir (Kaletra)	GI: **diarrhea** 14–24%, nausea 2–16%. More diarrhea with q24h dosing.	Lipid abnormalities in up to 20–40%. Possible increased risk of MI with cumulative exposure. ↑ PR interval, 2º or 3º heart block described. Post-marketing reports of ↑ QTc and torsades: avoid use in congenital QTc prolongation or in other circumstances that prolong QTc or increase susceptibility to torsades. Hepatitis, with hepatic decompensation; caution especially in those with pre-existing liver disease. Pancreatitis. Inflammatory edema of legs. Stevens-Johnson syndrome & erythema multiforme reported. Note high drug concentration in oral solution. Toxic potential of oral solution (contains ethanol and propylene glycol) in neonates.
Ritonavir (Norvir) (Currently, primary use is to enhance levels of other anti-retrovirals, because of ↑ toxicity/ interactions with full-dose ritonavir)	GI: bitter aftertaste ↓ by taking with chocolate milk, Ensure, or Advera; nausea 23%, ↓ by initial dose esc (titration) regimen; vomiting 13%; diarrhea 15%. Circumoral paresthesias 5–6%. Dose >100 mg bid assoc. with ↑ GI side effects & ↑ in lipid abnormalities.	**Black Box** warning relates to many important drug-drug interactions—inhibits P450 CYP3A & CYP2 D6 system—may be life-threatening. Several cases of iatrogenic Cushing's syndrome reported with concomitant use of ritonavir and corticosteroids, including dosing of the latter by inhalation, epidural injection or a single IM injection. Rarely Stevens-Johnson syndrome, toxic epidermal necrolysis anaphylaxis. Primary A-V block (and higher) and pancreatitis have been reported. Hepatic reactions, including fatalities. Monitor LFTs carefully during therapy, especially in those with pre-existing liver disease, including HBV and HCV.
Fusion Inhibitor		
Enfuvirtide (T20, Fuzeon)	Local injection site reactions (98% at least 1 local ISR, 4% dc because of ISR) (pain & discomfort, induration, erythema, nodules & cysts, pruritus, & ecchymosis). Diarrhea 32%, nausea 23%, fatigue 20%.	↑ Rate of bacterial pneumonia (3.2 pneumonia events/100 pt yrs), **hypersensitivity reactions** ≤1% (rash, fever, nausea & vomiting, chills, rigors, hypotension, & ↑ serum liver transaminases); can occur with reexposure. Cutaneous amyloid deposits containing enfuvirtide peptide reported in skin plaques persisting after discontinuation of drug.
CCR5 Co-receptor Antagonists		
Maraviroc (Selzentry)	With ARV background: Cough 13%, fever 12%, rash 10%, abdominal pain 8%. Also, dizziness, myalgia, arthralgias. ↑ Risk of URI, HSV infection.	**Black box warning-Hepatotoxicity.** May be preceded by allergic features (rash, ↑eosinophils or ↑IgE levels). Use with caution in pt with HepB or C. Cardiac ischemia/infarction in 1.3%. May cause ↓BP, orthostatic syncope, especially in patients with renal dysfunction. Significant interactions with CYP3A inducers/inhibitors. Long-term risk of malignancy unknown. Stevens-Johnson syndrome reported post-marketing. Generally favorable safety profile during trial of ART-naïve individuals.

TABLE 14D (4)

DRUG NAME(S): GENERIC (TRADE)	MOST COMMON ADVERSE EFFECTS	MOST SIGNIFICANT ADVERSE EFFECTS
Integrase Inhibitors		
Bictegravir (part of Biktarvy)	Reported in at least 5% of patients: nausea, diarrhea, headache. May increase serum creatinine 0.1-0.15 mg/dL due to inhibition of proximal tubular secretion of creatinine (does not reflect a decrease in GFR).	**Black Box Warning:** possible severe hepatitis B exacerbation in co-infected patients who discontinue therapy. Monitor for IRIS if treating an ARV-naive patient with a lower CD4 cell count (<150/microliter).
Cabotegravir (Vocabria); also co-packaged with IM rilpivirine as Cabenuva	All <1%: headache, nausea, abnormal dreams, anxiety, insomnia.	Hypersensitivity reaction (rash, fever, malaise, fatigue, myalgia, arthralgia, blisters, mucosal involvement, conjunctivitis, facial edema, hepatitis, eosinophilia, angioedema, dyspnea), hepatotoxicity, depressive disorders.
Dolutegravir (Tivicay)	Insomnia and headache (2-4%)	Rash, liver injury reported. Increased ALT/AST in 203%. Competition with creatinine for tubular secretion increased serum creatinine by a mean of 0.1 mg/dL with no change in GFR.
Elvitegravir+ Cobicistat (Stribild)	Nausea and diarrhea are the two most common AEs. Increased serum creatinine 0.1-0.15 mg/dL due to inhibition of prox. tubular enzymes by cobicistat with no decrease in GFR.	**Same Black Box warnings as ritonavir and tenofovir (TDF and TAF)**. Rare lactic acidosis syndrome. Owing to renal toxicity, should not initiate Rx when pre-Rx eGFR is <70 cc/min. Follow serial serum creatinine and urinary protein and glucose. Discontinue drug if serum Cr rises >0.4 mg/dl above baseline value.
Raltegravir (Isentress)	Diarrhea, headache, insomnia, nausea. LFT ↑ may be more common in pts co-infected with HBV or HCV.	Hypersensitivity reactions can occur. Rash, Stevens-Johnson syndrome, toxic epidermal necrolysis reported. Hepatic failure reported. ↑CK, myopathy and rhabdomyolysis reported. ↑ of preexisting depression reported in 4 pts; all could continue raltegravir after adjustment of psych. meds. Chewable tablets contain phenylalanine.
Attachment Inhibitors		
Fostemsavir (Rukobia)	Headache, rash, nausea, vomiting, diarrhea, fatigue, lack of energy.	IRIS, QT-interval prolongation, elevations in liver transaminases in patients with HBV or HCV co-infection, potential for drug interactions.
Ibalizumab-uiyk (Trogarzo)	Diarrhea, dizziness, nausea, rash.	Watch for IRIS.
Capsid Inhibitor		
Lenacapavir (Sunlenca)	Injection site reactions, nausea, IRIS	Many drug-drug interactions

TABLE 14E – HEPATITIS A & HBV TREATMENT

Hepatitis A Virus (HAV)

1. Outbreaks in homeless populations. Vaccination is primary defense.
2. **Drug/Dosage:** No therapy recommended. If within 2 wks of exposure, prophylactic IVIG 0.1 mL per kg IM times 1 protective. Hep A vaccine equally effective as IVIG in randomized trial and is emerging as preferred Rx.
3. **HAV Superinfection:** 40% of pts with chronic Hepatitis C virus (HCV) infection who developed superinfection with HAV developed fulminant hepatic failure. Similarly, patients with chronic Hepatitis B virus (HBV) infection can suffer acute hepatic failure with HAV superinfection. **Hence, need to vaccinate all HBV and HCV pts with HAV vaccine.**

Hepatitis B Virus (HBV): Treatment

HBeAg Status	HBV DNA (Viral Load)	ALT	Fibrosis*	Treatment**	Comments
Pos	>20,000	<2x ULN	F0-F2	Observe	Low efficacy with current Rx; biopsy helpful in determining whether to Rx. Lean toward Rx if older age or + Family Hx HCC
Pos	>20,000	<2x ULN	F3-F4	Treat: IFN or NUC	**No IFN if decompensated cirrhosis**
Pos	>20,000	>2x ULN	Any	Treat: IFN or NUC	IFN has higher chance of seroconversion to HBeAg Negative and HBsAg Negative status.
Neg	<2000	<1x ULN	Any	Observe	Might Treat if F4; **No IFN if decompensated cirrhosis**
Neg	2,000-20,000	<2x ULN	F0-F2	Observe	
Neg	2,000-20,000	<2x ULN	F3-F4	Treat: NUC (or IFN)	NUCs favored if HBeAg negative; Treatment duration ill-defined. Certainly > 1 year, likely chronic Rx (indefinitely)
Neg	>20,000	>2x ULN	Any	Treat: NUC or IFN	NUCs favored if HBeAg negative; Treatment duration chronic / indefinite

References: *AASLD HBV Treatment Guidelines (www.aasld.org); Hepatology 50:1, 2009 and WHO Guidelines, 2024.*
* Liver Biopsy or fibrosure assay is helpful in determining when and how to treat.
** Treatment Regimens listed below.

HBV Treatment Regimens. Single drug therapy is usually sufficient; combination therapy recommended for HIV co-infection.

	Drug/Dose	Comments
Preferred Regimens	**Pegylated-Interferon-alpha 2a** 180 μg sc once weekly OR **Entecavir** 0.5 mg po once daily OR **Tenofovir alafenamide (TAF/ Vemlidy)** 25 mg po once daily **Tenofovir disoproxil (TDF)** 300 mg po once daily	PEG-IFN: Treat for 48 weeks Entecavir: Do not use Entecavir if Lamivudine resistance present. Entecavir/Tenofovir: Treat for at least 48 weeks after seroconversion from HBeAg to anti-HBe (if no mod-adv fibrosis present). Indefinite chronic therapy for HBeAg negative patients. Renal impairment dose adjustments necessary.
Alternative Regimens	**Lamivudine** 100 mg po once daily OR **Telbivudine** 600 mg po once daily OR **Emtricitabine** 200 mg po once daily (investigational) OR **Adefovir** 10 mg po once daily	These alternative agents are rarely used except in combination. When used, restrict to short term therapy owing to high rates of development of resistance. Not recommended as first-line therapy. Use of Adefovir has been replaced by Tenofovir-based regimens.
Preferred Regimen for HIV-HBV Co-Infected Patient	**Truvada** (TDF + FTC) OR **Descovy** (TAF + FTC) po once daily + another anti-HIV drug	ALL patients if possible as part of a fully suppressive anti-HIV/anti-HBV regimen. Continue therapy indefinitely.

TABLE 14F – HCV TREATMENT REGIMENS AND RESPONSE

1. **Hepatitis C virus (HCV) indications for Treatment.** Treatment is indicated for **all patients** with chronic HCV. Rx should be initiated urgently for those with more advanced fibrosis (F3 / F4) and those with underlying co-morbid conditions due to HCV. Type and duration of Rx is based on genotype and stage of fibrosis. Pegylated interferon (Peg-IFN) is no longer a recommended regimen; all DAA regimens with or without ribavirin are the preferred choice. Treatment also indicated for acute HCV infection with DAA agents potentially with shorter duration of therapy.

2. **Definitions of Response to Therapy.**

End of Treatment Response (ETR)	Undetectable at end of treatment.
Relapse	Undetectable at end of therapy (ETR) but rebound (detectable) virus within 24 weeks after therapy stopped.
Sustained Virologic Response (SVR)	CURE! Still undetectable at end of therapy and beyond 12-24 weeks after therapy is stopped.

3. **HCV Treatment Regimens.**
   - Biopsy is a 'gold standard' for staging HCV infection and is helpful in some settings to determine the ideal choice, dose and duration of HCV treatment. When bx not obtained, "non-invasive" tests are usually employed to assess the relative probability of advanced fibrosis or cirrhosis. Fibroscan (elastography) is a preferred means of assessing liver fibrosis. Elastography values of >10 kPa (Kilopascals) correlates with significant fibrosis (F3 or F4 disease).
   - Resistance tests: Genotypic resistance assays are available that can determine polymorphisms associated with reduction in susceptibility to some DAAs (e.g., protease inhibitors). **However, resistance tests are recommended only for those who have failed treatment with a prior NS5A or protease inhibitor regimen.**
   - **Patients with decompensated cirrhosis should only be treated by hepatologists owing to the risk of rapid clinical deterioration while receiving treatment for HCV.**
   - **Black Box Warning for ALL Direct Acting Agents (DAA):** Cases of HBV reactivation, occasionally fulminant, during or after DAA therapy have been reported in HBV/HCV coinfected patients who were not already on HBV suppressive therapy. **For HCV/HBV coinfected patients who are HBsAg+ and are not already on HBV suppressive therapy, monitoring HBV DNA levels during and immediately after DAA therapy for HCV is recommended and antiviral treatment for HBV should be given.** *See HBV treatment.*

CURRENT DRUGS FOR INITIAL TREATMENT FOR PATIENTS WITH CHRONIC HCV

- Drugs and regimens are evolving. For updates go to: web.sanfordguide.com and *www.hcvguidelines.org*

Agents/Abbreviation	Tradename	Formulation/Dosing Specifics
Daclatasvir (DCV)	Daklinza	60 mg tab po once daily. Note: decrease dose to 30 mg/d when co-administered with a strong CYP3A inhibitor, e.g., several ARV drugs; increase dose to 90 mg/d when co-administered with a mild-moderate CYP3A inducer. Contraindicated when co-administered with a strong CYP3A inducer.
Elbasvir + **Grazoprevir**	Zepatier	Fixed dose combination (Elbasvir 50 mg + Grazoprevir 100 mg) 1 tab po once daily
Glecaprevir + **Pibrentasvir**	Mavyret	Fixed dose combination (Glecaprevir 100 mg + Pibrentasvir 40 mg) 3 tabs once daily with food
Paritaprevir/ritonavir + **Ombitasvir** (PrO)	Technivie	Fixed dose combination (Paritaprevir 150 mg/ritonavir 100 mg + Ombitasvir 25 mg) 1 tab once daily
Paritaprevir/ritonavir + **Ombitasvir** + **Dasabuvir** (PrOD)	Viekira Pak	Fixed dose combination [(Paritaprevir 150 mg/ritonavir 100 mg + Ombitasvir 25 mg) 1 tab once daily + Dasabuvir 250 mg] 1 tab twice daily with food
	Viekira XR	Extended release fixed dose combination [(Dasabuvir 200 mg + Paritaprevir 50 mg/ritonavir 33.3 mg + Ombitasvir 8.33 mg) 3 tabs once daily with food
Simeprevir (SMV)	Olysio	150 mg tab po once daily with food
Sofosbuvir (SOF)	Sovaldi	400 mg tab po once daily
Sofosbuvir + **Ledipasvir**	Harvoni	Fixed dose combination (Sofosbuvir 400 mg + Ledipasvir 90 mg) 1 tab po once daily
Sofosbuvir + **Velpatasvir**	Epclusa	Fixed dose combination (Sofosbuvir 400 mg + Velpatasvir 100 mg): 1 tab po once daily
Sofosbuvir + **Velpatasvir** + **Voxilaprevir**	Vosevi	Fixed dose combination (Sofosbuvir 400 mg + Velpatasvir 100 mg + Voxilaprevir 100 mg): 1 tab po once daily with food
Ribavirin	Ribavirin, Copegus	Weight-based daily dosing: 1000 mg (Wt <75 kg) or 1200 mg (Wt >75 kg). Low dose: 600 mg/day. Taken with food
Pegylated interferon (alfa 2a)	Roferon, Intron-A, Peg-Intron, Pegasys	180 mcg sc per week (rarely used any more)

TABLE 14F (2)

HCV RECOMMENDED TREATMENT REGIMENS (P = Primary regimen, A = Alternative regimen, Regimens from prior page)

HCV Mono Infection				
Genotype	**Regimen**	**Cirrhosis**	**Duration**	**Comments**
1-6	**Epclusa** 1 tab po once daily	With or without	12 weeks	Pan-genotypic DAAs
	Mavyret 3 tabs po once daily	Without	8 weeks	
		With	12 weeks	
1a	**Epclusa** 1 tab po once daily	With or without	12 weeks	
	Harvoni 1 tab po once daily	Without*	8 weeks	* If patient is HIV-uninfected, non-cirrhotic, and HCV RNA <6 million c/mL
		With**	12 weeks	** If patient is HIV-co-infected, compensated cirrhosis, or HCV RNA >6 million c/mL
	Mavyret 3 tabs po once daily	With or Without	8 weeks	
	Zepatier 1 tab po once daily	With or without	12 weeks	If no baseline high-fold NS5A resistance associated mutations
1b	**Epclusa** 1 tab po once daily	With or without	12 weeks	
	Harvoni 1 tab po once daily	Without*	8 weeks	* If patient is HIV-uninfected, non-cirrhotic, and HCV RNA <6 million c/mL
		With**	12 weeks	** If patient is HIV-co-infected, compensated cirrhosis, or HCV RNA >6 million c/mL
	Mavyret 3 tabs po once daily	Without	8 weeks	
		With	12 weeks	
	Zepatier 1 tab po once daily	With or without	12 weeks	
2	**Epclusa** 1 tab po once daily	With or without	12 weeks	
	Mavyret 3 tabs po once daily	With or Without	8 weeks	
3	**Epclusa** 1 tab po once daily	With or without	12 weeks	Do not use in cirrhosis if RAV Y93H is present
	Mavyret 3 tabs po once daily	With or Without	8 weeks	
	Vosevi 1 tab po once daily	With	12 weeks	(RAS) Y93H is present. Alternative regimen.
4	**Epclusa** 1 tab po once daily	With or without	12 weeks	
	Harvoni 1 tab po once daily	With or without	12 weeks	
	Mavyret 3 tabs po once daily	With or without	8 weeks	
	Zepatier 1 tab po once daily	With or without	12 weeks	
5 & 6	**Epclusa** 1 tab po once daily	With or without	12 weeks	
	Harvoni 1 tab po once daily	With or without	12 weeks	
	Mavyret 3 tabs po once daily	Without	8 weeks	
		With	12 weeks	

TABLE 14F (3)

Genotype	Regimen	Cirrhosis	Duration	Comments
HCV-HIV Co-infection				
1a & 1b	Same as for HCV Mono Infection		8-12 weeks*	Watch for drug-drug interactions. * 8 weeks ONLY in HCV Rx naive co-infected patients receiving **Mavyret**; otherwise, minimum 12 weeks with any other regimen
2	Same as for HCV Mono Infection		8- 12 weeks*	Watch for drug-drug interactions. * 8 weeks ONLY in HCV Rx naive co-infected patients receiving **Mavyret**; otherwise, minimum 12 weeks with any other regimen
3	Same as for HCV Mono Infection			Watch for drug-drug interactions.
4, 5, 6	Same as for HCV Mono Infection			
Post-Liver Transplant				
1-6	**Mavyret** 3 tabs po once daily	With or Without	12 weeks	
	Epclusa 1 tab po once daily	With or Without	12 weeks	

TABLE 15A – ANTIMICROBIAL PROPHYLAXIS FOR SELECTED BACTERIAL INFECTIONS*

CLASS OF ETIOLOGIC AGENT/DISEASE/CONDITION	PROPHYLAXIS AGENT/DOSE/ROUTE/DURATION	COMMENTS
Group B streptococcal disease (GBS), neonatal: Approaches to management (CDC Guidelines, *MMWR 59 (RR-10):1, 2010; CID 2017;65(S2):S143*)		
Pregnant women—intrapartum antimicrobial prophylaxis procedures: 1. Screen all pregnant women with vaginal & rectal swab for GBS at 35–37 wks gestation (unless other indications for prophylaxis exist: GBS bacteriuria during this pregnancy or previously delivered infant with invasive GBS disease; even then cultures may be useful for susceptibility testing). Use transport medium; GBS survive at room temp. up to 96 hrs. **Rx during labor if swab culture positive.** 2. Rx during labor if previously delivered infant with invasive GBS infection, or if any GBS bacteriuria during this pregnancy. 3. Rx if GBS status unknown but if any of the following are present: (a) delivery at <37 wks gestation [*see MMWR 59 (RR-10): 1, 2010* algorithms for preterm labor and preterm premature rupture of membranes]; or (b) duration of ruptured membranes ≥18 hrs; or (c) intrapartum temp. ≥100.4°F (≥38.0°C). If amnionitis suspected, broad-spectrum antibiotic coverage should include an agent active vs. group B streptococci. 4. Rx if positive intra-partum NAAT for GBS. 5. Unless other conditions exist, Rx not indicated if: negative vaginal/rectal cultures at 35-37 wks gestation or C-section performed before onset of labor with intact amniotic membranes (use standard surgical prophylaxis).		**Regimens for prophylaxis against early-onset group B streptococcal disease in neonate used during labor:** **Pen G** 5 million Units IV (initial dose) then 2.5 to 3 million Units IV q4h until delivery Alternative: **AMP** 2 gm IV (initial dose) then 1 gm IV q4h until delivery Penicillin-allergic patients: • Patient not at high risk for anaphylaxis: **Cefazolin** 2 gm IV (initial dose) then 1 gm IV q8h until delivery • Patient at high risk for anaphylaxis from β-lactams: ○ If organism is both clindamycin- and erythromycin-susceptible, **or** is erythromycin-resistant, but clindamycin-susceptible confirmed by D-zone test (or equivalent) showing lack of inducible resistance: **Clinda** 900 mg IV q8h until delivery ○ If susceptibility of organism unknown, lack of inducible resistance to clindamycin has not been excluded, or patient is allergic to clindamycin: **Vanco** 1 gm IV q12h until delivery
Neonate of mother given prophylaxis	*See detailed algorithm in MMWR 59 (RR-10):1, 2010.*	
Preterm, premature rupture of the membranes: Grp B strep-negative women Cochrane Database Rev *12:CD00:1058, 2013; Obstet Gyn 124:515:2014; Am J Ob-Gyn 207:475. 2012.*	Primary Regimens: No antibiotic allergy. **Azithro** 1 gm po x 1 + **AMP** 2 gm IV q6h x 48h, then **Amox** 250 mg po q8h x 5 days Alternative Regimens: If mild pen allergy: **Azithro** 1 gm po x 1 + **Cefazolin** 1 gm IV q8h x 48 h, then **Cephalexin** 500 mg po q 6h x 5 days If IgE mediated allergy to penicillin (anaphylaxis): **Azithro** 1 gm po x 1 + **Clinda** 900 mg IV q 8h x 48h + **Gent** 5 mg/kg IV q 24h x two doses, then **Clinda** 300 mg po q 8h x 5 days If IgE mediated penicillin allergy plus clinda resistant gp B streptococci: **Azithro** 1 gm po x 1 + **Vanco** 20 mg/kg IV q 8h (max 2 g dose) x 48h	
Post-splenectomy bacteremia. Usually encapsulated bacteria: pneumococci, meningococci, H. flu type B; bacteremia: Enterobacter, S. aureus, Capnocytophaga, P. aeruginosa. Also at risk for fatal malaria, severe babesiosis. Asplenia review *(Chest 2016,150:1394)*	Antibiotic Prophylaxis: Child age < 5 years: **Amox** 20 mg/kg/day or **Pen VK** 125 mg bid Age > 5 years: **Pen VK** 250 mg bid x at least 1 year post-splenectomy Some recommend prophylaxis for a minimum of 3 years or until at least age 18 years. All ages: Maintain immunizations PLUS If not taking daily prophylaxis: self-administer **Amox-clav** with any febrile illness while seeking physician assistance. Sickle cell disease: Child age < 5 years: **Pen VK** 125 mg po bid Age > 5 years: **Pen VK** 250 mg po bid or **Amox** 20 mg/kg/day Alternative Regimens: Alternative for self-administered therapy at onset of fever: Cefuroxime axetil can be used in the penicillin-allergic patient who is not allergic to cephalosporins. Alternatively, respiratory **FQ** can be considered in beta-lactam-allergic patient in appropriate populations. If Penicillin allergy: **TMP-SMX** or **Clarithro** are options, but resistance in Strep. pneumoniae may be significant in some areas, particularly among penicillin-resistant isolates.	

TABLE 15A (2)

CLASS OF ETIOLOGIC AGENT/DISEASE/CONDITION	PROPHYLAXIS AGENT/DOSE/ROUTE/DURATION	COMMENTS
Sexual Exposure		
Sexual assault survivor [likely agents and risks, *see CDC Guidelines at MMWR 64(RR-3):1, 2015]*. For review of overall care: *NEJM 365:834, 2011.*	Primary Regimens for Sexual assault, anatomic female: (**Ceftriaxone** 500 mg IM) + (**Metro** 500 mg po bid x 7 days) + [(Doxy 100 mg po bid x 7 days)]. *See Comments.* Anatomic male: (**Ceftriaxone** 500 mg IM) or (**Cefixime** 400 mg po single dose)] + (**Metro** 2 gm po single dose) + [(**Doxy** 100 mg po bid for 7 days)]. Give 1 g IM **Ceftriaxone** if >150 kg HIV and/or Hep B post-exposure prophylaxis as appropriate Sexual contact, to cover gonococci and chlamydia: (*Ceftriaxone* 500 mg IM once) for Gonococci + (**Doxy** 100 mg po bid x 7 days) for Chlamydia Give 1 gm **Ceftriaxone** if >150 kg Syphilis, post-exposure prophylaxis: Open label randomized study in men that have sex with men *(Lancet Infect Dis 2018;18:308)*. **Doxy** 200 mg po x 1 dose within 72hrs of exposure. 73% decrease in development of syphilis	• Obtain expert individualized advice re: forensic exam and specimens, pregnancy (incl. emergency contraception), physical trauma, psychological support • Test for chlamydia and gonococci at sites of penetration or attempted penetration by NAATs. Obtain molecular tests for trichomonas and check vaginal secretions for BV and candidiasis. • Serological evaluation for syphilis, HIV, HBV, HCV • Initiate post-exposure protocols for HBV vaccine, HIV post-exposure prophylaxis as appropriate • HPV vaccine recommended for females 9-26 or males 9-21, if not already immunized • Follow-up in 1 week to review results, repeat negative tests in 1-2 weeks to detect infections not detected previously, repeat syphilis testing 4-6 weeks and 3 months, repeat HIV testing 6 weeks and 3-6 months. • Check for anogenital warts at 1-2 months. Notes: If ceftriaxone not available, can use cefixime 400 mg po once in its place for prevention of gonorrhea, but the latter is less effective for pharyngeal infection and against strains with reduced susceptibility to cephalosporins. For non-pregnant individuals who cannot receive cephalosporins, treatment with (Gemifloxacin 320 mg po once + azithro 2 gm po once) or (Gentamicin 240 mg IM once + azithro 2 gm po once) can be substituted for ceftriaxone/azithro.
Contact with specific sexually transmitted diseases. *See comprehensive guidelines for specific pathogens in MMWR 64(RR-3):1, 2015.*		
Syphilis exposure		Presumptive rx for exposure within 3 mos., as tests may be negative. *See Table 1, page 26.* If exposure occurred >90 days prior, establish dx or treat empirically.
Sickle-cell disease. Likely agent: S. pneumoniae *(see post-splenectomy, above)* Ref.: *NEJM 376: 1561, 2017*	Children <5 yrs: **Pen V** 62.5 to 125 mg po bid ≥5 yrs: **Pen V** 250 mg po bid (Alternative in children: **Amox** 20 mg/kg/day)	Start prophylaxis by 2 mos. *(Pediatrics 106:367, 2000);* continue until at least age 5. When to d/c must be individualized. Age-appropriate vaccines, including pneumococcal, Hib, influenza, meningococcal. Treating infections, consider possibility of penicillin non-susceptible pneumococci. May need malaria prophylaxis entire life.

TABLE 15B – ANTIBIOTIC PROPHYLAXIS TO PREVENT SURGICAL INFECTIONS IN ADULTS*

2013 Guidelines: Am J Health Syst Pharm 70:195, 2013; Med Lett 58:63, 2016

General Comments:
- To be optimally effective, antibiotics must be started within 60 minutes of the surgical incision. Vancomycin and FQs may require 1-2 hr infusion time, so start dose 2 hrs before the surgical incision.
- Most applications employ a single preoperative dose or continuation for less than 24 hrs.
- For procedures lasting >2 half-lives of prophylactic agent, intraoperative supplementary dose(s) may be required.
- Dose adjustments may be desirable in pts with BMI >30.
- Prophylaxis does carry risk: e.g., C. difficile colitis, allergic reactions
- Active S. aureus screening, decolonization & customized antimicrobial prophylaxis demonstrated efficacious in decreasing infections after hip, knee & cardiac surgery *(JAMA 313:2131 & 2162, 2015)*.
- See additional details for prevention of surgical site infections by CDC *(JAMA Surg 152: 784, 2017)* and Am Coll Surg/Surg Infect Soc *(J Am Coll Surg 224: 59, 2016)*. Both support no further antibiotics once surgical wound is closed, although latter includes possible exceptions: breast reconstruction, joint arthroplasty, and cardiac procedures.

Use of Vancomycin:
- For many common prophylaxis indications, vancomycin is considered an alternative to β-lactams in pts allergic to or intolerant of the latter.
- Vancomycin use may be justifiable in centers where rates of post-operative infection with methicillin-resistant staphylococci are high or in pts at high risk for these.
- Unlike β-lactams in common use, vancomycin has no activity against gram-negative organisms. **When gram-negative bacteria are a concern following specific procedures, it may be necessary or desirable to add a second agent with appropriate in vitro activity.** This can be done using cefazolin with vancomycin in the non-allergic pt, or in pts intolerant of β-lactams using vancomycin with another ram-negative agent (e.g., aminoglycoside, fluoroquinolone, possibly aztreonam, if pt not allergic; local resistance patterns and pt factors would influence choice).
- Infusion of vancomycin, especially too rapidly, may result in hypotension or other manifestations of histamine release (vancomycin infusion reaction). Does not indicate an allergy to vancomycin.

TYPE OF SURGERY	PROPHYLAXIS	COMMENTS
Cardiovascular Surgery		
Antibiotic prophylaxis in cardiovascular surgery has been proven beneficial in the following procedures: • Reconstruction of abdominal aorta • Procedures on the leg that involve a groin incision • Any vascular procedure that inserts prosthesis/ foreign body • Lower extremity amputation for ischemia • Cardiac surgery • Permanent Pacemakers *(Circulation 121:458, 2010)* • Heart transplant • Implanted cardiac defibrillators	**Cefazolin** 1–2 gm (Wt <120 kg) or 3 gm (Wt >120 kg) IV as a single dose or q8h for 1–2 days or **Cefuroxime** 1.5 gm IV as a single dose or q12h for total of 6 gm or **Vanco** 1 gm IV as single dose or q12h for 1–2 days. For pts weighing >90 kg, use vanco 1.5 gm IV as a single dose or q12h for 1-2 days. Re-dose cefazolin q4h if CrCl>30 mL/min or q8h if CrCl ≤30 mL/min Consider **intranasal Mupirocin** evening before, day of surgery & bid for 5 days post-op in pts with pos. nasal culture for S. aureus. Mupirocin resistance has been encountered.	**Timing & duration:** Single infusion just before surgery as effective as multiple doses. No prophylaxis needed for cardiac catheterization. For prosthetic heart valves, customary to stop prophylaxis either after removal of retrosternal drainage catheters or just a 2nd dose after coming off bypass. **Vanco** may be preferable in hospitals with ↑ freq of MRSA, in high-risk pts, those colonized with MRSA or for Pen-allergic pts. **Clindamycin** 900 mg IV is another alternative for Pen-allergic or Vanco-allergic pt. Implanted devices ref: *JAC 70:325, 2015.* For insertion of ventricular assist devices, prophylaxis same as for cardiac surgery (e.g., cefazolin ± vancomycin) *(CID 64: 222, 2017)*.
Gastric, Biliary and Colonic Surgery		
Gastroduodenal/Biliary		
Gastroduodenal, includes percutaneous endoscopic gastrostomy (high risk only), pancreaticoduodenectomy (Whipple procedure)	**Cefazolin** (1-2 gm IV) or **Cefoxitin** (1-2 gm IV) or **Cefotetan** (1-2 gm IV) or **Ceftriaxone** (2 gm IV) as a single dose (some give additional doses q12h for 2–3 days*). See Comment*	Gastroduodenal (PEG placement): High-risk is marked obesity, obstruction, ↓ gastric acid or ↓ motility. Re-dose Cefazolin q4h and Cefoxitin q2h if CrCl >30 mL/min; q8h and q4h, respectively, if CrCl ≤30 mL/min
Biliary, includes laparoscopic cholecystectomy	Low risk, laparoscopic: No prophylaxis Open cholecystectomy: **Cefazolin, Cefoxitin, Cefotetan**	Biliary high-risk or open procedure: age >70, acute cholecystitis, non-functioning gallbladder, obstructive jaundice or common duct stones. With cholangitis, treat as infection, not prophylaxis.
Endoscopic retrograde cholangiopancreatography	No rx without obstruction. If obstruction: **CIP** 500–750 mg po or 400 mg IV 2 hrs prior to procedure or **Pip-tazo** 4.5 gm IV 1 hr prior to procedure	Most studies show that **achieving adequate drainage** will prevent post-procedural cholangitis or sepsis and no further benefit from prophylactic antibiotics; greatest benefit likely when complete drainage cannot be achieved. *See Gastroint Endosc 81: 81, 2015 for American Society of Gastrointestinal Endoscopy recommendations for ERCP; Gut 58:868, 2009.*

TABLE 15B (2)

TYPE OF SURGERY	PROPHYLAXIS	COMMENTS
Gastric, Biliary and Colonic Surgery *(continued)*		
Colorectal, elective colectomies Recommend combination of: • Mechanical bowel prep • po antibiotic *(See Comment)* • IV antibiotic Ref: *Ann Surg 2015;261:1034; Dis Colon Rectum 2019;62:3*	*Parenteral (emergency or elective surgery):* **Cefazolin** 1-2 gm IV + **Metro** 0.5 gm IV. Some experts routinely use cefazolin 2 gm with an increase to 3 gm if patient is >120 kg. Need to repeat the cefazolin dose 4 hrs. after the initial pre-op dose. NOTE: cefazolin and metronidazole can be mixed together in same IV bag (sometimes referred to as "cefanidazole"). **Cefoxitin** 2 gm IV or **Cefotetan** 2 gm IV (if available). NOTE: Increasing resistance of pertinent anaerobes to both cefoxitin and cefotetan. Further, the short half-life of cefoxitin requires frequent re-dosing. **Amp-Sulb** 3 gm IV. Many centers experiencing increasing resistance of aerobic gram-negatives to Amp-Sulb. No longer recommended for empiric therapy of peritonitis. **Ceftriaxone** 2 gm IV + **Metro** 500 mg IV. NOTE: This regimen may be useful in centers with high rates of resistance to first and second generation cephalosporins. **Erta** 1 gm IV	**Oral regimens: Neomycin + Erythro**. Pre-op day: (1) 10 am 4 L polyethylene glycol electrolyte solution (Colyte, GoLYTELY) po over 2 hr. (2) Clear liquid diet only. (3) 1 pm, 2 pm & 11 pm, Neomycin 1 gm + Erythro base 1 gm po. (4) NPO after midnight. Alternative regimens have been less well studied; GoLYTELY 1–6 pm, then Neomycin 2 gm po + Metronidazole 2 gm po at 7 pm & 11 pm. **Beta lactam allergy: Clinda** 900 mg IV + (**Gent** 5 mg/kg or **Aztreonam** 2 gm IV or **CIP** 400 mg IV)
Ruptured viscus: *See Peritoneum/Peritonitis, Secondary, Table 1, page 52.*		
Head and Neck Surgery		
	Cefazolin 2 gm IV (Single dose) (some add **Metro** 500 mg IV) OR **Clinda** 600-900 mg IV (single dose) ± **Gent** 5 mg/kg IV (single dose) *(See Table 10C for weight-based dose calculation)*.	Antimicrobial prophylaxis in head & neck surg appears efficacious only for procedures involving oral/ pharyngeal mucosa (e.g., laryngeal or pharyngeal tumor) but even with prophylaxis, wound infection rate can be high. **Clean, uncontaminated head & neck surg does not require prophylaxis.** Re-dose cefazolin q4h if CrCl>30 mL/min or q8h if CrCl ≤30 mL/min
Neurosurgical Procedures		
Clean, non-implant; e.g., elective craniotomy	**Cefazolin** 2 gm IV as single dose for clean procedures with prosthesis (repeat dose for procedures longer than 4 hours) (**Cefazolin** 2 gm IV or **Cefuroxime** 1.5 gm IV) as a single dose (repeat dose for procedures longer than 4 hours) + **Metro** 500 mg IV as a single dose for clean-contaminated procedures **Amp-sulb** 3 gm IV as a single dose for clean-contaminated procedures; repeat dose for procedures longer than 2 hours	Clindamycin 900 mg IV is alternative for vanco-allergic or beta-lactam allergic pt. Re-dose cefazolin q4h if CrCl>30 mL/min or q8h if CrCl ≤30 mL/min
Clean, contaminated (cross sinuses, or naso/oropharynx)	**Clinda** 900 mg IV (single dose)	British recommend Amoxicillin-Clavulanate 1.2 gm IV[NUS] or (Cefuroxime 1.5 gm IV + Metronidazole 0.5 gm IV)
CSF shunt surgery, intrathecal pumps:	**Cefazolin** 1-2 gm (Wt <120 kg) or 3 gm (Wt >120 kg) IV once. Alternative: **Vanco** 1 gm IV once; for pts weighing >90 kg, use vanco 1.5 gm IV as single dose OR **Clinda** 900 mg IV.	Randomized study in a hospital with high prevalence of infection due to methicillin-resistant staphylococci showed Vancomycin was more effective than cefazolin in preventing CSF shunt infections *(J Hosp Infect 69:337, 2008)*. Re-dose cefazolin q4h if CrCl >30 mL/min or q8h if CrCl ≤30 mL/min

TABLE 15B (3)

TYPE OF SURGERY	PROPHYLAXIS	COMMENTS
Obstetric/Gynecologic Surgery		
Vaginal or abdominal hysterectomy	**Cefazolin** 2 gm or **Cefoxitin** 2 gm or **Cefotetan** 2 gm or **Amp-sulb** 3 gm IV 30 min. before surgery.	Alternative: (**Clinda** 900 mg IV or **Vanco** 1 gm IV) + (**Gent** 5 mg/kg x 1 dose or **Aztreonam** 2 gm IV or **CIP** 400 mg IV) OR (**Metro** 500 mg IV + **CIP** 400 mg IV)
Cesarean section for premature rupture of membranes or active labor	**Cefazolin** 2 gm IV x 1 dose Alternative: **Clinda** 900 mg IV + (**Gent** 5 mg/kg IV or **Tobra** 5 mg/kg IV) x 1 dose. Increased risk of infection vs. cefazolin *(Obstet Gyn 2018;132:948)*.	Administering prophylaxis before the skin incision reduces surgical site infections. **In non-elective C-section,** addition of **Azithro** 500 mg IV in addition to standard antibiotics significantly decreased endometritis and wound infections *(NEJM 375: 1231, 2016)*. **In obesity**, give standard pre-op prophylaxis, then (Cephalexin 500 mg po q8h + Metro 500 mg po q8h) x 18 hrs *(JAMA 2017;318:1012 & 1026)*
Surgical Abortion (1st trimester)	1st trimester: **Doxy** 300 mg po: 100 mg 1 hr before procedure + 200 mg post-procedure.	Meta-analysis showed benefit of antibiotic prophylaxis in all risk groups.
Ophthalmic Surgery	(**Neomycin-Gent-Polymyxin B** or **Gati** or **Moxi**) eye drops, 1 drop q5-15 min x 5 doses	Some add **Cefazolin** 100 mg under conjunctiva at end of surgery.
Orthopedic Surgery		
Hip arthroplasty, spinal fusion	Same as cardiac surgery	Customarily stopped after "Hemovac" removed. 2013 Guidelines recommend stopping prophylaxis within 24 hrs of surgery *(Am J Health Syst Pharm 70:195, 2013)*.
Total joint replacement (other than hip)	Primary Regimens: *Repair of hip fracture, spine surgery, and joint replacements:* **Cefazolin** 2 gm IV as a single dose (3 gm IV if weight ≥ 120 kg) ADD **Vanco** 1 gm IV as single dose (use 1.5 gm IV if >90 kg), if patient is colonized with MRSA (also suggested for joint replacement in institutions with high rates of MRSA infection) If additional doses are preferred, use appropriate therapeutic dosing for no more than 24h	2013 Guidelines recommends stopping prophylaxis within 24 hrs of surgery (*Am J Health Syst Pharm 70:195, 2013)*. Usual to administer before tourniquet inflation. Intranasal mupirocin if colonized with S. aureus.
Open reduction of closed fracture with internal fixation	**Ceftriaxone** 2 gm IV once	3.6% (ceftriaxone) vs 8.3% (for placebo) infection found in Dutch trauma trial *(Ln 347:1133, 1996)*. Several alternative antimicrobials can ↓ risk of infection *(Cochrane Database Syst Rev 2010: CD 000244)*.
Prophylaxis to protect prosthetic joints from hematogenous infection related to distant procedures (patients with plates, pins and screws only are not considered to be at risk)	• A prospective, case-control study concluded that antibiotic prophylaxis for dental procedures did not decrease the risk of hip or knee prosthesis infection *(Clin Infect Dis 50:8, 2010)*. • An expert panel of the American Dental Association concluded that, in general, prophylactic antibiotics are not recommended prior to dental procedures to prevent prosthetic joint infection *(J Amer Dental Assoc 146: 11, 2015)*. • Individual circumstances should be considered; when there is planned manipulation of tissues thought to be actively infected, antimicrobial therapy for the infection is likely to be appropriate.	
Peritoneal Dialysis Catheter Placement	**Vanco** single 1 gm IV dose 12 hrs prior to procedure	Effectively reduced peritonitis during 14 days post-placement in 221 pts: Vanco 1%, Cefazolin 7%, placebo 12% (p=0.02) *(Am J Kidney Dis 36:1014, 2000)*.

TABLE 15B (4)

TYPE OF SURGERY	PROPHYLAXIS	COMMENTS
Urologic Surgery/Procedures • See *Best Practice Policy Statement* of Amer. Urological Assoc. (AUA) *(J Urol 179:1379, 2008)* and 2013 Guidelines *(Am J Health Syst Pharm 70:195, 2013)*. • Selection of agents targeting urinary pathogens may require modification based on local resistance patterns; ↑ TMP-SMX and/or fluoroquinolone (FQ) resistance among enteric gram-negative bacteria is a concern.		
Cystoscopy	• Prophylaxis generally not necessary if urine is sterile (however, AUA recommends FQ or TMP-SMX for those with several potentially adverse host factors (e.g., advanced age, immunocompromised state, anatomic abnormalities, etc.) • Treat patients with UTI prior to procedure using an antimicrobial active against pathogen isolated	
Cystoscopy with manipulation	**CIP** 500 mg po (**TMP-SMX** 1 DS tablet po may be an alternative in populations with low rates of resistance)	Procedures mentioned include ureteroscopy, biopsy, fulguration, TURP, etc. Treat UTI with targeted therapy before procedure if possible.
Transrectal prostate biopsy	**CIP** 500 mg po 12 hrs prior to biopsy and repeated 12 hrs after 1st dose. *See Comment.*	Bacteremia 7% with **CIP** vs 37% with **Gent** *(JAC 39:115, 1997)*. **Levofloxacin** 500 mg 30-60 min before procedure was effective in low risk pts; additional doses were given for ↑ risk (J Urol 168:1021, 2002). Serious bacteremias due to FQ-resistant organisms have been encountered in patients receiving FQ prophylaxis. Screening stool cultures pre-procedure for colonization with FQ-resistant organisms is increasingly utilized to inform choice of prophylaxis (Clin Infect Dis 60: 979, 2015). One study showed non-significant decrease in risk of infection with culture-directed antimicrobial prophylaxis (Urology 146: 11, 2015). Pre-operative prophylaxis should be determined on an institutional basis based on susceptibility profiles of prevailing organisms. Although 2nd or 3rd generation Cephalosporins or addition of single-dose gentamicin has been suggested, infections due to ESBL-producing and gent-resistant organisms have been encountered *(Urol 74:332, 2009)*. Meta-analysis found fosfomycin trometamol more effective than FQ in preventing infection after transrectal prostate biopsy *(World J Urol: 36: 323, 2018)*.
Other		
Breast surgery, herniorrhaphy, thoracotomy	**Cefazolin** 1-2 gm IV x 1 dose or **Amp-sulb** 3 gm IV x 1 dose or **Clinda** 900 mg IV x 1 dose or **Vanco** 1 gm IV x 1 dose (1.5 gm if wt >90 kg)	*Am J Health Syst Pharm 70:195, 2013.*
Vascular surgery: aneurysm repair, revascularization	**Cefazolin** 2 gm IV x 1 dose	

TABLE 15C – ANTIMICROBIAL PROPHYLAXIS FOR THE PREVENTION OF BACTERIAL ENDOCARDITIS IN PATIENTS WITH UNDERLYING CARDIAC CONDITIONS*

Reference for updated AHA guidelines: *Circulation. 2021;143:e963-e978*

- Antibiotic prophylaxis for dental procedures is now directed at individuals who are likely to suffer the most devastating consequences should they develop endocarditis. Prophylaxis to prevent endocarditis is no longer specified for gastrointestinal or genitourinary procedures. The following is adapted from and reflects the new AHA recommendations. *See original publication for explanation and precise details.*

SELECTION OF PATIENTS FOR ENDOCARDITIS PROPHYLAXIS				
FOR PATIENTS WITH ANY OF THESE HIGH-RISK CARDIAC CONDITIONS ASSOCIATED WITH ENDOCARDITIS:	**WHO UNDERGO DENTAL PROCEDURES INVOLVING:**	**WHO UNDERGO INVASIVE RESPIRATORY PROCEDURES INVOLVING:**	**WHO UNDERGO INVASIVE PROCEDURES OF THE GI OR GU TRACTS:**	**WHO UNDERGO PROCEDURES INVOLVING INFECTED SKIN AND SOFT TISSUES:**
Prosthetic heart valves Previous infective endocarditis Congenital heart disease with any of the following: • Completely repaired cardiac defect using prosthetic material (Only for 1st 6 months) • Partially corrected but with residual defect near prosthetic material • Uncorrected cyanotic congenital heart disease • Surgically constructed shunts and conduits Valvulopathy following heart transplant [Benefit unclear in pt with ventricular assist device *(CID 64: 222, 2017)*.]	Any manipulation of gingival tissue, dental periapical regions, or perforating the oral mucosa. **PROPHYLAXIS RECOMMENDED‡** *(see Dental Procedures Regimens table below)* (Prophylaxis is *not* recommended for routine anesthetic injections (unless through infected area), dental x-rays, shedding of primary teeth, adjustment of orthodontic appliances or placement of orthodontic brackets or removable appliances.)	Incision of respiratory tract mucosa **CONSIDER PROPHYLAXIS** *(see Dental Procedures Regimens table)* OR For treatment of established infection **PROPHYLAXIS RECOMMENDED** *(see Dental Procedures Regimens table for oral flora,* but include anti-staphylococcal coverage when *S. aureus* is of concern)	PROPHYLAXIS is no longer recommended solely to prevent endocarditis, **but the following approach is reasonable:** For patients with enterococcal UTIs • treat before elective GU procedures • include enterococcal coverage in perioperative regimen for non-elective procedures† For patients with existing GU or GI infections or those who receive perioperative antibiotics to prevent surgical site infections or sepsis • it is reasonable to include agents with anti-enterococcal activity in perioperative coverage†	Include coverage against staphylococci and β-hemolytic streptococci in treatment regimens

† Agents with anti-enterococcal activity include penicillin, ampicillin, amoxicillin, vancomycin and others. Check susceptibility if available. *(See Table 5 for highly resistant organisms.)*
‡ 2008 AHA/ACC focused update of guidelines on valvular heart disease use term "is reasonable" to reflect level of evidence *(Circulation 118:887, 2008)*.

PROPHYLACTIC REGIMENS FOR DENTAL PROCEDURES		
SITUATION	**AGENT**	**REGIMEN[1]**
Usual oral prophylaxis	**Amox**	Adults 2 gm, children 50 mg per kg; orally, 1 hour before procedure
Unable to take oral medications	**AMP[2]**	Adults 2 gm, children 50 mg per kg; IV or IM, within 30 min before procedure.
Allergic to penicillins	**Cephalexin[3]**	Adults 2 gm, children 50 mg per kg; orally, 1 hour before procedure
	Azithro or **Clarithro**	Adults 500 mg, children 15 mg per kg; orally, 1 hour before procedure
Allergic to penicillins and unable to take oral medications	**Cefazolin[3]** or **Ceftriaxone**	Adults 1 gm, children 50 mg per kg; IV or IM, within 30 min before procedure

[1] Children's dose should not exceed adult dose. AHA document lists all doses as 30-60 min before procedure.
[2] AHA lists Cefazolin or Ceftriaxone (at appropriate doses) as alternatives here.
[3] Cephalosporins should not be used in individuals with immediate-type hypersensitivity reaction (urticaria, angioedema, or anaphylaxis) to penicillins or other β-lactams. AHA proposes ceftriaxone as potential alternative to cefazolin; and other 1st or 2nd generation cephalosporin in equivalent doses as potential alternatives to cephalexin.

TABLE 15D – MANAGEMENT OF EXPOSURE TO HIV-1 AND HEPATITIS B AND C*

OCCUPATIONAL EXPOSURE TO BLOOD, PENILE/VAGINAL SECRETIONS OR OTHER POTENTIALLY INFECTIOUS BODY FLUIDS OR TISSUES WITH RISK OF TRANSMISSION OF HEPATITIS B/C AND/OR HIV-1 (E.G., NEEDLESTICK INJURY)

Free consultation for occupational exposures, call (PEPline) 1-888-448-4911. *[Information also available at www.aidsinfo.nih.gov]*

General steps in management:

1. Wash clean wounds/flush mucous membranes immediately (use of caustic agents or squeezing the wound is discouraged; data lacking regarding antiseptics).
2. Assess risk by doing the following: (a) Characterize exposure; (b) Determine/evaluate source of exposure by medical history, risk behavior, & testing for hepatitis B/C, HIV; (c) Evaluate and test exposed individual for hepatitis B/C & HIV.

Hepatitis B Occupational Exposure Prophylaxis *MMWR 67:1-31, 2018 (https://www.cdc.gov/mmwr/volumes/67/rr/rr6701a1.htm)*

Exposed Person Vaccine Status	Exposure Source		
	HBs Ag+	**HBs Ag–**	**Status Unknown or Unavailable for Testing[†]**
Unvaccinated	Give HBIG 0.06 mL per kg IM & initiate HB vaccine	Initiate HB vaccine	Initiate HB vaccine
Vaccinated (antibody status unknown)	Do anti-HBs on exposed person: If titer ≥10 milli-International units per mL, no rx If titer <10 milli-International units per mL, give HBIG + 1 dose HB vaccine**	No rx necessary	Do anti-HBs on exposed person: If titer ≥10 milli-International units per mL, no rx § If titer <10 milli-International units per mL, give 1 dose of HB vaccine**

§ Persons previously infected with HBV are immune to reinfection and do not require postexposure prophylaxis.

For known vaccine series responder (titer ≥10 milli-International units per mL), monitoring of levels or booster doses not currently recommended. Known non-responder (<10 milli-International units per mL) to 1º series HB vaccine & exposed to either HBsAg+ source or suspected high-risk source—rx with HBIG & re-initiate vaccine series **or** give 2 doses HBIG 1 month apart. For non-responders after a 2nd vaccine series, 2 doses HBIG 1 month apart is preferred approach to new exposure.

HEPSILAV (recombinant, adjuvanted HBV) vaccine preferred for 2nd vaccine series among those who did not respond to first vaccination series.

If known high risk source, treat as if source were HBsAG positive.

** Follow-up to assess vaccine response or address completion of vaccine series.

Hepatitis B Non-Occupational Exposure & Reactivation of Latent Hepatitis B

Non-Occupational Exposure

- Exposure to blood or sexual secretion of HBsAg-positive person
  - Percutaneous (bite, needlestick)
  - Sexual assault
- Initiate immunoprophylaxis within 24 hrs or sexual exposure & no more than 7 days after parenteral exposure
- Use Guidelines for occupational exposure for use of HBIG and HBV vaccine

Reactivation of Latent HBV *(AnIM 164:30 & 64, 2016)*

- Patients requiring administration of anti-CD 20 monoclonal antibodies as part of treatment selected malignancies, rheumatoid arthritis and vasculitis are at risk for reactivation of latent HBV
- Use of two FDA-approved anti-CD 20 drugs: ofatumumab (Arzerra) & rituximab (Rituxan) put patients at risk
- Prior to starting anti-CD 20 drug, test for latent HBV with test for HBsAg and Anti IgG HB core antibody & perhaps HIV PCR. Positive HBsAg and/or Anti IgG HBc AB = occult Hepatitis B
- **If pt has latent (occult) HBV & anti-CD 20 treatment is necessary, treatment should include an effective anti-HBV drug** *(see Table 14E)*

Hepatitis C Exposure *(MMWR July 24, 2020 / 69(6);1-8)*

- Determine HCV status for both exposed person &, if possible, exposure source (index patients).
  - If source + or unknown and exposed person negative: re-check follow-up HCV testing for HCV RNA 3 - 6 weeks post-exposure (detectable in blood in 1-3 weeks)
  - If remains negative: re-check at 6 months (this coincides with repeat HBV testing) with anti-HCV Antibody, and if positive, reflex to HCV RNA
- A positive HCV RNA test should be referred for treatment with DAA Rx as per Acute HCV Infection guidelines
- NO Post-Exposure prophylaxis is indicated

A. HIV OCCUPATIONAL EXPOSURE

The decision to initiate post-exposure prophylaxis (PEP) is a clinical judgment made in concert with the exposed individual and is based on three factors:

1. Type of exposure
   a. Potentially infectious substances include: blood, unfixed tissues, CSF; semen and vaginal secretions (these have not been implicated in occupational transmission of HIV); synovial, pleural, peritoneal, ascitic, and amniotic fluids; other visibly bloody fluids.
   b. Fluids of low or negligible risk for transmission, unless visibly bloody include: urine, sweat, vomitus, stool, saliva, nasal secretions, tears, and sputum. **PEP is not indicated.**
   c. If the exposure occurred to intact skin, regardless of whether the substance is potentially infectious or not, and regardless of the HIV status of the source patient, **PEP is not indicated.**
   d. If the exposure occurred to mucous membranes (e.g., blood splash to the eye) or non-intact skin (e.g., abraded skin, open wound, dermatitis) or occurred percutaneously as a consequence of a needle stick, scalpel, or other sharps injury or cut, then **PEP may be indicated.** Human bites resulting in a break in the skin could theoretically transmit HIV, particularly if oral blood is present, although these have not been implicated in occupational transmission of HIV.

2. Likelihood that the source patient is HIV infected
   a. If the exposure constitutes a risk of HIV transmission as described above and the source patient is **known positive for HIV**, then **PEP should be instituted** immediately, within hours of exposure (Animal studies show PEP less effective when started >72h post-exposure but interval after which PEP not beneficial is unknown; initiation of PEP after a longer interval may be considered if exposure risk of transmission is high).
   b. If exposure constitutes a risk of HIV transmission, and the HIV status is **unknown**, but patient is **likely to be HIV infected** or there is a **reasonable suspicion** for infection based on HIV risk factors, then **PEP should be initiated pending confirmation of the source patient's HIV status.**
      i. If a rapid HIV test of the source patient can be performed, it is reasonable to withhold therapy pending results of this test and initiating PEP if the test is positive.
      ii. If rapid testing cannot be performed, PEP should be initiated pending results of source patient testing and discontinued if the test returns negative.
      iii. NOTE: Antibody testing is sufficient to rule out HIV infection, unless the source patient has suspected acute retroviral syndrome, in which case HIV viral load testing is recommended.
   c. If the **source is unknown** or the source is known but status and risk cannot be determined, the decision to initiate PEP should be made on a case-by-case basis in **consultation with an expert** (PEPline at *http://www.nccc.ucsf.edu/about_nccc/pepline/*) (1-888-448-4911), guided by the severity of the exposure and epidemiologic likelihood of HIV exposure.

3. Adverse effects and potential for drug interactions with the PEP regimen
   a. Newer agents are better tolerated and should allow a higher proportion of exposed healthcare providers to complete the prescribed four-week course of therapy. Doses of some agents may need to be adjusted based on renal function.
   b. Information about drug interactions is available in Tables 16A and 16B, in the package insert and on-line at *hivinsite.ucsf.edu*
   c. Breast feeding and pregnancy are not contraindications to PEP.

PEP Algorithm

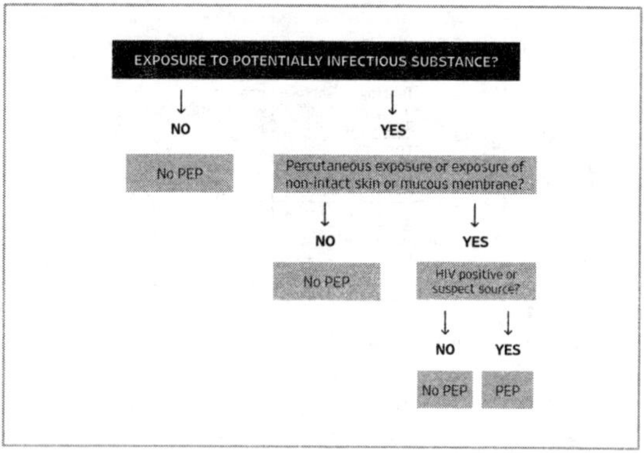

REGIMENS FOR PEP: a 4-week course of 3 or more drugs now routinely recommended for all PEP

Preferred	• **Descovy** (FTC 200 mg + TAF)(but not recommended if CrCl <30 mL/min) po once daily + (**Raltegravir** 1200 mg (two 600 tabs) once daily or **Dolutegravir** 50 mg orally daily); OR **Bictegravir** (FTC + TAF fixed dose formulation) one tab once daily • Creatinine clearance < 30 ml/min: [**Tenofovir disoproxil fumarate** (TDF) 300 mg q72-96h + **Emtricitabine** (FTC) 200 mg q72-96h + (**Dolutegravir** 50 mg po once daily OR **Raltegravir** 400 mg po twice daily]
Alternative	**Descovy** po once daily + ([DRV 800 mg po once daily + RTV 100 mg po once daily] or [**Prezcobix** (DRV 800 mg + Cobi 150 mg) one tab once daily])
	Descovy po once daily + **Lopinavir-Ritonavir** 800/200 mg po once daily
	Creatinine clearance < 30 ml/min: Renally adjusted doses of **Zidovudine** + **Lamivudine** + **Darunavir** 800 mg po once daily + **Ritonavir** 100 mg po once daily

1. Abacavir, efavirenz, enfuvirtide, maraviroc should be used only in consultation with an expert.
2. Didanosine, nelfinavir, tipranavir, stavudine (d4T) and nevirapine (contraindicated) are not recommended.
3. If transmission of drug resistant virus is suspected, the regimen should be appropriately modified in consultation with an expert to include agents to which it is likely to be susceptible.
4. **Descovy is the preferred substitute for Truvada** given lower potential for renal injury and osteomalacia for TAF vs. TDF. Note that Descovy is not recommended for CrCl <30 mL/min.

FOLLOW-UP

1. Complete blood count, renal and hepatic panels recommended at baseline and repeated at 2 weeks with further testing if results are abnormal.
2. HIV antibody testing to monitor seroconversion should be performed at baseline, 6 weeks, 12 weeks, and 6 months post-exposure.
3. If a 4th generation p24 antigen-HIV antibody test is used, testing may be terminated at 4 months.
4. Extended follow-up for 12 months is recommended if HCV conversion occurred upon exposure to an HIV-HCV co-infected patient.

B. HIV NON-OCCUPATIONAL EXPOSURE

- Risk of transmission of HIV via sexual contact or needle sharing may reach or exceed that of occupational needlestick exposure, thus HIV post-exposure prophylaxis (PEP) not later than 72 hours (and ideally within a few hours) of the exposure is recommended for HIV-negative persons non-occupationally exposed to blood or other potentially infected fluids from an HIV+ source.
- Substantial risk of HIV acquisition from HIV+ source
  - Exposure of vagina, rectum, eye, mouth, mucous membrane, non-intact skin, percutaneous contact
  - With blood semen, vaginal secretions, rectal secretions, breast milk, or anybody visibly contaminated with blood
- Negligible risk of HIV acquisition regardless of HIV status for any exposure to
  - Urine, nasal secretions, saliva, sweat, or tears if not visibly contaminated with blood
- PEP not effective and not recommended if ≥72 hours after an exposure.
- 4-week course of 3 ARV drugs is recommended for PEP.

Preferred Regimens

Age	Regimen
Age ≥13 years	**Descovy** (Emtricitabine [FTC] 200 mg + Tenofovir alafenamide fumerate [TAF]) + (**Dolutegravir** 50 mg po once daily OR **Raltegravir** 400 mg po twice daily) OR **Bictegravir** (FTC + TAF fixed dose formulation) one tab once daily (*See comments*; not recommended if CrCl is <30 ml/min). Bictegravir not recommended in pregnancy.
Age ≥13 years (includes pregnant women), CrCl <30 ml/min	**Tenofovir disoproxil fumarate** (TDF) 300 mg q72-96h + **Emtricitabine** (FTC) 200 mg q72-96h + (**Dolutegravir** 50 mg po once daily OR **Raltegravir** 1200 po once daily)
Children aged 2-12 years	**TDF** + **FTC** + **Raltegravir**, each dose adjusted for age and weight
Children aged 4 weeks to <2 years	**Zidovudine** + **Lamivudine** + (**Raltegravir** OR **Lopinavir-Ritonavir**) each as an oral solution dose adjusted for age and weight
Children aged birth to 27 days	Consult a pediatric HIV specialist

Alternative Regimens

Age	Regimen
Age ≥13 years (in pregnancy use TDF 300 mg + FTC 200 mg instead of Descovy), CrCl ≥30 ml/min	**Descovy** (FTC 200 mg + Tenofovir alafenamide fumerate [TAF]) + **Darunavir** 800 mg po once daily + **Ritonavir** 100 mg po once daily (See comments; not recommended if creatinine clearance is <30 ml/min).
Age ≥13 years (includes pregnant women), CrCl <30 ml/min	Renally adjusted doses of **Zidovudine** + **Lamivudine** + **Darunavir** 800 mg po once daily + Ritonavir 100 mg po once daily
Children aged 2-12 years	**Zidovudine** + **Lamivudine** + (**Raltegravir** OR **Lopinavir-Ritonavir**) once daily each dose adjusted for age and weight OR **TDF** + **FTC** + (**Lopinavir-Ritonavir** OR [**Darunavir** + **Ritonavir**]) each dose adjusted for age and weight
Children aged 4 weeks to <2 years	**Zidovudine** + **FTC** + (**Raltegravir** OR [**Lopinavir-Ritonavir**]) each as an oral solution dose adjusted for age and weight

TABLE 15E – PREVENTION OF SELECTED OPPORTUNISTIC INFECTIONS IN HUMAN HEMATOPOIETIC CELL TRANSPLANTATION (HCT) OR SOLID ORGAN TRANSPLANTATION (SOT) IN ADULTS WITH NORMAL RENAL FUNCTION

General comments: Medical centers performing transplants will have detailed protocols for the prevention of opportunistic infections which are appropriate to the infections encountered, patients represented and resources available at those sites. Regimens continue to evolve and protocols adopted by an institution may differ from those at other centers. Care of transplant patients should be guided by physicians with expertise in this area.

References:
For HCT: Expert guidelines endorsed by the IDSA, updating earlier guidelines *(MMWR 49 (RR-10):1, 2000)* in: *Biol Blood Marrow Transpl 15:1143, 2009*. These guidelines provide recommendations for prevention of additional infections not discussed in this table and provide more detailed information on the infections included here.
For SOT: The Third International Consensus Guidelines on the Management of Cytomegalovirus in Solid-organ Transplantation *(Transplantation 102(6):p 900-931, June 2018)*.

OPPORTUNISTIC INFECTION	TYPE OF TRANSPLANT	PROPHYLACTIC REGIMENS
CMV (Recipient + **or** Donor +/Recipient –) Ganciclovir resistance: risk, detection, management *(CID 68:1420, 2019; Clin Transplant, 33: e13512, 2019)*	SOT	Primary Regimens, Prophylaxis: **Valganciclovir** 900 mg po daily, **Letermovir** 480 mg IV/po daily (approved for kidney transplant) Duration of CMV Primary Prophylaxis by Organ and Donor/Recipient CMV Serostatus (Recommendations based on Clin Transplant 2019) **Also consider preemptive therapy** (monitor weekly for CMV viremia by PCR (or antigenemia) for 3-6 months post transplant. If viremia detected, start Valganciclovir 900 mg po bid or Ganciclovir 5 mg/kg IV q12h until clearance of viremia, but for not less than 2 weeks followed by secondary prophylaxis or preemptive approach. Prophylaxis vs pre-emptive rx compared: *CID 58:785, 2014*. CMV hyper IVIG is as adjunct to prophylaxis in high-risk lung, heart/lung, heart, or pancreas organ transplant recipients. Dosing: 150 mg/kg within 72 hrs of transplant and at 2, 4, 6 and 8 weeks; then 100 mg/kg at weeks 12 and 16.
	HCT	Preemptive Strategy: Monitor weekly for CMV viremia by PCR (or antigenemia) for 3-6 months post transplant with consideration for more prolonged monitoring in patients at risk for late-onset CMV disease (chronic GVHD, requiring systemic treatment, patients receiving high-dose steroids, T-cell depleted or cord blood transplant recipients, and CD4 <100 cells/mL). Start treatment with identification of CMV viremia or antigenemia as above. Consider prophylaxis (beginning post-engraftment) with **Valganciclovir** 900 mg po q24h or **Letermovir** 480 mg po/IV once daily. Letermovir is not active against HSV or VZV so addition of another agent for HSV/VZV prophylaxis is required. *National Comprehensive Cancer Network Guidelines on Prevention and Treatment of Cancer-Related Infections, Version 2021.*
Hepatitis B	SOT	Primary Regimens *Hepatic transplant recipients (HBV infected):* Recipient HBsAg+: HBIg (see below) + **Entecavir** 0.5 mg daily Recipient HBsAg-/HBcAb+/HBsAb+/-: Monitor q1-3 mo HBV DNA *Hepatic transplant recipients (HBV uninfected):* Donor HBsAg+: Transplant generally contraindicated Donor HBsAg-/HBcAb+/HBsAb+/-: **Entecavir** 0.5 mg daily if recipient HBsAb-; Consider monitoring for loss of HBsAb, in HBsAb+ recipients *Non-hepatic transplant recipients (HBV infected):* Recipient HBsAg+: HBIG (see below) + **Entecavir** 0.5 mg daily Recipient HBsAg-/HBcAb+/HBsAb+/-: Monitor q1-3 mo HBV DNA, LFTs, HBsAg *Non-hepatic transplant recipients (HBV uninfected):* Donor HBsAg+: Transplant generally contraindicated Donor HBsAg-/HBcAb+/HBsAb+/-: **Entecavir** 0.5 mg daily if recipient HBsAb-; Consider monitoring for loss of HBsAb, in HBsAb+ recipients Alternative Regimens **Tenofovir** 300 mg po daily (particularly if on Lamivudine pre-transplant) Emtricitabine/tenofovir 200/300 mg daily (if on pre-transplant)
	HCT	Patients who are anti-HBC positive and anti-HBs positive, but without evidence of active viral replication, can be monitored for ↑LFTs and presence of +HBV-DNA, and given pre-emptive therapy at that time. Alternatively, prophylactic anti-viral therapy can be given, commencing before transplant. **Entecavir** 0.5 mg daily is recommended as an antiviral.
Herpes simplex	SOT	**Acyclovir** 400 mg po bid, starting early post-transplant *(Clin Microbiol Rev 10:86, 1997)*.
	HCT	**Acyclovir** 250 mg/m² IV bid **or Acyclovir** 400 mg to 800 mg po bid, from conditioning to engraftment or resolution or mucositis. For those requiring prolonged suppression of HSV, the higher dose (Acyclovir 800 mg po bid) is recommended to minimize the risk of emerging resistance. Alternative: **valacyclovir** 500 mg po 2-3x/day; **famciclovir** 250 mg po 2x/day

TABLE 15E (2)

OPPORTUNISTIC INFECTION	TYPE OF TRANSPLANT	PROPHYLACTIC REGIMENS
Aspergillus spp.	SOT	Lung and heart/lung transplant: Inhaled **Ampho B** and/or a mold active oral azole are commonly used, but optimal regimen not defined. Aerosolized **Ampho B** 6 mg q8h (or 25 mg/day) OR aerosolized **LAB** 25 mg/day OR **Vori** 200 mg po bid OR **Itra** 200 mg po bid. 59% centers employ universal prophylaxis for 6 months in lung transplant recipients with 97% targeting Aspergillus. Most use Voriconazole alone or in combination with inhaled Amphotericin B *(Am J Transplant 11:361, 2011)*. Consider restarting prophylaxis during periods of intensified immune suppression. Liver transplant: Consider only in high-risk, re-transplant and/or those requiring renal-replacement therapy. Recommendations on aspergillus prophylaxis in SOT can be found at *(Clin Transplant, 33: e13544, 2019)*.
	HCT/Heme malignancy	Indications for prophylaxis against aspergillus include AML and MDS with neutropenia and HCT with GVHD. Posaconazole 200 mg po tid approved this indication *(NEJM 356:335, 2007 and NEJM 356:348,2007)*. Posaconazole ER tablets, also approved for prophylaxis (300 mg po BID x 1 day, then 300 daily). Retrospective analysis suggests that Voriconazole would have efficacy in steroid-treated patients with GVHD *(Bone Marrow Transpl 45:662, 2010)*, but is not approved for this indication. Caspofungin is more effective than fluconazole in preventing invasive fungal infection *(JAMA 322;1673,2019)*. Amphotericin B and echinocandins are alternatives as well.
Candida spp.	SOT	Consider in select, high risk patients (liver, small bowel, pancreas): Consider in select, high-risk patients (re-transplants, dialysis). **Flu** 400 mg daily for 4 weeks post-transplant *(Clin Transplant 33: e13623, 2019)*. Recipient of organ from donor, no active infection: o Lung transplant recipients: **Flu** 400 mg once daily, indefinitely. o Other organ recipients: **Flu** 400 mg once daily x 1 year; then 200 mg once daily indefinitely. Recipient residing in an endemic area who underwent an organ transplant (primary prevention): **Flu** 200 mg once daily x 6-12 months post transplantation *(Clin Infect Dis 63:e112, 2016)*.
	HCT/Heme malignancy	Recipient with no active infection at time of transplant: **Flu** 400 mg once daily x 1 year; then 200 mg once daily indefinitely. Acute leukemia undergoing intensive induction or re-induction during neutropenia. Autologous hematopoietic cell transplant recipients with mucositis pre-engraftment. Allogeneic hematopoietic cell transplant (HCT) recipients until engraftment when mold-active prophylaxis is not felt to be indicated. Fluconazole 400 mg po/IV q24h until recovery of neutropenia
Coccidioides immitis	Any	**Flu** 200-400 mg po q24h *(Transpl Inf Dis 5:3, 2003; Clin Transplant, 33:e13553, 2019)* for approach at one center in endemic area; e.g., for positive serology without evidence of active infection, Flu 400 mg q24h for first year post-transplant, then 200 mg q24h thereafter.
Pneumocystis jirovecii	SOT	**TMP-SMX:** 1 single-strength tab po q24h or 1 double-strength tab po once daily for 3 to 7 days per week. Duration: kidney: 6 mos to 1 year; heart, lung, liver: ≥1 year to life-long *(Clin Transplant 33: e13587, 2019)*.
	HCT	**TMP-SMX:** 1 single-strength tab po q24h or 1 double-strength tab po once daily or once a day for 3 days per week, from engraftment to ≥ 6 mos post transplant.
Toxoplasma gondii	SOT	<u>Primary Prophylaxis:</u> CD4 < 100/µL & IgG antibody to toxoplasmosis, continue until CD4 count >200 cells/µL for 3 months **TMP-SMX-DS** or **TMP-SMX-SS** po once daily (also effective prophylaxis for PJP) **Dapsone** 50 mg po q24h + **Pyrimethamine** 50 mg po q/week + **Folinic acid** 25 mg po q/week Once weekly: **Dapsone** 200 mg po + **Pyrimethamine** 75 mg po + **Folinic acid** 25 mg po *(JAIDS 15:104, 1997)* **Atovaquone** 1500 mg po q24h <u>Secondary Prophylaxis:</u> after treatment of cerebral toxoplasmosis, continue suppression until CD4 count > 200 cells/µL for 6 months **Sulfadiazine** 500-1000 mg po qid + **Pyrimethamine** 25-50 mg po q24h + **Folinic acid** 10-25 mg po q24h (prevents PJP and Toxoplasmosis) **Clinda** 300-450 mg po q6-8h + **Pyrimethamine** 25-50 mg po q24h + **Folinic acid** 10-25 mg po q24h (does not prevent PJP) **Atovaquone** 750 mg po q6-12h
	HCT	**TMP-SMX:** 1 single-strength tab po q24h or 1 double-strength tab po once daily or once a day for 3 days per week, from engraftment to ≥ 6 mos post transplant for seropositive allogeneic transplant recipients.
Trypanosoma cruzi	Heart	May be transmitted from organs or transfusions *(CID 48:1534, 2009)*. Inspect peripheral blood of suspected cases for parasites *(MMWR 55:798, 2006)*. Risk of reactivation during immunosuppression is variable *(JAMA 298:2171, 2007; JAMA 299:1134, 2008; J Cardiac Fail 15:249, 2009)*. If known Chagas disease in donor or recipient, contact CDC for treatment options *(phone 770-488-7775 or in emergency 770-488-7100)*. *Am J Transplant 11:672, 2011.*

TABLE 16 – PEDIATRIC DOSING (AGE >28 DAYS)

Groups/Drugs	Dose (Age >28 Days)	Max/Day
Antibacterials		
Aminoglycosides		
Amikacin	15-20 mg/kg/day (once daily) 5-7.5 mg/kg q8h	-
Gentamicin	5-7 mg/kg/day (once daily) 2.5 mg/kg q8h	-
Neomycin	HE: 50-100 mg/kg/day (divided q6-8hr) x5-6 days Seek safer alternative for longer use	-
Netilmicin	Safety and efficacy not established	-
Plazomicin	Safety and efficacy not established	-
Spectinomycin	Safety and efficacy not established	-
Tobramycin	5-7 mg/kg/day (once daily) 2.5 mg/kg q8h	-
Antifolates		
TMP-SMX (UTI, other)	8-10 mg TMP/kg/day (divided q12h)	-
TMP-SMX (PJP)	15-20 mg TMP/kg/day (divided q6-8h)	-
Trimethoprim	4 mg/kg/day (divided q12h)	-
Beta-Lactams		
Carbapenems		
Doripenem	Safety and efficacy not established	-
Ertapenem	30 mg/kg/day (divided q12h)	1 gm
Imipenem	Age <1 wk, wt ≥1.5 kg: 25 mg/kg q12h Age 1 wk to 4 wks, wt ≥1.5 kg: 25 mg/kg q8h Age 4 wks to 3 mon, wt ≥1.5 kg: 25 mg/kg q6h Age ≥3 mon: 15-25 mg/kg q6h	4 gm
Imipenem-cilastatin-relebactam	Safety and efficacy not established	-
Meropenem (standard)	60 mg/kg/day (divided q8h)	-
Meropenem (meningitis, CF)	120 mg/kg/day (divided q8h)	6 gm
Meropenem-vaborbactam	Safety and efficacy not established	-
Cephalosporins (po)		
1st generation:		
Cefadroxil	30 mg/kg/day (divided q12h)	2 gm
Cephalexin	25-100 mg/kg/day (divided q6h)	4 gm
2nd generation:		
Cefaclor	20-40 mg/kg/day (divided q8-12h)	1 gm
Cefprozil	15-30 mg/kg/day (divided q12h) (use 30 for AOM)	-
Cefuroxime axetil	Pharyngitis: 20 mg/kg/day (div q12h) AOM/ABS/impetigo: 30 mg/kg/day (div q12h)	1 gm
Loracarbef	15-30 mg/kg/day (divided q12h)	800 mg
3rd generation:		
Cefdinir	14 mg/kg/day (divided q12-24h)	-
Cefditoren pivoxil	Age >12 yrs: 200-400 mg q12h	-
Cefixime	8 mg/kg/day (divided q12-24h)	-
Cefpodoxime proxetil	10 mg/kg/day (divided q12h)	400 mg
Ceftibuten	9 mg/kg/day (divided q12-24h)	1 gm
Cephalosporins (IV)		
1st generation:		
Cefazolin	50-150 mg/kg/day (divided q6-8h)	6 gm
2nd generation:		
Cefmetazole	Safety and efficacy not established	-
Cefotetan	60-100 mg/kg/day (divided q12h)	6 gm
Cefoxitin	80-160 mg/kg/day (divided q6-8h)	-
Cefuroxime (standard)	150 mg/kg/day (divided q8h)	-
Cefuroxime (meningitis)	240 mg/kg/day (divided q8h)	-
3rd, 4th, advanced generation:		
Cefepime	Usual: 100 mg/kg/day (div q8h) Pseudomonas: 150 mg/kg/day (div q8h)	-
Cefepime-enmetazobactam	Safety and efficacy not established	-
Cefiderocol	Safety and efficacy not established	-
Cefoperazone	50-200 mg/kg/day (divided q8-12h) (divided q12h if age <8 days)	12 gm
Cefoperazone-sulbactam (standard)	40-80 mg/kg/day (divided q6-12h) (20-40 mg/kg/day cefoperazone using 1:1 ratio)	-

Groups/Drugs	Dose (Age >28 Days)	Max/Day
Antibacterials/Cephalosporins *(continued)*		
Cefoperazone-sulbactam (serious infection)	160 mg/kg/day (divided q6-12h) (80 mg/kg/day cefoperazone using 1:1 ratio) OR 240 mg/kg/day (divided q6-12h) (160 mg/kg/day cefoperazone using 1:2 ratio)	-
Cefotaxime (standard)	Age 0-7 days: 100 mg/kg/day (divided q12h) Age 8-28 days: 150 mg/kg/day (divided q8h) Age >28 days: 150-200 mg/kg/day (divided q6-8h)	-
Cefotaxime (meningitis)	Age 0-7 days: 100-150 mg/kg/day (divided q8-12h) Age 8-28 days: 150-200 mg/kg/day (divided q6-8h) Age >28 days: 225-300 mg/kg/day (divided q6-8h)	-
Cefpirome	Safety and efficacy not established	-
Ceftaroline	Age 0 to <2 mon (skin only): 6 mg/kg q8h (GA ≥34 wk, postnatal ≥12 days) Age 2 mon to <2 yrs: 8 mg/kg q8h Age 2 yrs to <18 yrs, ≤33 kg: 12 mg/kg q8h Age ≥2 yrs to <18 yrs, >33 kg: 400 mg q8h or 600 mg q12h	-
Ceftazidime (standard)	150-200 mg/kg/day (divided q8h)	6 gm
Ceftazidime (CF)	300 mg/kg/day (divided q8h)	6 gm
Ceftazidime-avibactam	Age 2 to <18 yrs: 62.5 (50/12.5) mg/kg q8h Age 6 mon to <2 yrs: 62.5 (50/12.5) mg/kg q8h Age 3 mon to <6 mon: 50 (40/10) mg/kg q8h	2.5 gm
Ceftizoxime	150-200 mg/kg/day (divided q6-8h)	-
Ceftobiprole medocaril	CAP, eGFR ≥50 mL/min/1.73 m^2 Age 3 mon to <12 yrs: 20 mg/kg (max 667 mg) q8h x7-14 days Age 12 yrs to <18 yrs: 13.3 mg/kg (max 667 mg) q8h x7-14 days CAP, eGFR <50 mL/min/1.73 m^2 Age 2 yrs to <6 yrs (by eGFR): 30 to <50: 13.3 mg/kg q12h (max 667 mg) 15 to <30: 13.3 mg/kg q24h (max 333 mg) <15: No data Age 6 yrs to <12 yrs (by eGFR): 30 to <50: 10 mg/kg (max 667 mg) q12h 15 to <30: 10 mg/kg (max 333 mg) q24h <15: No data Age 12 yrs to <18 yrs (by eGFR): 30 to <50: 10 mg/kg (max 667 mg) q12h 15 to <30: 10 mg/kg (max 333 mg) q12h <15: No data	-
Ceftolozane-tazobactam	Safety and efficacy not established	-
Ceftriaxone (standard)	50-100 mg/kg q24h	-
Ceftriaxone (meningitis)	50 mg/kg q12h Meningococcal proph, age <15: 125 mg IM x1	-
Monobactams		
Aztreonam	90-120 mg/kg/day (divided q8h)	8 gm
Aztreonam-avibactam	Safety and efficacy not established	-
Penicillins		
Aminopenicillins		
Amoxicillin (standard)	25-50 mg/kg/day (divided q8h)	-
Amoxicillin (AOM, pneumonia)	80-100 mg/kg/day (divided q8-12h; q12h for AOM)	-
Amoxicillin-clavulanate (7:1 formulation)	45 mg/kg/day (divided q12h)	-
Amoxicillin-clavulanate (14:1 formulation, for AOM)	90 mg/kg/day (divided q12h) for wt <40 kg	-
Amoxicillin-clavulanate (IV, 5:1 formulation)	Age <3 mon or <4 kg: 25 mg/5 mg per kg q12h Age ≥3 mon: 25 mg/5 mg per kg q8h	-
Ampicillin (oral)	50-100 mg/kg/day (divided q6h)	2 gm
Ampicillin (IV, standard)	200 mg/kg/day (divided q6h)	8 gm
Ampicillin (IV, meningitis)	300-400 mg/kg/day (divided q4h)	12 gm
Ampicillin-sulbactam	100-300 mg/kg/day (divided q6h)	-
Antipseudomonal penicillins		
Piperacillin	400 mg/kg/day (divided q6h)	-
Piperacillin-Tazobactam	DOSING BASED ON PIPERACILLIN COMPONENT 300-400 mg/kg/day (divided q6h) Mfr recs as of 12/2022 (wt ≤40 kg): Appendicitis/peritonitis, 2 to 9 mon: 80 mg/kg q8h Appendicitis/peritonitis, >9 mon: 100 mg/kg q8h Nosocomial pneumonia, 2 to 9 mon: 80 mg/kg q6h Nosocomial pneumonia, >9 mon: 100 mg/kg q6h	-
Antistaphylococcal penicillins		
Cloxacillin	50-200 mg/kg/day (divided q6h)	-
Dicloxacillin (mild-moderate infection)	12.5-25 mg/kg/day (divided q6h)	-
Dicloxacillin (osteoarticular infection)	100 mg/kg/day (divided q6h)	-

Groups/Drugs	Dose (Age >28 Days)	Max/Day
Antibacterials/Penicillins/Antistaphylococcal penicillins *(continued)*		
Flucloxacillin	Age <2 yrs: (62.5 mg po or 62.5-125 mg IV) q6h Age 2-10 yrs: (125 mg po or 125-250 mg IV) q6h	-
Nafcillin	150-200 mg/kg/day (divided q6h)	-
Oxacillin	150-200 mg/kg/day (divided q6h)	-
Natural penicillins		
Penicillin G	150,000-300,000 units/kg/day (divided q4-6h)	-
Penicillin VK	25-75 mg/kg/day (divided q6-8h)	-
Other penicillins		
Pivmecillinam	US: Safety and efficacy not established Outside US (Age >6 yrs, wt >40 kg): 20-40 mg/kg/day (div q8h)	1200 mg
Sulbactam + durlobactam (co-packaged)	Safety and efficacy not established	-
Temocillin	50 mg/kg/day (divided q12h)	-
Fluoroquinolones		
Ciprofloxacin[1] (po)	20-40 mg/kg/day (divided q12h)	1.5 gm
Ciprofloxacin[1] (IV)	20-30 mg/kg/day (divided q12h)	1.2 gm
Delafloxacin	Safety and efficacy not established	-
Gatifloxacin	Safety and efficacy not established	-
Levofloxacin[1] (IV/po)	16-20 mg/kg/day (divided q12h)	750 mg
Gemifloxacin	Safety and efficacy not established	-
Moxifloxacin	Safety and efficacy not established	-
Norfloxacin	Safety and efficacy not established	-
Ofloxacin	Safety and efficacy not established	-
Prulifloxacin	Safety and efficacy not established	-
Fusidanes		
Fusidic acid	Age <1 yr: 50 mg/kg/day (divided q8h) Age 1-5 yrs: 250 mg q8h Age 6-12 yrs: 250-500 mg q8h Age >12 yrs: adult dosing	-
Glyco-, Glycolipo-, Lipopeptides		
Dalbavancin	CrCl ≥30 mL/min/m²: Age 0 to <6 yrs: 22.5 mg/kg x1 dose Age 6 to <18 yrs: 18 mg/kg x1 dose CrCl <30 mL/min/m²: Not recommended	1500 mg
Daptomycin (cSSSI)	Age 12-17 yrs: 5 mg/kg (over 30 min) q24h Age 7-11 yrs: 7 mg/kg (over 30 min) q24h Age 2-6 yrs: 9 mg/kg (over 60 min) q24h Age 1 to <2 yrs: 10 mg/kg (over 60 min) q24h (Duration for all: ≤14 days)	-
Daptomycin (S. aureus bacteremia)	Age 12-17 yrs: 7 mg/kg (over 30 min) q24h Age 7-11 yrs: 9 mg/kg (over 30 min) q24h Age 1-6 yrs: 12 mg/kg (over 60 min) q24h (Duration for all: ≤42 days)	-
Oritavancin	Safety and efficacy not established	-
Teicoplanin	Age 0 to ≤2 mon: 16 mg/kg IV x1 dose, then 8 mg/kg IV q24h Age 2 mon to 12 yrs: 10 mg/kg IV q12h x3 doses, then 6-10 mg/kg IV q24h	-
Telavancin	Safety and efficacy not established	-
Vancomycin (IV)	60-80 mg/kg/day (divided q6-8h) Target AUC 400-600 μg/mL×hr, or trough 10-15 μg/mL	-
Vancomycin (po, C. difficile)	40 mg/kg/day (divided q6h)	-
Glycylcyclines		
Tigecycline	Avoid, but if necessary: Age 8-11 yrs: 1.2 mg/kg q12h Age 12-17 yrs: 50 mg q12h	100 mg
Ketolides		
Telithromycin	Safety and efficacy not established	-
Lincosamides		
Clindamycin (po)	30-40 mg/kg/day (divided q6-8h)	-
Clindamycin (IV)	20-40 mg/kg/day (divided q6-8h)	-
Lincomycin	10-20 mg/kg/day (divided q8-12h)	-
Macrolides		
Azithromycin (po)	5-12 mg/kg/day (once daily)	-
Azithromycin (IV)	10 mg/kg/day (once daily)	-
Clarithromycin	15 mg/kg/day (divided q12h)	1 gm
Erythromycin (po, IV)	40-50 mg/kg/day (divided q6h)	-
Fidaxomicin	Oral suspension, age >6 mon: 4 to <7 kg: 80 mg (2 mL) bid 7 to <9 kg: 120 mg (3 mL) bid 9 to <12.5 kg: 160 mg (4 mL) bid ≥12.5 kg: 200 mg (5 ml) bid (or use tabs)	-

Groups/Drugs	Dose (Age >28 Days)	Max/Day
Antibacterials *(continued)*		
Nitroimidazoles		
Metronidazole (po)	30-40 mg/kg/day (divided q6-8h) Giardiasis: 15 mg/kg/day (divided q8h) x7-10 days (max 250 mg/dose) Acute amebic dysentery: 35-50 mg/kg/day (divided q8h) x10 days Amebic liver abscess: 50 mg/kg/day (divided q8h) x7 days	2.25 gm
Metronidazole (IV)	22.5-40 mg/kg/day (divided q6-8h) ≤34 wks EGA, age 0-4 weeks: 15 mg/kg load then 7.5 mg/kg q12h Term infant, age 0-7 days: 15 mg/kg load then 7.5 mg/kg q8h Term infant, age 1-4 wks: 15 mg/kg load then 7.5 mg/kg q6h Appendicitis, age >1 month: 30 mg/kg/day (divided q6-8h)	2.25 gm
Secnidazole	Age ≥12 yrs: 2 gm po x1	2 gm
Oxazolidinones		
Linezolid	Age ≤28 days: GA <34 wk, PNA ≤7 days: 20 mg/kg/day (div q12h) All others: 30 mg/kg/day (div q8h) Age >28 days, all indications except uncomp SSTI: ≤11 yrs: 30 mg/kg/day (div q8h) >11 yrs: 600 mg q12h Age >28 days, uncomplicated SSTI: <5 yrs: 30 mg/kg/day (div q8h) 5 to 11 years: 20 mg/kg/day (div q12h) >11 years: 600 mg q12h	1200 mg
Tedizolid phosphate	6 mg/kg/day (divided q12h)	200 mg
Pleuromutilins		
Lefamulin	Safety and efficacy not established	-
Retapamulin	Age ≥9 mon: apply q12h x5 days (max area up to 2% BSA)	-
Polymyxins		
Colistin (polymyxin E) (standard)	2.5-5 mg/kg/day (divided q6-12h)	-
Colistin (polymyxin E) (CF)	3-8 mg/kg/day (divided q8h)	-
Polymyxin B (systemic)	Age ≥2 yrs: use adult dosing Age <2 yrs: 1.5-4.5 mg/kg/day (divided q12h)	-
Polymyxin B (intrathecal)	Age ≥2 yrs: use adult dosing Age <2 yrs: 2 mg q24h x3-4 days, then 2.5 mg q48h for ≥2 weeks	-
Rifamycins		
Rifampin (H. influenzae prophylaxis)	20 mg/kg q24h x4 days	600 mg
Rifampin (N. meningitidis prophylaxis)	Age <1 mon: 5 mg/kg q12h x4 doses Infants, children: 10 mg/kg q12h x4 doses	600 mg
Rifamycin SV	Safety and efficacy not established	-
Rifaximin	Safety and efficacy not established	-
Streptogramins		
Pristinamycin	50-100 mg/kg/day (divided q8h)	-
Quinupristin-dalfopristin	Safety and efficacy not established	-
Tetracyclines		
Doxycycline	2.2-4.4 mg/kg/day (divided q12h)	200 mg
Eravacycline	Safety and efficacy not established	-
Minocycline	Age >8 yrs: 4 mg/kg/day po (divided q12h)	-
Omadacycline	Safety and efficacy not established	-
Sarecycline	Age >9 yrs: Wt 33-54 kg: 60 mg po q24h Wt 55-84 kg: 100 mg po q24h Wt 85-136 kg: 150 mg po q24h	-
Tetracycline	Age >8 yrs: 25-50 mg/kg/day (divided q6h)	2 gm
Other		
Anthrax immune globulin	Wt-based dosing, single-dose: <10 kg: 60 units (1 vial) 10 to <18 kg: 120 units (2 vials) 18 to <25 kg: 180 units (3 vials) 25 to <35 kg: 240 units (4 vials) 35 to <50 kg: 300 units (5 vials) 50 to <60 kg: 360 units (6 vials) ≥60 kg: 420 units (7 vials)	-
Bezlotoxumab	Age ≥1 yr: 10 mg/kg IV (single dose) over 1 hr	-
Chloramphenicol	50-100 mg/kg/day IV (divided q6h)	2-4 gm
Fosfomycin IV	Prem neonate (GA+PNA <40 wk): 100 mg/kg/day (div q12h) Neonate (GA+PNA 40-44 wk): 200 mg/kg/day (div q8h) Age 1-12 mon, wt ≤10 kg: 200-300 mg/kg/day (div q8h) Age 1-12 years, wt 10-40 kg: 200-400 mg/kg/day (div q6-8h) Age ≥12 years, wt >40 kg: dose as adult	-
Fosfomycin PO	2 gm once	-

Groups/Drugs	Dose (Age >28 Days)	Max/Day
Antibacterials/Other *(continued)*		
Methenamine	Hippurate: Age 6-12 yrs: 0.5-1 gm q12h Age >12 yrs: 1 gm q12h Mandelate: Age <6 yrs: 50-75 mg/kg/day (divided q6-8h) Age 6-12 yrs: 500 mg q6h Age >12 yrs: 1 gm q6h	-
Mupirocin (topical)	2% cream (age >3 mon): apply q8h x10 days 2% oint (age >2 mon): apply q8h x10 days	-
Nitrofurantoin (cystitis)	5-7 mg/kg/day (divided q6h)	-
Nitrofurantoin (UTI prophylaxis)	1-2 mg/kg/day (once daily)	-
Obiltoxaximab	Wt ≤15 kg: 32 mg/kg Wt >15 to 40 kg: 24 mg/kg Wt >40 kg: 16 mg/kg	-
Pylera	Safety and efficacy not established	-
Raxibacumab	Wt ≤15 kg: 80 mg/kg Wt 15 to 50 kg: 60 mg/kg Wt >50 kg: 40 mg/kg	-
Sulopenem etzadroxil-probenecid	Safety and efficacy not established	-
Talicia	Safety and efficacy not established	-
Voquezna	Safety and efficacy not established	-
Antimycobacterials		
Bedaquiline	Age ≥5 yrs: Wt 15 to <30 kg: 200 mg q24h for wks 1-2, then 100 mg 3x/wk for wks 3-24 Wt ≥30 kg: 400 mg q24h for wks 1-2, then 200 mg 3x/wk for wks 3-24	-
Capreomycin	15-30 mg/kg/day (divided q12-24h)	1 gm
Clofazimine	Age 10-14 yrs: 150 mg once monthly + 50 mg on alternate days Age <10 yrs or wt <40 kg: 100 mg once monthly + 50 mg twice weekly	-
Cycloserine	10-15 mg/kg/day (divided q12h)	1 gm
Delamanid	Safety and efficacy not established	-
Ethambutol	15-25 mg/kg/day (once daily)	2.5 gm
Ethionamide	15-20 mg/kg/day (divided q12h)	1 gm
Isoniazid (INH) (daily dosing)	10-15 mg/kg/day (once daily)	300 mg
Isoniazid (INH) (twice weekly dosing)	20-30 mg/kg twice weekly	900 mg
Kanamycin	15-30 mg/kg/day (once daily)	1 gm
Para-aminosalicylic acid (PAS)	200-300 mg/kg/day (divided q6-12h)	-
Pretomanid	Safety and efficacy not established	-
Pyrazinamide (daily)	30-40 mg/kg/day (once daily)	2 gm
Pyrazinamide (twice weekly)	50 mg/kg twice weekly	4 gm
Rifabutin (MAC prophylaxis)	5 mg/kg/day (once daily)	300 mg
Rifabutin (active TB)	10-20 mg/kg/day (once daily)	300 mg
Rifampin (active TB)	10-20 mg/kg/day (once daily)	600 mg
Rifapentine (active TB)	Age ≥12 yrs: Initial phase 600 mg twice weekly x2 mon Continuation phase 600 mg once weekly x4-7 mon	-
Rifapentine (LTBI)	Age ≥2 yrs: Wt 10-14 kg: 300 mg once weekly Wt 14.1-25 kg: 450 mg once weekly Wt 25.1-32 kg: 600 mg once weekly Wt 32.1-50 kg: 750 mg once weekly Wt >50 kg: 900 mg once weekly	900 mg/wk
Streptomycin	Age ≥2 yrs: 20-40 mg/kg/day (once daily)	1 gm
Thalidomide	Safety and efficacy not established	-
Antifungals		
Amphotericin B (deoxycholate)	0.3-1.0 mg/kg/day (once daily)	-
Amphotericin B (lipid complex)	5 mg/kg/day (once daily)	-
Amphotericin B (liposomal)	3-5 mg/kg/day (once daily)	-
Anidulafungin	1.5-3 mg/kg load, then 0.75-1.5 mg/kg/day (once daily)	-
Caspofungin	Age >3 mon: 70 mg/m^2 load, then 50 mg/m^2 q24h	70 mg
Efinaconazole	Age ≥6 yrs: Apply to affected toenails once daily x48 wks	-
Fluconazole	6-12 mg/kg/day (once daily)	-
Flucytosine	Safety and efficacy not established	-
Griseofulvin (tinea capitis)	Age >2 yrs: Microsize susp 20-25 mg/kg/day Ultramicrosize tabs 10-15 mg/kg/day Treat ≥6 weeks, continue until clinically clear	-
Griseofulvin (tinea corporis)	Age >2 yrs: Microsize susp 10-20 mg/kg/day x2-4 weeks	-
Griseofulvin (tinea pedis)	Age >2 yrs: Microsize susp 10-20 mg/kg/day x4-8 weeks	-
Ibrexafungerp	VVC in post-menarchal females: 300 mg q12h x2 doses To reduce incidence of RVVC: 300 mg q12h x2 doses, repeat qmon x6 mon[3]	-

Groups/Drugs	Dose (Age >28 Days)	Max/Day
Antifungals *(continued)*		
Isavuconazonium sulfate	Injection: Age 1 to <3 yrs, wt <18 kg: 15 mg/kg q8h x6 doses, then q24h Age 3 to <18 yrs, wt <37 kg: 10 mg/kg q8h x6 doses, then q24h Age 3 to <18 yrs, wt ≥37 kg: 372 mg q8h x6 doses, then q24h Capsules, age 6 to <18 yrs: Wt 16 to <18 kg: 149 mg q8h x6 doses, then q24h Wt 18 to <25 kg: 223.5 mg q8h x6 doses, then q24h Wt 25 to <32 kg: 298 mg q8h x6 doses, then q24h Wt ≥32 kg: 372 mg q8h x6 doses, then q24h	Any individual loading or daily maintenance dose: 372 mg
Itraconazole	5-10 mg/kg/day (divided q12-24h)	600 mg
Ketoconazole	3.3-6.6 mg/kg/day (once daily)	400 mg
Micafungin (candidiasis)	Age >4 mon: 2 mg/kg q24h	100 mg
Micafungin (esophageal candidiasis)	Age >4 mon: Wt ≤30 kg: 3 mg/kg q24h Wt >30 mg: 2.5 mg/kg q24h	150 mg
Micafungin (prophylaxis, HSCT)	Age >4 mon: 1 mg/kg q24h	50 mg
Nystatin	Adolescents, children: 500,000 units (5 mL) q6h Infants: 200,000 units (2 mL) q6h Premature infants: 100,000 units (1 mL) q6h	-
Oteseconazole	Contraindicated in females of reproductive potential Safety and efficacy in pre-menarche not established	-
Posaconazole (OPC, refractory OPC)	Oral susp (age 13 to <18 yrs): OPC: 100 mg q12h x2 doses, then 100 mg q24h x14 days Refractory OPC: 400 mg q12h	-
Posaconazole (prophylaxis)	Oral susp (age 13 to <18 yrs): 200 mg q8h Delayed-rel tabs (age ≥2 yrs, wt >40 kg): 300 mg q12h x2 doses, then 300 mg q24h Delayed-rel oral susp (age 2 to <18 yrs, wt 10 to 40 kg): Wt 10 to <12 kg: 90 mg bid x2 doses, then 90 mg qd Wt 12 to <17 kg: 120 mg bid x2 doses, then 120 mg qd Wt 17 to <21 kg: 150 mg bid x2 doses, then 150 mg qd Wt 21 to <26 kg: 180 mg bid x2 doses, then 180 mg qd Wt 26 to <36 kg: 210 mg bid x2 doses, then 210 mg qd Wt 36 to 40 kg: 240 mg bid x2 doses, then 240 mg qd Injection (age 2 to <18 yrs): 6 mg/kg IV q12h x2 doses, then 6 mg/kg IV q24h	-
Rezafungin	Safety and efficacy not established	-
Terbinafine (tinea capitis)	Age >2 yrs (4-6 mg/kg/day): Wt 10-20 kg: 62.5 mg q24h Wt 20-40 kg: 125 mg q24h Wt >40 kg: 250 mg q24h Duration: 2 wks for T. tonsurans, 4 wks for M. canis	-
Terbinafine (onychomycosis)	Age >2 yrs (4-6 mg/kg/day): Wt 10-20 kg: 62.5 mg q24h Wt 20-40 kg: 125 mg q24h Wt >40 kg: 250 mg q24h Duration: 6 wks for fingernails, 12 wks for toenails	-
Voriconazole*	IA, serious Candida, Scedo, Fusarium: LD: 9 mg/kg IV q12h x2 doses MD: 8 mg/kg IV q12h OR 9 mg/kg po q12h Esophageal candidiasis: LD: not evaluated MD: 4 mg/kg IV q12h OR 9 mg/kg po q12h	700 mg
Antiparasitic drugs		
Albendazole*	WHO recommendations: Age >2 yrs: Adult dosing Age 1-2 yrs: Safe (at reduced dosage)	-
Antimony, pentavalent	20 mg Sb^V/kg/day (div q24h) IV/IM Dur: 28 days (ML/VL), 10-20 days (CL) Dose may require adjustment in some children. Seek expert advice.	-
Artemether-lumefantrine	<2 mon, <5 kg: not recommended 5 to <15 kg: 1 tab now, then 1 tab after 8 hr, then 1 tab q12h x2 days (6 tabs total). 15 to <25 kg: 2 tabs now, then 2 tabs after 8 hr, then 2 tabs q12h x2 days (12 tabs total). 25 to <35 kg: 3 tabs now, then 3 tabs after 8 hr, then 3 tabs q12h x2 days (18 tabs total). ≥35 kg: adult dosing (24 tabs total).	-
Artesunate (AS)	Wt <20 kg: 2.4 mg/kg IV at 0,12,24 hrs then q24h (7 days max). WHO recommended dose of 3 mg/kg is model-based and does not meet GRADE criteria.	-

Groups/Drugs	Dose (Age >28 Days)	Max/Day
Antiparasitic drugs *(continued)*		
Atovaquone	Age ≤12 yrs: safety and efficacy not established Suggested dosing: Babesiosis: 20 mg/kg q12h (w/azithro) PJP treatment, mild-moderate disease: Age 1-3 mon: 30-40 mg/kg q24h Age 4-24 mon: 45 mg/kg q24h Age >2 yrs to 12 yrs: 30-40 mg/kg q24h Age ≥13 yrs: 750 mg q12h PJP primary prophylaxis: Age 1-3 mon: 30-40 mg/kg q24h Age 4-24 mon: 45 mg/kg q24h Age >2 yrs to 12 yrs: 30-40 mg/kg q24h Age ≥13 yrs: 1500 mg q24h	1500 mg
Atovaquone-Proguanil	Malaria prevention (1-2 days before, during, x7 days post-exposure) Wt 5-8 kg: 1/2 pediatric tab q24h Wt 9-10 kg: 3/4 pediatric tab q24h Wt 11-20 kg: one pediatric tab q24h Wt 21-30 kg: two pediatric tabs q24h Wt 31-40 kg: three pediatric tabs q24h Wt >40 kg: one adult tab q24h Malaria treatment: Wt 5-8 kg: two pediatric tabs q24h x3 days Wt 9-10 kg: three pediatric tabs q24h x3 days Wt 11-20 kg: one adult tab q24h x3 days Wt 21-30 kg: two adult tabs q24h x3 days Wt 31-40 kg: three adult tabs q24h x3 days Wt >40 kg: four adult tabs q24h x3 days	-
Benznidazole	Age <12 yrs: 7.5 mg/kg/day (divided q12h) x60 days	-
Chloroquine phosphate	Varies with indication, see specific malaria topic for dosing	-
Dapsone	PJP prophylaxis: 2 mg/kg q24h	100 mg
Diethylcarbamazine	No data	-
Dihydroartemisinin-piperaquine*	Age >6 mon: Wt 5 to <7 kg: DHA 10 mg/PPQ 80 mg q24h x3 days Wt 7 to <13 kg: DHA 20 mg/PPQ 160 mg q24h x3 days Wt 13 to <24 kg: DHA 40 mg/PPQ 320 mg q24h x3 days Wt 24 to <36 kg: DHA 80mg/PPQ 640 mg q24h x3 days Wt 36 to <75 kg: DHA 120 mg/PPQ 960 mg q24h x3 days Wt 75 to 100 kg: DHA 160 mg/PPQ 1280 mg q24h x3 days Wt >100 kg: No data	
Diloxanide furoate	Wt >25 kg: 20 mg/kg/day (divided q8h) x10 days	1.5 gm
Eflornithine	For T. brucei gambiense: 400 mg/kg/day IV (divided q12h) x7 days (on WHO Essential Medicines list for age ≤12 yrs)	-
Fexinidazole	Age ≥6 yr, wt ≥20 kg: use adult dose	-
Fumagillin	No data	-
Hydroxychloroquine sulfate	Chloroquine-sensitive malaria: 10 mg base/kg po, then 5 mg base/kg at 6, 24, and 48 hrs	-
Iodoquinol	40 mg/kg/day (divided q8h) Max 650 mg per dose	-
Ivermectin*	Wt-based dosing to provide 200 µg/kg: <15 kg: Safe use unclear 15-24 kg: 3 mg single-dose 25-35 kg: 6 mg single-dose 36-50 kg: 9 mg single-dose 51-65 kg: 12 mg single-dose 66-79 kg: 15 mg single-dose ≥80 kg: 200 µg/kg	-
Mebendazole*	WHO recommendations: Age >2 yrs: Adult dosing Age 1-2 yrs: Safe (at reduced dosage)	-
Mefloquine	Weight-based dosing: <9 kg: 5 mg/kg weekly 10-19 kg: 62.5 mg (1/4 tab) weekly 20-30 kg: 125 mg (1/2 tab) weekly 31-45 kg: 187.5 mg (3/4 tab) weekly >45 kg: 250 mg (1 tab) weekly	-
Melarsoprol	No data	-
Miltefosine	Age >12 yrs, wt 30-44 kg: 50 mg po q12h	-
Moxidectin	Age ≥12 yrs: 8 mg (four 2 mg tabs) single-dose	-
Niclosamide	Fish, dog, beef, pork tapeworm: 50 mg/kg single dose (max 2 gm) Rat (H. diminuta) or human (H. nana) tapeworm: Wt 11-34 kg: 1 gm on day 1, then 500 mg q24h x6 days Wt >34 kg: 1.5 gm on day 1, then 1 gm q24h x6 days	-

Groups/Drugs	Dose (Age >28 Days)	Max/Day
Antiparasitic drugs *(continued)*		
Nifurtimox	Newborn (wt ≥2.5 kg) to <18 years: Wt ≥40 kg: 8-10 mg/kg/day (divided tid) x60 days Wt <40 kg: 10-20 mg/kg/day (divided tid) x60 days	-
Nitazoxanide*	Age 1-3 yrs: 100 mg susp q12h x3 days Age 4-11 yrs: 200 mg susp q12h x3 days Age ≥12 yrs: 500 mg q12h x3 days (tab or susp)	-
Paromomycin	E. histolytica, D. fragilis: 25-35 mg/kg/day (divided q8h) x7 days G. duodenalis: 30 mg/kg/day (divided q8h) x5-10 days	-
Pentamidine	PJP treatment: 4 mg/kg/day IM/IV (div q24h) PJP prophylaxis: 300 mg by aerosol q-month	-
Praziquantel	Age >4 yrs: dose as adult Age <4 yrs: not FDA approved. No harm in mass prevention campaigns.	-
Primaquine	Relapse prevention: 0.5 mg/kg base q24h x14 days Primary prophylaxis (day 1 before until 7 days after exposure): 0.5 mg/kg base q24h	-
Pyrantel pamoate	Age >1 yr: Pinworm: 11 mg/kg base x1 dose (may repeat in 2 weeks)	1 gm
Pyrimethamine	Adolescents: dose as adults	-
Pyronaridine-artesunate	Wt 5-7 kg: 1 sachet q24h x3 days Wt 8-14 kg: 2 sachets q24h x3 days Wt 15-19 kg: 3 sachets q24h x3 days (1 sachet = Pyr tetraphos 60 mg, AS 20 mg)	-
Quinacrine	6 mg/kg/day (divided q8h)	300 mg
Quinine sulfate	10 mg/kg (salt) po q8h x3 or x7 days (may require a compounding pharmacy)	-
Quinine dihydrochloride	20 mg/kg (salt) IV load, then 10mg/kg q8h Infuse doses over 4 hr to avoid hypotension	-
Spiramycin	Not applicable	-
Sulfadiazine	120-150 mg/kg/day (divided q4-6h)	6 gm
Sulfadoxine-pyrimethamine	Malaria treatment, age >2 mon (partner with an artemisinin drug): Wt >45 kg: 3 tabs single-dose Wt 31-45 kg: 2 tabs single-dose Wt 21-30 kg: 1.5 tabs single-dose Wt 11-20 kg: 1 tab single-dose Wt 5-10 kg: 0.5 tab single-dose	-
Suramin	20 mg/kg IV on days 1, 3, 7, 14, 21 (start with 2 mg/kg IV test dose)	1 gm
Tafenoquine	Safety and efficacy (age <16 yrs) not established Initial data, age <16: Lancet Child Adolesc Health 2022;6:86	-
Tinidazole (giardiasis)	Age >3 yrs: 50 mg/kg single dose	2 gm
Tinidazole (amebic liver abscess)	Age >3 yrs: 50 mg/kg q24h x3-5 days	2 gm
Tinidazole (intestinal amebiasis)	Age >3 yrs: 50 mg/kg q24h x3 days	2 gm
Triclabendazole	Age ≥6 years: 10 mg/kg po q12h x2 doses	-
Antiretrovirals		
Abacavir (ABC)	Oral solution: Age 0 to <1 mon: 2 mg/kg q12h Age ≥1 to <3 mon, full-term: 4 mg/kg q12h Age ≥3 mon: 8 mg/kg q12h OR 16 mg/kg q24h Tablets: Wt 14 to <20 kg: 150 mg q12h (300 mg q24h ok) Wt ≥20 to <25 kg: 150 mg qAM, 300 mg qPM (450 mg q24h ok) Wt ≥25 kg: 300 mg q12h (600 mg q24h ok) [source: *HHS panel, April 2023*]	600 mg
Atazanavir (ATV) (powder)	Age <3 mon: Not recommended Age ≥3 mon: 5 to <15 kg: ATV 200 mg q24h + RTV 80 mg q24h 15 to <25 kg: ATV 250 mg q24h + RTV 80 mg q24h ≥25 kg: ATV 300 mg q24h + RTV 100 mg q24h	-
Atazanavir (ATV) (capsules)	Age <6 yrs: not recommended Age ≥6 yrs: <15 kg: not recommended 15 to <35 kg: ATV 200 mg q24h + RTV 100 mg q24h ≥35 kg: ATV 300 mg q24h + RTV 100 mg q24h (may use cobicistat 150 mg q24h instead of RTV) Age ≥13 yrs, wt ≥40 kg, ART-naive, cannot tolerate RTV, not on TAF or TDF: ATV 400 mg q24h	-
Cabotegravir (CAB)[5] (IM, PrEP)	Age ≥12 yr, wt ≥35 kg: 600 mg q mon x2, then 600 mg q2 mon	-
Cabotegravir (CAB) (oral)	Age ≥12 yr, wt ≥35 kg: 30 mg q24h	-
Cobicistat (COBI or c)	Wt ≥35 kg: 150 mg po q24h with ATV 300 mg po q24h Wt ≥40 kg: 150 mg po q24h with DRV 800 mg po q24h	-

Groups/Drugs	Dose (Age >28 Days)	Max/Day
Antiretrovirals *(continued)*		
Darunavir (DRV)	Neonate: not approved Age <3 or wt <10 kg: avoid use Age ≥3 yr, tx naive or exp ± one or more DRV mutations: 10 to <11 kg: 200 mg (+ RTV 32 mg) q12h 11 to <12 kg: 220 mg (+ RTV 32 mg) q12h 12 to <13 kg: 240 mg (+ RTV 40 mg) q12h 13 to <14 kg: 260 mg (+ RTV 40 mg) q12h 14 to <15 kg: 280 mg (+ RTV 48 mg) q12h 15 to <30 kg: 375 mg (+ RTV 48 mg) q12h 30 to <40 kg: 450 mg (+ RTV 100 mg) q12h ≥40 kg: 600 mg (+ RTV 100 mg) q12h Adolescent (age ≥12 yrs): ≥30 to <40 kg, tx naive/exp ± ≥1 DRV mut: 450 mg (+ RTV 100 mg) q12h ≥40 kg, tx naive/exp, no DRV mut: 800 mg (+ RTV 100 mg) q24h (may sub cobicistat 150 mg q24h for the RTV) ≥40 kg, tx exp, ≥1 DRV mut: 600 mg (+ RTV 100 mg) q12h	-
Dolutegravir (DTG)[7]	Film-coated tabs (if feasible): 14 to <20 kg: 40 mg q24h ≥20 kg: 50 mg q24h Dispersible tabs, age ≥4 weeks: 3 to <6 kg: 5 mg q24h 6 to <10 kg: 15 mg q24h 10 to <14 kg: 20 mg q24h 14 to <20 kg: 25 mg q24h ≥20 kg: 30 mg q24h	-
Doravirine (DOR)	Age ≥12 yr, wt ≥35 kg: 100 mg q24h	-
Efavirenz (EFV)	Neonates: not approved for use Age 3 mon to <3 yrs, wt ≥3.5 kg: not recommended (variable PK) Age ≥3 yrs, wt ≥10 kg: 10 to <15 kg, 200 mg q24h 15 to <20 kg, 250 mg q24h 20 to <25 kg, 300 mg q24h 25 to <32.5 kg, 350 mg q24h 32.5 to <40 kg, 400 mg q24h ≥40 kg, 600 mg q24h	-
Emtricitabine (FTC)	Oral solution: 0 to ≤3 mon, 3 mg/kg q24h 3 mon to 17 yr: 6 mg/kg (max 240 mg) q24h ≥18 yr, 240 mg q24h Caps, wt >33 kg: 200 mg q24h	-
Enfuvirtide (ENF/T20)	Age <6 yrs: not approved for use Age 6-16 yr: 2 mg/kg (max 90 mg) sc q12h Age >16 yr: 90 mg sc q12h	-
Etravirine (ETR)	Neonate/infant: not approved Child <2 yrs: not approved Age 2-18 yr, wt ≥10 kg: Wt 10 to <20 kg, 100 mg q12h Wt 20 to <25 kg, 125 mg q12h Wt 25 to <30 kg, 150 mg q12h Wt ≥30 kg, 200 mg q12h	-
Fosamprenavir (FPV)	Age 6 mon to 18 yrs, ARV naive/experienced, by wt: <11 kg: 45 mg/kg (+ RTV 7 mg/kg) q12h 11 to <15 kg: 30 mg/kg (+ RTV 3 mg/kg) q12h 15 to <20 kg: 23 mg/kg (+ RTV 3 mg/kg) q12h ≥20 kg: 18 mg/kg (+ RTV 3 mg/kg) q12h Adolescents, ART naive: 700 mg (+ RTV 100 mg) q12h, OR 1400 mg (+ RTV 100-200 mg) q24h Adolescents, ARV experienced: 700 mg (+ RTV 100 mg) q12h	-
Fostemsavir (FTR)	Safety and efficacy not established	-
Ibalizumab-uiyk (IBA)	Safety and efficacy not established	-
Indinavir (IDV)	Neonate/infant/children: not approved for use Adolescent: 800 mg (+ RTV 100-200 mg) q12h	-

Groups/Drugs	Dose (Age >28 Days)	Max/Day
Antiretrovirals *(continued)*		
Lamivudine (3TC)	Oral solution 10 mg/mL: Age 0 to <4 wks: 2 mg/kg q12h Age ≥4 wks to <3 mon: 4 mg/kg q12h Age ≥3 mon to <3 yrs: 5 mg/kg (max 150 mg) q12h Age ≥3 yr: 5 mg/kg (max 150 mg) q12h, OR 10 mg/kg (max 300 mg) q24h Wt-band dosing, oral solution 10 mg/mL: 3 to <6 kg: 30 mg q12h 6 to <10 kg: 40 mg q12h 10 to <14 kg: 60 mg q12h Wt-band dosing, tabs: 14 to <20 kg: 75 mg q12h (or 150 mg q24h) ≥20 to <25 kg: 75 mg qam + 150 mg qpm (or 225 mg q24h) ≥25 kg: 150 mg q12h (or 300 mg q24h)	-
Lenacapavir (LEN)	Safety and efficacy not established	-
Maraviroc (MVC)	Full-term infants, tx-exp children/adolescents, no interacting drugs: 2 to <4 kg: 30 mg (1.5 mL) q12h (oral solution) 4 to <6 kg: 40 mg (2 mL) q12h (oral solution) 6 to <10 kg: 100 mg (5 mL) q12h (oral solution or tabs) 10 to <14 kg: 150 mg (7.5 mL) q12h (oral solution or tabs) 14 to <30 kg: 200 mg (10 mL) q12h (oral solution or tabs) 30 to <40 kg: 300 mg (15 mL) q12h (oral solution or tabs) ≥40 kg: 300 mg (15 mL) q12h (oral solution or tabs) Given w/potent CYP3A inhibitors (± CYP3A inducer), incl all PIs: 2 to <10 kg: not recommended 10 to <20 kg: 50 mg (2.5 mL) q12h (oral solution or tabs) 20 to <30 kg: 75-80 mg (4 mL) q12h (oral solution or tabs) 30 to <40 kg: 100 mg (5 mL) q12h (oral solution or tabs) ≥40 kg: 150 mg (7.5 mL) q12h (oral solution or tabs) Given w/potent CYP3A inducers, without a CYP3A inhibitor: no data	-
Nelfinavir (NFV)	Age <2 yrs: Not recommended Age ≥2 yrs: 45-55 mg/kg q12h Adolescent: 1250 mg q12h	-
Nevirapine (NVP) (immediate-release tabs, oral susp)	GA 32 to <34 wks: Birth to age 2 wks: 2 mg/kg q12h (no lead-in) Age 2 to 4 wks: 4 mg/kg q12h Age 4 to 6 wks: 6 mg/kg q12h Age >6 wks: 200 mg/m^2 q12h GA 34 to <37 wks: Birth to age 1 wk: 4 mg/kg q12h (no lead-in) Age 1 to 4 wks: 6 mg/kg q12h Age >4 wks: 200 mg/m^2 q12h GA ≥37 wks to age of <1 mon: Birth to age 4 wks: 6 mg/kg q12h (no lead-in) Age >4 wks: 200 mg/m^2 q12h Age ≥1 mon to <8 yrs: 200 mg/m^2 q12h (after lead-in). Age ≥8 yrs: 120-150 mg/m^2 q12h (after lead-in)	400 mg
Nevirapine (NVP) (XR tabs)	Age ≥6 yrs (no lead-in if already on immediate-release q12h): BSA 0.58 to 0.83 m^2: 200 mg q24h BSA 0.84 to 1.16 m^2: 300 mg q24h BSA ≥1.17 m^2: 400 mg q24h Adolescents, adults: 400 mg q24h (after lead-in)	400 mg

Groups/Drugs	Dose (Age >28 Days)	Max/Day
Antiretrovirals *(continued)*		
Raltegravir (RAL)	Preterm or low birth weight: no data Neonates (full-term), oral suspension: 0-1 wk, 2 to <3 kg: 4 mg (0.4 mL) q24h 0-1 wk, 3 to <4 kg: 5 mg (0.5 mL) q24h 0-1 wk, 4 to <5 kg: 7 mg (0.7 mL) q24h 1-4 wk, 2 to <3 kg: 8 mg (0.8 mL) q12h 1-4 wk, 3 to <4 kg: 10 mg (1 mL) q12h 1-4 wk, 4 to <5 kg: 15 mg (1.5 mL) q12h Infant >4 weeks, children ≥3 to <20 kg, oral suspension: 3 to <4 kg: 25 mg (2.5 mL) q12h 4 to <6 kg: 30 mg (3 mL) q12h 6 to <8 kg: 40 mg (4 mL) q12h 8 to <10 kg: 60 mg (6 mL) q12h 10 to <14 kg: 80 mg (8 mL) q12h 14 to <20 kg: 100 mg (10 mL) q12h Children (≥3 kg) and adolescents, chewable tablets: 3 to <6 kg: 25 mg q12h 6 to <10 kg: 50 mg q12h 10 to <14 kg: 75 mg q12h 14 to <20 kg: 100 mg q12h 20 to <28 kg: 150 mg q12h 28 to <40 kg: 200 mg q12h ≥40 kg: 300 mg q12h Children and adolescents, film-coated tablets: ≥25 kg: 400 mg q12h ≥40 kg, tx-naive or suppr on 400 mg q12h: 1200 mg q24h	-
Rilpivirine (RPV)	Age ≥2 years: Wt 14 to <20 kg: 12.5 mg q24h (dispersible tabs) Wt 20 to <25 kg: 15 mg q24h (dispersible tabs) Wt ≥25 kg: 25 mg q24h (film-coated tab)	-
Ritonavir (RTV)	350-400 mg/m^2 q12h (not recommended) Used as pharmacologic enhancer	-
Saquinavir (SQV)	Adolescent: 1000 mg (+ RTV 100 mg) q12h	-
Stavudine (d4T)	(NOTE: The DHHS Pediatric Guidelines Panel does not recommend d4T in children because of a higher rate of adverse effects compared to other NRTIs) Age 0-13 days: 0.5 mg/kg q12h Age ≥14 days, wt <30 kg: 1 mg/kg q12h Wt ≥30 kg: 30 mg q12h	-
Tenofovir disoproxil fumarate (TDF)	Age ≥2 to <12 yr, wt ≥10 kg: 8 mg/kg (max 300 mg) q24h Oral powder, weight-based: 10 to <12 kg: 2 scoops (80 mg) q24h 12 to <14 kg: 2.5 scoops (100 mg) q24h 14 to <17 kg: 3 scoops (120 mg) q24h 17 to <19 kg: 3.5 scoops (140 mg) q24h 19 to <22 kg: 4 scoops (160 mg) q24h 22 to <24 kg: 4.5 scoops (180 mg) q24h 24 to <27 kg: 5 scoops (200 mg) q24h 27 to <29 kg: 5.5 scoops (220 mg) q24h 29 to <32 kg: 6 scoops (240 mg) q24h 32 to <34 kg: 6.5 scoops (260 mg) q24h 34 to <35 kg: 7 scoops (280 mg) q24h ≥35 kg: 7.5 scoops (300 mg) q24h Tablets, weight-based: 17 to <22 kg: 150 mg q24h 22 to <28 kg: 200 mg q24h 28 to <35 kg: 250 mg q24h ≥35 kg: 300 mg q24h	-
Tipranavir (TPV)	Age <2 yrs: Not approved for use Age ≥2 to 18 yrs (not recommended if tx-naive): By BSA: 375 mg/m^2 (+ RTV 150 mg/m^2) q12h By wt: 14 mg/kg (+ RTV 6 mg/kg) q12h	500 mg (+ RTV 200 mg) q12h

Groups/Drugs	Dose (Age >28 Days)	Max/Day
Antiretrovirals *(continued)*		
Zidovudine (ZDV/AZT)	Premature infant, EGA <30 wks: Age 0-4 weeks: 2 mg/kg po q12h Age 4-8 weeks: 3 mg/kg po q12h Age >8 weeks: 12 mg/kg po q12h Premature infant, EGA ≥30 to <35 wks: Age 0-2 weeks: 2 mg/kg po q12h Age 2-6 weeks: 3 mg/kg po q12h Age >6 weeks: 12 mg/kg po q12h Neonate, EGA ≥35 wks: Age 0-4 wks: 4 mg/kg po q12h Infant/child/adolescent (EGA ≥35 wks, age ≥4 wks): Wt 4 to <9 kg: 12 mg/kg po q12h Wt 9 to <30 kg: 9 mg/kg po q12h Wt ≥30 kg: 300 mg po q12h Dosing by BSA: 180-240 mg/m^2 po q12h	-
Antiretroviral combination products		
Atripla (EFV/FTC/TDF)	Age ≥12 yr, wt ≥40 kg: one tab q24h	-
Biktarvy (BIC/FTC/TAF)	Age <2 yr, wt <14 kg: no data, studies ongoing Age ≥2 yr, wt 14 to <25 kg: BIC 30/FTC 120/TAF 15 mg q24h Wt ≥25 kg: BIC 50/FTC 200/TAF 25 mg q24h	-
Cabenuva (CAB/RPV)[6]	Age ≥12 yr, wt ≥35 kg Monthly injections: 600 mg/900 mg IM, then 400 mg/600 mg monthly Every two month injections: 600 mg/900 mg IM, repeat in 1 mon, then every 2 months	-
Cimduo, Temixys (3TC/TDF)	Wt ≥35 kg: one tab q24h	-
Combivir (3TC/ZDV)	Age ≥12 yr, wt ≥30 kg: one tab q12h	-
Complera/Eviplera (RPV/FTC/TDF)	Age ≥12 yr, wt ≥35 kg: one tab q24h	-
Delstrigo (DOR/3TC/TDF)	Wt ≥35 kg: one tab q24h	-
Descovy (FTC/TAF)	Wt ≥14 to <25 kg: FTC 120 mg/TAF 15 mg q24h (+ NNRTI or INSTI only) Wt 25 to <35 kg: FTC 200 mg/TAF 25 mg q24h (+ NNRTI or INSTI only) Wt ≥35 kg: FTC 200 mg/TAF 25 mg q24h (+ NNRTI, INSTI, or boosted PI)	-
Dovato (DTG/3TC)	Safety and efficacy of combination tablet not established	
Epzicom/Kivexa (ABC/3TC)	Wt ≥25 kg: one tab q24h	-
Evotaz (ATV/cobi)	Wt ≥35 kg: one tab q24h	-
Genvoya (EVG/cobi/FTC/TAF)	Wt 14 to <25 kg: limited data, studies ongoing Wt ≥25 kg: one tab q24h	-
Juluca (DTG/RPV)	Safety and efficacy of combination tablet not established	
Kaletra (LPV/RTV)	Age <14 days: avoid use Age 14 days to 12 mon: 300 mg/75 mg per m^2 q12h Age >12 mon to 18 yrs, tx experienced: 300 mg/75 mg per m^2 q12h If using 100 mg/25 mg tabs: 15-20 kg: 2 tabs q12h >20 to 30 kg: 3 tabs q12h >30 to 45 kg: 4 tabs q12h >45 kg: 4 tabs q12h (5 tabs q12h if on NVP, EFV, FPV, or NFV) Age >12 mon to 18 yrs, tx naive: 230 mg/57.5 mg per m^2 q12h If using 100 mg/25 mg tabs: 15-25 kg: 2 tabs q12h >25 to 35 kg: 3 tabs q12h >35 to 45 kg: 4 tabs q12h >45 kg: 4 tabs q12h	-
Odefsey (RPV/FTC/TAF)	Age ≥12 yr, wt ≥35 kg: one tab q24h	-
Prezcobix (DRV/cobi)	Wt ≥40 kg: one tab q24h	-
Stribild (EVG/cobi/FTC/TDF)	Age ≥12 yr, wt ≥35 kg: one tab q24h	-
Symfi, Symfi Lo (EFV/3TC/TDF)	Symfi (wt ≥40 kg): one tab q24h Symfi Lo (wt ≥35 kg): one tab q24h	
Symtuza (DRV/cobi/FTC/TAF)	Wt ≥40 kg: one tab q24h	-
Triumeq (DTG/3TC/ABC)	Wt 10 to <14 kg: 4 PD tabs q24h Wt 14 to <20 kg: 5 PD tabs q24h Wt 20 to <25 kg: 6 PD tabs q24h Wt ≥25 kg: one regular tab q24h	-
Trizivir (ABC/3TC/ZDV)	Wt ≥30 kg: one tab q12h (FDA approved wt is ≥40 kg)	-
Truvada (FTC/TDF)	Wt 17 to <22 kg: FTC 100 mg/TDF 150 mg q24h Wt 22 to <28 kg: FTC 133 mg/TDF 200 mg q24h Wt 28 to <35 kg: FTC 167 mg/TDF 250 mg q24h Wt ≥35 kg: FTC 200 mg/TDF 300 mg q24h	-

Groups/Drugs	Dose (Age >28 Days)	Max/Day
Antivirals		
Antivirals (coronavirus)		
Bamlanivimab + Etesevimab	Coadminister as a single IV infusion according to wt: ≥40 kg: Bam 700 mg + Ete 1400 mg <20 kg to <40 kg: Bam 350 mg + Ete 700 mg >12 kg to 20 kg: Bam 175 mg + Ete 350 mg 1 kg to 12 kg: Bam 12 mg/kg + Ete 24 mg/kg	-
Baricitinib (JAK inhibitor)	Age ≥9 years: 4 mg q24h Age 2 to <9 years: 2 mg q24h Age <2 years: not authorized	-
Bebtelovimab	Age ≥12 yr, wt ≥40 kg: 175 mg IV	-
Casirivimab + Imdevimab	Age ≥12 yr, wt ≥40 kg: Casirivimab 600 mg IV, Imdevimab 600 mg IV	-
Molnupiravir	Safety and efficacy not established	-
Nirmatrelvir/RTV	Age ≥12 yr, wt ≥40 kg: Nirmatrelvir/RTV 300 mg/100 mg q12h x5 days	-
Pemivibart	Age ≥12 yr, wt ≥40 kg: 4500 mg IV (may repeat q3 months)	-
Remdesivir	Age <28 days, wt ≥1.5 kg: 2.5 mg/kg day 1, then 1.25 mg/kg q24h Age ≥28 days, wt 1.5 to <3 kg: 2.5 mg/kg day 1, then 1.25 mg/kg q24h Age ≥28 days, wt 3 to <40 kg: 5 mg/kg day 1, then 2.5 mg/kg q24h Wt ≥40 kg: 200 mg day 1, then 100 mg q24h Treatment duration: 5 days (not on mech vent/ECMO) 10 days (if on mech vent/ECMO)	-
Sotrovimab	Age ≥12 yr, wt ≥40 kg: 500 mg IV	-
Tixagevimab + Cilgavimab	Age ≥12 yr, wt ≥40 kg: Tix 150 mg IM + Cil 150 mg IM	-
Tocilizumab (anti IL-6 MoAb)	Age ≥2 yr, wt <30 kg: 12 mg/kg IV Age ≥2 yr, wt ≥30 kg: 8 mg/kg IV	800 mg
Tofacitinib	COVID study pts were ≥18 yrs of age (NEJM 2021;385:406)	-
Vilobelimab	Safety and efficacy not established	-
Antivirals (Ebola virus)		
Ansuvimab-zykl	50 mg/kg IV single infusion (over 60 min)	-
Inmazeb	50 mg/kg (all 3 MoAbs) IV single infusion	-
Antivirals (hepatitis B)		
Adefovir	Age ≥12 yrs: 10 mg q24h	-
Entecavir (treatment-naive)	Age ≥2 yrs, oral solution: Wt 10-11 kg: 0.15 mg q24h >11 to 14 kg: 0.2 mg q24h >14 to 17 kg: 0.25 mg q24h >17 to 20 kg: 0.3 mg q24h >20 to 23 kg: 0.35 mg q24h >23 to 26 kg: 0.4 mg q24h >26 to 30 kg: 0.45 mg q24h >30 kg: 0.5 mg q24h	-
Entecavir (lamivudine-experienced)	Age ≥2 yrs, oral solution: Wt 10-11 kg: 0.3 mg q24h >11 to 14 kg: 0.4 mg q24h >14 to 17 kg: 0.5 mg q24h >17 to 20 kg: 0.6 mg q24h >20 to 23 kg: 0.7 mg q24h >23 to 26 kg: 0.8 mg q24h >26 to 30 kg: 0.9 mg q24h >30 kg: 1 mg q24h	-
Telbivudine	Age ≥16 yrs: 600 mg q24h (not available in US)	-
Tenofovir alafenamide fumarate (TAF)	Age ≥6 yrs: 25 mg po q24h	-
Antivirals (hepatitis C)		
Daclatasvir	Safety and efficacy not established	-
Ribavirin (with sofosbuvir, Epclusa, Harvoni)	Wt <47 kg: 15 mg/kg/day (divided q12h) 47-49 kg: 600 mg/day (200 mg in am, 400 mg in pm) 50-65 kg: 800 mg/day (400 mg q12h) 66-80 kg: 1000 mg/day (400 mg in am, 600 mg in pm) >80 kg: 1200 mg/day (divided q12h)	-
Simeprevir	Safety and efficacy not established (not available in US)	-
Sofosbuvir	Age ≥3 years: Wt ≥35 kg: 400 mg q24h Wt 17 to <35 kg: 200 mg q24h Wt <17 kg: 150 mg q24h Geno 2, tx-naive/exp, no cirr or comp=12 wks (with ribavirin) Geno 3, tx-naive/exp, no cirr or comp=24 wks (with ribavirin).	-

Groups/Drugs	Dose (Age >28 Days)	Max/Day
Antivirals/Antivirals (hepatitis C combinations)		
Elbasvir/Grazoprevir (Zepatier)	Age ≥12 yrs, wt ≥30 kg: 1 tab po q24h	
Glecaprevir/Pibrentasvir (Mavyret)	Age 3 to <12 yrs: <20 kg: 150 mg/60 mg (3 packets) q24h 20 to <30 kg: 200 mg/80 mg (4 packets) q24h 30 to <45 kg: 250 mg/100 mg (5 packets) q24h Age ≥12 yrs, wt ≥45 kg: 300 mg/120 mg (3 tabs) q24h	-
Ledipasvir/Sofosbuvir (Harvoni)	Age ≥3 yrs, wt ≥35 kg: 90 mg/400 mg q24h Age ≥3 yrs, wt 17 kg to <35 kg: 45 mg/200 mg q24h Age ≥3 yrs, wt <17 kg: 33.75 mg/150 mg q24h Duration: Geno 1, tx-naive, no cirr or comp: 12 wks Geno 1, tx-exp, no cirr: 12 wks Geno 1, tx-exp with comp: 24 wks Geno 1, tx-naive/exp with decomp cirr:12 wks (+ribavirin) Geno 1/4, tx-naive/exp LT recipients, no cirr or comp: 12 wks (+ribavirin) Geno 4/5/6, tx-naive/exp, no cirr or comp: 12 wks	-
Ombitasvir/Paritaprevir/RTV (Technivie)	Safety and efficacy not established (not available in US)	-
Ombitasvir + Paritaprevir/RTV + Dasabuvir (Viekira Pak)	Safety and efficacy not established (not available in US)	-
Sofosbuvir/velpatasvir (Epclusa)	Age ≥3 years: Wt <17 kg: 150 mg/37.5 q24h (oral pellets) Wt 17 to <30 kg: 200 mg/50 mg q24h (oral pellets or tablets) Wt ≥30 kg: 400 mg/100 mg q24h (oral pellets or tablets)	-
Velpatasvir/Sofosbuvir/ Voxilaprevir (Vosevi)	Safety and efficacy not established	
Antivirals (herpesvirus)		
Acyclovir (neonatal HSV)	60 mg/kg/day (divided q8h)	-
Acyclovir (HSV encephalitis)	Age >3 mon: 30-45 mg/kg/day (divided q8h)	-
Acyclovir (varicella, immunocompromised)	Age <1 year: 30 mg/kg/day (divided q8h) Age >1 year: 30 mg/kg/day or 1500 mg/m²/day (divided q8h)	-
Acyclovir (HSV, immunocompromised)	30 mg/kg/day (divided q8h)	-
Cidofovir	Induction 5 mg/kg once weekly Suppressive therapy 3 mg/kg once weekly (all with hydration + probenecid)	-
Famciclovir	Safety and efficacy not established	-
Foscarnet	120-180 mg/kg/day (divided q8-12h)	-
Ganciclovir	Symptomatic congenital CMV: 12 mg/kg/day (divided q12h) CMV tx or first 2 weeks after SOT: 10 mg/kg/day (divided q12h) Suppressive tx or prophylaxis: 5 mg/kg/day (once daily)	-
Letermovir	Safety and efficacy not established	-
Maribavir	Age ≥12 yr, wt ≥35kg: 400 mg po q12h (same as adults)	-
Penciclovir (topical)	Age ≥12 yr: Apply q2h (while awake) x4 days	-
Trifluridine (1% oph soln)	1 drop q2h until corneal re-epithelialization, then 1 drop q4h x7 days (min 5 drops/day)[9]	9 drops
Valacyclovir (herpes labialis)	Age ≥12 yrs: 2 gm q12h x1 day	-
Valacyclovir[8] (chickenpox)	Age 2 to <18 yrs: 60 mg/kg/day (divided q8h) x5 days	3 gm
Valganciclovir	Symptomatic congenital CMV: 32 mg/kg/day (divided q12h) po x6 mon. Prevention of CMV after SOT: (7 mg x BSA x CrCl) po q24h (use Schwartz formula for CrCl; if calculated CrCl >150, use 150 to avoid overdosage)	-
Antivirals (human papillomavirus)		
Imiquimod (5% cream)	Genital warts (age ≥12 yrs): Apply 3x/week, max 16 weeks (wash off after 6-10 hrs)	-
Podofilox (0.5% gel, soln)	Safety and efficacy not established	-
Sinecatechins (15% ointment)	Safety and efficacy not established	-
Antivirals (influenza)		
Amantadine	Age 1 to <9 years: 4.4-8.8 mg/kg (max 150 mg) po q24h Age ≥9 years: use adult dose	-
Baloxavir marboxil	Age ≥5 yrs: <20 kg: 2 mg/kg (oral susp) x1 dose 20 to <80 kg: 40 mg (tab or oral susp) x1 dose ≥80 kg: 80 mg (tab or oral susp) x1 dose	-
Favipiravir	Safety and efficacy not established	-
Laninamivir	Treatment or prophylaxis: Age <10 yrs: 20 mg inhaled (single dose) Age ≥10 yrs: 40 mg inhaled (single dose)	-
Oseltamivir (treatment)	Infants 2 wks-11 mons: 3 mg/kg bid x5 days ≤15 kg: 30 mg bid x5 days >15 to 23 kg: 45 mg bid x5 days >23 to 40 kg: 60 mg bid x5 days >40 kg: 75 mg bid x5 days	-

Groups/Drugs	Dose (Age >28 Days)	Max/Day
Antivirals/Antivirals (influenza) *(continued)*		
Oseltamivir (prophylaxis)	Infants <3 mons: not recommended Infants 3-11 mons: 3 mg/kg qd x10 days ≤15 kg: 30 mg qd x10 days >15 to 23 kg: 45 mg qd x10 days >23 to 40 kg: 60 mg qd x10 days >40 kg: 75 mg qd x10 days	-
Peramivir	Age 6 mon to 12 yrs: 12 mg/kg IV x1 Age 13-18 yrs: 600 mg IV x1	600 mg
Rimantadine	Age 1 to <10 years: 5 mg/kg (max 150 mg) po q24h Age ≥10 years: use adult dose	-
Zanamivir (treatment)	Age ≥7 yrs: 10 mg (two 5-mg inhalations) q12h x5 days	-
Zanamivir (prophylaxis)	Age ≥5 yrs: 10 mg (two 5-mg inhalations) q24h x10 days	-
Antivirals (poxviruses)		
Brincidofovir	Wt <10 kg: 6 mg/kg on days 1 and 8 Wt 10 to <48 kg: 4 mg/kg on days 1 and 8 Wt ≥48 kg: 200 mg on days 1 and 8	-
Tecovirimat (po dosing)	Wt 13 to <25 kg: 200 mg q12h x14 days Wt 25 to <40 kg: 400 mg q12h x14 days Wt ≥40 to <120 kg: 600 mg q12h x14 days Wt ≥120 kg; 600 mg q8h x14 days	-
Tecovirimat (IV dosing)	Wt 3 to <35 kg: 6 mg/kg q12h x14 days Wt 35 to <120 kg: 200 mg q12h x14 days Wt ≥120 kg: 300 mg q12h x14 days	-
Antivirals (RSV)		
Nirsevimab-alip	Neonates, infants born during or entering their first RSV season: Wt <5 kg: 50 mg IM x1 Wt ≥5 kg: 100 mg IM x1 Children up to 24 mon of age who remain vulnerable to severe disease through their second RSV season: 200 mg IM x1 (given as two 100 mg injections). For children undergoing cardiac surgery with cardiopulmonary bypass, an additional dose is recommended when the child is stable after surgery: - First RSV season: if surgery is within 90 days after receiving nirsevimab-alip, base additional dose on body weight. If >90 days have elapsed, the additional dose should be 50 mg. - Second RSV season: if surgery is within 90 days after receiving nirsevimab-alip, the additional dose should be 200 mg. If >90 days have elapsed, the additional dose should be 100 mg.	-
Palivizumab	15 mg/kg IM qmonth throughout RSV season	-

1 Approved only for CF, anthrax, and complicated UTI
2 LD = loading dose, MD = maintenance dose
3 VVC = vulvovaginal candidiasis, RVVC = recurrent vulvovaginal candidiasis
4 BSA = body surface area
5 Consider oral lead-in (CAB x1 mon) to assess tolerability
6 Consider oral lead-in (CAB/RPV x1 mon) to assess tolerability
7 If certain drugs that induce UGT1A or CYP3A are coadministered, administered DTG twice daily
8 Use extemporaneous oral suspension formulation
9 Administer eyedrops while awake

TABLE 17A – DOSAGE OF ANTIMICROBIAL DRUGS IN ADULT PATIENTS WITH RENAL IMPAIRMENT

- For listing of drugs with NO need for adjustment for renal failure, *see Table 17B*.
- Adjustments for renal failure are based on an estimate of creatinine clearance (CrCl) which reflects the glomerular filtration rate.
- **Different methods for calculating estimated CrCl are suggested for underweight, normal weight, overweight, and obese patients.**
  - Calculations for ideal body weight (IBW) in kg:
    - *Men:* 50 kg plus 2.3 kg/inch over 60 inches height.
    - *Women:* 45.5 kg plus 2.3 kg/inch over 60 inches height.
  - Obese is defined as body mass index (BMI) >30

- Calculations of estimated CrCl *(Nephron 1976;16:31)*
  - Calculate ideal body weight (IBW) in kg (as above)-
  - Use the following formula to determine estimated CrCl

$$\frac{(140 \text{ minus age})(\text{weight in kg})}{72 \times \text{serum creatinine}} = \text{CrCl in mL/min for men. Multiply answer by 0.85 for women (estimated)}$$

Use the following body weights in the above formula *(Pharmacotherapy 2012;32:604)*:

- Underweight pt (BMI <18.5 kg/m²): use actual weight
- Normal weight pt (BMI 18.5-24.9 kg/m²): use IBW
- Overweight pt (BMI 25-29.9 kg/m²): use adjusted weight*
- Obese pt (BMI >30 kg/m²): use adjusted weight

*adjusted weight = IBW + 0.4(actual BW - IBW)

Estimated CrCl is the most common method used for FDA-approved dose adjustments for renal insufficiency. The bulk of the data in this table are based on calculated estimates of CrCl. **Emerging methods use calculations designed to estimate the glomerular filtration rate (eGFR).** Going forward the FDA may require that renal dosing adjustments be based on estimated CrCl and/or eGFR. See *Adv Chronic Kid Dis 2018,25:14*.

Sources for drug dose adjustment for renal impairment: 1) Drug Prescribing in Renal Failure, 5th ed., Aronoff, et al *(eds)(Am College Physicians, 2007)*; 2) package inserts; 3) *AAC 63:e00583, 2019.*

- For slow or sustained extended daily dialysis **(SLEDD)** over 6-12 hours, adjust doses as for CRRT. For details, *see CID 49:433, 2009; CCM 39:560, 2011.*
- **SLED:** Limited data on dose adjustment for sustained low efficiency dialysis (SLED)*(Can J Kidney Health Dis 2018;5:1)*.

TABLE 17A (2)

Groups/Drugs	Half-life, hrs (renal function normal)	Half-life, hrs (ESRD)	Dose (renal function normal)	CrCl or eGFR	Hemodialysis	CAPD	CRRT	SLED
Antibacterials								
Aminoglycosides								
Amikacin[1,2] (conventional)	2-3	30-70	7.5 mg/kg IM/IV q12h	CrCl >50: No dosage adjustment CrCl 10-50: 7.5 mg/kg q24h CrCl <10: 7.5 mg/kg q48h	7.5 mg/kg q48h (+ extra 3.75 mg/kg AD)	For peritonitis only: 2 mg/kg IP once daily	7.5 mg/kg q24h	No data
Amikacin[3] (extended interval)	2-3	30-70	15 mg/kg q24h	CrCl 60-80: 12 mg/kg q24h CrCl 40-60: 7.5 mg/kg q24h CrCl 30-40: 4 mg/kg q24h CrCl 20-30: 7.5 mg/kg q48h CrCl 10-20: 4 mg/kg q48h CrCl <10: 3 mg/kg q72h	3 mg/kg q72h (dose AD)	No data	No data	No data
Gentamicin[1,2] (conventional)	2-3	30-70	1.7-2.0 mg/kg IM/IV q8h	CrCl >50: No dosage adjustment CrCl 10-50: 1.7-2.0 mg/kg q12-24h CrCl <10: 1.7-2.0 mg/kg q48h	1.7-2.0 mg/kg q48h (+ extra 0.85-1.0 mg/kg AD)	For peritonitis only: 0.6 mg/kg IP once daily	1.7-2.0 mg/kg q24h	6 mg/kg IV q48h Begin 30 min before start of SLED *(AAC 2010; 54:3635)*
Gentamicin[3] (extended interval)	2-3	30-70	5.1 mg/kg q24h	CrCl 60-80: 4 mg/kg q24h CrCl 40-60: 3.5 mg/kg q24h CrCl 30-40: 2.5 mg/kg q24h CrCl 20-30: 4 mg/kg q48h CrCl 10-20: 3 mg/kg q48h CrCl <10: 2 mg/kg q72h	2 mg/kg q72h (dose AD)	No data	No data	No data
Isepamicin (extended interval)	2-3	30-70	8 mg/kg q24h	CrCl >40: No dosage adjustment CrCl 20-40: 8 mg/kg q48h CrCl 10-20: 8 mg/kg q72h CrCl <10: 8 mg/kg q96h	8 mg/kg q96h (dose AD)	No data	No data	No data
Kanamycin[3] (extended interval)	2-3	30-70	15 mg/kg q24h	CrCl 60-80: 12 mg/kg q24h CrCl 40-60: 7.5 mg/kg q24h CrCl 30-40: 4 mg/kg q24h CrCl 20-30: 7.5 mg/kg q48h CrCl 10-20: 4 mg/kg q48h CrCl <10: 3 mg/kg q72h	3 mg/kg q72h (dose AD)	No data	No data	No data
Neomycin (oral, non-absorbed)	2-3	30-70	1 gm po x3 (prior to surgery)	No dosage adjustment for renal impairment	No dosage adjustment	No data	No data	No data
Netilmicin[1,2] (conventional)	2-3	30-70	1.7-2.0 mg/kg IM/IV q8h	CrCl >50: No dosage adjustment CrCl 10-50: 1.7-2.0 mg/kg q12-24h CrCl <10: 1.7-2.0 mg/kg q48h	1.7-2.0 mg/kg q48h (+ extra 0.85-1.0 mg/kg AD)	For peritonitis only: 0.6 mg/kg IP once daily	1.7-2.0 mg/kg q24h	No data

TABLE 17A (3)

Groups/Drugs	Half-life, hrs (renal function normal)	Half-life, hrs (ESRD)	Dose (renal function normal)	CrCl or eGFR	Hemodialysis	CAPD	CRRT	SLED
Antibacterials/Aminoglycosides *(continued)*								
Netilmicin[3] (extended interval)	2-3	30-70	6.5 mg/kg q24h	CrCl 60-80: 5 mg/kg q24h CrCl 40-60: 4 mg/kg q24h CrCl 30-40: 2 mg/kg q24h CrCl 20-30: 3 mg/kg q48h CrCl 10-20: 2.5 mg/kg q48h CrCl <10: 2 mg/kg q72h	2 mg/kg q72h (dose AD)	No data	No data	No data
Plazomicin (extended interval)	3.5	No data	15 mg/kg IV q24h	CrCl ≥60: No dosage adjustment CrCl ≥30 to <60: 10 mg/kg q24h CrCl ≥15 to <30: 10 mg/kg q48h CrCl <15: No data	No data	No data	No data	No data
Spectinomycin (single-dose)	1.5-2	No data	2 gm IM x1	No dosage adjustment for renal impairment	No dosage adjustment	No data	No data	No data
Streptomycin[3] (extended interval)	2-3	30-70	15 mg/kg q24h	CrCl 60-80: 12 mg/kg q24h CrCl 40-60: 7.5 mg/kg q24h CrCl 30-40: 4 mg/kg q24h CrCl 20-30: 7.5 mg/kg q48h CrCl 10-20: 4 mg/kg q48h CrCl <10: 3 mg/kg q72h	3 mg/kg q72h (dose AD)	No data	No data	No data
Tobramycin[1,2] (conventional)	2-3	30-70	1.7-2.0 mg/kg IM/IV q8h	CrCl >50: No dosage adjustment CrCl 10-50: 1.7-2.0 mg/kg q12-24h CrCl <10: 1.7-2.0 mg/kg q48h	1.7-2.0 mg/kg q48h (+ extra 0.85-1.0 mg/kg AD)	For peritonitis only: 0.6 mg/kg IP once daily	1.7-2.0 mg/kg q24h	No data
Tobramycin[3] (extended interval)	2-3	30-70	5.1 mg/kg q24h	CrCl 60-80: 4 mg/kg q24h CrCl 40-60: 3.5 mg/kg q24h CrCl 30-40: 2.5 mg/kg q24h CrCl 20-30: 4 mg/kg q48h CrCl 10-20: 3 mg/kg q48h CrCl <10: 2 mg/kg q72h	2 mg/kg q72h (dose AD)	No data	No data	No data
Beta-Lactams								
Carbapenems								
Doripenem	1	18	500 mg IV q8h	CrCl >50: No dosage adjustment CrCl 30-50: 250 mg q8h CrCl 10-30: 250 mg q12h CrCl <10: No data	No data	No data	500 mg q8h (JAC 69:2508, 2014)	No data
Ertapenem	4	>4	1 gm IV q24h	CrCl >30 mL/min/1.73 m^2: No dosage adjustment CrCl ≤30 mL/min/1.73 m^2: 500 mg q24h	500 mg q24h (+150 mg AD if given ≤6 hr bef HD), OR 500 mg 3x/wk AD[6]	500 mg q24h	0.5-1 gm q24h	1 gm q24h[13]

TABLE 17A (4)

Groups/Drugs	Half-life, hrs (renal function normal)	Half-life, hrs (ESRD)	Dose (renal function normal)	CrCl or eGFR	Hemodialysis	CAPD	CRRT	SLED
Antibacterials/Carbapenems *(continued)*								
Imipenem-cilastatin	1	4	Variable	If target dose 500 mg q6h: CrCl ≥90: No dosage adjustment CrCl 60 to <90: 400 mg q6h CrCl 30 to <60: 300 mg q6h CrCl 15 to <30: 200 mg q6h If target dose 1 gm q8h: CrCl ≥90: No dosage adjustment CrCl 60 o <90: 500 mg q6h CrCl 30 to <60: 500 mg q8h CrCl 15 to <30: 500 mg q12h If target dose 1 gm q6h: CrCl ≥90: No dosage adjustment CrCl 60 to <90: 750 mg q8h CrCl 30 to <60: 500 mg q6h CrCl 15 to <30: 500 mg q12h	If target dose 500 mg q6h: Give 200 mg q6h (dose AD) If target dose 1 gm q8h: Give 500 mg q12h (dose AD) If target dose 1 gm q6h: Give 500 mg q12h (dose AD)	No data	0.5-1 gm q12h *(AAC 49:2421, 2005)*	No data
Imipenem-cilastatin-relebactam	1 (imi)	4 (imi)	1.25 gm IV q6h	CrCl ≥90: No dosage adjustment CrCl 60-89: 1 gm q6h CrCl 30-59: 0.75 gm q6h CrCl 15-29: 0.5 gm q6h CrCl <10: No data	0.5 gm q6h (dose AD)	No data	No data	No data
Meropenem	1	10	1 gm IV q8h	CrCl >50: No dosage adjustment CrCl 26-50: 1 gm q12h CrCl 10-25: 0.5 gm q12h CrCl <10: 0.5 gm q24h	0.5 gm q24h (AD on dialysis days)	0.5 gm q24h	CVVH, CVVHD: 0.75-1 gm IV q8h[29]	0.5 gm q8h[30]
Meropenem-vaborbactam	Mer 1.2 Vab 1.7	Mer 10 Vab ND	2 gm/2 gm IV q8h	eGFR ≥50: No dosage adjustment eGFR 30-49: 1 gm/1 gm q8h eGFR 15-29: 1 gm/1 gm q12h eGFR <15: 0.5 gm/0.5 gm q12h	0.5 gm/0.5 gm q12h (AD)	No data	No data	No data
Cephalosporins, IV, 1st gen								
Cefazolin	2	40-70	1-2 gm IV q8h	CrCl >50: No dosage adjustment CrCl 10-50: 0.5-2 gm q8-12h CrCl <10: 0.5-1 gm q24h	0.5-1 gm q24h (AD on dialysis days). Outpts: 2 gm AD MW, 3 gm AD Fri *(CID 2007;44:190)*.	0.5 gm q12h	1-2 gm q12h	No data
Cephalosporins, IV, 2nd gen								
Cefmetazole	1-1.5	29	2 gm IV q8-12h	CrCl >90: No dosage adjustment CrCl 50-90: 1-2 gm q12h CrCl 30-49: 1 gm q12h CrCl 10-29: 1-2 gm q24h CrCl <10: 1-2 gm q48h	1-2 gm q48h (AD on dialysis days)	No data	No data	No data

TABLE 17A (5)

Groups/Drugs	Half-life, hrs (renal function normal)	Half-life, hrs (ESRD)	Dose (renal function normal)	CrCl or eGFR	Hemodialysis	CAPD	CRRT	SLED
Antibacterials/Cephalosporins, IV, 2nd gen *(continued)*								
Cefotetan	3-4.6	12-30	1-2 gm IV q12h	CrCl >30: No dosage adjustment CrCl 10-30: 1-2 gm q24h CrCl <10: 1-2 gm q48h	1-2 gm q24h (+ extra 1 gm AD)	1 gm q24h	1-2 gm q24h	No data
Cefoxitin[4]	0.8	13-23	2 gm IV q8h	CrCl >50: No dosage adjustment CrCl 10-50: 2 gm q8-12h CrCl <10: 2 gm q24-48h	2 gm q24-48h (+ extra 1 gm AD)	1 gm q24h	2 gm q8-12h	No data
Cefuroxime	1.5	17	0.75-1.5 gm IV q8h	CrCl >50: No dosage adjustment CrCl 10-50: 0.75-1.5 gm q8-12h CrCl <10: 0.75-1.5 gm q24h	0.75-1.5 gm q24h (AD on dialysis days)	0.75-1.5 gm q24h	0.75-1.5 gm q8-12h	No data
Cephalosporins, IV, 3rd gen, Non-Antipseudomonal								
Cefotaxime	1.5	15-35	2 gm IV q8h	CrCl >90: No dosage adjustment CrCl >50-90: 2 gm q8-12h CrCl 10-50: 2 gm q12-24h CrCl <10: 2 gm q24h	2 gm q24h (+ extra 1 gm AD)	0.5-1 gm q24h	2 gm q12-24h	No data
Ceftizoxime	1.7	15-35	2 gm IV q8h	CrCl >90: No dosage adjustment CrCl >50-90: 2 gm q8-12h CrCl 10-50: 2 gm q12-24h CrCl <10: 2 gm q24h	2 gm q24h (+ extra 1 gm AD)	0.5-1 gm q24h	2 gm q12-24h	No data
Ceftriaxone*	8	Unchanged	1-2 gm IV q12-24h	No dosage adjustment for renal impairment	No dosage adjustment	No dosage adjustment	No dosage adjustment	No data
Cephalosporins, IV, Antipseudomonal								
Cefepime	2	18	2 gm IV q8h	CrCl >60: No dosage adjustment CrCl 30-60: 2 gm q12h CrCl 11-29: 2 gm q24h CrCl <10: 1 gm q24h	1 gm q24h AD	2 gm q48h	2 gm q12-24h	No data
Cefepime-enmetazobactam	Cefepime 2.7 Enmetazo-bactam 2.6	No data	2.5 gm (over 2 hr) q8h	eGFR ≥130: 2.5 gm (over 4 hr) q8h eGFR 60-129: 2.5 gm (over 2 hr) q8h eGFR 30-59: 1.25 gm (over 2 hr) q8h eGFR 15-29: 1.25 gm (over 2 hr) q12h eGFR <15: 1.25 gm, then 0.625 gm (over 2 hr) q24h	1.25 gm, then 0.625 gm (over 2 hr) q24h (dose AD)	No data	No data	No data
Cefiderocol	2-3	No data	2 gm IV q8h	CrCl ≥120: 2 gm q6h CrCl 60-119: 2 gm q8h CrCl 30-59: 1.5 gm q8h CrCl 15-29: 1 gm q8h CrCl <15: 0.75 gm q12h	0.75 gm q12h (dose AD)	No data	Effluent flow rate: ≤2 L/hr: 1.5 gm q12h 2.1 to 3 L/hr: 2 gm q12h 3.1 to 4 L/hr: 1.5 gm q8h ≥4.1 L/hr: 2 gm q8h	No data

TABLE 17A (6)

Groups/Drugs	Half-life, hrs (renal function normal)	Half-life, hrs (ESRD)	Dose (renal function normal)	CrCl or eGFR	Hemodialysis	CAPD	CRRT	SLED
Antibacterials/Cephalosporins, IV, Antipseudomonal *(continued)*								
Cefoperazone[5]	1.7-2.0	No change	1-2 gm IV q12h	No dosage adjustment for renal impairment (if GFR <18, do not exceed 4 gm/day)	No dosage adjustment (AD on dialysis days)	No data	No data	No data
Cefoperazone-sulbactam[5, 17]	Cefoperazone: 1.7-2.0 Sulbactam: 1.0	Cefoperazone: No change Sulbactam: 6.9-9.7	2-4 gm/day (divided q12h) (i.e., cefoperazone 1-2 gm/day)	Adjustment necessary for the sulbactam: CrCl ≥30: No dosage adjustment CrCl 15-30: Sulbactam 1 gm q12h CrCl <15: Sulbactam 500 mg q12h	Sulbactam 500 mg q12h (AD on dialysis days)	No data	Sulbactam 1 gm q8h	No data
Cefpirome	2	14.5	2 gm IV q12h	CrCl >50: No dosage adjustment CrCl 10-50: 1 gm q12h CrCl <10: 1 gm q24h	1 gm q24h (AD on dialysis days)	0.5 gm 3x/wk	2 gm load, then 1 gm q12h	No data
Ceftazidime	1.9	13-25	1-2 gm IV q8-12h	CrCl >50: No dosage adjustment CrCl 10-50: 1-2 gm q12-24h CrCl <10: 1-2 gm q24h	0.5-1 gm q24h (AD on dialysis days)	No data	1-2 gm q8-12h *(Pharmacother 2009;29:562)*	1-2 gm q8-12h *(Can J Kidney Health Dis 2018;5:1)*
Ceftazidime-avibactam	ceftaz 2.8, avi 2.7	ceftaz 13-25	2.5 gm IV q8h	CrCl >50: No dosage adjustment CrCl 31-50: 1.25 gm q8h CrCl 16-30: 0.94 gm q12h CrCl 6-15 (± HD): 0.94 gm q24h CrCl ≤5 (± HD): 0.94 gm q48h	CrCl ≤15 on HD (AD on dialysis days)	No data	CVVH: 1.25 gm q8h *(AAC 2017; 61:e00464-17)*	No data
Ceftolozane-tazobactam	ceftolozane 3.1	ceftolozane 40	IAI/UTI: 1.5 gm IV q8h HAP/VAP: 3 gm IV q8h	CrCl >50: No dosage adjustment CrCl 30-50: IAI/UTI: 750 mg q8h HAP/VAP: 1.5 gm q8h CrCl 15-29: IAI/UTI: 375 mg q8h HAP/VAP: 750 mg q8h CrCl <15 on HD: *See HD recommendations*	IAI/UTI: 750 mg load, 150 mg q8h (dose AD) HAP/VAP: 2.25 gm load, 450 mg q8h (dose AD)	No data	CVVHDF: 3 gm x1, then 750 mg q8h[23]	No data
Cephalosporins, IV, Anti-MRSA								
Ceftaroline	2.7	No data	600 mg IV q12h	CrCl >50: No dosage adjustment CrCl 30-50: 400 mg q12h CrCl 15-30: 300 mg q12h CrCl <15: 200 mg q12h	200 mg q12h	No data	70 kg pt, effluent flow rate 3 L/hr: 400 mg q12h *(Pharmacother 2021;41:205)*	No data

TABLE 17A (7)

Groups/Drugs	Half-life, hrs (renal function normal)	Half-life, hrs (ESRD)	Dose (renal function normal)	CrCl or eGFR	Hemodialysis	CAPD	CRRT	SLED
Antibacterials/Cephalosporins, IV, Anti-MRSA *(continued)*								
Ceftobiprole medocaril	3.3	21	667 mg IV q8h	CrCl >150: 667 mg q6h CrCl ≥50 to 150: No dosage adjustment CrCl 30 to <50: SAB: 667 mg q8h days 1-8, then q12h ABSSSI, CAP: 667 mg q12h CrCl 15 to <30: SAB: 333 mg q8h days 1-8, then q12h ABSSSI, CAP: 333 mg q12h CrCl <15: 333 mg q24h	333 mg q24h (AD on dialysis days)	No data	No data	No data
Cephalosporins, Oral, 1st gen								
Cefadroxil	1.5	20	1 gm po q12h	CrCl >50: No dosage adjustment CrCl 10-50: 1 gm, then 500 mg q12-24h CrCl <10: 1 gm, then 500 mg q36h	1 gm, then 1 gm AD	500 mg q24h	No data	No data
Cephalexin	0.5-1.2	5-30	250-1000 mg po q6h	CrCl >50: No dosage adjustment CrCl 10-50: 250-1000 mg q8-12h CrCl <10: 250-1000 mg q24-48h	250-500 mg q12-24h (AD on dialysis days)	250-500 mg q12-24h	No data	No data
Cephalosporins, Oral, 2nd gen								
Cefaclor	0.8	3	500 mg po q8h	CrCl ≥10: No dosage adjustment CrCl <10: 500 mg q12h	500 mg q12h (give one of the dialysis day doses AD)	500 mg q12h	No data	No data
Cefprozil	1.5	5-6	500 mg po q12h	CrCl >50: No dosage adjustment CrCl 10-50: 500 mg q24h CrCl <10: 250 mg q12h	250 mg q12h (give one of the dialysis day doses AD)	250 mg q24h	No data	No data
Cefuroxime axetil	1.5	17	250-500 mg po q12h	CrCl ≥30: No dosage adjustment CrCl 10-29: 250-500 mg q24h CrCl <10: 250-500 mg q48h	250-500 mg q48h (give extra 250-500 mg AD)	250-500 mg q24h	No data	No data
Loracarbef	1.2	32	200-400 mg po q12h	CrCl ≥50: No dosage adjustment CrCl 10-49: 200-400 mg q24h CrCl <10: 200-400 mg q3-5 days	200-400 mg q3-5 days (give extra 200-400 mg AD)	No data	No data	No data
Cephalosporins, Oral, 3rd gen								
Cefdinir	1.7	16	300 mg po q12h	CrCl ≥30: No dosage adjustment CrCl <30: 300 mg q24h	300 mg q48h (AD on dialysis days)	No data	No data	No data
Cefditoren pivoxil	1.6	5	400 mg po q12h	CrCl >50: No dosage adjustment CrCl 10-50: 200 mg q12h CrCl <10: 200 mg 24h	200 mg q24h (AD on dialysis days)	200 mg q24h	No data	No data
Cefixime	3	12	400 mg po q24h	CrCl ≥60: No dosage adjustment CrCl 21-60: 260 mg q24h (use susp) CrCl ≤20: 200 mg q24h	260 mg q24h (use susp) (AD on dialysis days)	200 mg q24h	No data	No data

TABLE 17A (8)

Groups/Drugs	Half-life, hrs (renal function normal)	Half-life, hrs (ESRD)	Dose (renal function normal)	CrCl or eGFR	Hemodialysis	CAPD	CRRT	SLED
Antibacterials/Cephalosporins, Oral, 3rd gen *(continued)*								
Cefpodoxime proxetil	2.3	10	200 mg po q12h	CrCl ≥10: No dosage adjustment CrCl <10: 200 mg q24h	200 mg q24h (AD on dialysis days)	200 mg q24h	No data	No data
Ceftibuten	2.5	13	400 mg po q24h	CrCl >50: No dosage adjustment CrCl 10-50: 200 mg q24h CrCl <10: 100 mg q24h	100 mg q24h (AD on dialysis days)	100 mg po q24h	No data	No data
Monobactams								
Aztreonam*	2	6-8	Varies with indication	CrCl ≥30: No dosage adjustment CrCl 10 to <30: 50% dosage reduction CrCl <10: 1-2 gm q24h	1-2 gm q24h (AD on dialysis days)	2 gm q24h	CVVH: 1-2 gm q12h CVVHD: 2 gm q12h CVVHDF: 2 gm q12h[25]	No data
Aztreonam-avibactam*	Az: 2-3 Avi: 2-3	Az: 6-8 Avi: no data	2 gm/0.67 gm IV load, then 1.5 gm/0.5 gm IV q6h	CrCl >50: No dosage adjustment CrCl >30 to 50: 2 gm/0.67 gm x1, then 0.75 gm/0.25 gm q6h CrCl >15 to 30: 1.35 gm/0.45 gm x1, then 0.675gm/0.225 gm q8h CrCl ≤15, no RRT: not recommended	1 gm/0.33 gm x1, then 0.675 gm/ 0.225 gm q12h (AD on dialysis days)	No data	No data	No data
Penicillins (Natural)								
Penicillin G	0.5	6-20	0.5-4 million U IV q4h	CrCl >50: No dosage adjustment CrCl 10-50: 0.5-4 million U q8h CrCl <10: 0.5-4 million U q12h	0.5-4 million U q12h (give one of the dialysis day doses AD)	0.5-4 million U q12h	1-4 million U q6-8h	No data
Penicillin VK	0.5	4.1	250-500 mg po q6-8h	No dosage adjustment for renal impairment	No dosage adjustment (give one or more doses AD)	No dosage adjustment	No data	No data
Penicillins (Aminopenicillins)								
Amoxicillin* (standard)	1.2	5-20	500 mg po q8h (or 875 mg po q12h)	CrCl >30: No dosage adjustment CrCl 10-30: 250-500 mg q12h CrCl <10: 250-500 mg q24h	250-500 mg q24h (+ extra dose AD)	250-500 mg q12h	250-500 mg q8-12h	No data
Amoxicillin (ER)	1.2-1.5	No data	775 mg po q24h	CrCl ≥30: No dosage adjustment CrCl <30: No data, avoid usage	No data	No data	No data	No data
Amoxicillin-clavulanate*	Amox: 1.4 Clav: 1	Amox: 5-20 Clav: 4	500 mg/125 mg po q8h 875 mg/125 mg po q12h 1000 mg/200 mg IV q8h	Oral: CrCl >30: No dosage adjustment CrCl 10-30: 250-500 mg (amox) q12h CrCl <10: 250-500 mg (amox) q24h IV: CrCl >30: No dosage adjustment CrCl 10-30: 1000 mg/200 mg x1, then 500 mg/100 mg q12h CrCl <10: 1000 mg/200 mg x1, then 500 mg/100 mg q24h	Oral: 250-500 mg (amox) q24h (+ extra dose AD) IV: 1000 mg/200 mg x1, then 500 mg/100 mg q24h (+ extra dose AD)	No data	No data	No data

TABLE 17A (9)

Groups/Drugs	Half-life, hrs (renal function normal)	Half-life, hrs (ESRD)	Dose (renal function normal)	CrCl or eGFR	Hemodialysis	CAPD	CRRT	SLED
Antibacterials/Penicillins (Aminopenicillins) *(continued)*								
Ampicillin	1.2	7-20	1-2 gm IV q4-6h	CrCl >50: No dosage adjustment CrCl 30-50: 1-2 gm q6-8h CrCl 10-30: 1-2 gm q8-12h	1-2 gm q12h (give one of the dialysis day doses AD)	500 mg - 1 gm q12h	1-2 gm q8-12h	No data
Ampicillin-sulbactam	Amp: 1.4 Sulb: 1.7	Amp: 7-20 Sulb: 10	1.5-3 gm IV q6h	CrCl ≥30: No dosage adjustment CrCl 15-29: 1.5-3 gm q12h CrCl 5-14: 1.5-3 gm q24h	1.5-3 gm q24h (AD on dialysis days)	3 gm q24h	1.5-3 gm q8-12h	3 gm q12h *(Can J Kidney Health Dis 2018;5:1)*
Penicillins (Antistaphylococcal)								
Cloxacillin	0.4	0.7	250-500 mg po q6h	No dosage adjustment for renal impairment	No data	No data	No data	No data
Dicloxacillin	0.7	No change	125-500 mg po q6h	No dosage adjustment for renal impairment	No data	No data	No data	No data
Flucloxacillin	0.75	No data	250-500 mg po q6h 1-2 gm IV q4-6h	Dosage recommendations not available Consider 50% reduction if CrCl <10 mL/min	No data (not significantly removed by HD)	No data	No data	No data
Nafcillin[5]	0.5-1	No change	2 gm IM/IV q4h	No dosage adjustment for renal impairment	No dosage adjustment	No dosage adjustment	No dosage adjustment	No data
Oxacillin[5]	0.5-0.7	No data	2 gm IV q4h	Dosage recommendations not available[20]	No data	No data	No data	No data
Penicillins (Antipseudomonal)								
Piperacillin	1	3-5	3-4 gm IV q4-6h	CrCl >50: No dosage adjustment CrCl 30-50: 3-4 gm q6-8h CrCl 10-30: 3-4 gm q8h	2 gm q8h (+ extra 1 gm AD)	3-4 gm q8h	3-4 gm q6-8h	No data
Piperacillin-Tazobactam (short infusion, non-Pseudomonas)	Pip: 1 Tazo: 1	Pip: 3-5 Tazo: 2.8	3.375 gm (over 30 min) q6h	CrCl >40: No dosage adjustment CrCl 20-40: 2.25 gm q6h CrCl <20: 2.25 gm q8h	2.25 gm q12h (+ extra 0.75 gm AD)	2.25 gm q12h	2.25 gm q6h	No data
Piperacillin-Tazobactam (short infusion, Pseudomonas)	Pip: 1 Tazo: 1	Pip: 3-5 Tazo: 2.8	4.5 gm (over 30 min) q6h	CrCl >40: No dosage adjustment CrCl 20-40: 3.375 gm q6h CrCl <20: 2.25 gm q6h	2.25 gm q8h (+ extra 0.75 gm AD)	2.25 gm q8h	MIC ≤16: 3.375 gm (over 30 min) q6h *(Clin J Am Soc Nephrol 2012;7:452)*; MIC >16 to 64: 4.5 gm (over 4 hr) q8h *(Pharmacother 2015;35:600)*	No data
Piperacillin-Tazobactam (prolonged infusion)	Pip: 1 Tazo: 1	Pip: 3-5 Tazo: 2.8	4.5 gm (over 30 min), then 3.375 gm (over 4 hr) q8h	CrCl ≥20: No dosage adjustment CrCl <20: 3.375 gm (over 4 hr) q12h	3.375 gm (over 4 hr) q12h	No data	4.5 gm (over 4 hr) q8h *(Pharmacother 2015;35:600)*	No data

TABLE 17A (10)

Groups/Drugs	Half-life, hrs (renal function normal)	Half-life, hrs (ESRD)	Dose (renal function normal)	CrCl or eGFR	Hemodialysis	CAPD	CRRT	SLED
Antibacterials *(continued)*								
Penicillins (Other)								
Pivmecillinam	1	No data	US: 185 mg po q8h	No dosage adjustment for renal impairment	No data	No data	No data	No data
Sulbactam + durlobactam (co-packaged)	Sul 2.15, Dur 2.52	No data	Sul, Dur: 1 gm q6h (both)	CrCl ≥130: Sul, Dur: 1 gm q4h (both) CrCl 45-129: Sul, Dur: 1 gm q6h (both) CrCl 30-44: Sul, Dur: 1 gm q8h (both) CrCl 15-29: Sul, Dur: 1 gm q12h (both) CrCl <15: Sul, Dur: 1 gm q12h x3 doses, then q24h (both)	Use CrCl <15 dosing (AD on dialysis days)	No data	No data	No data
Temocillin	4	No data	1-2 gm IV q12h	CrCl >50: No dosing adjustment CrCl 30-50: 1-2 gm q24h CrCl 10-30: 1 gm q48h	1 gm q48h (AD on dialysis days)	1 gm q48h	No data	No data
Fluoroquinolones								
Ciprofloxacin (po (not XR))	3-4	6-9	250-750 mg po q12h	CrCl >50: No dosage adjustment CrCl 30-50: 250-500 mg q12h CrCl 5-29: 500-750 mg q24h	250-500 mg q24h (AD on dialysis days)	250-500 mg q24h	250-500 mg q12h	No data
Ciprofloxacin (po (XR))	5-7	6-9	Cystitis 500 mg po q24h Pyelo/cUTI 1 gm po q24h	CrCl ≥30: No dosage adjustment CrCl 5-29: 500 mg q24h (all)	500 mg q24h (all) (AD on dialysis days)	500 mg q24h (all)	Cystitis: 500 mg q24h Pyelo/cUTI: no data	No data
Ciprofloxacin (IV)	4	6-9	200-400 mg IV q8-12h	CrCl ≥30: No dosage adjustment CrCl 5-29: 200-400 mg q18-24h	200-400 mg q24h (AD on dialysis days)	200-400 mg q24h	200-400 mg q12h	No data
Delafloxacin[16]	4.2-8.5	No data	450 mg po q12h 300 mg IV q12h	Oral: eGFR ≥15: No dosage adjustment eGFR <15: Not recommended (no data) IV: eGFR ≥30: No dosage adjustment eGFR 15-29: 200 mg IV q12h eGFR <15: Not recommended (no data)	Not recommended (no data)	No data	No data	No data
Gatifloxacin (NUS)	7-8	11-40	400 mg po/IV q24h	CrCl >50: No dosage adjustment CrCl 10-50: 400 mg, then 200 mg q24h CrCl <10: 400 mg, then 200 mg q24h	200 mg q24h (AD on dialysis days)	200 mg q24h	400 mg, then 200 mg q24h	No data
Gemifloxacin	7	>7	320 mg po q24h	CrCl >50: No dosage adjustment CrCl 10-50: 160 mg q24h CrCl <10: 160 mg q24h	160 mg q24h (AD on dialysis days)	160 mg q24h	No data	No data
Levofloxacin	7	76	750 mg po/IV q24h	CrCl >50: No dosage adjustment CrCl 20-49: 750 mg q48h CrCl <20: 750 mg x1, then 500 mg q48h	750 mg x1, then 500 mg q48h	750 mg x1, then 500 mg q48h	750 mg x1, then 500 mg q48h	No data
Moxifloxacin	10-14	Unchanged	400 mg po/IV q24h	No dosage adjustment for renal impairment	No dosage adjustment	No dosage adjustment	No dosage adjustment	No dosage adjustment

TABLE 17A (11)

Groups/Drugs	Half-life, hrs (renal function normal)	Half-life, hrs (ESRD)	Dose (renal function normal)	CrCl or eGFR	Hemodialysis	CAPD	CRRT	SLED
Antibacterials/Fluoroquinolones *(continued)*								
Norfloxacin	3-4	8	400 mg po q12h	CrCl >50: No dosage adjustment CrCl 30-49: 400 mg q12h CrCl 10-30: 400 mg q24h	400 mg q24h	400 mg q24h	Not applicable	No data
Ofloxacin	7	28-37	200-400 mg po q12h	CrCl >50: No dosage adjustment CrCl 10-50: 200-400 mg q24h CrCl <10: 200 mg q24h	200 mg q24h (AD on dialysis days)	200 mg q24h	200-400 mg q24h	No data
Prulifloxacin (NUS)	10.6-12.1	No data	600 mg po q24h	CrCl ≥60: No dosage adjustment CrCl <60: No data	No data	No data	No data	No data
Glycopeptides, Lipoglycopeptides, Lipopeptides								
Dalbavancin	147-258 (terminal)	No data	1 gm IV x1 then 500 mg IV in 7 days, OR 1.5 gm IV x1	CrCl ≥30: No dosage adjustment CrCl <30 (no regular HD): 750 mg x1 then 375 mg in 7 days, OR 1125 mg x1	No dosage adjustment	No data	No data	No data
Daptomycin	8-9	30	6-10 mg/kg IV q24h	CrCl ≥30: No dosage adjustment CrCl <30: 6-10 mg/kg q48h	6-10 mg/kg q48h (AD); if next planned dialysis is 72 hrs away, give 9-15 mg/kg[26]	6-10 mg/kg q48h	6-8 mg/kg q24h[27]	No data
Oritavancin	245 (terminal)	No data	1200 mg IV x1	No dosage adjustment in mild-moderate impairment Not studied in severe impairment	Not removed by hemodialysis	No data	No data	No data
Teicoplanin (NUS)	70-100	up to 230	6-12 mg/kg IV q12h x3 doses (load), then 6-12 mg/kg IV q24h	CrCl >80: No dosage adjustment CrCl 30-80: Load, then 6-12 mg/kg q48h CrCl <30: Load, then 6-12 mg/kg q72h	Not removed by HD	No data	Load, then 6-12 mg/kg q48h	No data
Telavancin	8.1	17.9	10 mg/kg IV q24h	CrCl >50: No dosage adjustment CrCl 30-50: 7.5 mg/kg q24h CrCl 10 to <30: 10 mg/kg q48h CrCl <10: No data	No data	No data	No data	No data

TABLE 17A (12)

Groups/Drugs	Half-life, hrs (renal function normal)	Half-life, hrs (ESRD)	Dose (renal function normal)	CrCl or eGFR	Hemodialysis	CAPD	CRRT	SLED
Antibacterials/Glycopeptides, Lipoglycopeptides, Lipopeptides *(continued)*								
Vancomycin[7, 15]	6	200-250	15-20 mg/kg IV q8-12h	CrCl >100: No dosage adjustment CrCl >50-100: 15-20 mg/kg q12h CrCl 20-50: 15-20 mg/kg q24h CrCl <20: 15-20 mg/kg q48h	POST-HD DOSING Low perm membrane: • Load: 25 mg/kg • Maint: 7.5 mg/kg AD High perm membrane: • Load: 25 mg/kg • Maint: 10 mg/kg AD INTRADIALYTIC DOSING Low perm membrane: • Load: 30 mg/kg • Maint: 7.5-10 mg/kg High perm membrane: • Load: 35 mg/kg • Maint: 10-15 mg/kg	7.5 mg/kg q48-96h	7.5-10 mg/kg q12h (effluent 20-25 mL/kg/hr)	No data
H pylori combination products								
Pylera	Bismuth: 120 Metronidazole: 6-14 Tetracycline: 6-12	Bismuth: >120 Metronidazole: 7-21 Tetracycline: 57-108	3 caps q6h x10 days	CrCl ≥30: No dosage adjustment CrCl <30: Contraindicated	No data	No data	No data	No data
Talicia	Omeprazole: 1 Amoxicillin: 1.4 Rifabutin: 34	Omeprazole: Unchanged Amoxicillin: 5-20 Rifabutin: Unchanged	4 caps q8h x14 days	CrCl ≥30: No dosage adjustment CrCl <30: Not recommended	No data	No data	No data	No data

TABLE 17A (13)

Groups/Drugs	Half-life, hrs (renal function normal)	Half-life, hrs (ESRD)	Dose (renal function normal)	CrCl or eGFR	Hemodialysis	CAPD	CRRT	SLED
Antibacterials/H pylori combination products *(continued)*								
Voquezna	Vonoprazan: 6.8 Amoxicillin: 1.4 Clarithromycin: 5-7	Vonoprazan: >6.8 Amoxicillin: 5-20 Clarithro-mycin: 22	Triple Pak (x14 days): - Vonoprazan 20 mg q12h - Amoxicillin 1 gm q12h - Clarithromycin 500 mg q12h Dual Pak (x14 days): - Vonoprazan 20 mg q12h - Amoxicillin 1 gm q8h	eGFR ≥30: No dosage adjustment eGFR <30: Not recommended	No data	No data	No data	No data
Macrolides, Azalides, Lincosamides, Ketolides								
Azithromycin	68	Unchanged	250-500 mg IV/po q24h	No dosage adjustment for renal impairment	No dosage adjustment	No dosage adjustment	No dosage adjustment	No data
Clarithromycin*	5-7	22	500 mg po q12h	CrCl >50: No dosage adjustment CrCl 10-50: 500 mg q12-24h CrCl <10: 500 mg q24h	500 mg q24h (AD on dialysis days)	500 mg q24h	500 mg q12-24h	No data
Clindamycin[5]	2.4	Unchanged	900 mg IV q8h 150-450 mg po q6h	No dosage adjustment for renal impairment	No dosage adjustment	No dosage adjustment	No dosage adjustment	No data
Erythromycin base, esters	2-4	5-6	250-500 mg po q6h	No dosage adjustment for renal impairment	No dosage adjustment	No dosage adjustment	No dosage adjustment	No data
Fidaxomicin	2	Unchanged	200 mg po q12h	No dosage adjustment for renal impairment	No data	No data	No data	No data
Lincomycin	5.4	No data	0.6-1 gm IV q8-12h	CrCl ≥30: No dosage adjustment CrCl <30: 25-30% of usual dose	Not removed by dialysis	Not removed by dialysis	No data	No data
Telithromycin[5]	10	15	800 mg po q24h	CrCl ≥30: No dosage adjustment CrCl <30: 600 mg q24h	600 mg q24h (AD on dialysis days)	No data	No data	No data
Miscellaneous Antibacterials								
Anthrax immune globulin	24-28 days	No data	420 units IV x1	No dosage adjustment for renal impairment	No data	No data	No data	No data
Chloramphenicol[5]	4.1	Unchanged	50-100 mg/kg/day po/IV (divided q6h)	No dosage adjustment for renal impairment	No dosage adjustment	No dosage adjustment	No dosage adjustment	No data

TABLE 17A (14)

Groups/Drugs	Half-life, hrs (renal function normal)	Half-life, hrs (ESRD)	Dose (renal function normal)	CrCl or eGFR	Hemodialysis	CAPD	CRRT	SLED
Antibacterials/Miscellaneous *(continued)*								
Fosfomycin IV	2.0	50	Varies with indication	Shown is % of normal daily dose. For loading dose, increase first dose by 100% (max 8 gm). CrCl >40: No dosage adjustment CrCl 40: 70% (divided q8-12h) CrCl 30: 60% (divided q8-12h) CrCl 20: 40% (divided q8-12h) CrCl 10: 20% (divided q12-24h)	2 gm q48h (give AD)	No data	CVVH: No dosage adjustment (based on limited data)	No data
Fosfomycin PO	5.7	50	3 gm po x1	CrCl ≥10: no dosage adjustment CrCl <10: Avoid use (poor urinary excretion)	No data	No data	No data	No data
Fusidic acid[5] (NUS)	8.9-11	Unchanged	500 mg po/IV q8h	No dosage adjustment for renal impairment	No data	No data	No data	No data
Methenamine	4	No data	Hippurate: 1 gm q12h Mandelate: 1 gm q6h	CrCl ≥50: No dosage adjustment CrCl <50: Avoid use	Avoid use	Avoid use	Avoid use	Avoid use
Metronidazole[5]	6-14	7-21	7.5 mg/kg IV/po q6h	CrCl ≥10: no dosage adjustment CrCl <10: 7.5 mg/kg q12h	7.5 mg/kg q12h (dose AD)	No dosage adjustment	No dosage adjustment	No data
Nitrofurantoin	1	No data	100 mg po q12h (Macrobid)	CrCl >30: No dosage adjustment CrCl ≤30: Avoid use	Avoid use	Avoid use	Avoid use	No data
Rifamycin SV	No data	No data	388 mg po q12h	No dosage adjustment for renal impairment	No data	No data	No data	No data
Rifaximin	2-5	Unchanged	200 mg po q8h	No dosage adjustment for renal impairment	No dosage adjustment	No dosage adjustment	No dosage adjustment	No data
Secnidazole	17	No data	2 gm single-dose	No dosage adjustment for renal impairment	No data	No data	No data	No data
Sulopenem etzadroxil-probenecid	Sulopenem: 1.3 Probenecid: 3.8	No data	1 tab q12h x5 days	CrCl ≥15: No dosage adjustment CrCl <15: Not recommended	Not recommended	No data	No data	No data
Tinidazole[5]	13	No data	2 gm po q24h x1-5 days	No dosage adjustment for renal impairment	No dosage adjustment (give an extra 1 gm AD if administered before dialysis)	No data	No data	No data
Trimethoprim	8-15	20-49	100-200 mg po q12h	CrCl >30: No dosage adjustment CrCl 10-30: 100-200 mg q18h CrCl <10: 100-200 mg q24h	100-200 mg q24h (AD on dialysis days)	100-200 mg q24h	100-200 mg q18h	No data

TABLE 17A (15)

Groups/Drugs	Half-life, hrs (renal function normal)	Half-life, hrs (ESRD)	Dose (renal function normal)	CrCl or eGFR	Hemodialysis	CAPD	CRRT	SLED
Antibacterials/Miscellaneous *(continued)*								
TMP-SMX*	TMP: 8-15 SMX: 10	TMP: 20-49 SMX: 20-50	Treatment: 5-20 mg/kg/day po/IV (div q6-12h) Prophylaxis: 1 DS tab po q24h or 3x/week	Treatment: CrCl ≥30: No dosage adjustment CrCl 10-29: 5-10 mg/kg/day (div q12h) CrCl <10: Not recommended (if used: 5-10 mg/kg q24h) Prophylaxis: No dosage adjustment for renal impairment	Treatment: Not recommended (if used: 5-10 mg/kg q24h, AD on dialysis days) Prophylaxis: No data	Treatment: Not recommended (if used: 5-10 mg/kg q24h) Prophylaxis: No data	Treatment: 5 mg/kg q8h Prophylaxis: No data	No data
Monoclonal antibodies								
Bezlotoxumab	19 days	No data	10 mg/kg IV x1	No dosage adjustment for renal impairment	No data	No data	No data	No data
Obiltoxaximab	≥16 days	No data	16 mg/kg IV x1	No dosage adjustment for renal impairment	No data	No data	No data	No data
Raxibacumab	16-19 days	No data	40 mg/kg IV x1	No dosage adjustment for renal impairment	No data	No data	No data	
Oxazolidinones								
Linezolid	5	6-8	600 mg po/IV q12h	No dosage adjustment for renal impairment (product labeling). Debated: 300 mg q12h for eGFR <60 *(Drugs RD 2024;24:109; AAC 2019;63:e00605-19)*.	No dosage adjustment (dose AD)	No dosage adjustment	No dosage adjustment	No data
Tedizolid	12	Unchanged	200 mg po/IV q24h	No dosage adjustment for renal impairment	No dosage adjustment	No dosage adjustment	No dosage adjustment	No data
Pleuromutilins								
Lefamulin	8	Unchanged	600 mg po q12h 150 mg IV q12h	No dosage adjustment for renal impairment	No dosage adjustment	No data	No data	No data
Retapamulin	No data	No data	Apply q12h x5 days	No dosage adjustment for renal impairment	No data	No data	No data	No data
Polymyxins								
Colistin (polymyxin E) *(Doses are mg CBA)*	6.3-12	≥48	Load: 4 x (pt wt in kg). Use lower of ideal or actual wt. Load may exceed 300 mg. Start maintenance 12 hrs later.	CrCl ≥90: 180 mg q12h CrCl 80 to <90: 170 mg q12h CrCl 70 to <80: 150 mg q12h CrCl 60 to <70: 137.5 mg q12h CrCl 50 to <60: 122.5 mg q12h CrCl 40 to <50: 110 mg q12h CrCl 30 to <40: 97.5 mg q12h CrCl 20 to <30: 87.5 mg q12h CrCl 10 to <20: 80 mg q12h CrCl 5 to <10: 72.5 mg q12h CrCl <5: 65 mg q12h	On non-HD days, give 65 mg IV q12h. On HD days, add 40-50 mg to the daily dose after a 3-4 hr session. Give this supplement with the next regular dose after the dialysis has ended.	No data	Add 13 mg per hour of CRRT to the baseline dose of 65 mg q12h.	Add 13 mg per hour of SLED to the baseline dose of 65 mg q12h.

TABLE 17A (16)

Groups/Drugs	Half-life, hrs (renal function normal)	Half-life, hrs (ESRD)	Dose (renal function normal)	CrCl or eGFR	Hemodialysis	CAPD	CRRT	SLED
Antibacterials/Polymyxins *(continued)*								
Polymyxin B	4.5-6 (old data)	Unchanged	2.5 mg/kg IV x1, then 1.5 mg/kg IV q12h	No dosage adjustment for renal impairment	No dosage adjustment	No dosage adjustment	No dosage adjustment	No data
Streptogramins								
Pristinamycin	PIA: 4.03 PIIA: 2.83	PIA: Unchanged PIIA: Unchanged	2-4 gm/day po (divided q8-12h)	No dosage adjustment for renal impairment	No data	No data	No data	No data
Quinupristin-dalfopristin[5]	Quin: 0.85 Dalfo: 0.7	Quin: Unchanged Dalfo: Unchanged	7.5 mg/kg IV q12h	No dosage adjustment for renal impairment	No dosage adjustment	No dosage adjustment	No dosage adjustment	No data
Tetracyclines, Glycylcyclines								
Doxycycline	18	Unchanged	100 mg po/IV q12h	No dosage adjustment for renal impairment	No dosage adjustment	No dosage adjustment	No dosage adjustment	No data
Eravacycline[5]	20	Unchanged	1 mg/kg IV q12h	No dosage adjustment for renal impairment	No dosage adjustment	No data	No data	No data
Minocycline	16	Unchanged	100 mg po/IV q12h	No dosage adjustment for renal impairment	No dosage adjustment	No dosage adjustment	No dosage adjustment	No data
Omadacycline	15.5-16.8	Unchanged	100 mg IV q24h 300 mg po q24h	No dosage adjustment for renal impairment	No dosage adjustment	No data	No data	No data
Sarecycline	21-22	No data	60-150 mg po q24h	No dosage adjustment for renal impairment (not studied in ESRD)	No data	No data	No data	No data
Tetracycline	6-12	57-108	250-500 mg po q6h	CrCl >90: No dosage adjustment CrCl >50-90: 250-500 mg q8-12h CrCl 10-50: 250-500 mg q12-24h CrCl <10: 250-500 mg q24h	250-500 mg q24h	250-500 mg q24h	250-500 mg q12-24h	No data
Tigecycline[5]	42	Unchanged	100 mg, then 50 mg IV q12h	No dosage adjustment for renal impairment	No dosage adjustment	No dosage adjustment	No dosage adjustment	No data
Antifungals								
Polyenes								
Amphotericin B	24 hrs-15 days	Unchanged	0.3-1.0 mg/kg/day (deoxycholate) 3-5 mg/kg/day (liposomal)	No dosage adjustment for renal impairment	No dosage adjustment	No dosage adjustment	No dosage adjustment	No dosage adjustment
Nystatin	No data	No data	500,000 units q6h	No dosage adjustment for renal impairment	No dosage adjustment	No dosage adjustment	No dosage adjustment	No dosage adjustment

TABLE 17A (17)

Groups/Drugs	Half-life, hrs (renal function normal)	Half-life, hrs (ESRD)	Dose (renal function normal)	CrCl or eGFR	Hemodialysis	CAPD	CRRT	SLED
Antifungals *(continued)*								
Antimetabolites								
Flucytosine[8]	3-5	75-200	25 mg/kg po q6h	CrCl >40: No dosage adjustment CrCl 21-40: 25 mg/kg q12h CrCl 10-20: 25 mg/kg q24h CrCl <10: 25 mg/kg q48h	25-50 mg/kg q48-72h (dose AD)	CCPD: 25 mg/kg q24h	No data	No data
Allylamines, Azoles								
Efinaconazole	29.9	No data	Topical q24h	No dosage adjustment for renal impairment	No dosage adjustment	No dosage adjustment	No dosage adjustment	No dosage adjustment
Fluconazole	20-50	100	100-400 mg IV/po q24h	CrCl >50: No dosage adjustment CrCl ≤50: 50-200 mg q24h	50-200 mg q24h on non-dialysis days, 100-400 mg (full dose) AD on dialysis days	50-200 mg q24h	At least 2x usual dose suggested[22]	No data
Isavuconazonium sulfate	130	Unchanged	372 mg po/IV q24h	No dosage adjustment for renal impairment	No dosage adjustment	No dosage adjustment	No dosage adjustment	SLED may ↓plasma conc *(AAC 2019; 63:e01162-19)*
Itraconazole[5]	35-40	Unchanged	100-200 mg po q12-24h (oral solution)	No dosage adjustment for renal impairment Avoid IV if CrCl <30 due to vehicle	No dosage adjustment	No dosage adjustment	No data	No data
Ketoconazole	8	Unchanged	200-400 mg po q24h	No dosage adjustment for renal impairment	No dosage adjustment	No dosage adjustment	No dosage adjustment	No data
Oteseconazole	138 days	No data	150 mg q-wk (after load)	eGFR ≥30: No dosage adjustment eGFR <30: Not recommended	Not recommended	No data	No data	No data
Posaconazole	20-66	Unchanged	Varies by formulation	No dosage adjustment for renal impairment Avoid IV if CrCl <50 due to vehicle	No dosage adjustment	No dosage adjustment	No dosage adjustment	No data
Terbinafine	36	No data	250 mg po q24h	CrCl >50: No dosage adjustment CrCl ≤50: No data	No data	No data	No data	No data
Voriconazole[5]	Dose-dependent	Dose-dependent	Varies by formulation	No dosage adjustment for renal impairment Avoid IV if CrCl <50 due to vehicle	No dosage adjustment	No dosage adjustment	No dosage adjustment	No data
Echinocandins								
Anidulafungin	26.5	Unchanged	50-100 mg IV q24h	No dosage adjustment for renal impairment	No dosage adjustment	No dosage adjustment	No dosage adjustment	No data
Caspofungin[5]	13	Unchanged	50 mg IV q24h	No dosage adjustment for renal impairment	No dosage adjustment	No dosage adjustment	No dosage adjustment	No data

TABLE 17A (18)

Groups/Drugs	Half-life, hrs (renal function normal)	Half-life, hrs (ESRD)	Dose (renal function normal)	CrCl or eGFR	Hemodialysis	CAPD	CRRT	SLED
Antifungals/Echinocandins *(continued)*								
Micafungin	15-17	Unchanged	100 mg IV q24h	No dosage adjustment for renal impairment	No dosage adjustment	No dosage adjustment	Consider 150-200 mg q24h *(Crit Care 2018;22:289)*	No data
Rezafungin	152 (terminal)	Unchanged	200 mg once weekly (400 mg load)	No dosage adjustment for renal impairment	No dosage adjustment	No data	No data	No data
Miscellaneous Antifungals								
Griseofulvin	9-24	No data	500-1000 mg q24h (microsize)	No dosage adjustment for renal impairment	No data	No data	No data	No data
Ibrexafungerp	20	No data	300 mg po q12h	No dosage adjustment for renal impairment	No data	No data	No data	No data
Antimycobacterials								
First line, tuberculosis								
Ethambutol	4	7-15	15-25 mg/kg po q24h	CrCl ≥30: No dosage adjustment CrCl <30: 15-25 mg/kg 3x/week	15-25 mg/kg 3x/wk (AD on dialysis days)[9]	15-25 mg/kg q48h	15-25 mg/kg q24-36h[9, 31]	No data
Isoniazid (INH)	0.7-4	8-17	5 mg/kg po q24h	No dosage adjustment for renal impairment	No dosage adjustment (AD on dialysis days)	No dosage adjustment	No dosage adjustment	No data
Pyrazinamide	10-16	26	25 mg/kg po q24h	CrCl >20: No dosage adjustment CrCl ≤20: 25 mg/kg q48h	25 mg/kg q48h (AD on dialysis days)	25 mg/kg q24h	25 mg/kg q24h	No data
Rifabutin[5]	32-67	Unchanged	300 mg po q24h	CrCl >50: No dosage adjustment CrCl ≤50: 150 mg q24h	No data	No data	No data	No data
Rifampin[5]	1.5-5	up to 11	600 mg po q24h	CrCl >50: No dosage adjustment CrCl ≤50: 300-600 mg q24h	300-600 mg q24h	300-600 mg q24h	300-600 mg q24h	No data
Rifapentine	13.2-14.1	Unchanged	600 mg po 1-2x/wk	No dosage adjustment for renal impairment	No dosage adjustment	No dosage adjustment	No dosage adjustment	No data
Streptomycin[1, 2]	2-3	30-70	15 mg/kg (max 1 gm) IM q24h	CrCl >50: No dosage adjustment CrCl 10-50: 15 mg/kg q24-72h CrCl <10: 15 mg/kg q72-96h	15 mg/kg q72-96h (+ extra 7.5 mg/kg AD)	20-40 mg lost per L of dialysate/day	15 mg/kg q24-72h	No data
Second line, tuberculosis								
Bedaquiline	24-30 (terminal 4-5 mo)	No data	400 mg q24h x2 wk, then 200 mg 3x/wk x22 wk	CrCl ≥10: No dosage adjustment CrCl <10: Use with caution	Use with caution	Use with caution	No data	No data

TABLE 17A (19)

Groups/Drugs	Half-life, hrs (renal function normal)	Half-life, hrs (ESRD)	Dose (renal function normal)	CrCl or eGFR	Hemodialysis	CAPD	CRRT	SLED
Antimycobacterials/Second line, tuberculosis *(continued)*								
Capreomycin	2-5	No data	15 mg/kg IM/IV q24h	CrCl ≥10: No dosage adjustment CrCl <10: 15 mg/kg 3x/wk	15 mg/kg 3x/wk (AD on dialysis days)	No data	No data	No data
Clofazimine	Up to 70 days	No data	50 mg q24h + 300 mg 1x/mon	No data	No data	No data	No data	No data
Cycloserine[10]	10	No data	250-500 mg po q12h	CrCl >50: No dosage adjustment CrCl 10-50: 250-500 mg q12h-24h CrCl <10: 500 mg q48h (or 3x/wk)	500 mg 3x/wk (AD on dialysis days)	No data	No data	No data
Delamanid	30-38	No data	100 mg po q12h	CrCl ≥30: No dosage adjustment CrCl <30: No data	No data	No data	No data	No data
Ethionamide	2	9	500 mg po q12h	CrCl ≥10: No dosage adjustment CrCl <10: 250 mg q12h	250 mg q12h	250 mg q12h	500 mg q12h	No data
Kanamycin[1,2]	2-3	30-70	7.5 mg/kg IM/IV q12h	CrCl >50: No dosage adjustment CrCl 10-50: 7.5 mg/kg q24h CrCl <10: 7.5 mg/kg q48h	7.5 mg/kg q48h (+ extra 3.25 mg/kg AD)	15-20 mg lost per L of dialysate/day	7.5 mg/kg q24h	No data
Para-aminosalicylic acid (PAS)	0.75-1.0	23	4 gm po q12h	CrCl >50: No dosage adjustment CrCl 10-50: 2-3 gm q12h CrCl <10: 2 gm q12h	2 gm q12h (AD on dialysis days)	No data	No data	No data
Pretomanid	17.4	No data	200 mg po q24h	No data	No data	No data	No data	No data
Other antimycobacterials								
Thalidomide	5.5-7.3	Unchanged	100-300 mg po q24h	No dosage adjustment for renal impairment	No dosage adjustment	No data	No data	No data
Antiparasitics								
Antimalarials								
Artemether-lumefantrine (20 mg-120 mg)	Art: 1.6-2.2 DHA: 1.6-2.2 Lum: 101-119	No data	4 tabs x1, 4 tabs in 8 hr, then 4 tabs q12h x2 days	No dosage adjustment for renal impairment (data limited, use caution)	No data	No data	No data	No data
Artesunate (AS)	0.3	No data	2.4 mg/kg IV at 0, 12, and 24 hrs	No dosage adjustment for renal impairment	No data	No data	No data	No data
Atovaquone-Proguanil (250 mg-100 mg)	Atova 48-72 Pro 12-21	No data	4 tabs q24h x3 days	CrCl ≥30: No dosage adjustment CrCl <30: Use with caution for treatment (contraindicated for prophylaxis)	No data	No data	No data	No data
Chloroquine phosphate	45-55 days (terminal)	No data	2.5 gm po over 3 days	CrCl ≥10: No dosage adjustment CrCl <10: Consider reducing dose 50%	Consider reducing dose 50%	No data	No data	No data
Dihydroartemisinin-piperaquine	DHA:1 hr PPQ: 22 days	No data	Varies with weight	No data	No data	No data	No data	No data
Hydroxychloroquine sulfate	40-50 days (terminal)	No data	800 mg, then 400 mg x3	CrCl ≥10: No dosage adjustment CrCl <10: Consider reducing dose 50%	Consider reducing dose 50%	No data	No data	No data

TABLE 17A (20)

Groups/Drugs	Half-life, hrs (renal function normal)	Half-life, hrs (ESRD)	Dose (renal function normal)	CrCl or eGFR	Hemodialysis	CAPD	CRRT	SLED
Antiparasitics/Antimalarials *(continued)*								
Mefloquine	13-24 days	No data	Tx: 750 mg, then 500 mg in 6-8 hr	No dosage adjustment for renal impairment	No data	No data	No data	No data
Primaquine	3.7-9.6	No data	Varies with indication	No dosage adjustment for renal impairment[19]	No data	No data	No data	No data
Pyronaridine-artesunate	Pyronaridine: 14-18 days Artesunate: 0.5 hr	No data	Varies with weight	CrCl ≥30: Use with caution CrCl <30: Avoid use	No data	No data	No data	No data
Quinine dihydrochloride	9.7-12.5	up to 16	10 mg/kg (of salt) IV q8h	CrCl >50: No dosage adjustment CrCl 10-50: 10 mg/kg q8-12h CrCl <10: 10 mg/kg q24h	10 mg/kg q24h (AD on dialysis days)	10 mg/kg q24h	10 mg/kg q8-12h	No data
Quinine sulfate	9.7-12.5	up to 16	648 mg po q8h	CrCl >50: No dosage adjustment CrCl 10-50: 648 mg q8-12h CrCl <10: 648 mg q24h	648 mg q24h (AD on dialysis days)	648 mg q24h	648 mg q8-12h	No data
Sulfadoxine-pyrimethamine	Sulfadoxine: 200 Pyrimethamine: 100	No data	3 tablets po x1	No data	No data	No data	No data	No data
Tafenoquine	15 days (terminal)	No data	Varies with indication	No data	No data	No data	No data	No data
Other								
Albendazole	8-12	No data	400 mg po q12-24h	No dosage adjustment for renal impairment	No data	No data	No data	No data
Antimony, pentavalent	elim 2 hr terminal 1-3 days	No data	20 mg/kg/day	Dosage adjustment advised (or select alternative treatment) Specific recommendation unavailable	No data	No data	No data	No data
Atovaquone	67-78	No data	750 mg po q12h	No data	No data	No data	No data	No data
Benznidazole	13.3	No data	5-7 mg/kg/day (div q12h)	No data Dosage reduction may be advised to reduce risk of adverse effects	No data	No data	No data	No data
Dapsone	10-50	No data	100 mg po q24h	No data	No data	No data	No data	No data
Diethylcarbamazine	9	No data	Varies with indication	Specific recommendation unavailable[20]	No data	No data	No data	No data
Diloxanide furoate	No data	No data	500 mg po q8h	No data	No data	No data	No data	No data
Eflornithine	3.3	No data	400 mg/kg/day IV	Dosage reduction advised Specific recommendation unavailable	No data	No data	No data	No data
Fexinidazole	15	No data	Varies by patient weight	No dosage adjustment for renal impairment	No data	No data	No data	No data
Fumagillin	No data	No data	20 mg po q8h	No data	No data	No data	No data	No data

TABLE 17A (21)

Groups/Drugs	Half-life, hrs (renal function normal)	Half-life, hrs (ESRD)	Dose (renal function normal)	CrCl or eGFR	Hemodialysis	CAPD	CRRT	SLED
Antiparasitics/Other *(continued)*								
Iodoquinol*	No data	No data	650 mg po q8h x20 days	No data	No data	No data	No data	No data
Ivermectin	20	No data	200 µg/kg/day po x1-2 days	No dosage adjustment for renal impairment	No data	No data	No data	No data
Mebendazole	3-6	No data	Varies with indication	No dosage adjustment for renal impairment	No dosage adjustment	No data	No data	No data
Melarsoprol	<0.5 (parent)	No data	2.2 mg/kg/day	No data	No data	No data	No data	No data
Miltefosine	7-31 days	No data	50 mg po q8h	No data	No data	No data	No data	No data
Moxidectin	23.3 days (terminal)	No data	8 mg po x1	CrCl ≥30: No dosage adjustment CrCl <30: No data	No data	No data	No data	No data
Niclosamide	No data	No data	2 gm po x1 dose (or q24h x7)	No dosage adjustment for renal impairment	No data	No data	No data	No data
Nifurtimox	2.4-3.6	No data	Varies with indication	No data	No data[24]	No data	No data	No data
Nitazoxanide	tizoxanide 1.3-1.8	No data	500 mg po q12h	No data	No data	No data	No data	No data
Paromomycin	2-3	No data	Varies with indication	No dosage adjustment for renal impairment	No data	No data	No data	No data
Pentamidine	3-12	73-118	4 mg/kg IM/IV q24h	CrCl ≥10: No dosage adjustment CrCl <10: 4 mg/kg q24-36h	4 mg/kg q48h (AD on dialysis days)	4 mg/kg q24-36h	4 mg/kg q24h	No data
Praziquantel[5]	0.8-1.5	Unchanged	Varies with indication	No dosage adjustment for renal impairment	No dosage adjustment	No dosage adjustment	No dosage adjustment	No data
Pyrantel pamoate*	No data	No data	11 mg/kg po	No data	No data	No data	No data	No data
Pyrimethamine	96	No data	Varies with indication	No dosage adjustment for renal impairment	No data	No data	No data	No data
Quinacrine	5-14 days	No data	100 mg po q8h	Dosage recommendations not available[20]	No data	No data	No data	No data
Spiramycin	4.5-6.2	No data	1 gm po q8h	No data	No data	No data	No data	No data
Sulfadiazine	10	No data	1-1.5 gm po q6h	CrCl ≥50: No dosage adjustment CrCl <50: Specific recommendation unavailable (consider 1-1.5 gm q12-24h)	Specific recommendation unavailable	No data	No data	No data
Suramin	44-54 days	No data	20 mg/kg (max 1 gm) q-wkly x5 wks	No data Avoid use in severe renal impairment	No data (not removed by HD)	No data	No data	No data
Triclabendazole	8	No data	10 mg/kg po q12h x2 doses	No data	No data	No data	No data	No data

TABLE 17A (22)

Groups/Drugs	Half-life, hrs (renal function normal)	Half-life, hrs (ESRD)	Dose (renal function normal)	CrCl or eGFR	Hemodialysis	CAPD	CRRT	SLED
Antivirals								
Coronavirus								
Bamlanivimab + Etesevimab	Bamlanivimab 17.6 days Etesevimab 25.1 days	No data	Bamlanivimab 700 mg x1 Etesevimab 1400 mg x1	No dosage adjustment for renal impairment	No data	No data	No data	No data
Baricitinib[16]	12	No data	2-4 mg po q24h	Age 2 to <9 years: eGFR ≥60: 2 mg q24h eGFR 30 to <60: 1 mg q24h eGFR <30: Not recommended Age ≥9 years: eGFR ≥60: 4 mg q24h eGFR 30 to <60: 2 mg q24h eGFR 15 to <30: 1 mg q24h eGFR <15: Not recommended	No data	No data	No data	No data
Bebtelovimab	11.5 days	No data	175 mg IV x1	No dosage adjustment for renal impairment	No data	No data	No data	No data
Casirivimab + Imdevimab	Casirivimab 31.8 days Imdevimab 26.9 days	No data	Casirivimab 600 mg IV x1 Imdevimab 600 mg IV x1	No dosage adjustment for renal impairment	No data	No data	No data	No data
Molnupiravir	3.3 (NHC)	No data	800 mg po q12h	No dosage adjustment for renal impairment	No data	No data	No data	No data
Nirmatrelvir/Ritonavir	6.05/6.15	No data	300 mg/100 mg q12h	eGFR ≥60: No dosage adjustment eGFR ≥30 to <60: 150 mg/100 mg q12h eGFR <30: Not recommended	No data	No data	No data	No data
Pemivibart	44.8 days	No data	4500 mg IV x1	No dosage adjustment for renal impairment	No data	No data	No data	No data
Remdesivir	1.0	No data	100 mg IV q24h	No dosage adjustment for renal impairment	No dosage adjustment	No data	No data	No data
Sotrovimab	No data	No data	500 mg IV x1	No dosage adjustment for renal impairment	No data	No data	No data	No data
Tofacitinib[16]	3	No data	10 mg po q12h	eGFR ≥50: No dosage adjustment eGFR <50: 5 mg q12h	No data	No data	No data	No data

TABLE 17A (23)

Groups/Drugs	Half-life, hrs (renal function normal)	Half-life, hrs (ESRD)	Dose (renal function normal)	CrCl or eGFR	Hemodialysis	CAPD	CRRT	SLED
Antivirals *(continued)*								
Hepatitis B								
Adefovir	7.5	15	10 mg po q24h	CrCl ≥50: No dosage adjustment CrCl 30-49: 10 mg q48h CrCl 10-29: 10 mg q72h CrCl <10, non-HD: No data	10 mg weekly (AD on dialysis days)	No data	No data	No data
Entecavir[14]	128-149	No data	Tx-naive: 0.5 mg q24h 3TC-refract, decomp liver dis: 1 mg q24h	CrCl ≥50: No dosage adjustment CrCl 30 to <50: - Tx-naive: 0.25 mg q24h - 3TC-refract, decomp liver dis: 0.5 mg q24h CrCl 10 to <30: - Tx-naive: 0.15 mg q24h - 3TC-refract, decomp liver dis: 0.3 mg q24h CrCl <10: - Tx-naive: 0.05 mg q24h - 3TC-refract, decomp liver dis: 0.1 mg q24h	Tx-naive: 0.05 mg q24h 3TC-refract, decomp liver dis: 0.1 mg q24h (AD on dialysis days)	Tx-naive: 0.05 mg q24h 3TC-refract, decomp liver dis: 0.1 mg q24h	No data	No data
Interferons	2-3	No data	Varies with indication	No dosage adjustment for renal impairment	No data	No data	No data	No data
Telbivudine	40-49	No data	600 mg po q24h	CrCl >50: No dosage adjustment CrCl 30-49: 600 mg q48h CrCl 10-30: 600 mg q72h CrCl <10: 600 mg q96h	600 mg q96h (AD on dialysis days)	No data	No data	No data
Tenofovir alafenamide (Vemlidy)	0.51	No data	25 mg po q24h	CrCl ≥15: No dosage adjustment CrCl <15, no chronic HD: Not recommended	No dosage adjustment (AD on dialysis days)	No data	No data	No data
Hepatitis C (Single Agents)								
Daclatasvir	12-15	No data	60 mg po q24h	No dosage adjustment for renal impairment	No data	No data	No data	No data
Ribavirin	44	No data	Varies with indication	CrCl >50: No dosage adjustment CrCl ≤50: Use with caution	No data	No data	No data	No data
Simeprevir	41	Unchanged	150 mg po q24h	CrCl >50: No dosage adjustment CrCl <30: Use with caution (no data)	No data	No data	No data	No data
Sofosbuvir[16]	0.5-0.75	Unchanged	400 mg po q24h	eGFR ≥30: No dosage adjustment eGFR <30: No data	No data	No data	No data	No data

TABLE 17A (24)

Groups/Drugs	Half-life, hrs (renal function normal)	Half-life, hrs (ESRD)	Dose (renal function normal)	CrCl or eGFR	Hemodialysis	CAPD	CRRT	SLED
Antivirals *(continued)*								
Hepatitis C (Fixed-Dose Combinations)								
Elbasvir/Grazoprevir (Zepatier)	Elbasvir 24 Grazoprevir 31	No data	1 tab po q24	No dosage adjustment for renal impairment	No dosage adjustment	No data	No data	No data
Glecaprevir/Pibrentasvir (Mavyret)	Glecaprevir 6 Pibrentasvir 13	No data	3 tabs po q24h	No dosage adjustment for renal impairment	No dosage adjustment	No data	No data	No data
Ledipasvir/Sofosbuvir (Harvoni)	Ledipasvir 47 Sofosbuvir 0.5-0.75	No data	1 tab po q24h	No dosage adjustment for renal impairment	No dosage adjustment	No data	No data	No data
Sofosbuvir/velpatasvir (Epclusa)	Sofosbuvir 0.5 Velpatasvir 15	No data	1 tab po q24h	No dosage adjustment for renal impairment	No dosage adjustment	No data	No data	No data
Velpatasvir/Sofosbuvir/ Voxilaprevir (Vosevi)	Velpatasvir 17 Sofosbuvir 0.5 Voxilaprevir 33	No data	1 tab po q24h	No dosage adjustment for renal impairment	No dosage adjustment	No data	No data	No data
Herpes Virus								
Acyclovir[11] (IV)	2.5 -3.5	20	5-12.5 mg/kg IV q8h	CrCl >50: No dosage adjustment CrCl 10-50: 5-12.5 mg/kg q12-24h CrCl <10: 2.5-6.25 mg/kg q24h	2.5-6.25 mg/kg q24h (AD on dialysis days)	2.5-6.25 mg/kg q24h	2.5-6.25 mg/kg q24h	No data
Acyclovir (po)	2.5 -3.5	20	800 mg po q4h (5x/day)	CrCl >25: No dosage adjustment CrCl 10-25: 800 mg q8h CrCl <10: 800 mg q12h	800 mg q12h (give extra dose AD)	800 mg q12h	No data	No data
Cidofovir	2.6	No data	Induction: 5 mg/kg IV q-wk x2 doses Maintenance: 5 mg/kg IV q-2wks	CrCl >55: No dosage adjustment CrCl ≤ 55: Contraindicated	Contraindicated	Contraindicated	Contraindicated	No data

TABLE 17A (25)

Groups/Drugs	Half-life, hrs (renal function normal)	Half-life, hrs (ESRD)	Dose (renal function normal)	CrCl or eGFR	Hemodialysis	CAPD	CRRT	SLED
Antivirals/Herpes Virus *(continued)*								
Famciclovir	penciclovir 2-3	penciclovir 10-22	Varies with indication	Recurrent genital herpes: CrCl ≥60: 1000 mg q12h x1 day CrCl 40-59: 500 mg q12h x1 day CrCl 20-39: 500 mg x1 dose CrCl <20: 250 mg x1 dose Recurrent herpes labialis: CrCl ≥60: 1500 mg x1 dose CrCl 40-59: 750 mg x1 dose CrCl 20-39: 500 mg x1 dose CrCl <20: 250 mg x1 dose Herpes zoster: CrCl ≥60: 500 mg q8h CrCl 40-59: 500 mg q12h CrCl 20-39: 500 mg q24h CrCl <20: 250 mg q24h Suppression of recurrent genital herpes: CrCl ≥40: 250 mg q12h CrCl 20-39: 125 mg q12h CrCl <20: 125 mg q24h Recurrent orolabial/genital herpes (HIV) CrCl ≥40: 500 mg q12h CrCl 20-39: 500 mg q24h CrCl <20: 250 mg q24h	Recurrent genital herpes: 250 mg x1 dose AD Recurrent herpes labialis: 250 mg x1 dose AD Herpes zoster: 250 mg after each dialysis Suppression of recurrent genital herpes: 125 mg after each dialysis Recurrent orolabial/ genital herpes (HIV): 250 mg after each dialysis	No data	No data	No data
Foscarnet (induction, special dosing scale)	3 (terminal 18-88)	Very long	90 mg/kg IV q12h OR 60 mg/ kg IV q8h (x2-3 wks)	CrCl above 1.4 ml/min/kg: 60 mg/kg IV q8h CrCl >1 to 1.4 mL/min/kg: 45 mg/kg q8h CrCl >0.8 to 1.0 mL/min/kg: 50 mg/kg q12h CrCl >0.6 to 0.8 mL/min/kg: 40 mg/kg q12h CrCl >0.5 to 0.6 mL/min/kg: 60 mg/kg q24h CrCl 0.4 to 0.5 mL/min/kg: 50 mg/kg q24h CrCl <0.4 mL/min/kg: Not recommended	No data	No data	No data	No data

TABLE 17A (26)

Groups/Drugs	Half-life, hrs (renal function normal)	Half-life, hrs (ESRD)	Dose (renal function normal)	CrCl or eGFR	Hemodialysis	CAPD	CRRT	SLED
Antivirals/Herpes Virus *(continued)*								
Foscarnet (maintenance, special dosing scale)	3 (terminal 18-88)	Very long	90-120 mg/kg IV q24h	CrCl above 1.4 ml/min/kg: 90-120 mg/kg IV q24h CrCl >1 to 1.4 mL/min/kg: 70-90 mg/kg q24h CrCl >0.8 to 1.0 mL/min/kg: 50-65 mg/kg q24h CrCl >0.6 to 0.8 mL/min/kg: 80-105 mg/kg q48h CrCl >0.5 to 0.6 mL/min/kg: 60-80 mg/kg q48h CrCl 0.4 to 0.5 mL/min/kg: 50-65 mg/kg q48h CrCl <0.4 mL/min/kg: Not recommended	No data	No data	No data	No data
Ganciclovir (IV induction)	3.5	30	5 mg/kg IV q12h	CrCl ≥70: No dosage adjustment CrCl 50-69: 2.5 mg/kg q12h CrCl 25-49: 2.5 mg/kg q24h CrCl 10-24: 1.25 mg/kg q24h CrCl <10: 1.25 mg/kg 3x/week	1.25 mg/kg 3x/week (AD on dialysis days)	1.25 mg/kg 3x/week	CVVHDF: 2.5 mg/kg q24h[21]	No data
Ganciclovir (IV maintenance)	3.5	30	5 mg/kg IV q24h	CrCl >90: No dosage adjustment CrCl >50-90: 2.5-5 mg/kg q24h CrCl 10-50: 0.625-1.25 mg/kg q24h CrCl <10: 0.625 mg/kg 3x/week	0.625 mg/kg 3x/week (AD on dialysis days)	0.625 mg/kg 3x/week	No data	No data
Ganciclovir (oral)	3.5	30	1 gm po q8h	CrCl >90: No dosage adjustment CrCl >50-90: 0.5-1 gm q8h CrCl 10-50: 0.5-1 gm q24h CrCl <10: 0.5 gm 3x/week	0.5 gm 3x/week (AD on dialysis days)	No data	No data	No data
Letermovir	12	No data	480 mg po/IV q24h	CrCl >10: No dosage adjustment CrCl ≤10: No data	No data	No data	No data	No data
Maribavir	4.3	No data	400 mg q12h	No dosage adjustment for renal impairment	No data	No data	No data	No data

TABLE 17A (27)

Groups/Drugs	Half-life, hrs (renal function normal)	Half-life, hrs (ESRD)	Dose (renal function normal)	CrCl or eGFR	Hemodialysis	CAPD	CRRT	SLED
Antivirals/Herpes Virus *(continued)*								
Valacyclovir	3	14	Varies with indication	Herpes labialis: CrCl ≥50: 2 gm q12h x2 doses CrCl 30-49: 1 gm q12h x2 doses CrCl 10-29: 500 mg q12h x2 doses CrCl <10: 500 mg x1 dose Genital herpes, initial episode: CrCl ≥50: 1 gm q12h CrCl 30-49: No dosage adjustment CrCl 10-29: 1 gm q24h CrCl <10: 500 mg q24h Genital herpes, recurrent episode: CrCl ≥50: 500 mg q12h CrCl 30-49: No dosage adjustment CrCl 10-29: 500 mg q24h CrCl <10: 500 mg q24h Genital herpes, suppression: CrCl ≥50: 1 gm q24h CrCl 30-49: No dosage adjustment CrCl 10-29: 500 mg q24h CrCl <10: 500 mg q24h Genital herpes, suppression, HIV-infected: CrCl ≥50: 500 mg q12h CrCl 30-49: No dosage adjustment CrCl 10-29: 500 mg q24h CrCl <10: 500 mg q24h Herpes zoster: CrCl ≥50: 1 gm q8h CrCl 30-49: 1 gm q12h CrCl 10-29: 1 gm q24h CrCl <10: 500 mg q24h	500 mg q24h (AD on dialysis days)	500 mg q24h	No data	No data
Valganciclovir (induction)	ganciclovir 4	ganciclovir 67	900 mg po q12h	CrCl ≥60: 900 mg q12h CrCl 40-59: 450 mg q12h CrCl 25-39: 450 mg q24h CrCl 10-24: 450 mg q48h CrCl <10: Not recommended	Not recommended	No data	No data	No data
Valganciclovir (maintenance)	ganciclovir 4	ganciclovir 67	900 mg po q24h	CrCl ≥60: 900 mg q24h CrCl 40-59: 450 mg q24h CrCl 25-39: 450 mg q48h CrCl 10-24: 450 mg 2x/week CrCl <10: Not recommended	Not recommended	No data	CVVHD: 450 mg q24h *(CID 2021;73:101)*	No data

TABLE 17A (28)

Groups/Drugs	Half-life, hrs (renal function normal)	Half-life, hrs (ESRD)	Dose (renal function normal)	CrCl or eGFR	Hemodialysis	CAPD	CRRT	SLED
Antivirals *(continued)*								
Influenza								
Amantadine	16	192	100 mg po q12h	CrCl >50: No dosage adjustment CrCl 30-50: 200 mg, then 100 mg q24h CrCl 15-29: 200 mg, then 100 mg q48h CrCl <15: 200 mg once weekly	200 mg once weekly	No data	No data	No data
Baloxavir marboxil	baloxavir 79.1	No data	40-80 mg po x1	CrCl ≥50: No dosage adjustment CrCl <50: No data	No data	No data	No data	No data
Favipiravir	5.6	No data	600 mg po bid	No data	No data	No data	No data	No data
Laninamivir	laninamivir 64.7	No data	40 mg (inhaled) x1	No dosage adjustment for renal impairment	No data	No data	No data	No data
Oseltamivir	carboxylate 6-10	carboxylate >20	Treatment: 75 mg po q12h x5 days Prophylaxis: 75 mg po q24h	Treatment: CrCl >60: No dosage adjustment CrCl >30-60: 30 mg q12h x5 days CrCl >10-30: 30 mg q24h x5 days CrCl ≤10, no HD: Not recommended Prophylaxis: CrCl >60: No dosage adjustment CrCl >30-60: 30 mg q24h CrCl >10-30: 30 mg q48h CrCl ≤10, no HD: Not recommended	Treatment: 30 mg x1, then 30 mg after every HD cycle. Prophylaxis: 30 mg x1, then 30 mg after alternate HD cycles. Pediatrics: For age >1 yr (after each HD): Wt ≤15 kg: 7.5 mg Wt 16-23 kg: 10 mg Wt 24-40 kg: 15 mg Wt >40 kg: 30 mg[12]	Treatment (CAPD): 30 mg x1. Prophylaxis (CAPD): 30 mg x1, then 30 mg q-week. Treatment (APD): 75 mg po x1[28]	No data	No data
Peramivir	20	No data	600 mg IV x1	Age ≥13 yrs: CrCl ≥50: No dosage adjustment CrCl 30-49: 200 mg x1 CrCl 10-29: 100 mg x1 Age 2-12 yrs: CrCl ≥50: No dosage adjustment CrCl 30-49: 4 mg/kg x1 CrCl 10-29: 2 mg/kg x1	Dose AD (HD removes 73-81%)	No data	No data	No data
Rimantadine[5]	25.4	Prolonged	100 mg po q12h	CrCl ≥30: No dosage adjustment CrCl <30: 100 mg q24h	100 mg q24h	No data	No data	No data
Zanamivir	2.5-5.1	No data	10 mg inhaled q12h	No dosage adjustment for renal impairment	No data	No data	No data	No data
Pox Viruses								
Brincidofovir	19.3	No data	Weight-based	No dosage adjustment for renal impairment	No dosage adjustment	No data	No data	No data
Tecovirimat	19-21	No data	Weight-based	Capsules: No dosage adjustment Injection: CrCl ≥30: No dosage adjustment CrCl <30: Contraindicated due to vehicle	Capsules: No dosage adjustment Injection: Contraindicated	No data	No data	No data

TABLE 17A (29)

Groups/Drugs	Half-life, hrs (renal function normal)	Half-life, hrs (ESRD)	Dose (renal function normal)	CrCl or eGFR	Hemodialysis	CAPD	CRRT	SLED
Antiretrovirals								
NRTIs								
Abacavir (ABC)[5]	1.5	No data	600 mg po q24h	No dosage adjustment for renal impairment	No data	No data	No data	No data
Didanosine (ddI) (delayed-release caps)	1.6	4.5	400 mg po q24h	CrCl ≥60, wt ≥60 kg: No dosage adjustment CrCl ≥60, wt <60 kg: 250 mg q24h CrCl 30-59, wt ≥60 kg: 200 mg q24h CrCl 30-59, wt <60 kg: 125 mg q24h CrCl 10-29, wt ≥60 kg: 125 mg q24h CrCl 10-29, wt <60 kg: 125 mg q24h CrCl <10, wt ≥60 kg: 125 mg q24h CrCl <10, wt <60 kg: Not recommended	Use CrCl <10 recommendations (no supplemental dose post HD required)	Use CrCl <10 recommendations	No data	No data
Didanosine (ddI) (pwd for oral solution)	1.6	4.5	200 mg po q12h (wt ≥60 kg)	CrCl ≥60, wt ≥60 kg: No dosage adjustment CrCl ≥60, wt <60 kg: 125 mg q12h CrCl 30-59, wt ≥60 kg: 200 mg q24h CrCl 30-59, wt <60 kg: 150 mg q24h CrCl 10-29, wt ≥60 kg: 150 mg q24h CrCl 10-29, wt <60 kg: 100 mg q24h CrCl <10, wt ≥60 kg: 100 mg q24h CrCl <10, wt <60 kg: 75 mg q24h	Use CrCl <10 recommendations (no supplemental dose post HD required)	Use CrCl <10 recommendations	No data	No data
Emtricitabine (FTC) (capsules)	10	>10	200 mg po q24h	CrCl >50: No dosage adjustment CrCl 30-49: 200 mg q48h CrCl 10-29: 200 mg q72h CrCl <10: 200 mg q96h	200 mg q96h	No data	No data	No data
Emtricitabine (FTC) (oral solution)	10	> 10	240 mg po q24h	CrCl >50: No dosage adjustment CrCl 30-49: 120 mg q24h CrCl 10-29: 80 mg q24h CrCl <10: 60 mg q24h	60 mg q24h	No data	No data	No data
Lamivudine (3TC)	5 - 7	15 - 35	300 mg po q24h (HIV dose)	CrCl >50: No dosage adjustment CrCl 10-50: 50-150 mg q24h CrCl <10: 25-50 mg q24h	25-50 mg q24h (AD on dialysis days) (HIV)	25-50 mg po q24h (HIV)	100 mg first day, then 50 mg q24h (HIV)	No data
Stavudine (d4T)	1.2-1.6	5.5-8	30-40 mg po q12h	CrCl >50: No dosage adjustment CrCl 10-50: 15-20 mg q12h CrCl <10, wt ≥60 kg: 20 mg q24h CrCl <10, wt <60 kg: 15 mg q24h	Use CrCl <10 recommendations (AD on dialysis days)	No data	30-40 mg q12h	No data
Tenofovir (TDF)	17	Prolonged	300 mg po q24h	CrCl >50: No dosage adjustment CrCl 30-49: 300 mg q48h CrCl 10-29: 300 mg q72-96h CrCl <10: No data	300 mg after every 3rd dialysis, or q7 days if no dialysis	No data	No data	No data

TABLE 17A (30)

Groups/Drugs	Half-life, hrs (renal function normal)	Half-life, hrs (ESRD)	Dose (renal function normal)	CrCl or eGFR	Hemodialysis	CAPD	CRRT	SLED
Antiretrovirals/NRTIs *(continued)*								
Zidovudine (ZDV/AZT)	0.5 - 3	1.3 - 3	300 mg po q12h	CrCl >50: No dosage adjustment CrCl 10-50: 300 mg q12h CrCl <10: 100 mg q8h	100 mg q8h (AD on dialysis days)	100 mg q8h	300 mg q12h	No data
NNRTIs								
Doravirine (DOR)	15	No data	100 mg po q24h	No dosage adjustment for renal impairment	Some removal by HD, but viral suppression maintained *(J Infect Chemother 2023;29:558)*	No data	No data	No data
Efavirenz (EFV)	40-55	No data	600 mg po q24h	No dosage adjustment for renal impairment	No data	No data	No data	No data
Etravirine (ETR)	41	No data	200 mg po q12h	No dosage adjustment for renal impairment	No dosage adjustment	No dosage adjustment	No data	No data
Nevirapine (NVP)	25-30	No data	200 mg po q12h	No dosage adjustment for renal impairment	Give extra 200 mg AD	No data	No data	No data
Rilpivirine (RPV)	45-50	No data	25 mg po q24h	CrCl ≥30: No dosage adjustment CrCl <30: Use with caution	No data	No data	No data	No data
PIs, Boosting Agents								
Atazanavir (ATV)[5]	≈7	No data	300 mg po q24h (if boosted)	No dosage adjustment for renal impairment	Do not use if ART-experienced	No data	No data	No data
Cobicistat (COBI or c)[*]	3-4	No data	150 mg po q24h	No dosage adjustment for renal impairment	No data	No data	No data	No data
Darunavir (DRV)	15	No data	600 mg po q12h (if boosted)	No dosage adjustment for renal impairment	No dosage adjustment	No data	No data	No data
Fosamprenavir (FPV)[5]	7.7	No data	700 mg po q12h (if boosted)	No dosage adjustment for renal impairment	No data	No data	No data	No data
Indinavir (IDV)[5]	1.2-2	No data	800 mg po q12h (if boosted)	No dosage adjustment for renal impairment	No data	No data	No data	No data
Nelfinavir (NFV)	3.5-5	No data	1250 mg po q12h	No dosage adjustment for renal impairment	No data	No data	No data	No data
Ritonavir (RTV)	3-5	No data	Used as booster (dosage varies)	No dosage adjustment for renal impairment	No data	No data	No data	No data
Saquinavir (SQV)	1-2	No data	1000 mg po q12h (if boosted)	CrCl ≥30: No dosage adjustment CrCl <30: No data	No data	No data	No data	No data
Tipranavir (TPV)	5.5-6	No data	500 mg po q12h (if boosted)	No dosage adjustment for renal impairment	No data	No data	No data	No data

Groups/Drugs	Half-life, hrs (renal function normal)	Half-life, hrs (ESRD)	Dose (renal function normal)	CrCl or eGFR	Hemodialysis	CAPD	CRRT	SLED
Antiretrovirals *(continued)*								
INSTIs								
Cabotegravir (CAB)	41	Unchanged	30 mg po q24h	CrCl ≥15: No dosage adjustment CrCl <15: No data	No data	No data	No data	No data
Dolutegravir (DTG)	14	No data	50 mg po q24h	INSTI-naive: No dosage adjustment for renal impairment INSTI-experienced: No dose adjustment for mild-moderate impairment Use with caution if CrCl <30 (DTG conc will be lower)	No data	No data	No data	No data
Raltegravir (RAL)	9	No data	400 mg po q12h	No dosage adjustment for renal impairment	No data	No data	No data	No data
Attachment Inhibitors								
Fostemsavir (FTR)	11	No data	600 mg po q12h	No dosage adjustment for renal impairment	No dosage adjustment	No data	No data	No data
Ibalizumab-uiyk (IBA)	Dose-dependent	No data	2 gm IV load, then 800 mg IV q2 weeks	No dosage adjustment for renal impairment	No data	No data	No data	No data
Capsid inhibitors								
Lenacapavir (LEN)	po: 10-12 days sc: 8-12 weeks	No data	Varies	CrCl ≥15: No dosage adjustment CrCl <15: No data	No data	No data	No data	No data
Entry Inhibitors								
Maraviroc (MVC)	14-18	No data	300 mg po q12h	CrCl >50: No dosage adjustment CrCl <50: No data	No data	No data	No data	No data
Fusion inhibitors								
Enfuvirtide (ENF/T20)	3.8	No data	90 mg sc q12h	No dosage adjustment for renal impairment	No dosage adjustment	No data	No data	No data
Fixed-Dose Combinations								
Atripla (EFV/FTC/TDF)	EFV: 40-55 FTC: 10 TDF: 17	EFV: No data FTC: >10 TDF: Prolonged	1 tab po q24h	CrCl ≥50: 1 tab q24h CrCl <50: Do not use	Do not use	Do not use	Do not use	Do not use

TABLE 17A (32)

Groups/Drugs	Half-life, hrs (renal function normal)	Half-life, hrs (ESRD)	Dose (renal function normal)	CrCl or eGFR	Hemodialysis	CAPD	CRRT	SLED
Antiretrovirals/Fixed-Dose Combinations *(continued)*								
Biktarvy (BIC/FTC/TAF)	BIC: 17.3 FTC: 10 TAF: 0.51	BIC: No data FTC: >10 TAF: No data	1 tab po q24h	CrCl ≥30: 1 tab q24h CrCl <30: Do not use (see HD)	On HD, virologically suppressed: 1 tab q24h (AD on dialysis days). On HD, not virologically suppressed: Do not use.	Do not use	Do not use	Do not use
Cabenuva (CAB/RPV) (IM)	CAB: 5.6-11.5 wks RPV: 13-28 wks	CAB: No data RPV: No data	CAB: 600 mg x1 then 400 mg q-mon RPV: 900 mg x1 then 600 mg q-mon	CrCl ≥30: No dosage adjustment CrCl <30: No dosage adjustment, monitor for toxicity	No data	No data	No data	No data
Cimduo, Temixys (3TC/TDF)	3TC: 5-7 TDF: 17	3TC: 15-35 TDF: Prolonged	1 tab po q24h	CrCl ≥50: 1 tab q24h CrCl <50: Do not use	Do not use	Do not use	Do not use	Do not use
Combivir (3TC/ZDV)	3TC: 5-7 ZDV: 0.5-3	3TC: 15-35 ZDV: 1.3-3	1 tab po q12h	CrCl ≥50: 1 tab q12h CrCl <50: Do not use	Do not use	Do not use	Do not use	Do not use
Complera / Eviplera (RPV/FTC/TDF)	RPV: 45-50 FTC: 10 TDF: 17	RPV: No data FTC: >10 TDF: Prolonged	1 tab po q24h	CrCl ≥50: 1 tab q24h CrCl <50: Do not use	Do not use	Do not use	Do not use	Do not use
Delstrigo (DOR/3TC/TDF)	DOR: 15 3TC: 5-7 TDF: 17	DOR: No data 3TC: 15-35 TDF: Prolonged	1 tab po q24h	CrCl ≥50: 1 tab q24h CrCl <50: Do not use	Do not use	Do not use	Do not use	Do not use
Descovy (FTC/TAF)	FTC: 10 TAF: 0.51	FTC: >10 TAF: No data	1 tab po q24h	CrCl ≥50: 1 tab q24h CrCl <50: Do not use	Do not use	Do not use	Do not use	Do not use
Dovato (DTG/3TC)	DTG: 14 3TC: 5-7	DTG: No data 3TC: 15-35	1 tab po q24h	CrCl ≥30: 1 tab q24h CrCl <30: Do not use	Do not use	Do not use	Do not use	Do not use
Dutrebis (3TC/RAL)	3TC: 5-7 RAL: 9	3TC: 15-35 RAL: No data	1 tab po q12h	CrCl ≥50: 1 tab q12h CrCl <50: Do not use	Do not use	Do not use	Do not use	Do not use
Epzicom / Kivexa (ABC/3TC)	ABC: 1.5 3TC: 5-7	ABC: No data 3TC: 15-35	1 tab po q24h	CrCl ≥50: 1 tab q24h CrCl <50: Do not use	Do not use	Do not use	Do not use	Do not use
Evotaz (ATV/Cobi)*	ATV: ≈7 Cobi: 3-4	ATV: No data Cobi: No data	1 tab po q24h	No dosage adjustment for renal impairment	Do not use in treatment-experienced patients	No data	No data	No data

TABLE 17A (33)

Groups/Drugs	Half-life, hrs (renal function normal)	Half-life, hrs (ESRD)	Dose (renal function normal)	CrCl or eGFR	Hemodialysis	CAPD	CRRT	SLED
Antiretrovirals/Fixed-Dose Combinations *(continued)*								
Genvoya (EVG/Cobi/FTC/TAF)	EVG: 12.9 Cobi: 3-4 FTC: 10 TAF: 0.51	EVG: No data Cobi: No data FTC: >10 TAF: No data	1 tab po q24h	CrCl ≥30: 1 tab q24h CrCl <30: Do not use	Do not use	Do not use	Do not use	Do not use
Juluca (DTG/RPV)	DTG: 14 RPV: 45-50	DTG: No data RPV: No data	1 tab po q24h	CrCl ≥30: 1 tab q24h CrCl <30: Use with caution	Use with caution	Use with caution	Use with caution	No data
Kaletra (LPV/RTV)	Lopinavir 6.9 Ritonavir 3-5	No data	2 tab po q12h (one tab: LPV 200 mg, RTV 50 mg)	No dosage adjustment for renal impairment	No data	No data	No data	No data
Odefsey (RPV/FTC/TAF)	RPV: 45-50 FTC: 10 TAF: 0.51	RPV: No data FTC: >10 TAF: No data	1 tab po q24h	CrCl ≥30: 1 tab q24h CrCl <30: Do not use	Do not use	Do not use	Do not use	Do not use
Prezcobix (DRV/Cobi)*	DRV: 15 Cobi: 3-4	DRV: No data Cobi: No data	1 tab po q24h	No dosage adjustment for renal impairment	Do not use	Do not use	Do not use	Do not use
Stribild (EVG/Cobi/FTC/TDF)	EVG: 12.9 Cobi: 3-4 FTC: 10 TDF: 17	EVG: No data Cobi: No data FTC: >10 TDF: Prolonged	1 tab po q24h	CrCl ≥70: 1 tab q24h CrCl <70 at start of tx: Do not use CrCl <50 during tx: Discontinue use	Do not use	Do not use	Do not use	Do not use
Symfi, Symfi Lo (EFV/3TC/TDF)	EFV: 40-55 3TC: 5-7 TDF: 17	EFV: No data 3TC: 15-35 TDF: Prolonged	1 tab po q24h	CrCl ≥50: 1 tab q24h CrCl <50: Do not use	Do not use	Do not use	Do not use	Do not use
Symtuza (DRV/Cobi/FTC/TAF)	DRV: 15 Cobi: 3-4 FTC: 10 TAF: 0.51	DRV: No data Cobi: No data FTC: >10 TAF: No data	1 tab po q24h	CrCl ≥30: 1 tab q24h CrCl <30: Do not use	Do not use	Do not use	Do not use	Do not use
Temixys (3TC/TDF)	3TC: 5-7 TDF: 17	3TC: 15-35 TDF: Prolonged	1 tab po q24h	CrCl ≥50: 1 tab q24h CrCl <50: Do not use	Do not use	Do not use	Do not use	Do not use
Triumeq (DTG/3TC/ABC)	DTG: 14 3TC: 5-7 ABC: 1.5	DTG: No data 3TC: 15-35 ABC: No data	1 tab po q24h	CrCl ≥30: 1 tab q24h CrCl <30: Do not use	Do not use	Do not use	Do not use	Do not use
Trizivir (ABC/3TC/ZDV)	ABC: 1.5 3TC: 5-7 ZDV: 0.5-3	ABC: No data 3TC: 15-35 ZDV: 1.3-3	1 tab po q12h	CrCl ≥50: 1 tab q12h CrCl <50: Do not use	Do not use	Do not use	Do not use	Do not use
Truvada (FTC/TDF)	FTC: 10 TDF: 17	FTC: >10 TDF: Prolonged	1 tab po q24h	CrCl ≥50: 1 tab q24h CrCl 30-49: 1 tab q48h CrCl <30: Do not use	Do not use	Do not use	Do not use	Do not use

[1] High flux HD membranes lead to unpredictable drug Cl; measure post-dialysis drug levels.
[2] Check levels with CAPD, PK highly variable. Usual method w/CAPD: 2L dialysis fluid replaced qid (Example amikacin: give 8L x 20 mg lost/L = 160 mg amikacin IV supplement daily).
[3] Extended-interval dosing recommendations for renal impairment: *Infect Dis Clin North Am 1989;3:517.*
[4] May falsely increase Scr by interference with assay.
[5] Dosage adjustment may be required in hepatic disease.
[6] *Antimicrob Agents Chemother 2019;63:e01427-19.*
[7] Hemodialysis recommendations assume HD 3x/week.
[8] Goal peak serum concentration: 25-100 µg/ml.
[9] Therapeutic drug monitoring recommended.
[10] Goal peak serum concentration: 20-35 µg/ml.
[11] Rapid infusion can increase SCr.
[12] Pediatric HD ref: *Clin Infect Dis 2010;50:1427.*
[13] *Can J Kidney Health Dis 2018;5:2054358118792229.*
[14] Use entecavir suspension for doses less than 0.5 mg
[15] HD, CRRT recommendations: *Am J Health Sys Pharm 2020;77:835-863.*
[16] eGFR: estimated glomerular filtration rate (mL/min/1.73 m^2).
[17] Administer extra cefoperazone separately as needed (cefoperazone does not require dosage adjustment in renal impairment).
[18] Dosing based on TMP component.
[19] *Indian J Pharmacol 2013;45:330.*
[20] Consider dosage adjustment for moderate to severe impairment.
[21] *Antimicrob Agents Chemother 2014;58:94.*
[22] *J Crit Care 2024;85:154924.*
[23] *Antimicrob Agents Chemother 2019;64:e01655-19.*
[24] Study suggests ↑ blood conc *(Eur J Clin Pharmacol 1992;42:671).*
[25] Loading dose for all CRRT modalities: 2 gm.
[26] *Ann Pharmacother 2013;47:1342.*
[27] *Pharmaceutics 2022;14:842.*
[28] APD reference: *Br J Clin Pharmacol 2015;79:624.*
[29] Attains 40% fT>4MIC, MIC=2, effluent rate 35 mL/kg/hr *(Blood Purif 2023;52:503).*
[30] Attains 40% fT>MIC, MIC=2 *(Crit Care 2018;22:25).*
[31] Expert opinion (no published data).

TABLE 17B – NO DOSAGE ADJUSTMENT WITH RENAL INSUFFICIENCY BY CATEGORY

Antibacterials		Antifungals	Anti-TBc	Antivirals		Antiparasitics
Azithromycin	Minocycline	Amphotericin B	Bedaquiline	Abacavir	Lopinavir	Albendazole
Ceftriaxone	Moxifloxacin	Anidulafungin	Isoniazid	Atazanavir	Mavyret	Artesunate
Chloramphenicol	Nafcillin	Caspofungin	Rifampin	Bamlanivimab-Etesevimab	Molnupiravir	Fexinidazole
Clindamycin	Omadacycline	Ibrexafungerp	Rifapentine	Bebtelovimab	Nelfinavir	Mefloquine
Dicloxacillin	Oritavancin	Isavuconazonium sulfate		Brincidofovir	Nevirapine	Paromomycin
Doxycycline	Pivmecillinam	Itraconazole oral solution		Casirivimab-Imdevimab	Raltegravir	Pyrimethamine
Eravacycline	Polymyxin B	Ketoconazole		Cobicistat	Remdesivir	
Erythromycin	Rifamycin SV	Micafungin[1]		Daclatasvir	Ribavirin	
Fidaxomicin	Rifaximin	Posaconazole, **po only**		Darunavir	Rilpivirine	
Fusidic acid	Secnidazole	Voriconazole, **po only**		Delavirdine	Ritonavir	
Lefamulin	Tedizolid			Dolutegravir	Saquinavir	
Linezolid[3]	Tigecycline			Efavirenz	Simeprevir[2]	
				Epclusa	Sofosbuvir	
				Etravirine	Sotrovimab	
				Fosamprenavir	Tecovirimat	
				Fostemsavir	Tipranavir	
				Harvoni	Vosevi	
				Ibalizumab-uiyk	Zepatier	
				Indinavir		
				Interferon-alfa 2a, 2b		

[1] Micafungin: consider dose increase in CRRT
[2] No data for CrCl <30 mL/min
[3] Increased risk of bone marrow toxicity

TABLE 17C – ANTIMICROBIAL DOSING IN OBESITY

The number of obese patients is increasing. Intuitively, the standard doses of some drugs may not achieve effective serum concentrations. Pertinent data on anti-infective dosing in the obese patient is gradually emerging. Though some of the data needs further validation, the following table reflects what is currently known. **Obesity is defined as ≥20% over Ideal Body Weight (Ideal BW) or Body Mass Index (BMI) >30. Dose =** suggested body weight (BW) for dose calculation in obese patient, or specific dose if applicable. In general, the absence of a drug in the table indicates a lack of pertinent information in the published literature.

Drug	Dose	Comments
Acyclovir	Use **Adjusted BW** *(see Comments)*	Unpublished data from 7 obese volunteers *(Davis, et al., ICAAC abstract, 1991)* suggested ideal BW, but newer and more convincing PK data suggest that adjusted BW better approximates drug exposure in normals *(AAC 60:1830, 2016)*.
Aminoglycosides	Use **Adjusted BW**	Adjusted BW = Ideal BW + 0.4(Actual BW – Ideal BW). Ref: *Pharmacother 27:1081, 2007.* Follow levels so as to lower dose once hemodynamics stabilizes.
Amphotericin B liposomal	Use **Adjusted BW**, but consider actual BW if critically ill	Recommendation based on a retrospective analysis evaluating clinical outcomes in 238 patients *(AAC 2021;65:e02366-20)*. Earlier data from a small PK study support a fixed dose in patients ≥100 kg (e.g., 500 mg for a target dose of 5 mg/kg), which similarly suggests that using actual BW in all obese patients is not the best strategy *(CID 2020;70:2213)*.
Anidulafungin	Data insufficient for a firm recommendation	Accumulating data suggest reduced echinocandin exposure in obesity, but evidence for the ideal dose adjustment strategy is limited *(Am J Health Syst Pharm 2023;80:503)*. PK modeling data suggest a 25% increase in loading and maintenance dose in patients >140 kg results in exposure comparable to non-obese patients receiving usual dosing *(AAC 2018;62:e00063-18)*. A retrospective cohort study (n=173) showed no difference in outcomes across BMI category in patients receiving standard dosing *(J Pharm Pract 2022;35:20)*.
Artemether-lumefantrine	No dose adjustment appears necessary	Data from a PK study in healthy volunteers (6 normal weight, 7 overweight [mean BMI 28.2], 3 obese [mean BMI 33.9]). Only one with BMI >35. Small numbers limit conclusions *(IJAA 2022;59:106482)*.
Caspofungin	Data insufficient for a firm recommendation	Accumulating data suggest reduced echinocandin exposure in obesity, but evidence for the ideal dose adjustment strategy is limited *(Am J Health Syst Pharm 2023;80:503)*. A weight-based regimen (2 mg/kg load, 1.25 mg/kg q24h) has been suggested *(AAC 2020;64:e00905-20)*.

Drug	Dose	Comments
Cefazolin (surgical prophylaxis in adults)	Data insufficient for a firm recommendation	Joint recommendation from ASHP/IDSA/SIS/SHEA is for 3 gm x1 if ≥120 kg, 2 gm x1 if <120 kg *(Am J Health Syst Pharm 2013;70:195)*. However, in a recent systematic review, 3/3 outcome studies and 9/15 PK studies found the 3 gm dose in patients ≥120 kg to be unnecessary *(Obes Surg 2022;32:3138)*.
Cefazolin (tx of active infection)	Data insufficient for a firm recommendation	PK considerably altered in obesity. Consider higher dose and/or continuous infusion in patients ≥120 kg with less susceptible gram-negative infection, critically ill, or immunocompromised *(IJAA 2023;61:107651)*.
Cefepime	Modest dose increase: 2 gm IV q8h instead of the usual q12h	Data from 10 patients (mean BMI 48) undergoing bariatric surgery; regimen yields free T > MIC of 60% for MIC of 8 µg/mL. Ref: *Obes Surg 22:465, 2012.*
Cefotetan	No dose adjustment appears necessary	No difference in surg wound infection rates between 2 and 3 gm prophylaxis doses in patients ≥120 kg, median BMI 42 kg/m² *(Surg Infect 19:504, 2018)*.
Cefoxitin (surgical prophylaxis)	Larger dose possibly required but data insufficient for a firm recommendation	Single 40 mg/kg perioperative dose in obese patients (based on actual BW; range 4-7.5 gm) resulted in suboptimal achievement of pharmacodynamic targets in both serum and tissue, although performance was better than a simulated 2 gm dose *(AAC 60:5885, 2016)*. A single 4 gm dose administered preop to 200 pts (mean BMI 45.8 kg/m²) failed to reach predefined PK/PD targets for most common pathogens *(AAC 2019;63:e01613-19)*.
Ceftaroline	No dose adjustment appears necessary	Based on PK simulations. Consider q8h dosing if targeting 50% fT>MIC for MRSA *(Pharmacotherapy 2023;43:226)*.
Ceftriaxone	**Larger dose possibly required** but data are insufficient for a conclusive recommendation	Retrospective cohort study suggests clinical failure more likely in obese patients treated with standard dosing; higher quality data are required before a recommendation is appropriate *(Diseases 2020;8:E27)*.
Ciprofloxacin	No dose adjustment appears necessary	No influence of obesity on ciprofloxacin plasma PK in a prospective clinical study (n=20, median BMI 45 kg/m²). Increased dosing may be required if target tissue penetration is known to be impaired in obesity, e.g., SSTI *(Clin Pharmacokinet 2022;61:1167)*.
Clindamycin	Consider **Actual BW**	Combined PK modeling data from three prospective trials in children suggests actual BW to be most appropriate; no clinical outcome data available *(AAC 61:e02014, 2016)*.
Colistin	Use **Ideal BW**	Maximum colistin base activity 360 mg/day to limit risk of nephrotoxicity. Clinical data in obese patients limited and difficult to interpret *(Pharmacotherapy 2023;43:226)*.
Dalbavancin	No dose adjustment appears necessary	Ref: *AAC 2024;68:e0171923*
Daptomycin	**Adjusted BW suggested**	Data from a retrospective study suggest similar outcomes using actual BW and adjusted BW *(Ther Adv Infectious Dis 2019;6:1)*. Other data suggest similar outcomes with ideal BW and actual BW *(AAC 58:88, 2014)*. Some recommend fixed, non-weight-based dosing in morbid obesity based on a recent PK study *(Pharmacother 2018;38:981)*.
Delafloxacin	No dose adjustment appears necessary	Data limited to skin infections *(AAC 2024;68:e0171923)*.
Eravacycline	No dose adjustment appears necessary	Standard dosing uses actual BW. A post hoc analysis of two RCTs demonstrates safety and efficacy in patients with BMI ≥30 kg/m² *(OFID 2020;7:ofaa548)*.
Ertapenem	Larger dose possibly required	PK data suggest that a modest dose increase may be appropriate, particularly in extreme obesity or when pathogen MICs are elevated *(AAC 2018;62:e00784-18; Eur J Clin Pharmacol 2019;75:711; Minerva Anestesiol 2014;80:1005; AAC 2006;50:1222)*. In a case report, 1.5 gm q24h provided adequate drug exposure for susceptible bacteria in a 250 kg patient with pneumonia *(Case Rep Crit Care 2017:5310768)*.
Ethambutol	Use lean body weight	ATS/CDC/IDSA recommendation *(CID 2016;63:e147)*
Fluconazole	Larger dose possibly required but data insufficient for a firm recommendation	Case reports suggest larger dose required in critically ill obese pts. Recent paper suggests that wt-based dosing (12 mg/kg load then 6 mg/kg/day using total BW) reaches desired PK/PD targets more reliably than fixed dosing; clinical validation required *(Pharmacother 17:1023, 1997; AAC 60:6550, 2016)*.
Flucytosine	Use **Ideal BW**	Data from one obese patient with cryptococcal disease. Ref: *Pharmacother 15:251, 1995.*
Fosfomycin IV	Data are insufficient for a firm recommendation	Limited data suggest ↓ exposure in obesity. If MIC ≤16 µg/mL, 8 gm IV q8h appears sufficient if CrCl ≤130 mL/min, regardless of obesity status or PK/PD index employed *(AAC 2022;66:e0230221; JAC 2019;74:2335)*.
Ganciclovir	Similar outcomes using actual BW and adjusted BW	No differences in safety or efficacy outcomes observed in a single-center retrospective cohort study. Larger, prospective studies focusing on specific patient subgroups are needed *(Transpl ID 2023;25:e14134)*.

Drug	Dose	Comments
Isavuconazole	No dose adjustment appears necessary	Similar AUC in obese (BMI >30 kg/m²) and non-obese patients. Data published in abstract form. Ref: *OFID 2016;3.* Available at *http://dx.doi.org/10.1093/ofid/ofw172.1498*
Levofloxacin	No dose adjustment appears necessary	Data from 13 obese patients; variability in study findings renders conclusion uncertain. Refs: *AAC 55:3240, 2011; JAC 66:1653, 2011.* A recent PK study (requiring clinical validation) in patients with BMI of 40 or more suggests that higher doses may be necessary to achieve adequate drug exposure *(Clin Pharmacokin 53:753, 2014).*
Linezolid	Newest data suggest standard dosing may be inadequate	In a PK/PD modeling study in 15 obese patients with MRSA pneumonia (MIC 1-4 µg/mL), standard dosing led to low probability of target attainment in patients age <65 years *(JAC 2019; 74:667).* Insufficient concentrations from standard dosing also suggested by PK studies in intraabdominal surgery patients *(J Clin Med 2020;9:1067)* and critically ill patients with skin and soft tissue infections *(AAC 2021;65:e01619).*
Metronidazole	No dose adjustment appears necessary	Insufficient evidence to support the use of higher doses in obesity *(AAC 2024;68:e0171923).* Use actual BW for weight-based dosing, max 4 gm/day.
Micafungin	Data insufficient for a firm recommendation	Accumulating data suggest reduced echinocandin exposure in obesity, but evidence for the ideal dose adjustment strategy is limited *(Am J Health Syst Pharm 2023;80:503).* A PK/PD study suggests 150 mg q24h adequate for C. albicans in pts ≤115 kg, 200 mg q24h in pts >115 kg. 200 mg q24h adequate for C. glabrata in pts ≤115 kg *(Crit Care 2018 Apr 15;22(1):94).* A more recent PK/PD study suggests 200 mg q24h in patients >125 kg with a Candida species that has an MIC of 0.016 µg/mL, and 300 mg q24h if the MIC is 0.032 µg/mL. A loading dose of 2x the maintenance dose is also suggested *(JAC 2019;74:978).*
Moxifloxacin	No dose adjustment appears necessary	Based on limited PK data *(AAC 2024;68:e0171923)*
Omadacycline	No dose adjustment appears necessary	Based on two post hoc analyses of clinical trial data *(Pharmacotherapy 2023;43:226).*
Oritavancin	Data insufficient for a recommendation	No available data *(AAC 2024;68:e0171923).*
Oseltamivir	No dose adjustment appears necessary Example: 75 mg po q12h	Data from 10 obese volunteers, unclear if applicable to patients >250 kg (OK to give 150 mg po q12h). Ref: *J Antimicrob Chemother 66:2083, 2011.* Newer data consistent *(AAC 58:1616, 2014).*
Piperacillin-tazobactam	4.5 gm IV (over 4 hr) q6-8h	Suggested dosing in obesity particularly for critically ill patients, if MICs ≥8 µg/mL, or CrCl >100 mL/min *(Pharmacotherapy 2023;43:226).*
Polymyxin B	Use **adjusted BW**	Max daily dose of 200-249 mg suggested to limit risk of nephrotoxicity (not clinically validated); may be insufficient if MIC >0.5 µg/mL *(Pharmacotherapy 2023;43:226).*
Posaconazole (IV)	**Consider increased treatment dose** (not prophylaxis) in patients >140 kg Example: 400 mg IV q24h	In a PK study, total body weight best predicted changes in drug clearance and Vd. For sufficient exposure, modeling suggests increasing the dose used for treatment to 400 mg IV q24h in patients weighing >140 kg. For prophylaxis, 300 mg IV q24h provides sufficient exposure in patients up to 190 kg. Ref: *JAC 2020;75:1006.*
Pyrazinamide	Use lean body weight	ATS/CDC/IDSA recommendation *(CID 2016;63:e147).*
Rezafungin	Data insufficient for a firm recommendation	Accumulating data suggest reduced echinocandin exposure in obesity, but evidence for the ideal dose adjustment strategy is limited *(Am J Health Syst Pharm 2023;80:503).* A sub-analysis of phase 2 trial data (abstract only) suggests dose adjustment in obesity unnecessary *(OFID 2020;7(suppl 1):S378-9).*
Tecovirimat	600 mg po q8h x14 days 300 mg IV q12h x14 days	Manufacturer PI recs for peds and adult pts weighing ≥120 kg. Infuse IV doses over 6 hours.
Tedizolid phosphate	**No dose adjustment** appears necessary	Based on limited data *(Pharmacotherapy 2023;43:226).*
Teicoplanin	Use **Actual BW**	Ref: *AAC 2024;68:e0171923.*
Telavancin	**750 mg IV q24h** probably adequate for most patients	Data suggest this dose achieves efficacy targets and minimizes risk of nephrotoxicity. If higher systemic exposure is desired, consider 10 mg/kg q24h based on adjusted BW, not to exceed 1000 mg q24h *(Pharmacotherapy 2023;43:226).*
Tigecycline	**No dose adjustment** appears necessary	Standard dosing recommended in obesity. However, for resistant Gram-negative bacteria, consider higher dose (200 mg, then 100 mg IV q12h) regardless of patient weight *(AAC 2024;68:e0171923).*
TMP-SMX	Use **Adjusted BW**	Based on extremely limited evidence *(AAC 2024;68:e0171923).*

Drug	Dose	Comments
Vancomycin	Use **Actual BW**	Vancomycin Vd increases with actual body weight, but not in a predictable or proportionate manner. Current guidelines suggest capping the loading dose at 3 gm, and individual maintenance doses at 2 gm. Daily maintenance doses above 4.5 gm should rarely be required. Early and frequent AUC_{24} monitoring is recommended *(Am J Health Syst Pharm 2020;77:835)*. Decreased AKI risk with AUC_{24} monitoring (compared to trough monitoring) in patients with BMI >30 *(AAC 2022;66:e0088621)*. Controversy continues: recent review suggests loading dose based on actual BW and maintenance dose based on adjusted BW *(Expert Opin Drug Metab Toxicol 2022;18:323)*.
Voriconazole	Use **Ideal BW**	Dosing using actual body weight may result in supratherapeutic concentrations, but published data are insufficient to recommend adjusted BW vs. ideal BW. Best approach for now is to use ideal BW and check serum concentrations to avoid underdosing *(AAC 2011;55:2601; CID 2011;53:745; CID 2016;63:286; AAC 2021;65:e02460-20)*.

TABLE 17D – NO DOSING ADJUSTMENT REQUIRED IN OBESITY

The pharmacokinetics of antibacterials in obese patients is emerging, but only selected drugs have been evaluated. Those drugs where data justifies a dose adjustment in the obese are summarized in *Table 17C*. Those drugs where data indicates **NO NEED** for dose adjustment are listed below.

Drug	Drug
Ceftazidime/avibactam Ceftolozane/tazobactam Doripenem	Imipenem/cilastatin Meropenem

Ref: *Pharmacotherapy 37:1415, 2017*

TABLE 18 – ANTIMICROBIALS AND HEPATIC DISEASE: DOSAGE ADJUSTMENT*

The following alphabetical list indicates antibacterials excreted/metabolized by the liver **wherein a dosage adjustment may be indicated** in the presence of hepatic disease. Space precludes details; consult the PDR or package inserts for details. List is **not** all-inclusive:

Antibacterials		Antifungals	Antiparasitics	Antivirals[§]	
Ceftriaxone	Nafcillin	Caspofungin	Benznidazole	Abacavir	Indinavir
Chloramphenicol	Rifabutin	Isavuconazole	Nifurtimox	Atazanavir	Lopinavir/Ritonavir
Clindamycin	Rifampin	Itraconazole	Praziquantel	Darunavir	Nelfinavir
Eravacycline	Telithromycin[**]	Voriconazole		Efavirenz	Rimantadine
Fusidic acid	Tigecycline			Fosamprenavir	Ritonavir
Isoniazid	Tinidazole				Tofacitinib (JAK inhibitor)
Lefamulin (IV)					
Metronidazole					

§ Ref. on antiretrovirals: *CID 40:174, 2005* ** Telithro: reduce dose in renal & hepatic failure

TABLE 19 – TREATMENT OF CAPD PERITONITIS IN ADULTS

(Adapted from Guidelines – Int'l Soc Peritoneal Dialysis, *Perit Dial Int 2022;42:110*)

Principles: Empiric antibiotic therapy

- Initiate antibiotics asap after collection of peritoneal fluid & blood for culture
- Empiric regimens should cover both gram-positive and gram-negative organisms, and be guided by local susceptibilities.
    - o Recommended: (Vancomycin or Cefazolin) + (3rd-generation cephalosporin or Aminoglycoside)
    - o Cefepime monotherapy may be an acceptable alternative
- Can treat by IP route or systemic IV therapy, but Guidelines favor IP therapy

Intraperitoneal (IP) therapy

- Can be either continuous (drugs in each exchange) or intermittent (once daily)
- If intermittent, need antibiotic-containing dialysis fluid to dwell for minimum 6 hrs
- Vanco, aminoglycosides, cephalosporins can be combined in same dialysis bag; penicillins and aminoglycosides **cannot** be combined

Specific recommendations

IP Antibiotic Dosing Recommendations for Treatment of Peritonitis		
	Intermittent (1 exchange daily)	**Continuous (all exchanges)**
Aminoglycosides:		
Amikacin	2 mg/kg daily	Not advised
Gentamicin	0.6 mg/kg daily	Not advised
Netilmicin	0.6 mg/kg daily	Not advised
Tobramycin	0.6 mg/kg daily	Not advised
Cephalosporins:		
Cefazolin	15 mg/kg daily (long dwell) 20 mg/kg daily (short dwell)	LD 500 mg/L, MD 125 mg/L[1]
Cefepime	1000 mg daily	LD 500 mg/L, MD 125 mg/L[1]
Cefoperazone	No data	LD 500 mg/L, MD 62.5-125 mg/L
Cefotaxime	0.5-1 gm daily	No data
Ceftazidime	1-1.5 gm daily (for long dwell) 20 mg/kg daily (for short dwell)	LD 500 mg/L, MD 125 mg/L[1]
Ceftriaxone	1000 mg daily	No data
Penicillins:		
Amoxicillin	No data	MD 150 mg/L
Ampicillin	4 gm daily[2]	MD 125 mg/L
Amp/sulb	No data	LD 1.5 gm, MD 200 mg/bag
Penicillin G	No data	LD 50,000 unit/L, MD 25,000 unit/L
Pip/tazo	No data	LD 4.5 gm, MD 1.125 gm/bag
Others:		
Aztreonam	2 gm daily	LD 500 mg/L, MD 250 mg/L
Ciprofloxacin	No data	MD 50 mg/L
Clindamycin	No data	MD 600 mg/bag
Daptomycin	300 mg daily	LD 100 mg/L, MD 20 mg/L
Fosfomycin	4 gm daily	No data
Imipenem	500 mg in alternate exch	LD 250 mg/L, MD 50 mg/L
Meropenem	500 mg daily (for long dwell in APD) 1 gm daily (for short dwell in CAPD)	MD 125 mg/L
Ofloxacin	No data	LD 200 mg/L, MD 25 mg/L
Polymyxin B	No data	MD 300,000 unit (30 mg)/bag
Teicoplanin	15 mg/kg every 5 days	LD 400 mg/bag, MD 20 mg/L
Vancomycin	15-30 mg/kg q5-7 days for CAPD[3] 15 mg/kg q4 days for APD[3]	LD 20-25 mg/kg, MD 25 mg/L
Antifungals:		
Fluconazole	150-200 mg q24-48h (po preferred)	No data
Voriconazole	2.5 mg/kg q24h (po preferred)	No data

LD = loading dose in mg; MD = maintenance dose in mg; IP = intraperitoneal
Ref: *Perit Dial Int 2022;42:110*

[1] Increase in doses by 25% may be needed for pts with residual kidney function
[2] IP ampicillin is not recommended for treatment of enterococcal peritonitis
[3] Supplemental doses may be need for APD pts and dwell time of min 6 hr preferred

Systemic dosing recommendations for treatment of CAPD peritonitis

- In general, IP dosing leads to high IP drug levels and, hence, IP is preferable to IV antibiotic administration
- See individual systemic drugs for dose recommendations for patients with end stage renal disease (ESRD)
- Do not co-administer the same drug IP and systemically (either po or IV)

Indications for removal of CAPD catheter

- Relapse with same organism within one month
- No clinical response within 5 days (failure)
- Infection at catheter exit site and/or catheter subcutaneous tunnel
- Fungal peritonitis
- Fecal flora peritonitis; sign of bowel wall erosion & perforation

TABLE 20A – ANTI-TETANUS PROPHYLAXIS, WOUND CLASSIFICATION, IMMUNIZATION

WOUND CLASSIFICATION		
Clinical Features	**Tetanus Prone**	**Non-Tetanus Prone**
Age of wound	>6 hours	≤6 hours
Configuration	Stellate, avulsion	Linear
Depth	>1 cm	≤1 cm
Mechanism of injury	Missile, crush, burn, frostbite	Sharp surface (glass, knife)
Devitalized tissue	Present	Absent
Contaminants (dirt, saliva, etc.)	Present	Absent

IMMUNIZATION SCHEDULE				
History of Tetanus Immunization	**Dirty, Tetanus-Prone Wound**		**Clean, non-Tetanus-Prone Wound**	
	Td[1,2]	Tetanus Immune Globulin	Td[1,2]	Tetanus Immune Globulin
Unknown or <3 doses[3]	Yes	Yes	Yes	No
3 or more doses	No[4]	No	No[5]	No

Ref: *MMWR 60:13, 2011; MMWR 61:468, 2012; MMWR 62:131, 2013 (pregnancy)*

[1] Td = Tetanus & diphtheria toxoids, adsorbed (adult). For adult who has not received Tdap previously, substitute one dose of Tdap for Td when immunization is indicated *(MMWR 61:468, 2012)*.
[2] For children <7 years, use DTaP unless contraindicated; for persons ≥7 years, Td is preferred to tetanus toxoid alone, but single dose of Tdap can be used if required for catch-up series.
[3] Individuals who have not completed vaccine series should do so.
[4] Yes, if >5 years since last booster.
[5] Yes, if >10 years since last booster.

TABLE 20B – RABIES POSTEXPOSURE PROPHYLAXIS

All wounds should be cleaned immediately & thoroughly with soap & water. This has been shown to protect 90% of experimental animals![1]

Exposure to animal saliva or nervous system tissue through a bite, scratch, or contamination of open wounds or mucous membranes *(www.cdc.gov/rabies/exposure/type.html)* or when such exposure cannot be reliably excluded (e.g., bat found in room of sleeping person).

Animal Type	Evaluation & Disposition of Animal	Recommendations for Prophylaxis
Dogs, cats, ferrets	Healthy & available for 10-day observation	Don't start unless animal develops sx, then immediately begin HRIG + vaccine
	Rabid or suspected rabid	Immediate HRIG + vaccine
	Unknown (escaped)	Consult public health officials
Skunks, raccoons, *bats, foxes, coyotes, most carnivores	Regard as rabid	Immediate prophylaxis unless brain of animal tests negative for rabies virus
Livestock, horses, rodents, rabbits; includes hares, squirrels, hamsters, guinea pigs, gerbils, chipmunks, rats, mice, woodchucks	Consider case-by-case	Consult public health officials. Bites of squirrels, hamsters, guinea pigs, gerbils, chipmunks, rats, mice, other small rodents, rabbits, and hares **almost never** require rabies post-exposure prophylaxis.

* Most recent cases of human rabies in U.S. due to contact (not bites) with silver-haired bats or rarely big brown bats but risk of acquiring rabies from non-contact bat exposure is exceedingly low.

Postexposure Rabies Immunization Schedule

IF NOT PREVIOUSLY VACCINATED

Treatment	Regimen[2]
Local wound cleaning	**All postexposure treatment should begin with immediate, thorough cleaning of all wounds with soap & water.** Then irrigate with a virucidal agent such as povidone-iodine solution if available.
Human rabies immune globulin (HRIG)	20 IU per kg body weight given once on day 0. If anatomically feasible, the full dose should be infiltrated around the wound(s), the rest should be administered IM in the gluteal area. If the calculated dose of HRIG is insufficient to inject all the wounds, it should be diluted with normal saline to allow infiltration around additional wound areas. HRIG should **not** be administered in the **same syringe, or** into the **same anatomical site** as vaccine, or more than 7 days after the initiation of vaccine. Because HRIG may partially suppress active production of antibody, no more than the recommended dose should be given.[3]
Vaccine	Human diploid cell vaccine (HDCV), rabies vaccine adsorbed (RVA), or purified chick embryo cell vaccine (PCECV) 1 mL **IM (deltoid area[4])**, one each day 0, 3, 7, 14[5].

IF PREVIOUSLY VACCINATED[6]

Treatment	Regimen[2]
Local wound cleaning	All postexposure treatment should begin with immediate, thorough cleaning of all wounds with soap **&** water. Then irrigate with a virucidal agent such as povidone-iodine solution if available.
HRIG	HRIG should **not** be administered
Vaccine	HDCV or PCEC, 1 mL **IM (deltoid area[4])**, one each on days 0 & 3

CORRECT VACCINE ADMINISTRATION SITES

Age Group	Administration Site
Children & adults	**DELTOID[4]** only (**NEVER** in gluteus)
Infants & young children	Outer aspect of thigh (anterolateral thigh) may be used (**NEVER** in gluteus)

[1] From *MMWR 48:RR-1, 1999; CID 30:4, 2000*; B. T. Matyas, Mass. Dept. of Public Health. *MMWR 57:1, 2008*

[2] These regimens are applicable for all age groups, including children.

[3] In most reported post-exposure treatment failures, only identified deficiency was failure to infiltrate wound(s) with HRIG *(CID 22:228, 1996)*. However, several failures reported from SE Asia in patients in whom WHO protocol followed *(CID 28:143, 1999)*.

[4] The **deltoid** area is the **only** acceptable site of vaccination for adults & older children. For infants & young children, outer aspect of the thigh (anterolateral thigh) may be used. Vaccine should **NEVER** be administered in gluteal area.

[5] Note that this is a change from previous recommendation of 5 doses (days 0, 3, 7, 14 & 28) based on new data & recommendations from ACIP. Note that the number of doses for persons with altered immunocompetence remains unchanged (5 doses on days 0, 3, 7, 14 & 28) and recommendations for pre-exposure prophylaxis remain 3 doses administered on days 0, 7 and 21 or 28 *(MMWR 59 (RR-2), 2010)*.

[6] Any person with a history of pre-exposure vaccination with HDCV, RVA, PCECV; prior post-exposure prophylaxis with HDCV, PCEC or rabies vaccine adsorbed (RVA); or previous vaccination with any other type of rabies vaccine & a documented history of antibody response to the prior vaccination.

TABLE 21 – DOSE/SCHEDULE SUMMARY FOR US TRAVEL VACCINES

Vaccine	Tradename (Manufacturer)	Age	Dose	Route	Schedule	Booster
Chikungunya, live attenuated	Ixchiq (Valneva)	≥18 yrs	0.5 mL	IM	1 dose	At least 3 yrs
Cholera, 103-HgR vaccine	Vaxchora (Bavarian Nordic)	2-64 yrs (use off-label for ≥65 yrs)	100 mL (reconstituted)	po	1 dose[1]	2 yrs (off-label D)[2]
Hepatitis A vaccine, inactivated	Havrix (GlaxoSmithKline)	1-18 yrs	0.5 mL (720 ELISA units)	IM	0, 6–12 mos	None
		≥19 yrs	1 mL (1,440 ELISA units)	IM	0, 6–12 mos	None
Hepatitis A vaccine, inactivated	Vaqta (Merck & Co., Inc.)	1-18 yrs	0.5 mL (25 U)	IM	0, 6–18 mos	None
		≥19 yrs	1 mL (50 U)	IM	0, 6–18 mos	None
Hepatitis B vaccine, recombinant with novel adjuvant	Heplisav-B (Dynavax Technologies Corp.)	≥18 yrs	0.5 mL (10 µg HBsAg) and 3,000 µg of adjuvant CPG 1018)	IM	0, 1 mo	None
Hepatitis B vaccine, recombinant	Engerix-B (GlaxoSmithKline)	0-19 yrs	0.5 mL (10 µg HBsAg)	IM	0, 1, 6 mos	None
		0-10 yrs (accelerated)	0.5 mL (10 µg HBsAg)	IM	0, 1, 2 mos	12 mos
		11-19 yrs (accelerated)	1 mL (20 µg HBsAg)	IM	0, 1, 2 mos	12 mos
		≥20 yrs[3] (primary)	1 mL (20 µg HBsAg)	IM	0, 1, 6 mos	None
		≥20 yrs (accelerated)	1 mL (20 µg HBsAg)	IM	0, 1, 2 mos	12 mos
Hepatitis B vaccine, recombinant	Recombivax HB (Merck & Co., Inc.)	0-19 yrs (primary)	0.5 mL (5 µg HBsAg)	IM	0, 1, 6 mos	None
		11-15 yrs (adolescent accelerated)	1 mL (10 µg HBsAg)	IM	0, 4-6 mos	None
		≥20 yrs (primary)	1 mL (10 µg HBsAg)	IM	0, 4-6 mos	None
Combined hepatitis A and hepatitis B vaccine	Twinrix (GlaxoSmithKline)	≥18 yrs (primary)	1 mL (720 ELU HAV + 20 µg HBsAg)	IM	0, 1, 6 mos	
		≥18 yrs (accelerated)	1 mL (720 ELU HAV + 20 µg HBsAg)	IM	0, 7, 21–30 days	12 mos
Japanese encephalitis vaccine, inactivated	Ixiaro (Valneva)	2 mos-2 yrs	0.25 mL	IM	0, 28 days	≥1 year after primary series[4]
		3-17 yrs	0.5 mL	IM	0, 28 days	≥1 year after primary series[4]
		18-65 yrs	0.5 mL	IM	0, 7-28 days	≥1 year after primary series[4]
		>65 yrs	0.5 mL	IM	0, 28 days	≥1 year after primary series[4]
Meningococcal Polysaccharide Tetanus Toxoid Conjugate (MenACWY-TT)[5]	Menquadfi (Sanofi Pasteur)	≥2 yrs (do not use <2 yrs of age)	0.5 mL	IM	Single dose (2 doses spaced by 8 wks for asplenia, complement deficiency, HIV and compromised)	If at continued risk (travel or compromised) one dose 5 yr after dose 1 (3 yrs after dose 1 if age <7), subsequents boosters q5 yr after 1st booster

TABLE 21 (2)

Vaccine	Tradename (Manufacturer)	Age	Dose	Route	Schedule	Booster
Meningococcal oligosaccharide diphtheria, CRM[197] conjugate vaccine (MenACWY-CRM)[5]	Menveo (GSK)	≥2 yrs *(see Menveo, Child <2 yrs for dosing)*	0.5 mL	IM	Single dose (2 doses spaced by 8 wks for asplenia, complement deficiency, HIV and compromised)	If at continued risk (travel or compromised) one dose 5 yr after dose 1 (3 yrs after dose 1 if age <7), subsequents boosters q5 yr after 1st booster
Polio vaccine, inactivated	Ipol (Sanofi Pasteur)	≥18 yrs	0.5 mL	SC or IM	1 dose if person has completed a pediatric series	Repeat boosters may be needed for long-term travelers to polio-affected countries
Rabies vaccine (human diploid embryo cell)	Imovax (Sanofi Pasteur)	Any	1 mL	IM	Pre-exposure series: days 0, 7.	1 mL IM one time, only if titer check done between 1-3 yr after primary series is <0.5 IU/ml. Option: empirically give 1 dose at 21 d to 3 yrs to avoid titer check after traveler returns from initial trip. Also, *see Rabies, Postexposure Prophylaxis*
Rabies vaccine (purified chick embryo cell)	RabAvert (Bavarian Nordic)	Any	1 mL	IM	Pre-exposure series: days 0, 7.	
Tickborne Encephalitis	TicoVac (Pfizer); Branded as FSMEImmun in Europe	1-15 yrs	0.25 mL	IM	1 dose at 0, 1-3 mos, and 5-12 mos after dose 2	3 yrs after third primary dose
		≥16 yrs	0.5 mL	IM	1 dose at 0, 14 days to 3 mos, and 5-12 mos after dose 2	3 yrs after third primary dose. If continued risk repeat q5 yrs for ages 16-49, q3 yrs for ≥50 yrs
Typhoid vaccine (oral, live, attenuated)	Vivotif (Bavarian Nordic)	≥6 yrs	1 capsule[6]	po	0, 2, 4, 6 days	Repeat primary series after 5 yrs
Typhoid vaccine (Vi capsular polysaccharide)	Typhim Vi (Sanofi Pasteur)	≥2 yrs	0.5 mL	IM	1 dose	2 yrs
Yellow fever						Not recommended for most itineraries[7,8]

Abbreviations: ACIP, Advisory Committee on Immunization Practices; ELU, ELISA units of inactivated HAV; HAV, hepatitis A virus; HBsAg, hepatitis B surface antigen; IM, intramuscular; U, units HAV antigen; SC, subcutaneous.

[1] Must be administered in a health care setting.
[2] Booster dose recommended off-label at 2 yrs after vaccination based on robust data showing antibody persistence in adolescents aged 12-17 yrs. FDA and ACIP have not yet considered this data.
[3] Consult the prescribing information for differences in dosing for hemodialysis and other immunocompromised patients.
[4] If potential for Japanese encephalitis virus exposure continues.
[5] MenABCWY (Penbraya) is an option when both MenB and MenACWY would be given on the same day as an initial dose of each but MenB is not indicated as a specific travel vaccine.
[6] Must be kept refrigerated at 35.6°F–46.4°F (2°C–8°C); administer with cool liquid no warmer than 98.6°F (37°C).
[7] Ages 6–8 months and ≥60 years are precautions and age <6 months is a contraindication to the use of yellow fever vaccine.
[8] YF Vax is available in single-dose and multiple-dose (5-dose) vials.

TABLE 22 – LIST OF GENERIC AND TRADE NAMES

GENERIC NAME: TRADE NAMES

Abacavir: Ziagen
Abacavir + Lamivudine: Epzicom
Abacavir + Lamivudine + Dolutegravir: Triumeq
Abacavir + Lamivudine + Zidovudine: Trizivir
Acyclovir: Zovirax
Adefovir: Hepsera
Albendazole: Albenza
Amantadine: Symmetrel
Amikacin: Amikin
Amikacin liposomal: Arikayce
Amoxicillin: Amoxil, Polymox
Amoxicillin extended release: Moxatag
Amox./clav.: Augmentin, Augmentin ES-600; Augmentin XR
Amphotericin B: Fungizone
Ampho B-liposomal: AmBisome
Ampho B-lipid complex: Abelcet
Ampicillin: Omnipen, Polycillin
Ampicillin + Sulbactam: Unasyn
Ansuvimab-zykl: Ebanga
Artemether + Lumefantrine: Coartem
Atazanavir: Reyataz
Atovaquone: Mepron
Atovaquone + Proguanil: Malarone
Azithromycin: Zithromax
Azithromycin ER: Zmax
Aztreonam: Azactam, Cayston
Baloxavir marboxil: Xofluza
Baricitinib: Olumiant
Bedaquiline: Sirturo
Benznidazole: Exeltis, Abarax
Bezlotoxumab: Zinplava
Bictegravir + FTC + TAF: Biktarvy
Brincidofovir: Tembexa
Cabotegravir + Rilpivirine: Cabenuva
Casirivimab + Imdevimab: REGEN-COV
Caspofungin: Cancidas
Cefaclor: Ceclor, Ceclor CD
Cefadroxil: Duricef
Cefazolin: Ancef, Kefzol
Cefdinir: Omnicef
Cefditoren pivoxil: Spectracef
Cefepime: Maxipime
Cefiderocol: Fetroja
Cefixime[NUS]: Suprax
Cefoperazone + Sulbactam: Sulperazon[NUS]
Cefotaxime: Claforan
Cefotetan: Cefotan
Cefoxitin: Mefoxin
Cefpodoxime proxetil: Vantin
Cefprozil: Cefzil
Ceftaroline: Teflaro
Ceftazidime: Fortaz, Tazicef, Tazidime
Ceftazidime + Avibactam: Avycaz
Ceftibuten: Cedax
Ceftizoxime: Cefizox
Ceftobiprole: Zeftera
Ceftolozane + Tazobactam: Zerbaxa
Ceftriaxone: Rocephin
Cefuroxime: Zinacef, Ceftin
Cephalexin: Keflex
Cephradine: Anspor, Velosef
Chloroquine: Aralen
Cidofovir: Vistide
Ciprofloxacin: Cipro, Cipro XR
Clarithromycin: Biaxin, Biaxin XL
Clindamycin: Cleocin
Clofazimine: Lamprene
Clotrimazole: Lotrimin, Mycelex
Cloxacillin: Tegopen
Colistimethate: Coly-Mycin M
Cycloserine: Seromycin
Daclatasvir: Daklinza
Daptomycin: Cubicin
Dalbavancin: Dalvance
Darunavir: Prezista
Darunavir + Cobi + FTC + TAF: Symtuza
Delafloxacin: Baxdela
Dicloxacillin: Dynapen
Diethylcarbamazine: Hetrazan
Diloxanide furoate: Furamide
Dolutegravir: Tivicay
Dolutegravir + Emtricitabine: Dovato
Dolutegravir + Rilpivirine: Juluca
Doravirine + 3TC + TDF: Delstrigo
Doripenem: Doribax
Doxycycline: Vibramycin
Efavirenz: Sustiva
Efavirenz + Emtricitabine + Tenofovir: Atripla
Elbasvir + Grazoprevir: Zepatier
Elvitegravir + Cobicistat + Emtricitabine + Tenofovir: Stribild
Elvitegravir + Cobicistat + Emtricitabine + Tenofovir AF: Genvoya
Emtricitabine: Emtriva
Emtricitabine + Tenofovir: Truvada
Emtricitabine + Tenofovir + Rilpivirine: Complera
Enfuvirtide (T-20): Fuzeon
Entecavir: Baraclude
Eravacycline: Xerava
Ertapenem: Invanz
Erythromycin(s): Ilotycin
Ethyl succinate: Pediamycin
Glucoheptonate: Erythrocin
Estolate: Ilosone
Erythro + Sulfisoxazole: Pediazole
Ethambutol: Myambutol
Ethionamide: Trecator
Etravirine: Intelence
Famciclovir: Famvir
Fidaxomicin: Dificid
Fluconazole: Diflucan
Flucytosine: Ancobon
Foscarnet: Foscavir
Fosfomycin: Monurol
Fostemsavir: Rukobia
Fusidic acid: Taksta
Ganciclovir: Cytovene
Gatifloxacin: Tequin
Gemifloxacin: Factive
Gentamicin: Garamycin
Grazoprevir + Elbasvir: Zepatier
Griseofulvin: Fulvicin
Halofantrine: Halfan
Ibalizumab-uiyk: Trogarzo
Ibrexafungerp: Brexafemme
Idoxuridine: Dendrid, Stoxil
Imipenem + Cilastatin: Primaxin, Tienam
Imiquimod: Aldara
Imipenem + cilastatin + relebactam: Recarbrio
INH + RIF: Rifamate
INH + RIF + PZA: Rifater
Interferon alfa: Intron A
Interferon, pegylated: PEG-Intron, Pegasys
Interferon + Ribavirin: Rebetron
Isavuconazonium sulfate: Cresemba
Itraconazole: Sporanox
Iodoquinol: Yodoxin
Ivermectin: Stromectol, Sklice, Mectizan
Ketoconazole: Nizoral
Lamivudine: Epivir, Epivir-HBV
Lamivudine + Abacavir: Epzicom
Ledipasvir + Sofosbuvir: Harvoni
Lefamulin: Xenleta
Lenacapavir: Sunlenca
Letermovir: Prevymis
Levofloxacin: Levaquin
Linezolid: Zyvox
Lopinavir + Ritonavir: Kaletra
Loracarbef: Lorabid
Mafenide: Sulfamylon
Maraviroc: Selzentry
Maribavir: Livtencity
Mebendazole: Vermox
Mefloquine: Lariam
Meropenem: Merrem
Meropenem + vaborbactam: Vabomere
Mesalamine: Asacol, Pentasa
Methenamine: Hiprex, Mandelamine
Metronidazole: Flagyl
Micafungin: Mycamine
Miltefosine: Impavido
Minocycline: Minocin
Molnupiravir: Lagevrio
Moxifloxacin: Avelox
Mupirocin: Bactroban
Nafcillin: Unipen
Nevirapine: Viramune
Nifurtimox: Lampit
Nirmatrelvir/r: Paxlovid
Nitazoxanide: Alinia
Nitrofurantoin: Macrobid, Macrodantin
Nystatin: Mycostatin
Ofloxacin: Floxin
Olysio: Simeprevir
Omadacycline: Nuzyra
Oritavancin: Orbactiv, Kimyrsa
Oseltamivir: Tamiflu
Oxacillin: Prostaphlin
Palivizumab: Synagis
Paritaprevir + Ritonavir + Ombitasvir: Technivie
Paritaprevir + Ritonavir + Ombitasvir + Dasabuvir: Viekira Pak
Paromomycin: Humatin
Pentamidine: NebuPent, Pentam 300
Peramivir: Rapivab
Piperacillin + Tazobactam: Zosyn, Tazocin
Piperazine: Antepar
Plazomicin: Zemdri
Podophyllotoxin: Condylox
Polymyxin B: Poly-Rx
Posaconazole: Noxafil
Praziquantel: Biltricide
Pretomanid: Pretomanid
Primaquine: Primachine
Proguanil: Paludrine
Prulifloxacin: Sword
Pyrantel pamoate: Antiminth
Pyrimethamine: Daraprim
Pyrimethamine + Sulfadoxine: Fansidar
Raltegravir: Isentress
Remdesivir: Veklury
Retapamulin: Altabax
Rezafungin: Rezzayo
Ribavirin: Virazole, Rebetol
Rifabutin: Mycobutin
Rifampin: Rifadin, Rimactane
Rifamycin: Aemcolo
Rifapentine: Priftin
Rifaximin: Xifaxan
Rilpivirine: Edurant
Rimantadine: Flumadine
Ritonavir: Norvir
Sarecycline: Seysara
Secnidazole: Solosec
Spectinomycin: Trobicin
Stibogluconate: Pentostam
Silver sulfadiazine: Silvadene
Simeprevir: Olysio
Sofosbuvir: Sovaldi
Sulfamethoxazole: Gantanol
Sulfasalazine: Azulfidine
Sulfisoxazole: Gantrisin
Suramin: Germanin
Tafenoquine: Krintafel, Arakoda
Tecovirimat: Tpoxx
Tedizolid: Sivextro
Telaprevir: Incivek
Telavancin: Vibativ
Telbivudine: Tyzeka
Telithromycin: Ketek
Temocillin: Negaban, Temopen
Tenofovir AF-FTC: Descovy
Tenofovir alafenamide: Vemlidy
Tenofovir DF: Viread
Terbinafine: Lamisil
Thalidomide: Thalomid
Thiabendazole: Mintezol
Tigecycline: Tygacil
Tinidazole: Tindamax
Tixagevimab + Cilgavimab: Evusheld
Tobramycin: Nebcin
Tocilizumab: Actemra
Tofacitinib: Xeljanz, Xeljanz XR
Triclabendazole: Egaten
Trifluridine: Viroptic
Trimethoprim: Primsol
Trimethoprim + Sulfamethoxazole: Bactrim, Septra
Valacyclovir: Valtrex
Valganciclovir: Valcyte
Vancomycin: Vancocin
Velpatasvir + Sofosbuvir: Epclusa
Voriconazole: Vfend
Zanamivir: Relenza
Zidovudine (ZDV): Retrovir
Zidovudine + 3TC: Combivir
Zidovudine + 3TC + Abacavir: Trizivir

TABLE 22 (2) – LIST OF TRADE AND GENERIC NAMES

TRADE NAMES: GENERIC NAME

Abelcet: Ampho B-lipid complex
Actemra: Tocilizumab
Albenza: Albendazole
Aldara: Imiquimod
Alinia: Nitazoxanide
Altabax: Retapamulin
AmBisome: Ampho B-liposomal
Amikin: Amikacin
Amoxil: Amoxicillin
Ancef: Cefazolin
Ancobon: Flucytosine
Anspor: Cephradine
Antepar: Piperazine
Antiminth: Pyrantel pamoate
Aralen: Chloroquine
Arakoda: Tafenoquine
Arikayce: Amikacin liposomal
Asacol: Mesalamine
Atripla: Efavirenz + Emtricitabine + Tenofovir
Augmentin, Augmentin ES-600 Augmentin XR: Amox./clav.
Avelox: Moxifloxacin
Avycaz: Ceftazidime + AvibactamAzactam: Aztreonam
Azulfidine: Sulfasalazine
Bactroban: Mupirocin
Bactrim: Trimethoprim + SMX
Baraclude: Entecavir
Baxdela: Delafloxacin
Biaxin, Biaxin XL: Clarithromycin
Biktarvy: Bictegravir + FTC + TAF
Biltricide: Praziquantel
Brexafemme: Ibrexafungerp
Cabenuva: Cabotegravir + Rilpivirine
Cancidas: Caspofungin
Cayston: Aztreonam (inhaled)
Ceclor, Ceclor CD: Cefaclor
Cedax: Ceftibuten
Cefizox: Ceftizoxime
Cefotan: Cefotetan
Ceftin: Cefuroxime axetil
Cefzil: Cefprozil
Cipro, Cipro XR: Ciprofloxacin & extended release
Claforan: Cefotaxime
Coartem: Artemether + Lumefantrine
Coly-Mycin M: Colistimethate
Combivir: Zidovudine + 3TC
Complera: Emtricitabine + Tenofovir + Rilpivirine
Cresemba: Isavuconazonium sulfate
Cubicin: Daptomycin
Cytovene: Ganciclovir
Daklinza: Daclatasvir
Dalvance: Dalbavancin
Daraprim: Pyrimethamine
Descovy: Tenofovir AF-FTC
Delstrigo: Doravirine + 3TC + TDF
Dificid: Fidaxomicin
Diflucan: Fluconazole
Doribax: Doripenem
Dovato: Dolutegravir + Emtricitabine
Duricef: Cefadroxil
Dynapen: Dicloxacillin
Ebanga: Ansuvimab-zykl
Edurant: Rilpivirine
Emtriva: Emtricitabine
Epclusa: Velpatasvir + Sofosbuvir
Epivir, Epivir-HBV: Lamivudine
Epzicom: Lamivudine + Abacavir
Evusheld: Tixagevimab + Cilgavimab
Exeltis: Benznidazole
Factive: Gemifloxacin
Famvir: Famciclovir
Fansidar: Pyrimethamine + Sulfadoxine
Fetroja: Cefiderocol
Flagyl: Metronidazole
Floxin: Ofloxacin
Flumadine: Rimantadine
Foscavir: Foscarnet
Fortaz: Ceftazidime
Fulvicin: Griseofulvin
Fungizone: Amphotericin B
Furadantin: Nitrofurantoin
Fuzeon: Enfuvirtide (T-20)
Gantanol: Sulfamethoxazole
Gantrisin: Sulfisoxazole
Garamycin: Gentamicin
Genvoya: Elvitegravir + Cobicistat + Emtricitabine + Tenofovir AF
Halfan: Halofantrine
Harvoni: Ledipasvir + Sofosbuvir
Hepsera: Adefovir
Herplex: Idoxuridine
Hiprex: Methenamine hippurate
Humatin: Paromomycin
Ilosone: Erythromycin estolate
Ilotycin: Erythromycin
Incivek: Telaprevir
Intelence: Etravirine
Intron A: Interferon alfa
Invanz: Ertapenem
Isentress: Raltegravir
Juluca: Dolutegravir + Rilpivirine
Kantrex: Kanamycin
Kaletra: Lopinavir + Ritonavir
Keflex: Cephalexin
Ketek: Telithromycin
Krintafel: Tafenoquine
Kimyrsa: Oritavancin
Lagevrio: Molnupiravir
Lamisil: Terbinafine
Lamprene: Clofazimine
Lariam: Mefloquine
Levaquin: Levofloxacin
Livtencity: Maribavir
Lorabid: Loracarbef
Macrodantin, Macrobid: Nitrofurantoin
Malarone: Atovaquone + Proguanil
Mandelamine: Methenamine mandelate
Maxipime: Cefepime
Mefoxin: Cefoxitin
Mepron: Atovaquone
Merrem: Meropenem
Minocin: Minocycline
Mintezol: Thiabendazole
Monurol: Fosfomycin
Moxatag: Amoxicillin extended release
Myambutol: Ethambutol
Mycamine: Micafungin
Mycobutin: Rifabutin
Mycostatin: Nystatin
Nafcil: Nafcillin
Nebcin: Tobramycin
NebuPent: Pentamidine
Nizoral: Ketoconazole
Norvir: Ritonavir
Noxafil: Posaconazole
Nuzyra: Omadacycline
Olysio: Simeprevir
Olumiant: Baricitinib
Omnicef: Cefdinir
Omnipen: Ampicillin
Orbactiv: Oritavancin
Paxlovid: Nirmatrelvir/r
Pediamycin: Erythro. ethyl succinate
Pediazole: Erythro. ethyl succinate + sulfisoxazole
Pegasys, PEG-Intron: Interferon, pegylated
Pentam 300: Pentamidine
Pentasa: Mesalamine
Polycillin: Ampicillin
Polymox: Amoxicillin
Poly-Rx: Polymyxin B
Pretomanid: Pretomanid
Prevymis: Letermovir
Prezista: Darunavir
Priftin: Rifapentine
Primaxin: Imipenem + Cilastatin
Primsol: Trimethoprim
Prostaphlin: Oxacillin
Rapivab: Peramivir
Rebetol: Ribavirin
Rebetron: Interferon + Ribavirin
Recarbrio: Imipenem + cilastatin + relebactam
REGEN-COV: Casirivimab + Imdevimab
Relenza: Zanamivir
Retin A: Tretinoin
Retrovir: Zidovudine (ZDV)
Reyataz: Atazanavir
Rezzayo: Rezafungin
Rifadin: Rifampin
Rifamate: INH + RIF
Rifater: INH + RIF + PZA
Rimactane: Rifampin
Rocephin: Ceftriaxone
Rukobia: Fostemsavir
Selzentry: Maraviroc
Septra: Trimethoprim + Sulfamethoxazole
Seromycin: Cycloserine
Silvadene: Silver sulfadiazine
Sirturo: Bedaquiline
Sivextro: Tedizolid
Sklice: Ivermectin lotion
Solosec: Secnidazole
Sovaldi: Sofosbuvir
Spectracef: Cefditoren pivoxil
Sporanox: Itraconazole
Stoxil: Idoxuridine
Stribild: Elvitegravir + Cobicistat + Emtricitabine + Tenofovir
Stromectol: Ivermectin
Sulfamylon: Mafenide
Sulperazon[NUS]: Cefoperazone + Sulbactam
Sunlenca: Lenacapavir
Suprax: Cefixime[NUS]
Sustiva: Efavirenz
Symmetrel: Amantadine
Symtuza: Darunavir + Cobi + TAF
Synagis: Palivizumab
Taksta: Fusidic acid
Talicia: Amoxicillin + Rifampin + Omeprazole
Tamiflu: Oseltamivir
Tazicef: Ceftazidime
Technivie: Paritaprevir + Ritonavir + Ombitasvir
Teflaro: Ceftaroline
Tegopen: Cloxacillin
Tequin: Gatifloxacin
Tembexa: Brincidofovir
Thalomid: Thalidomide
Tienam: Imipenem
Tinactin: Tolnaftate
Tindamax: Tinidazole
Tivicay: Dolutegravir
Tpoxx: Tecovirimat
Trogarzo: Ibalizumab-uiyk
Trecator SC: Ethionamide
Triumeq: Abacavir + Lamivudine + Dolutegravir
Trizivir: Zidovudine + 3TC + Abacavir
Trobicin: Spectinomycin
Truvada: Emtricitabine + Tenofovir
Tygacil: Tigecycline
Tyzeka: Telbivudine
Unasyn: Ampicillin/sulbactam
Unipen: Nafcillin
Vabomere: Meropenem + vaborbactam
Valcyte: Valganciclovir
Valtrex: Valacyclovir
Vancocin: Vancomycin
Vantin: Cefpodoxime proxetil
Veklury: Remdesivir
Velosef: Cephradine
Vemlidy: Tenofovir alafenamide
Vermox: Mebendazole
Vfend: Voriconazole
Vibativ: Telavancin
Vibramycin: Doxycycline
Viekira Pak: Paritaprevir + Ritonavir + Ombitasvir + Dasabuvir
Viramune: Nevirapine
Virazole: Ribavirin
Viread: Tenofovir
Vistide: Cidofovir
Xenleta: Lefamulin
Xerava: Eravacycline
Xifaxan: Rifaximin
Xofluza: Baloxavir marboxil
Yodoxin: Iodoquinol
Zemdri: Plazomicin
Zerit: Stavudine
Zeftera: Ceftobiprole
Xeljanz, Xeljanz XR: Tofacitinib
Zepatier: Elbasvir + Grazoprevir
Zerbaxa: Ceftolozane + Tazobactam
Ziagen: Abacavir
Zinacef: Cefuroxime
Zinplava: Bezlotoxumab
Zithromax: Azithromycin
Zmax: Azithromycin ER
Zovirax: Acyclovir
Zosyn: Piperacillin + Tazobactam
Zyvox: Linezolid

INDEX

D

E